FIRST AID FOR COLLEGES AND UNIVERSITIES

NINTH EDITION

Keith J. Karren
BRIGHAM YOUNG UNIVERSITY

Brent Q. Hafen
LATE OF BRIGHAM YOUNG UNIVERSITY

Daniel Limmer
YORK COUNTY COMMUNITY COLLEGE

Joseph J. Mistovich
YOUNGSTOWN STATE UNIVERSITY

PEARSON

Benjamin Cummings

San Francisco   Boston   New York
Cape Town   Hong Kong   London   Madrid   Mexico City
Montreal   Munich   Paris   Singapore   Sydney   Tokyo   Toronto

Acquisitions Editor: Sandra Lindelof

Project Editors: Barbara Yien, Nicole George-O' Brien

Development Manager: Claire Alexander

Editorial Assistant: Amy Yu

Managing Editor: Deborah Cogan

Production Supervisor: Beth Masse

Production Management and Compositor: Jeanine Furino/GGS Book Services

Copyeditor: Suzanne Ingrao

Interior Designer: Seventeenth Street Studios

Cover Designer: Yvo Riezebos Design

Photographer: Carl Leet

Director, Image Resource Center: Melindia Patelli

Image Rights and Permissions Manager: Zina Arabia

Manufacturing Buyer: Stacy Wong

Marketing Manager: Neena Chandra

Text printer: RR Donnelley and Sons, Willard

Cover printer: Phoenix Color

Cover Photo Credit: Amy and Chuck Wiley/Wales/IndexStock

Credits can be found on page 541, which constitutes a continuation of this copyright page.

ISBN-10: 0-8053-4625-2

ISBN-13: 978-08053-4625-1

NOTICE ON CARE PROCEDURES

It is the intent of the authors and publisher that this textbook be used as part of a formal First Aid education program taught by a qualified instructor. The procedures described in the textbook are based on consultation with First Aid, First Responder, and medical authorities. The authors and publisher have taken care to make certain that these procedures reflect currently accepted practices; however, they cannot be considered absolute recommendations.

The material in the textbook contains the most current information available at the time of publication. However, federal, state, and local guidelines concerning first aid practices—including, without limitation, those governing infection control and universal precautions—change rapidly. The reader should note, therefore, that new regulations may require changes in some procedures.

It is the responsibility of the reader to become familiar with the policies and procedures set by national, state, and local agencies as well as the institution or agency where the reader is being trained. It is the reader's responsibility to stay informed of any new changes or recommendations made by any of these agencies. The authors and the publisher of this textbook and supplements written to accompany it disclaim any liability, loss, or risk resulting directly or indirectly from the suggested procedures and theory, from any undetected errors, or from the reader's misunderstanding of the text.

Library of Congress Cataloging-in-Publication Data

First aid for colleges and universities / Keith J. Karren . . . [et al.].—9th ed.
　　p. cm.
　ISBN 978-0-8053-4625-1 (alk paper)
　　1. First aid in illness and injury. 2. Medical emergencies. I.　Karren, Keith J.

RC86.7.H339 2008
616.02'52-dc22   2006101113

PEARSON

Benjamin
Cummings

- **In memory of Brent Q. Hafen, Ph.D.**
  Dr. Brent Hafen was a man of great conviction. He was dedicated to his family, his students, and to First Aid and Emergency Care Education. This first aid text and others co-authored by Dr. Hafen have had a tremendous influence on first aid training nationally and internationally. He is deeply missed and fondly remembered.

- This text is dedicated to all Good Samaritans who have a great desire to help others in distress, and who desire proper preparation so that their first aid care is correct and helpful.
  KJK

- To Stephanie, Sarah Katherine, and Theo
  DL

- To my beautiful wife, Andrea, for her love and encouragement, and for being my best friend. To my girls, Katie, Kristyn, Chelsea, Morgan, and Kara, for their unconditional love and the constant hugs, kisses, smiles, and laughter that make life worth living to its fullest. In memory of my father, Paul, who is, without any doubt, my hero in life.
  JJM

Contents

chapter. Extensive coverage and illustration of the body systems familiarizes you with anatomical features and physiological concepts that are essential for successful first aid.

- Chapter 12, "Common Sport and Recreational Injuries," discusses the most likely mechanisms of injury in sports and recreational activities, lists the most common signs and symptoms, and outlines valuable first aid techniques that can prevent further injury.

- Chapter 27, "Wilderness Emergencies," gives valuable information on how to care for victims when you are far from the safety of the 9-1-1 system and in a potentially hostile environment. This important chapter also describes how to prevent problems in the wilderness setting, covers the basics of survival, and details common wilderness problems. Finally, it describes special considerations in assessing and caring for victims when you have limited equipment and supplies.

- An innovative learning technique, SQ3R Plus (survey, question, read, recite, review, plus write and reflect), has been incorporated into every chapter to encourage active participation in learning, studying, and reviewing, and to reinforce the key points in each chapter.

- A running glossary defines key terms where they first appear in the text, assuring understanding of the material as it is presented.

The SQ3R Plus System

The SQ3R Plus system provides structured learning aids throughout each chapter that can boost your effectiveness, enhance your learning, and increase your retention. The following learning aids form the SQ3R Plus system:

- Learning Objectives, presented at the beginning of each chapter, are used to organize the text and focus on major concepts. These objectives are repeated in the chapter to introduce the material to which they refer.

- Progress Checks at the end of each major section of the chapter immediately reinforce the material just covered and check your comprehension.

- A Self-Test at the end of each chapter provides a review of the material by testing your retention, and provides an excellent study tool for exams.

We've structured the Ninth Edition so that you can use the SQ3R Plus system—*survey, question, read, recite, review*, plus *write* and *reflect*—as you study the material.

The following steps will help you get the most out of this text.

- **Survey.** Before you start reading a chapter, take a few minutes to scan it. Read the case study that begins each chapter to get a sense of how the principles apply to real-life examples. Then flip through the pages, reading the section headings and subheadings. Finally, look at the illustrations and tables. When you're finished, you'll have a good idea of what lies ahead.

- **Question.** Write down some questions you'd like answered by the material you'll study in each chapter. Need help? Look at the detailed learning objectives listed at the beginning of each chapter and the Progress Checks at the end of each section. You might also turn section headings or subheadings into questions. Developing your own list of questions makes the information more relevant and interesting. And because you have a goal, it gets you more involved!

- **Read.** Now read the text and find the answers to the questions you wrote down. Use the Learning Objectives as prompts and pointers—they'll guide you to information and key terms. As you read, pause often to determine how the material is personally relevant.

- **Recite.** Each time you finish reading the material under a heading, stop and *recite*. How? Mentally rehearse what you just read—this time, in your own words. Think of your own examples and metaphors.

- **Review.** To begin, look at your list of questions; answer them from memory. Now look at the list of learning objectives; write a summary for each from memory. Next, look at the list of key terms at the end of each chapter; write a definition for each from memory. Finally, take the Self-Test at the end of the chapter. These give you immediate feedback on how well you learned the key concepts. If you're unsure about some of the questions, go back and study those sections in the chapter again.

- **Write and Reflect.** You've already started writing a summary of what you've learned; make sure you really understand the material and that you've covered all the key points. As a final step, reflect on how you personally can use this information and apply what you've learned. Write down the specifics to make them more meaningful and to increase your involvement in what you've studied.

Supplements

The following instructor supplements are available for this text.

About the Authors

Keith J. Karren. Ph.D., EMT-B, is professor of Health Sciences at Brigham Young University. He is also the director of Emergency Medical Services, an educational service that offers continuing education for EMS personnel. He has been involved in higher education for 37 years and is the author of numerous EMS publications.

Daniel Limmer, NREMT-P, is a faculty member at York County Community College in Wells, Maine. He has been involved in EMS and law enforcement for 28 years and practices as a paramedic with Kennebunk Fire Rescue in Kennebunk, Maine. Dan is a frequent lecturer at conferences and colleges nationwide. He is a co-author of several textbooks, including *Emergency Care, Essentials of Emergency Care, Advanced Medical Life Support, and First Responder—A Skills Approach.*

Joseph J. Mistovich, M.Ed, NREMT-P, is chairperson of the Department of Health Professions and a professor at Youngstown State University in Youngstown, Ohio. He has more than 22 years of experience as an educator in emergency medical services and multidisciplinary health care. He received a Master of Education degree from Kent State University, a Bachelor of Science in Applied Science degree and an Associate in Applied Science degree in Emergency Medical Services, both from Youngstown State University. He has authored several EMS textbooks and numerous EMS articles. He is a frequent speaker at state and national conferences.

Preface

Why Study First Aid?

How people respond to an emergency before medical help arrives often determines how well a victim recovers. In extreme cases, it can spell the difference between life and death. Since you might be the person to respond first at the scene of an emergency, you need to know how to recognize emergencies and how to respond in a way that best protects and aids the victim. This text, along with your course, will prepare you to make appropriate decisions regarding first aid care and to act skillfully and effectively.

Approach

Meeting and often exceeding the standards of Red Cross, National Safety Council, and all other first aid training courses, *First Aid for Colleges and Universities,* Ninth Edition, provides the most complete coverage of certification-level instruction. Written particularly with college and university courses in mind, this comprehensive text is the only first aid text on the market that contains enough material to fill a semester-long college course in first aid. It also serves as a valuable resource after completion of a first aid training course.

Obtaining American Red Cross Certification

You can use what you learn in *First Aid for Colleges and Universities,* Ninth Edition, to obtain an American Red Cross First Aid/CPR certificate. Study the text and test yourself by taking the Chapter Self-Test at the end of each chapter. Then contact the local branch of the American Red Cross (local chapter information is available on the American Red Cross web site ttp://www.crossnet.org) and request an appointment with the Health and Safety Director to take a challenge test. Once you successfully complete the skills and written test, the American Red Cross will issue you a certificate.

What's New in This Edition?

Along with offering the most complete coverage of certification-level instruction in first aid, the Ninth Edition has been thoroughly updated as follows:

- The CPR section has been updated to meet the 2005 American Red Cross standards for adults a pediatric patients, including new guidelines for ratio of compressions to ventilations.

- A table on the inside front cover of the text summarizes the variations between the latest America Red Cross and American Heart Association guidelines for CPR.

- New Critical Thinking Exercises at the end of each chapter challenge students to apply what they have learned to realistic case scenarios.

- Chapter 2: "Anatomy and Physiology of Body Systems" has been extensively revised for a more concise presentation.

- Thirty new photos have been added to Chapter 3: Victim Assessment.

- Pages are now perforated so that end-of-chapter Self-Tests can be easily detached.

- Each chapter has been carefully updated in response to reviewer feedback.

This text also retains the following key features:

- Complete and practical coverage of victim assessment and care, designed to provide students with the critical information they need to pass the first aid course and to function effectively in emergencies as First Aiders.

- Detailed coverage of topics minimally covered in most first aid books, including pediatrics, geriatrics, and multiple casualty situations.

- Realistic chapter opening scenarios ("On the Scene") that introduce students to the chapter at hand.

- An author team with a combined 75+ years of experience in emergency medical practice and education.

What's Unique in This Text?

- Chapter 2, "Anatomy and Physiology of Body Systems," is an expanded anatomy and physiology

INSTRUCTOR'S MANUAL AND TEST BANK
(ISBN 0-321-49772-4)

The *Instructor's Manual* includes learning objectives, critical chapter information, suggestions for teaching aids and equipment, suggested skill activities, key questions, key terms, and room for notes. The *Instructor's Manual* also provides perforated copies of the skills assessment sheets available in the main text, which can be torn out and photocopied, and hypothetical scenario worksheets that can be used for student assignments. The *Test Bank* contains matching and true/false questions for each chapter. Both the *Instructor's Manual* and the *Test Bank* have been completely revised for the Ninth Edition.

COMPUTERIZED TEST BANK
(ISBN 0-321-49771-6)

Available on a user-friendly cross-platform CD-ROM, the *Computerized Test Bank* provides all the questions available in the print version of the *Test Bank,* as well as the capability to add new questions and modify existing ones. Instructors can pick and choose to create custom-made tests and quizzes that fit the specific needs of their course.

COMPLETION CERTIFICATES
(ISBN 0-321-49177-7)

Wallet-sized completion certificates allow instructors to provide recognition to all the students who complete their course.

FILMS FOR THE HUMANITIES VIDEOS

Videos on topics such as basic first aid, home safety, and treating medical emergencies are available to qualified adopters. Please contact your local Benjamin Cummings sales representative for more information. To locate a sales representative, visit: www.aw-bc.com.

Acknowledgments

We would like to thank the following reviewers for their valuable suggestions and input into the Ninth Edition: Jay Bradley, Indiana University-Purdue University, Indianapolis; Anna Bustamante, Palo Alto College; Julie Calvery, University of Arkansas-Fort Smith; Nick Dicicco, Camden County College; Mike Davey, Western Illinois University; Cecile Grasfeder, University of Tennessee-Martin; Michael Klinkner, Fox Valley Technical College; Sarah Lee, South Piedmont Community College; Daniel Pray, Shoreline Community College; and Ron Timberlake, Volunteer State Community College.

We would also like to thank Carl Leet, photographer, from Youngstown State University, for his expertise, creative work, and continued support; as well as models James Hasson, AAS, NREMT-P, and Will Cohen, NREMT-P.

We gratefully acknowledge the work of Mike Helbock, who succeeded in creating clear and pedagogically sound supplements.

Finally, we thank the editorial, production, and marketing teams at Benjamin Cummings for their work on the Ninth Edition.

1

Introduction to First Aid Care

Learning Objectives

When you have mastered the material in this chapter, you will be able to

1 Identify the need for properly prepared First Aiders

2 Identify the principal aims of first aid

3 Identify skills performed by a First Aider

4 Understand the legal aspects of first aid and emergency medical care

5 Explain the factors that constitute negligence on the part of a First Aider

6 Understand how infections are transmitted

7 Identify the infectious diseases that are of concern in an emergency setting

8 Describe ways to prevent the spread of AIDS and other infectious diseases in an emergency setting

On the Scene

I remember the first serious victim I ever cared for. I had been trained in first aid at my local community college. A friend and I were driving down a country road and observed an older lady standing by her parked car, frantically waving to us. As we pulled closer I saw a man slumped in the front seat. My mind began racing: "Would I remember everything from class? What if the man is unconscious? Worse yet, what if he needs CPR?"

As we rolled to a stop behind the parked car, the woman came to us and said that her husband was experiencing terrible chest pain. He looked pale and ashen and had broken out in a sweat. Recognizing these as signs of a possible heart attack, we hurried to the parked car.

I felt myself rushing, losing my concentration. Fortunately, I remembered my first aid instructor's words: "Sometimes it feels like you're going to lose it. If that happens, stop briefly. Recite the letters A, B, C, D a few times to yourself." He said it would keep me from jumping in too fast and losing the big picture. He also said it would remind me of my priorities in caring for any victim. It worked.

I introduced myself to the victim. He had all the classic signs of a heart attack (myocardial infarction). I tried to reassure him. He was clutching his chest and told me that he felt like there was a huge band pulling tightly around it. I began taking vital signs, and I sent my friend to call 9-1-1 and get paramedics on their way.

When the paramedics arrived, we were ready for them with a complete set of vitals, information on the victim's complaint, and a medical history. I gave all the information to the ambulance crew chief. The patient was now theirs, but my friend and I stuck around to help until he was wheeled into the ambulance.

Although it was my first serious call, it went pretty well. Since then, there have been many opportunities to give first aid. I've learned that being prepared to give first aid is important: Giving early first aid at the scene of an emergency not only helps injured victims, it also saves lives—A First-Aider.

A
mong the most critical and visible health problems in America today are catastrophic accidents and illnesses and the resultant disabilities and/or sudden loss of life. More than 70 million Americans receive hospital emergency care each year. One American in three suffers a nonfatal injury (see Figure 1-1).

Too often, those who arrive first at the scene of an accident are not trained sufficiently to give proper, on-the-scene first aid care or in-transit emergency assistance. Often, too much time passes before proper emergency care is given, and victims who might have been saved die as a result.

> Learning Objective 1 Identify the need for properly prepared First Aiders.

The first people on the scene, the First Aiders, can initiate various life-saving procedures:

- Airway and respiratory intervention
- Cardiopulmonary resuscitation
- Bleeding control
- Special wound care
- Stabilization of spinal injuries
- Splinting of fractures

As a First Aider, you become an important part of the emergency care team, prepared with the knowledge and the skills to render appropriate life-saving care.

1.1 What Is First Aid?

> Learning Objective 2 Identify the principal aims of first aid.

First aid is the temporary and immediate care given to a person who is injured or who suddenly becomes ill. First aid includes recognizing life-threatening conditions and taking effective action to keep the injured or ill person alive and in the best possible condition until medical treatment can be obtained.

First aid does *not* replace the physician, nurse, or paramedic. In fact, one of the primary principles of first aid is to activate the EMS system in all cases of serious injury.

The principal aims of first aid are to

- Recognize life-threatening situations
- Activate the EMS system
- Supply artificial ventilation and circulation when needed
- Control bleeding
- Care for other life-threatening conditions
- Minimize further injury and complications
- Prevent infection
- Make the victim as comfortable as possible

Your first aid training will be of obvious benefit to those you treat—from your friends and family members to coworkers and strangers. It will be of particular

> **first aid** The temporary and immediate care given to a person who is injured or who suddenly becomes ill.

FIGURE 1–1. First Aiders provide vital care to patients with injury or illness before EMS arrives.

value when you use it to help those who will not have access to medical care for an extended period—such as someone camping in the wilderness or working on a remote farm. But it will also be of tremendous benefit to you, as you will be able to provide immediate care for your own sudden injuries and illnesses.

As a First Aider, you need to be able to take charge of a situation, keep calm while working under pressure, and organize others to do the same. By demonstrating competence and using well-chosen words of encouragement, First Aiders should win the confidence of others nearby so that they can do everything possible to reassure the victim.

PROGRESS CHECK

1. First aid is the _____ care given to a person who is injured or suddenly becomes ill. *(first/basic/temporary)*

2. One of the primary principles of first aid is to _____. *(activate the EMS system/drive the patient to the hospital/care for all wounds yourself)*

3. A goal of first aid is to minimize _____. *(complications/pain/need for additional care)*

1.2 General Procedures

Being involved in a sudden injury or illness situation requires fast thinking and action. Consider the following plan of action:

1. Observe the accident scene as you approach it.

2. Keep yourself and others at the scene safe; if necessary, assign a bystander to direct traffic away from the accident scene, position safety flares, keep bystanders at a safe distance, turn off any engines that are still running, and so on.

3. Gain access to the victim(s) and determine any immediate threats to life.

4. Provide basic life support to those whose lives are threatened; always give first aid to the most seriously injured victims first.

5. Summon more advanced medical help if needed. You should activate the EMS system for any serious or potentially serious conditions, including childbirth; if a victim has been drowned, electrocuted, burned, or poisoned; if you suspect heart attack or spinal injury; or if the victim is bleeding profusely, has

difficulty breathing, is choking, has any paralysis, has an altered level of consciousness, or has more than one seizure. If in doubt, activate the EMS system.

Arranging for Medical Assistance (Activating the EMS System)

During the first minutes after an accident, it is essential that the Emergency Medical Services (EMS) system be activated. In most areas of the United States, you can activate the EMS system by dialing 9-1-1; learn how to access the system in your area (see Figure 1-2). Give the following information to the dispatcher:

- The exact location of the victim—for example, the complete address and, if applicable, the number of the floor or office in the building

- The phone number where you can be reached

- Any information about the victim that will help the dispatcher send appropriate personnel and equipment

If at all possible, send a responsible bystander to telephone with the above information. If you're alone, activate the EMS system immediately after you determine unresponsiveness in an adult; in the case of an unconscious infant or child, provide 2 minutes of rescue support before you activate the EMS system.

If no telephone is available, continue giving first aid care until a bystander is available to activate the EMS system.

FIGURE 1-2. By dialing the emergency response system, 9-1-1, you activate Emergency Medical Services.

1. You should provide basic life support first to _____. *(victims of cardiac arrest/ victims who are bleeding/the most seriously injured)*

2. During the first few minutes after an accident, you should activate _____. *(bystanders/the EMS system/additional caregivers)*

3. If you are alone, you should provide rescue support to a child for _____ before telephoning for help. *(1 minute/2 minutes/ 5 minutes)*

1.3 Aspects of First Aid

First Aider Skills

Learning Objective **3** Identify skills performed by a First Aider.

When you have finished the first aid course, you should be able to

- Control an accident scene to prevent further injury

- Gain access to victims in the easiest and safest ways possible

- Open a victim's airway

- Perform rescue breathing

- Provide one- and two-rescuer cardiopulmonary resuscitation.

- Control bleeding by direct pressure, elevation, pressure points, and tourniquets

- Detect and care for shock

- Detect and care for soft-tissue and internal injuries

- Perform basic dressing and bandaging techniques

- Detect and care for open and closed fractures

- Detect and care for poisoning, including poisoning by alcohol or drugs

- Detect and care for heart attack, stroke, diabetic coma, insulin shock, and seizures

- Detect and care for facial and head injuries and chest injuries (including fractured ribs, flail chest, and penetrating chest wounds)

- Detect and care for superficial, partial-thickness and full-thickness burns, and smoke inhalation

- Detect and care for heat- and cold-related injuries

- Assist in childbirth and care of the newborn

- Give psychological support to victims of crises and disasters

- Perform emergency and nonemergency moves

Legal Aspects of First Aid

Learning Objective **4** Understand the legal aspects of first aid and emergency medical care.

First Aiders are bound by the same legal statutes as other Emergency-Care Providers. Every state has laws that govern these providers; find out what the laws are in your state.

Basically, the First Aider's duty can be legally defined as follows:

- The First Aider should not interfere with the first aid being given by others.

- The First Aider should follow the directions of a police officer and do what a reasonable First Aider would do under the circumstances.

- The First Aider should not force help on a victim who is unwilling to be treated unless the situation is life-threatening.

- Once a First Aider has *voluntarily* started care, he or she should not leave the scene or stop the care until relieved by a qualified and responsible person *who renders care at the same or a higher level of care.* Otherwise, leaving the scene or stopping care is legally considered *abandonment* and places the First Aider at risk of litigation.

- The First Aider should follow accepted and recognized first aid care procedures taught in first aid texts.

- The First Aider should respect the victim's privacy and should disclose confidential information—such as a victim's medical condition, injury, physical condition, or medications—only to those with a medical need to know.

- Any First Aider involved with a victim at a crime scene should document and preserve evidence and should comply with state laws requiring the reporting of specific criminal incidents (such as abuse, rape, and gunshot wounds).

DUTY TO ACT

Duty to act means there is a legal obligation to give aid or perform first aid care. This legal obligation may exist in the following situations:

- When you have a preexisting responsibility—you have an already established relationship that legally binds you to give aid, such as the relationship between driver and passenger or between parent and child.

- When your employment requires it—this includes occupations such as school teachers, park rangers, lifeguards, and police and fire personnel.

- When first aid has begun—once you have started, you must continue administering first aid until you have done all you can do.

As part of the duty to act, a First Aider must follow guidelines for the standard of care. Essentially, a First Aider is legally expected to provide the level and type of care consistent with his or her training. A First Aider has a different standard of care, for example, than a physician or an emergency medical technician.

Good Samaritan Laws

> Learning Objective **5** Explain the factors that constitute negligence on the part of a First Aider.

To protect health care personnel from being sued, many states have enacted **Good Samaritan laws.** In essence, these protect you as a First Aider unless you are found guilty of **negligence**—carelessness, inattention, disregard, inadvertence, or oversight that was accidental but avoidable. In order to establish negligence, the court must decide that

- The victim was injured

- Your actions or lack of action caused or contributed to the injury

- You had a duty to act

- You acted in an unusual, unreasonable, or imprudent way

"REASONABLE-MAN" TEST

Your defense against a charge of negligence is the **"reasonable-man" test**—did you act the same way a normal, prudent person with your same background and training would have acted under the same circumstances? Essentially, the burden of proof is on the victim; you can be prosecuted only if the victim can prove

that you are guilty of gross negligence, recklessness, willful or wanton conduct, or causing intentional injury.

RIGHT TO REFUSE CARE

A competent adult has the right to refuse emergency care and/or transportation for himself or herself or a minor in need of such care. If the victim or guardian refuses to consent, *you may not give first aid care or forcibly transport the victim.* If you do, you can be legally charged with battery. Generally, law enforcement personnel are the only people who can touch, restrain, or transport someone against his or her will.

There are four different kinds of consent:

1. **Actual consent.** The consent must be informed; you need to explain the care you will provide. Oral consent is valid.

2. **Implied consent.** If a victim is unconscious, the law assumes he or she would consent to care if conscious.

3. **Minor's consent.** The right to consent is usually given to the parent or guardian of a minor.

4. **Consent of the mentally ill.** The right to consent is usually given to the parent, guardian, or permanent caregiver of the mentally ill.

If a victim or guardian will not give consent and you believe that a life is at stake, summon the police. If injuries are serious but not life-threatening, explain the possible consequences of refusing treatment and try to persuade the victim to consent; enlist the help of family members or friends if necessary. If the victim still refuses, make sure there are witnesses who can verify that the victim refused care. Police and EMS personnel should make the final decision about care and transport.

> **duty to act** The legal obligation to give aid or perform first aid care
>
> **Good Samaritan laws** Laws that protect health care personnel and provide guidelines for care
>
> **negligence** Acting with carelessness, inattention, disregard, inadvertence, or avoidable oversight
>
> **"reasonable-man" test** Did the First Aider act the same way a normal, prudent person with similar training would have acted under the same circumstances?
>
> **actual consent** Informed consent
>
> **implied consent** Assumption that a victim of life-threatening injury or illness would give consent
>
> **minor's consent** The right of consent given to a parent or guardian

Controversies in First Aid Care

The first aid and emergency-care procedures in this text are accepted practices in the United States. However, there are still some areas of controversy in first aid care. When controversies exist, you should follow local protocol as outlined by your instructor.

PROGRESS CHECK

1. Duty to act means you have a _____ to give aid. *(responsibility/legal obligation/choice)*

2. The "reasonable-man" test shows that you acted as a normal, prudent person would have acted under the _____. *(same circumstances/law)*

3. _____ means you acted with carelessness, inattention, disregard, or oversight. *(Imprudence/Negligence/Recklessness)*

4. Every competent adult has the right to give _____ to treatment. *(approval/permission/consent)*

1.4 Infectious Disease Transmission

An **infectious**, or communicable, **disease** is one that can be transmitted from one person to another or from an infected animal or the environment to a person. *All body fluids should be considered infectious,* including saliva, blood, vaginal secretions, semen, amniotic fluid (the fluid that surrounds a fetus in the uterus), and fluids that lubricate the brain, spine, lungs, heart, abdominal organs, and joints and tendons.

Transmission of Infectious Disease

Learning Objective **6** Understand how infections are transmitted.

For disease to spread, three things must happen:

1. Infecting organisms, such as bacteria and viruses, must survive outside their host—an infected person, an animal, or an insect. Bacteria and viruses can also survive on inert objects, such as surfaces in the environment or discarded needles.

2. The infecting organism must then move from one place to another. Some organisms, such as cold viruses, are easily transmitted; others, such as tuberculosis bacteria, are relatively difficult to transmit (see Figure 1-3).

3. The infecting organism must then invade a new person's body and begin to multiply there. Inadequate nutrition, poor hygiene, crowded or unsanitary conditions, and stress can all increase a person's susceptibility to infection.

Identifying Infectious Diseases

A victim with any of the following should be considered infectious:

A rash or skin lesion
An open sore
Diarrhea
Vomiting
Coughing or sneezing
Draining or oozing wounds
Profuse sweating
Abdominal pain
Headache with stiff neck
Yellowish skin or eyes

Not all patients who are infectious will show outward signs of disease. You should avoid all contact with all body fluids from all patients—regardless of whether they appear sick.

Diseases of Concern in the Emergency Setting

Learning Objective **7** Identify the infectious diseases that are of concern in an emergency setting.

BLOODBORNE PATHOGENS

Of greatest concern to First Aiders and others in emergency settings are *bloodborne pathogens,* or diseases that are caused by microorganisms that are carried in the blood. You can be exposed to these any time you come in contact with a victim's blood or any other body fluid that contains blood; you can minimize your risk by using protective equipment, such as protective gloves, to avoid contact with the victim's blood.

Three bloodborne pathogens are of particular concern:

- **Hepatitis B.** The most common type of hepatitis, Hepatitis B, is a viral infection of the liver; symptoms

infectious disease A disease that can be transmitted from one person to another or from an insect or animal to a person

HOW INFECTIOUS DISEASES CAN SPREAD

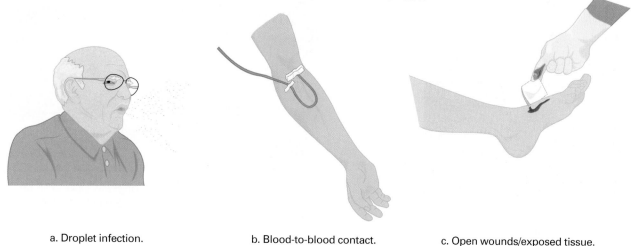

a. Droplet infection.   b. Blood-to-blood contact.   c. Open wounds/exposed tissue.

FIGURE 1–3. You can pick up and spread infections through physical contact with blood and other body fluids.

may resemble those of the flu, but many victims do not have symptoms at all. Even those without symptoms can still pass the infection on to others, however. The infection causes inflammation of the liver and can in some cases lead to permanent liver damage or even cancer of the liver. A vaccine for Hepatitis B is available, and is recommended for all those who may come in contact with the blood of others.

- **Hepatitis C.** Caused by a different virus than Hepatitis B, Hepatitis C can also lead to permanent liver damage or cancer of the liver. Like Hepatitis B, it may not cause symptoms, but the victim remains contagious even without symptoms. There is currently no effective treatment for or vaccine against Hepatitis C.

- **HIV.** The HIV virus suppresses the immune system and interferes with the body's ability to defend itself against other diseases. People infected with HIV may develop AIDS, which is fatal. HIV is spread by contact with infected blood or blood products, needles, urine, feces, or by sexual contact. People infected with HIV may have no symptoms, but even symptom-free victims can pass the virus to others. There is no vaccine against HIV, and there is no effective way of removing the virus from the body. The best defense against HIV is to avoid infection; always wear protective equipment, such as gloves, when caring for victims. Because the virus lives only a few hours in a dry environment and can be killed by common disinfectants, you should always be especially careful to clean any areas or equipment that have been contaminated by body fluids.

Several other diseases are of particular concern to First Aiders and others in an emergency setting.

- **Herpes.** A highly contagious viral infection of the skin and mucous membranes, herpes is spread through contact with active lesions. Genital herpes is also spread through contact with active lesions.

- **Tuberculosis.** Tuberculosis is a severe lung infection spread through the air or through direct contact with nasal or oral secretions. You can be infected by someone who is coughing, spitting, or simply speaking.

- **Meningitis.** Meningitis is an infection of the membranes lining the brain and spinal cord that is spread through infected water, food, air, or direct contact.

Protecting Yourself from Risk of Infection

Learning Objective **8** Describe ways to prevent the spread of AIDS and other infectious diseases in an emergency setting.

The following guidelines will help you avoid being infected by contact with blood, body fluids, secretions, sores, droplets, and bites.

- Make sure your immunizations are up to date. Adults who may render first aid should have the MMR (measles, mumps, rubella), DPT (diphtheria, pertussis, tetanus), varicella (chicken pox), Hepatitis B, and influenza immunizations.

- Wear disposable protective gloves whenever you have direct contact with a victim (see Figure 1-4). Do not use gloves that are discolored, brittle, punctured, or torn.

FIGURE 1–4. An Emergency-Care Provider using protective gloves for infectious disease protection. Victims or First Aiders can be allergic to latex. Because of the potential for serious latex allergies, many ambulances are totally latex-free, and most gloves are now vinyl or another protective material.

FIGURE 1–5. An Emergency-Care Provider should wear infection-control gear while treating a victim with an infectious disease.

- If there is risk of significant body fluid contact, wear additional disposable protective gear, such as a face mask, protective eyewear, and a gown (see Figure 1-5.)

- Wash your hands thoroughly with soap and hot water or an antibacterial agent immediately after providing care, even if you were wearing gloves; be sure to scrub under your fingernails.

- Avoid touching your mouth, nose, or eyes or any personal items (such as a comb, car keys, or food) until you have washed your hands.

- Cover any abrasions or skin conditions you have with protective clothing and/or protective gloves.

FIGURE 1–6. Pocket masks with one-way valves can be used to reduce the risk of cross-contamination. Many disposable types are also available.

- Use a pocket mask if possible when giving mouth-to-mouth resuscitation (Figure 1-6.)

- Report all incidents of exposure to body fluids to your physician or campus health service.

If you are required to clean up spills of blood or body fluid, wear the same protective equipment you would wear when treating a patient. Use paper towels or absorbent wipes to pick up all visible fluids. Then use a 1:100 bleach-to-water solution to clean the area. Allow to air dry. Dispose of all cleaning products in a manner that will not cause additional exposure to others and as required by local rules.

> ### PROGRESS CHECK
>
> 1. To prevent the risk of bloodborne infection, you should always wear _____ when caring for a victim. *(a face mask/a gown/ protective gloves)*
>
> 2. Use a _____ when giving mouth-to-mouth resuscitation. *(face mask/pocket mask/face shield)*
>
> 3. The best protection you have against disease is to _____ after giving treatment. *(wash your hands/take an antibiotic/use antiseptic)*

1.5 Safety at the Scene

One of the first things you will need to deal with at many scenes is safety—not just for the victim, but for you and for bystanders at the scene. *Staying safe is your first priority;* you won't be able to help someone else if you become a victim yourself.

As soon as you arrive at a scene, assess the situation from a safety standpoint. Do not enter an unsafe situation unless you have been properly trained and have proper protective equipment. In addition to activating the EMS for a victim, you might need to send for specialized personnel who can move wreckage, take care of downed power lines, put out a fire, and so on.

Fire

Immediately call the fire department, regardless of how small the fire is—fire of any size can get out of control, threatening life and property. Unless you have been specifically trained, never approach a burning building or a burning vehicle; stay a safe distance away, upwind from any smoke or fumes, until the fire has been contained.

Unstable Structures

An unstable structure is defined as one in which you may become trapped or injured because of weak floors or ceilings, partially collapsed walls, debris, hazardous gases in the air, or the threat of explosion or fire. And instability is not limited to buildings—it can also involve wells, trenches, silos, vats, pits, and mines, in which you could be buried or trapped. Call the fire department for help; in the meantime, figure out the probable location of any victims so you can offer help as soon as the structure is stabilized.

Motor Vehicle Accidents

One of the greatest threats related to a motor vehicle accident is that posed by oncoming traffic. As soon as you arrive at the scene, park where you will not interfere with an ambulance and where you will be least likely to cause increased traffic problems. Assign a bystander to direct traffic as far away from the accident as possible. If they are available, place safety flares or reflectors well beyond the accident in both directions.

Other safety threats at the site of an accident include spilled gasoline (which can cause fire or explosion), hazardous materials, and unstable wreckage. Methods of stabilizing a vehicle and extricating a victim from wreckage are discussed in Chapter 30.

People who transport or store hazardous materials are required by law to post placards on their vehicles identifying the hazardous materials. Even if you do not see such a placard, you may suspect the presence of a hazardous material because of leaking containers or an unusual odor, liquid, or vapor. If you suspect a hazardous

material, alert the fire department or a HAZMAT team, then wait a safe distance upwind and take care not to create sparks.

Electrical Hazards

Look for downed power lines at the scene of *every* motor vehicle accident, and always consider downed power lines to be "live." Immediately notify the local power company and fire department, and wait for trained personnel to shut off the power source before you get close to the wires. *Never try to move downed wires yourself.*

Never touch a vehicle, body of water, or metal object that is in contact with a downed wire. If power lines are touching a vehicle, tell victims—even those who seem seriously injured—to stay inside until help arrives. Keep all bystanders a safe distance from downed wires; live wires can whip and lash about, so as a general rule, stay at a distance at least twice as long as the span of wire.

Water

Never enter the water or venture out onto ice to rescue someone unless you have been specifically trained in water rescue—and, even then, do it only as a last resort. Call for help, then follow these guidelines while you wait for help to arrive:

- If the victim is near enough to reach you, hold out your hand, a pole, a branch, or some other object; once the victim grabs it, pull the victim to shore. Make sure your footing is stable so that you are not pulled into the water.

- If you can not reach the victim, tie a buoyant object to the end of a rope and throw the object to the victim. You can use an ice chest, a milk jug, an inflated toy, a branch, a life jacket, or anything else that floats. Tell the victim to hold on to the floating object, then tow the victim to shore. Again, check your own footing to avoid being pulled into the water.

Hostility and Violence

Stay a safe distance from a hostile victim while you calmly explain who you are and what you want to do to help; if possible, enlist the help of a family member or friend to try to defuse the situation. If a victim remains hostile, retreat and call for help. *Never* approach a hostile crowd; call the police and wait until the situation is under control.

Never approach a victim of violence—even one with life-threatening injuries—until you are sure that the perpetrator has left the scene. Likewise, never approach an armed person who is threatening suicide.

Immediately call the police and wait for them to secure the scene; do not touch anything or disturb any evidence while you wait.

PROGRESS CHECK

1. Your first priority at the scene of an accident is _____. *(reaching the victim/staying safe/preventing further injury to the victim)*

2. You should call the fire department in case of _____. *(any fire/a fire that is out of control/a fire that is creating toxic fumes)*

3. One of the greatest threats to safety from a motor vehicle accident is _____. *(fire/gasoline fumes/oncoming traffic)*

4. You can touch a downed power line _____. *(with a stick/if you are wearing rubber-soled boots/only after the power company has turned off the power)*

5. If a victim is hostile, _____. *(restrain the victim yourself/have bystanders help you restrain the victim/call the police)*

Summary

- First Aid is temporary and immediate care given to a person who is injured or who suddenly becomes ill; it does not replace the care of a physician, nurse, or paramedic.

- A primary principle of first aid is to activate the EMS system in all cases of serious injury.

- First Aiders should be able to recognize life-threatening problems, supply artificial ventilation and circulation, control bleeding, prevent further injury, and minimize complications.

- You should always provide care to the most seriously injured victims first.

- You have a duty to act—the legal obligation to give aid or perform first aid care—if you have a preexisting responsibility, your employment requires it, or you have already started first aid.

- As a First Aider, you are protected under the law as long as you act the same way that a normal, prudent person with your background and training would have acted under the same circumstances.

- Any competent adult has the right to refuse first aid care and/or transportation; you must obtain consent before beginning treatment.

- Infectious diseases—especially Hepatitis B, meningitis, tuberculosis, and AIDS—are of particular concern in the emergency setting.

- You can minimize your risk of infection by wearing protective gloves; wearing other protective gear as appropriate; using a pocket mask during mouth-to-mouth resuscitation; and washing your hands thoroughly after any contact with a victim.

Key Terms

Make sure you understand the following key terms:

first aid	actual consent
duty to act	implied consent
Good Samaritan laws	minor's consent
negligence	infectious disease
"reasonable-man" test	

Critical Thinking Exercise

You are on campus and observe a young man fall down a flight of stairs. He tries to get up as you approach. After asking your companion to alert campus police and EMS, you identify yourself as being trained in first aid and offer your help. The patient tells you "I think I sprained my ankle, but I'm OK. I'm just going to walk it off."

You observed the patient's fall and realize he could be hurt worse than he thinks. An abrasion above his eye leads you to think he also hit his head. He is still refusing any help.

1. Should you call to cancel campus security and EMS? Why or why not?

2. Should this patient be examined by EMS? Why or why not?

3. If you decided that the patient does require further care, how could you convince this patient to stay in place and await EMS?

1 Chapter 1 Self-Test

Part 1   True/False

If you believe the statement is true, circle the T. If you believe the statement is false, circle the F.

T   F   **1.** One in five Americans is injured each year.

T   F   **2.** Two important words in a definition of first aid are *immediate* and *temporary*.

T   F   **3.** Activating the EMS system is an important part of first aid.

T   F   **4.** The first thing to do for an injured person is to control bleeding.

T   F   **5.** One of the main concerns of a First Aider is to prevent added injury or death.

T   F   **6.** You should not activate the EMS system until you have rendered all possible first aid care.

T   F   **7.** A person who receives first aid training is required by law to stop and help at an accident scene.

T   F   **8.** You have to receive a person's consent for treatment before you can render first aid care.

T   F   **9.** A First Aider should take specific precautions against infectious disease.

T   F   **10.** If you wear protective gloves while treating a victim, you don't need to wash your hands.

Part 2   Multiple Choice

For each item, circle the correct answer or the phrase that best completes the statement.

1. First aid is the immediate action taken to
   a. care for the injured until medical help is available
   b. supplement proper medical or surgical treatment
   c. preserve vitality and resistance to disease
   d. rescue and transport the injured

2. When administering first aid, the condition that should be cared for first is
   a. the most painful one
   b. the most life-threatening one
   c. the most obvious one
   d. bleeding

3. The most correct definition of first aid is
   a. immediate care given to someone who is ill or injured
   b. care given in the ambulance
   c. rescue and transport of ill or injured people
   d. all of the above

4. Under normal circumstances, the best first contact for help in case of accident is
   a. the hospital emergency room
   b. the first response department
   c. the police or highway patrol
   d. the Emergency Medical Services (EMS) system

5. The "reasonable-man" test is
   a. given to First Aiders to test their skills
   b. given to First Aiders to test personality traits
   c. used to ascertain whether a First Aider provided care that was fair, reasonable, and unbiased
   d. used to ascertain whether a First Aider acted as a normal, prudent person with first aid training would have acted

6. Infectious disease is a disease that
   a. always causes permanent disability or death
   b. can be spread from one person to another
   c. must be reported to state or federal agencies
   d. cannot be prevented

Match the terms on the right with their proper definition.

A. In a true emergency, the law assumes an unconscious person would give consent.

B. The right to consent is given to the parent or guardian.

C. An informed consent.

Actual consent _____

Implied consent _____

Minor's consent _____

2

Anatomy and Physiology of Body Systems

Learning Objectives

When you have mastered the material in this chapter, you will be able to

1 Define and use the common anatomical terms of body position

2 Define and use the common topographical terms of direction and location

3 Describe the main structures and functions of the skeletal system

4 Describe the main structures and functions of the muscular system

5 Describe the main structures and functions of the circulatory system

6 Describe the main structures and functions of the respiratory system

7 Describe the main structures and functions of the digestive system

8 Describe the main structures and functions of the urinary system

9 Describe the main structures and functions of the endocrine system

10 Describe the main structures and functions of the nervous system

11 Describe the main structures and functions of the skin

On the Scene

Jim Stewart was a volunteer in a first aid station during a bike marathon. Shortly after the race began, he received a report of a fall. It occurred close to his station, so he went to check it out. The course was partially on paved road and partially on special bike trails, which were not wide enough for cars. Jim took his bicycle and first aid kit.

When Jim arrived, a few of the riders were gathered around the woman who had fallen, so he sent one of them to activate the EMS system and another to the head of the trail to direct the ambulance to them.

The woman had somehow lost control of her bike, gone off the trail, and hit a tree. She was alert, but complained of pain in several places. Jim had one of the onlookers keep her head and cervical spine in a neutral in-line position without removing the helmet she was wearing, while he continued to evaluate her other injuries.

Jim found the woman in a face-up (supine) position, though she had fallen on her left side. She complained of pain in her lower ribs and left arm. She also had numerous abrasions and one laceration approximately 2 inches long on the inner (medial) aspect of her left lower leg, which was still bleeding. Jim applied a dressing and had a bystander apply pressure to the wound so he could check the woman's vital signs.

Jim was concerned about the pain in the woman's upper left abdomen (upper left quadrant)—which could indicate a potentially serious injury. He continued to monitor her vital signs closely. He also had time to dress and bandage the laceration on her leg while waiting.

When the EMS crew arrived, they removed the victim's helmet, performed an assessment, applied oxygen by a mask, splinted her arm, immobilized her on a backboard, and otherwise made her ready for transport. Jim walked beside them on the way to the ambulance, wheeling both of the bikes. He assured the victim that he would notify family members who were waiting for her at the end of the course and give them her bike.

To render first aid effectively, you need to have a knowledge of the basic structures of the human body. A cell is the basic unit of all living tissue, and *tissues* are collections of similar cells. A *system* is a group of organs that work together to perform a specific function. *Anatomy* deals with the structure of the body and the relationship of its parts to each other. *Physiology* deals with the function of the living body and its parts—in other words, how the body works.

2.1 Anatomical Terminology

When you seek medical assistance, you need to use correct anatomical terms to describe the victim's position, direction, and location—a practice that eliminates confusion and helps you communicate the extent of injury more effectively.

Terms of Position

Learning Objective 1 Define and use the common anatomical terms of body position.

The terms of position include

- **Anatomical position**—The victim is standing erect, arms down to the sides, palms facing forward. "Right" and "left" refer to the victim's right and left.
- **Supine position**—The victim is lying face up (on the back) (see Figure 2–1).
- **Prone position**—The victim is lying face down (on the stomach) (see Figure 2–2).
- **Lateral recumbent position**—The victim is lying on the left or right side with the lower arm in front of the body, head dependent, with no excess pressure on the chest. This is also known as the recovery, or coma, position (see Figure 2–3 and 2–4).

anatomical position Standing erect with the arms down at the sides, the palms facing forward

supine position Lying face up on the back

prone position Lying face down on the stomach (face down)

lateral recumbent (recovery, or coma) position Lying on the right or left side with the lower arm in front of the body, with the head dependent

FIGURE 2–1. Supine position

FIGURE 2–2. Prone position

FIGURE 2–3. Right lateral recumbent position, also known as the recovery, or coma, position

FIGURE 2–4. Left lateral recumbent position, also known as the recovery, or coma, position

FIGURE 2–5. Modified HAINES recovery position

- **Modified HAINES recovery position**—If the victim has a suspected injury to the spine, is unresponsive, and has a possible airway compromise due to a large amount of blood, vomitus, or secretions, place the victim in a modified HAINES recovery position. Extend the victim's arm above the head, logroll him into his side so his head rests on the extended arm. Bend the legs at the knees to stabilize his position.

Terms of Direction and Location

Learning Objective **2** Define and use the common topographical terms of direction and location.

Terms of direction and location (see Figure 2–6) include

- **Superior**—above, or higher than a point of reference (e.g., the knee is superior to the ankle)
- **Inferior**—below, or lower than a point of reference (e.g., the wrist is inferior to the elbow)
- **Anterior**—toward the front
- **Posterior**—toward the back
- **Medial**—toward the midline or center of the body
- **Lateral**—to the right or left of the midline; away from the midline
- **Superficial**—near the surface

modified HAINES recovery position Extend the arm, logroll the victim on his side, rest his head on the extended arm, bend the knees to stabilize his body.

superior Above, or higher than, a point of reference

inferior Below, or lower than, a point of reference

anterior Toward the front

posterior Toward the back

medial Toward the midline (center) of the body

lateral To the right or left of the midline (center) of the body; away from the midline

superficial Near the surface

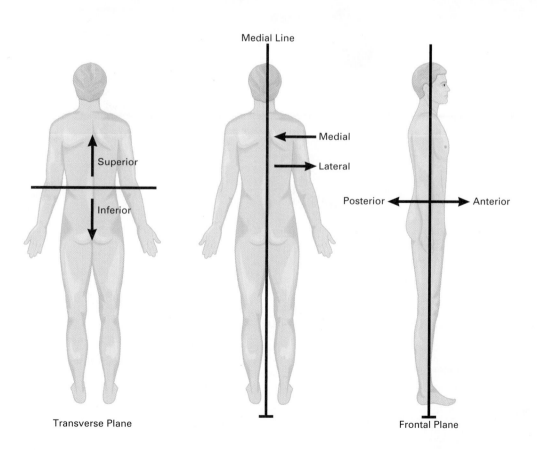

Medial Line

Superior

Inferior

Medial

Lateral

Posterior ← → Anterior

Transverse Plane

Frontal Plane

FIGURE 2–6. Anatomical planes and terms

- **Deep**—remote from the surface
- **Internal**—inside
- **External**—outside

1. A victim lying on his or her back is in the _____ position. *(supine/prone/lateral)*

2. A victim lying on her or his stomach is in the _____ position. *(supine/prone/lateral)*

3. _____ means above a point of reference. *(superior/anterior/posterior)*

4. _____ means below a point of reference. *(superior/inferior/posterior)*

5. A wound near the surface is a _____ wound. *(internal/external/superficial)*

2.2 The Body's Framework

The Skeletal System

Learning Objective **3** Describe the main structures and functions of the skeletal system.

The human body (see Figure 2–7) is shaped by a framework of bones held together by ligaments that connect bone to bone; layers of muscles; tendons, which connect muscles to bones or other structures; and various connective tissues. Bones and their adjacent tissues help to move, support, and protect the vital organs.

deep Remote from the surface
internal Inside
external Outside

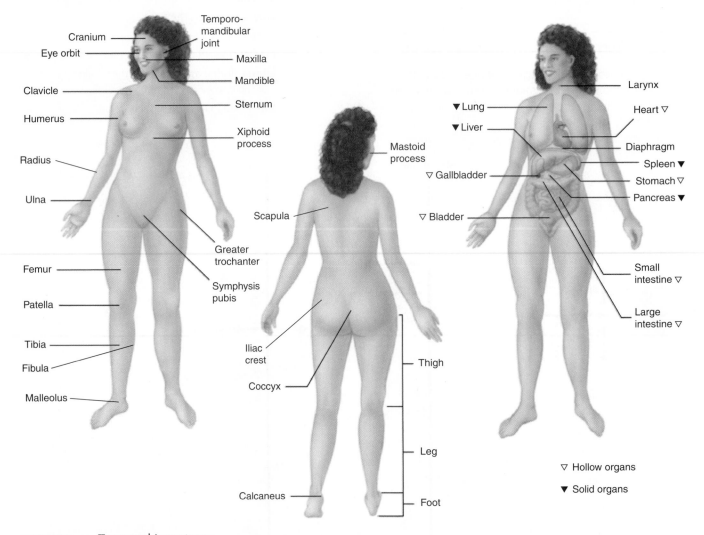

FIGURE 2–7. Topographic anatomy

The skeleton (see Figure 2–8) is

- Strong, to provide support and protection
- Jointed, to permit motion
- Flexible, to withstand stress

Bones are richly supplied by nerves and blood vessels. When fractured, some bones, like the pelvis and femur, can bleed excessively from the bone itself. Thus, fractures to the femur and pelvis are considered critical injuries.

SKULL

The skull, also known as the cranium, is a very tough bone that protects the brain. At the bottom of the skull is the largest opening (foramen magnum). The brain exits this opening and continues as the spinal cord.

SPINAL COLUMN

The spinal column contains 33 bones called vertebrae. The vertebrae lie on top of each other and form the bony spinal column. Inside the bony spinal column is the spinal cord. One of the functions of the spinal column is to protect the spinal cord. The spinal cord is responsible for carrying impulses to and away from the brain. Like the brain tissue, if the spinal cord is injured or compressed, it usually will not function below the point of injury. This results in a possible loss of sensation and movement to the areas below the site of injury.

There are five sections of the spinal column:

1. Cervical
2. Thoracic
3. Lumbar
4. Sacrum
5. Coccyx

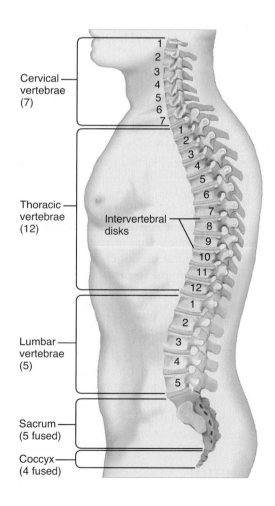

FIGURE 2–8. The skeletal system

It is important to understand that a victim can have an injured or fractured spinal column with no injury to the spinal cord.

THORAX

The thorax is made up of the ribs and sternum in the front (anteriorly) and the spinal column in the back (posteriorly). The sternum, or breastbone, is located in the center of the chest. The chest is made up of 12 pairs of ribs, which are all attached to the spinal column on the back (posterior) side. The first 10 anterior ribs are connected to the sternum either directly or by cartilage. The last two ribs are called floating ribs. They are only attached to the spine and are free floating and not connected to the sternum.

The clavicles, also known as the collarbones, are easily felt at the top of the chest. The clavicle can be fractured and results in severe pain and gross deformity.

PELVIS

The pelvis contains organs such as the urinary bladder and some of the reproductive organs. The pelvic bone contains a very rich blood supply. A fracture to the pelvis can result in excessive internal bleeding. A suspected fractured pelvis is a critical injury.

LOWER EXTREMITIES

The lower extremities are composed of the femur, which is also commonly known as the thigh bone. The femur fits into the pelvis, forming a ball-and-socket joint that allows for movement. The femur is the longest and strongest bone of the body. It takes a significant amount of force to fracture the femur. The femur, like the pelvis, contains a very rich blood supply. If fractured, the femur can lead to serious blood loss. A fracture to the femur usually results in gross deformity to the thigh and extreme pain to the victim. Due to the potential for blood loss, a fractured femur is a critical injury.

The knee is the strongest joint of the body. The kneecap (patella) can be fractured or dislocated.

The lower leg is made up of the tibia and fibula. The tibia, which is commonly referred to as the shin bone, is larger than the fibula. It is located in front of (interior to) and in the middle of (medial) the lower leg. The upper portion of the tibia forms the knee joint where it meets with the femur. The lowest portion of the tibia forms the ankle joint.

The ankle contains the tarsals. The metatarsals form the foot. The toes are also called the phalanges.

UPPER EXTREMITIES

The long bone in the arm is the humerus. The humerus fits into the socket of the shoulder blade (scapula) allowing for movement in many directions. A common injury

is a dislocation where the head of humerus pulls out of the socket of the scapula.

The forearm is made up of two bones that lie alongside each other. The radius is the bone located on the thumb side and the ulna is located on the little finger side of the forearm.

The wrist is composed of the carpals. The carpals meet with the radius and ulna to form the wrist. The hand is made up of the metacarpals. The bones in the fingers are referred to as the phalanges.

JOINT MOVEMENTS

A joint is where two bone ends **articulate**, or fit into each other. Joints can be immovable (such as those of the skull), slightly movable (such as those of the spinal column), or freely movable (such as the knee or elbow). Joints typically allow for movement and may result in dislocations of bones when injured.

The most common emergency involving the skeletal system is a **fracture,** a break in the continuity of the bone. A fracture can not only cause injury to the bone and surrounding muscle, but can damage adjacent nerves, blood vessels, and organs. When blood vessel damage occurs, a fracture can also cause potentially serious internal bleeding.

The Muscular System

Learning Objective **4** Describe the main structures and functions of the muscular system.

The muscles give the body its ability to move.

There are three basic kinds of muscles in the body (see Figure 2–9):

1. **Skeletal muscle**, or **voluntary muscle**, is under a person's conscious control and makes possible actions such as walking, chewing, swallowing, smiling, frowning, talking, and moving the eyeballs. Skeletal muscle helps give the body its shape. Most skeletal muscles are attached to the bone by tendons.

2. **Smooth muscle**, or **involuntary muscle**, is muscle over which a person has little or no conscious control. Smooth muscle is found in the walls of some organs, ducts, blood vessels, bronchioles in

articulate To fit into each other

fracture A break in the bone

skeletal (voluntary) muscle Muscle that is under direct voluntary control of the brain

smooth muscle The muscles found in the walls of the internal organs and blood vessels, generally not under voluntary control

involuntary muscle Smooth muscle over which a person has no voluntary or conscious control

FIGURE 2–9. There are three types of muscle. Skeletal muscle, also called voluntary muscle, is found throughout the body. Cardiac muscle is limited to the heart. Smooth muscle, occasionally called involuntary muscle, is found in many structures, including the intestines, arterioles, and bronchioles.

the respiratory tract, and the intestines. Smooth muscle has the ability to contract and relax.

3. **Cardiac muscle** forms the heart. Cardiac muscle receives stimulation from the nervous system; however, it is able to stimulate contractions without a signal from the nervous system.

PROGRESS CHECK

1. The largest bone in the body is the
   _____ . *(tibia/humerus/femur)*

2. Dislocations will occur at _____ .
   (muscle attachments/joints/tendons)

3. Deliberate acts, such as walking and talking,
   depend on _____ muscle.
   (skeletal/smooth/cardiac)

4. The movement of the intestines depends on
   _____ muscle. *(skeletal/smooth/cardiac)*

2.3 The Body's Organ Systems

The Circulatory System

Learning Objective **5** Describe the main structures and functions of the circulatory system.

The circulatory system (see Figure 2–10 on page 20) is made up of two major transportation systems: The cardiovascular system, which consists of the heart, blood vessels, and blood, carries oxygen and nutrients to body cells and transports waste from body cells and kidneys. The lymphatic system provides drainage for tissue fluid, called *lymph.*

HEART

The heart alternately contracts and relaxes to pump blood through the lungs, where it is oxygenated, and then through the vast network of blood vessels. About the size of a man's fist, the heart is located in the left center of the chest, just behind the sternum (breastbone). The heart has four chambers. The two upper chambers are called the *atria* and the two lower chambers are called the *ventricles.* The left ventricle, which pumps blood through the body, is the strongest and thickest part of the heart. Since the heart is a muscle, a continuous supply of oxygen and nutrients is necessary for it to function properly.

BLOOD VESSELS

The arteries carry oxygenated blood from the heart to the cells of the body. The exchange of fluid, oxygen, and carbon dioxide between the blood and the tissue cells takes place through the capillaries. The veins carry oxygen-depleted blood back to the heart (see Figure 2–11 on page 21), where the cycle begins again. Coronary arteries supply oxygenated blood and nutrients to the heart.

PULSE

Every time the heart contracts, the flow of blood can be felt as a pulse wherever an artery passes over a bone near the surface of the skin. Major pulses can be felt in the wrist on the thumb side (radial), upper arm between the bicep and tricep muscles (brachial), thigh (femoral), ankle (posterior tibial), and neck (carotid).

BLOOD

The blood is composed of red blood cells, white blood cells, platelets, and plasma. The red blood cells are responsible for carrying oxygen to the tissues and cells

cardiac muscle The muscle that makes up the heart

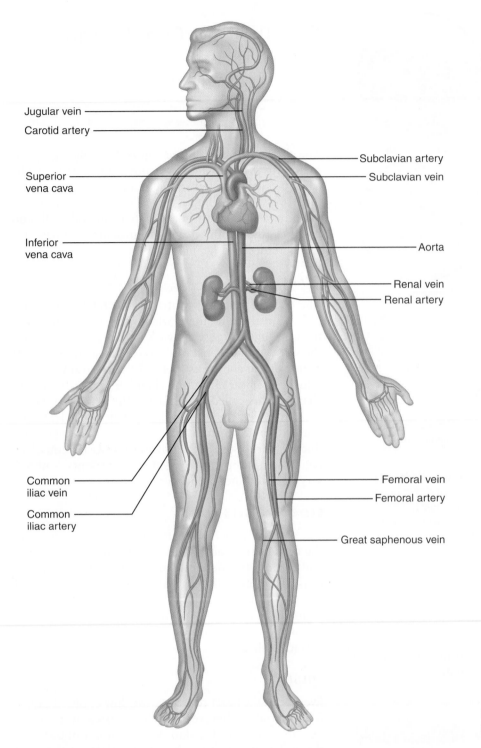

Jugular vein

Carotid artery

Superior
vena cava

Inferior
vena cava

Subclavian artery

Subclavian vein

Aorta

Renal vein

Renal artery

Common
iliac vein

Common
iliac artery

Femoral vein

Femoral artery

Great saphenous vein

FIGURE 2–10. The circulatory system

throughout the body. The white blood cells play a role in fighting infection. The platelets are a component in the clotting process. Plasma is the liquid portion of the blood that is responsible for suspending and transporting the red blood cells, white blood cells, and platelets.

Emergencies involving the circulatory system occur when there is uncontrolled bleeding, when circulation is impaired, or when the heart loses its ability to pump.

The Respiratory System

Learning Objective **6** Describe the main structures and functions of the respiratory system.

The body depends on a constant supply of oxygen, which is made available to the blood through the respiratory system (see Figure 2–12) on page 22.

Superior vena cava

Right pulmonary artery

Aorta

Pulmonary semilunar valve

Right atrium

Right AV valve

Right ventricle

Inferior vena cava

Left pulmonary artery

Pulmonary trunk

Left pulmonary veins

Left atrium

Aortic semilunar valve

Left AV valve

Left ventricle

Chordae tendineae

Papillary muscles

Septum

FIGURE 2–11. The heart

The mechanical process of moving air into and out of the lungs is called **ventilation**. During **inhalation** (or **inspiration**), air enters the lungs through the nose, mouth, trachea, bronchi, and bronchioles; the air is warmed, moistened, and filtered before it reaches the lungs. The lungs expand and fill the alveoli. Blood circulating through the lungs is oxygenated. **Respiration** is the exchange of oxygen and carbon dioxide between the alveoli and the blood. Oxygen moves into the blood from the alveoli, and carbon dioxide moves into the alveoli from the blood.

During **exhalation** (or **expiration**), the muscles of the chest relax, decreasing the size of the chest, and releasing air from the lungs. The exhaled breath carries with it carbon dioxide and other waste products.

The average breathing rate at rest is 12 to 20 breaths per minute in adults, 15 to 30 breaths per minute in children, and 25 to 50 breaths per minute in infants.

Emergencies involving the respiratory system include obstruction (choking), difficulty breathing, respiratory distress, and respiratory arrest. Airway obstruction is more common among infants and children because their respiratory structures are much smaller.

The Digestive System

Learning Objective 7 Describe the main structures and functions of the digestive system.

The digestive system (see Figure 2–13 on page 23) consists of the alimentary tract (the food passageway) and the accessory organs of digestion—the mouth, esophagus, stomach, pancreas, liver, spleen, gallbladder, small intestine, and large intestine. Following are the main functions of the digestive system:

- Ingest and carry food
- Digest food
- Absorb nutrients
- Eliminate wastes

Emergency care is required for any blunt or penetrating injury to the abdomen. Internal bleeding in the abdomen is also a critical injury.

ventilation The mechanical process of moving (breathing) air into and out of the lungs

inhalation The act of breathing in (inspiration), or the drawing of air or other gases into the lungs

inspiration The act of breathing in (inhalation)

respiration Exchange of oxygen and carbon dioxide in the lungs

exhalation (**expiration**) The act of breathing air out of the lungs

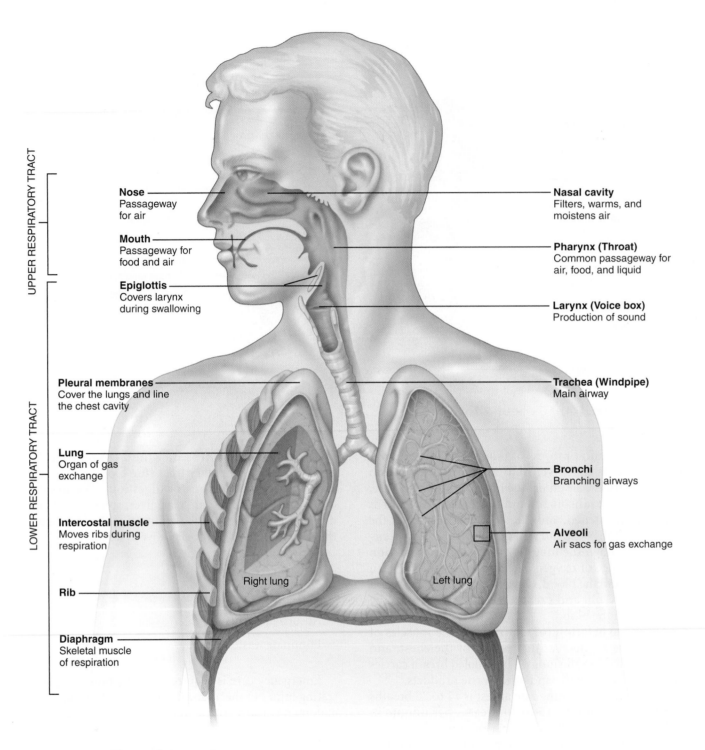

UPPER RESPIRATORY TRACT

LOWER RESPIRATORY TRACT

Nose
Passageway
for air

Mouth
Passageway for
food and air

Epiglottis
Covers larynx
during swallowing

Pleural membranes
Cover the lungs and line
the chest cavity

Lung
Organ of gas
exchange

Intercostal muscle
Moves ribs during
respiration

Rib

Diaphragm
Skeletal muscle
of respiration

Nasal cavity
Filters, warms, and
moistens air

Pharynx (Throat)
Common passageway for
air, food, and liquid

Larynx (Voice box)
Production of sound

Trachea (Windpipe)
Main airway

Bronchi
Branching airways

Alveoli
Air sacs for gas exchange

Right lung   Left lung

FIGURE 2–12. The respiratory system

The Urinary System

Learning Objective **8** Describe the main structures and functions of the urinary system.

The urinary system (see Figure 2–14 on page 24) filters
and excretes waste from the body; it consists of two kidneys, two ureters (which carry urine from the kidneys

to the bladder), one urinary bladder, and one urethra
(which carries urine from the bladder out of the body).
  The urinary system

- Helps maintain the delicate balance of water and
  other chemicals needed for survival
- Removes wastes from the bloodstream
- Returns useful products to the blood

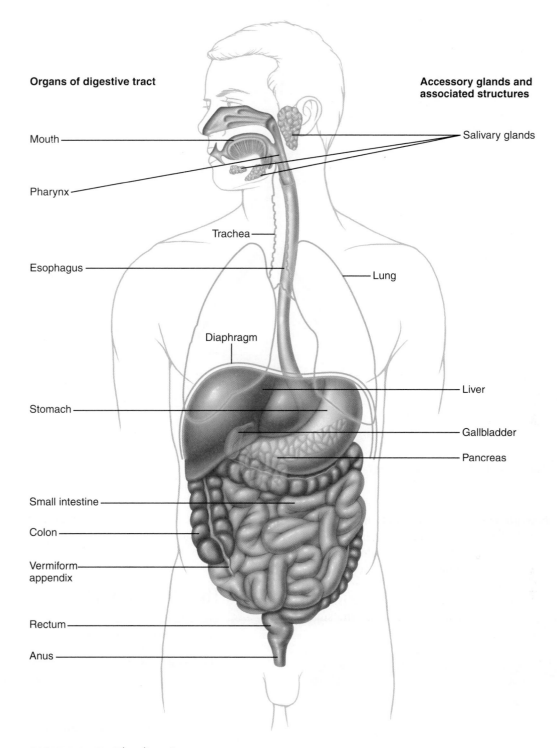

Organs of digestive tract

Accessory glands and associated structures

Mouth

Pharynx

Trachea

Esophagus

Salivary glands

Lung

Diaphragm

Stomach

Liver

Gallbladder

Pancreas

Small intestine

Colon

Vermiform appendix

Rectum

Anus

FIGURE 2–13. The digestive system

Emergency care is required for any blunt or penetrating injury to the lower abdomen or genitals, any significant injury to any quadrant of the abdomen, any injury to the external genitals, and any forceful injury to the area of the back below the rib cage.

The Endocrine System

Learning Objective **9** Describe the main structures and functions of the endocrine system.

Inferior vena cava
Abdominal aorta
Adrenal gland
(part of the endocrine system)

Kidney
Renal hilus
Renal artery
Renal vein
Ureter

Bladder
Neck of bladder
Urethra

FIGURE 2–14. The urinary system

The **endocrine glands** regulate the body by secreting hormones that affect physical strength, mental ability, stature, maturity, reproduction, and behavior.

Endocrine glands, which have no ducts, secrete hormones directly into the bloodstream. The adrenal gland secretes adrenalin (epinephrine). The islets of Langerhans play a major role in regulating the sugar level in the blood.

Emergency care is required for diabetics who have had too much or too little insulin.

<table>
<tr><td>2.4</td><td>

The Nerves and Skin

</td></tr>
</table>

The Nervous System

Learning Objective **10** Describe the common structures and functions of the nervous system.

The nervous system (see Figure 2–15) has two major functions: communication and control. The nervous system

- Enables the person to be aware of the environment
- Enables the person to react to the environment
- Coordinates responses of the body to stimuli
- Keeps body systems working together

PROGRESS CHECK

1. The circulatory system has two major fluid transportation systems: the cardiovascular and the _____ . *(cardiopulmonary/ genitourinary/lymphatic)*

2. The mechanical process of moving air into and out of the lungs is called _____ . *(inspiration/ventilation/expiration)*

3. The urinary system filters and _____ body wastes. *(breaks down/metabolizes/ eliminates)*

4. Endocrine glands, which have no ducts, secrete _____ directly into the bloodstream. *(hormones/chemicals/fluids)*

endocrine glands The ductless glands that regulate the body by secreting hormones

THE BRAIN

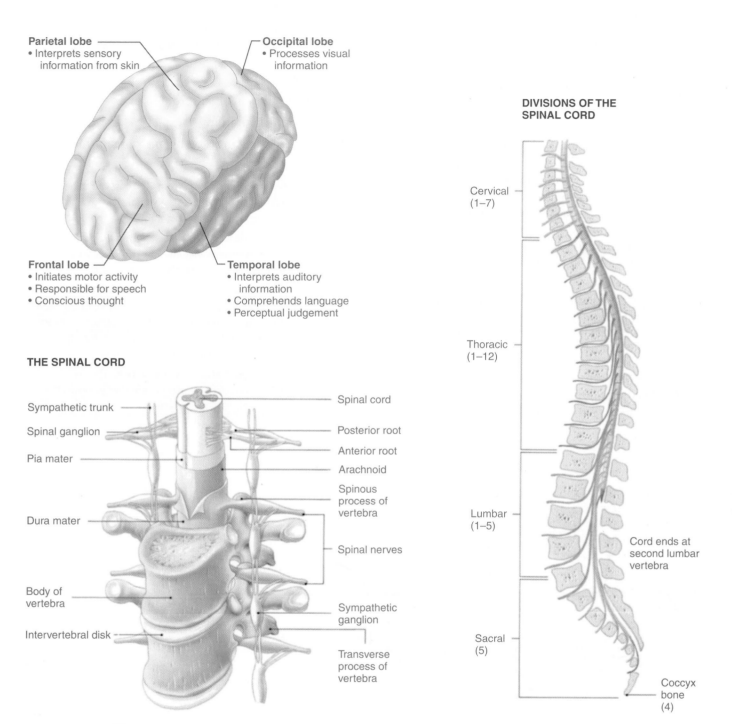

Parietal lobe
• Interprets sensory information from skin

Occipital lobe
• Processes visual information

Frontal lobe
• Initiates motor activity
• Responsible for speech
• Conscious thought

Temporal lobe
• Interprets auditory information
• Comprehends language
• Perceptual judgement

THE SPINAL CORD

Sympathetic trunk

Spinal ganglion

Pia mater

Dura mater

Body of vertebra

Intervertebral disk

Spinal cord

Posterior root

Anterior root

Arachnoid

Spinous process of vertebra

Spinal nerves

Sympathetic ganglion

Transverse process of vertebra

DIVISIONS OF THE SPINAL CORD

Cervical (1–7)

Thoracic (1–12)

Lumbar (1–5)

Sacral (5)

Cord ends at second lumbar vertebra

Coccyx bone (4)

FIGURE 2–15. The nervous system

The nervous system consists of nerve centers (most of them in the brain and spinal cord) and nerves that branch off from those centers, leading to body tissues and organs.

There are two main structural divisions of the nervous system: The **central nervous system** consists of the brain and spinal cord; the **peripheral nervous system** consists of nerves located outside the brain and spinal cord.

central nervous system The part of the nervous system that consists of the brain and the spinal cord

peripheral nervous system Structures of the nervous system (especially nerve endings) that lie outside the brain and spinal cord

There are also two functional divisions of the nervous system: The **voluntary nervous system** is responsible for voluntary movements throughout the body; the **autonomic nervous system**, influences the involuntary muscles, glands, and organs.

The autonomic nervous system (see Figure 2–16), which regulates unconscious, involuntary body functions, is further divided into two systems:

- The **sympathetic nervous system** regulates heart rate and force of contraction, supply of blood to the arteries, secretions of ductless glands, smooth muscle action in the digestive tract and bronchioles, and action of other internal organs. The sympathetic nervous system causes the release of adrenalin epinephrine from the adrenal glands. This system responds to stress, pain, injury, and blood loss with the classic "fight-or-flight" syndrome.

- The **parasympathetic nervous system** opposes the sympathetic nervous system and has the opposite effect on organs, vessels, glands, and other structures.

Emergency care is required for any loss of consciousness, head injury, brain injury, spinal injury, and any loss of sensory or motor function.

The Skin

Learning Objective 11 Describe the main structures and functions of the skin.

The skin

- Protects internal organs from injury
- Prevents dehydration
- Protects against invasion by microorganisms

voluntary nervous system The part of the nervous system that influences activity of the voluntary muscles and movements throughout the body

autonomic nervous system The part of the nervous system that influences the activities of involuntary muscles, glands, and organs

sympathetic nervous system The part of the autonomic nervous system that causes blood vessels to constrict, stimulates sweating, increases the heart rate, causes the sphincter muscles to contract, and prepares the body to respond to stress

parasympathetic nervous system The part of the autonomic nervous system that opposes the sympathetic nervous system.

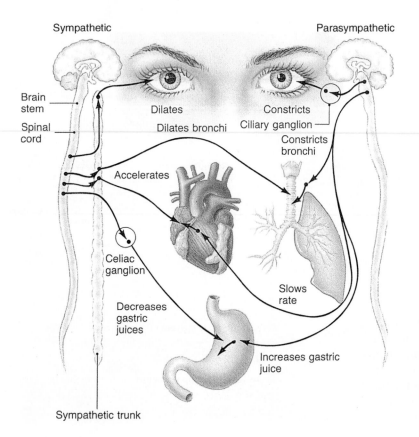

FIGURE 2–16. The autonomic nervous system is subdivided into the sympathetic and the parasympathetic nervous systems. The effects are opposite of each system

- Regulates body temperature
- Aids in elimination of water and various salts
- Acts as the receptor organ for touch, pain, heat, and cold

The skin consists of two layers (see Figure 2–17). The outermost layer is the **epidermis**. The **dermis**, the inner layer, contains a vast network of blood vessels and other structures. Just below the dermis is a layer of fatty tissue.

Body Cavities

The body has six different cavities that contain organs and structures. Injury can occur to the organs and structures within any of these cavities, producing internal bleeding. The cavities are

- **cranial cavity**—contains the brain
- **spinal cavity**—contains the spinal cord
- **thoracic cavity**—contains the heart, trachea, lungs, large vessels, and esophagus
- **pericardial cavity**—the tough fibrous covering that contains the heart

---

epidermis The outermost layer of the skin

dermis The inner layer of skin

cranial cavity Contains the brain

spinal cavity Contains the spinal cord

thoracic cavity Contains the heart, trachea, lungs, large vessels, and esophagus

pericardial cavity The tough fibrous covering that contains the heart

---

FIGURE 2–17. The anatomy of the skin. The outermost layer of the skin is the epidermis. The dermis or second layer of skin contains the network of blood vessels, hair follicles, sweat and oil glands, and sensory nerves. The hypodermis is a layer of fatty tissue that is beneath the dermis and serves as a body insulator

- **abdominal cavity**—contains the liver, spleen, gallbladder, small and large intestine, pancreas, appendix, and stomach
- **pelvic cavity**—contains the reproductive organs, urinary bladder, urethra, and rectum

The abdominal cavity is separated from the thoracic cavity by the diaphragm. The diaphragm is a major muscle responsible for breathing.

> **abdominal cavity** Contains the liver, spleen, gallbladder, small and large intestine, pancreas, appendix, and stomach
>
> **pelvic cavity** Contains the reproductive organs, urinary bladder, urethra, and rectum

Summary

- Using proper anatomical terms to describe position, direction, and location lets you more accurately communicate the victim's condition and extent of injury.
- The skeletal system serves as the framework of the body, providing support, protection, motion, and flexibility.
- There are three different kinds of muscles: skeletal, which control voluntary movement; smooth, which control involuntary movement; and cardiac, which make up the heart.
- The circulatory system consists of two major fluid transportation systems, one for blood and one for lymphatic fluid.
- The respiratory system provides oxygen to the blood.
- The digestive system ingests food, carries it so it can be digested and absorbed, and eliminates waste.
- The urinary system helps maintain the delicate balance of water and various chemicals in the body and removes wastes from the bloodstream.
- The endocrine glands secrete hormones directly into the bloodstream for the regulation of various body functions.
- The nervous system, which provides communication and control, consists mainly of the nerve centers in the brain and spinal cord and the peripheral nerves that branch out to all body tissues and organs.
- The skin, which consists of two layers, protects the internal organs from infection and helps regulate body temperature and aids in elimination.
- There are six body cavities: cranial, spinal, thoracic, pericardial, abdominal, and pelvic.

Key Terms

Make sure you understand the following key terms:

anatomical position	superficial
supine position	deep
prone position	internal
lateral recumbent position	external
modified HAINES recovery position	articulate
	fracture
superior	skeletal (voluntary)
inferior	muscle
anterior	smooth muscle
posterior	involuntary muscle
medial	cardiac muscle
lateral	ventilation

inhalation

inspiration

respiration

exhalation (expiration)

endocrine glands

central nervous system

peripheral nervous system

voluntary nervous system

autonomic nervous system

sympathetic nervous system

parasympathetic nervous
   system

epidermis

dermis

cranial cavity

spinal cavity

thoracic cavity

pericardial cavity

abdominal cavity

pelvic cavity

Critical Thinking Exercise

You are called by a neighbor to provide care to a young
boy who fell off of his bicycle while riding down the road.
As you approach the boy, you note that his left thigh is
grossly deformed. He is crying uncontrollably and is in
severe pain.

1. What bone would you likely expect to be fractured?

2. What are the possible complications of the fracture?

3. Based on the function of bones, what might be other
   signs that the bone is fractured?

4. What other structures might be injured in addition to
   the bone?

2 Chapter 2 Self-Test

Student: _____   Date: _____

Course: _____   Section #: _____

Part 1   True/False

If you believe the statement is true, circle the T. If you believe the statement is false, circle the F.

T   F   **1.** In the supine position, the victim is lying face down.

T   F   **2.** The location of a joint determines how much it is able to move.

T   F   **3.** Smooth muscle is also known as voluntary muscle.

T   F   **4.** Cardiac muscle can generate its own impulse to contract even without the nervous system.

T   F   **5.** An important function of the skin is to regulate body temperature.

Part 2   Multiple Choice

For each item, circle the correct answer or the phrase that best completes the statement.

1. The longest bone in the body is the
   a. tibia
   b. humerus
   c. radius
   d. femur

2. Because of the possibility of severe blood loss, a fracture of what bone would be considered a critical injury?
   a. cranium
   b. pelvis
   c. fibula
   d. tarsals

3. Which is an example of an involuntary muscle?
   a. the eye muscle
   b. intestinal muscle
   c. heart muscle
   d. leg muscle

4. The mechanical process of moving air into and out of the lungs is known as
   a. inhalation
   b. ventilation
   c. respiration
   d. exhalation

5. Which system permits the body to eliminate certain waste materials filtered from the blood?
   a. endocrine system
   b. lymphatic system
   c. exocrine system
   d. urinary system

6. The peripheral nervous system is made up of
   a. nerves within the spinal cord
   b. special ganglia within the cerebrum
   c. the pons and medulla
   d. nerves located outside the brain and spinal cord

7. Which of the following is the outer layer of the skin?
   a. dermis
   b. sebaceous gland
   c. endodermis
   d. epidermis

8. A victim lying flat with face up is in which position?
   a. lateral recumbent
   b. anatomical
   c. prone
   d. supine

9. The front of the body is also referred to as
   a. anterior
   b. medial
   c. posterior
   d. lateral

Match the terms on the right with their definitions.

1. _____ Superior
2. _____ Inferior
3. _____ Anterior
4. _____ Posterior
5. _____ Medial
6. _____ Lateral
7. _____ Superficial
8. _____ Deep
9. _____ Internal
10. _____ External
11. _____ Supine
12. _____ Prone
13. _____ Lateral recumbent

A. Lower
B. Inside
C. Front
D. To the right or left of center
E. Near the surface
F. Back
G. Above or higher
H. Outside
I. Remote from the surface
J. Toward midline
K. Lying face down
L. Lying on left/right side
M. Lying face up

3

Victim Assessment

Learning Objectives

When you have mastered the material in this chapter, you will be able to

1 Understand how to properly assess a victim

2 Describe how to establish rapport with the victim

3 Explain how to survey and control the scene

4 Describe and conduct a primary survey

5 Know how to conduct a neurologic exam

6 Explain how to determine the chief complaint

7 Understand the significance of vital signs (pulse, respiration, and relative skin temperature)

8 Explain how to take a history

9 Understand the sequence and practical application of a secondary survey

On the Scene

Elaine Smith was preparing the soil in her flowerbeds for a new planting of Martha Washington geraniums. As she rounded the corner of her house, she saw her 82-year-old neighbor, Bessie Johnson, lying on the concrete patio, crying softly.

"Please help me," Bessie whispered. "My leg—oh, it hurts so much! I think I've broken my hip!" As Elaine knelt at her side, she asked what happened. "I don't quite know," Bessie said. "I felt so dizzy. . . ."

As the older woman guarded her hip, Elaine looked at her carefully. Her breathing was labored. When Elaine placed the back of her hand against Bessie's pale cheek, she found it to be cool and moist.

Elaine realized that, coupled with her dizziness, Bessie's other symptoms strongly suggested the possibility of a heart attack—even though the woman's chief complaint was the pain in her hip. Elaine called out to a third neighbor who was washing his car to call 9-1-1, then helped Bessie into a more comfortable position and monitored her vital signs while waiting for the ambulance to arrive.

Assessing the victim is one of the most important and critical parts of first aid. The assessment is conducted to identify and care for immediate life threats to the airway, breathing, and circulation.

Some injuries are obvious; others are hidden. A conscious victim may be able to guide you to the problem—but an unconscious victim will be of no help at all.

This chapter provides detailed information on assessment and gives you an assessment routine that will help you

- Get the victim's consent for first aid care
- Win the victim's confidence and ease the victim's anxiety
- Rapidly identify the victim's problem(s)
- Quickly determine which problem is a priority for care
- Obtain information that will help emergency personnel

As you assess the victim, your main goals are to

- Protect yourself from injury
- Identify and correct life-threatening problems
- Render proper first aid care
- Prepare the victim for transport

3.1 The Victim Assessment Routine

Learning Objective 1 Understand how to properly assess a victim.

In most cases, conduct victim assessment in this order:

1. Conduct a scene size-up.
2. Establish rapport and control.
3. Conduct a primary survey.
4. Conduct a brief neurologic (i.e., "neuro") exam.
5. Determine the chief complaint.
6. Assess vital signs.
7. Look for medical information devices.
8. Take a SAMPLE history.
9. Conduct a secondary survey.

You may need to adapt or change the sequence, depending on your experience and the specific emergency situation.

Conduct a Scene Size-Up

The first priority when preparing to perform first aid is to ensure your own personal safety. Never risk your own safety. Next, you will ensure the safety of the victim and any bystanders at the scene. The scene can also provide clues to whether the victim is injured or ill, the number of victims you may need to provide care for, and what resources will be needed to effectively manage the victims and the scene. There are five components of the scene size-up:

1. Take body substance isolation precautions, by using personal protective equipment (PPE) if possible.
2. Assess the safety of the scene.
3. Determine if the victim is injured or ill.
4. Determine the number of victims.
5. Determine the resources needed.

If at all possible, put on protective gloves to guard against exposure to any blood or body fluids. Prior to approaching the victim, quickly scan the scene for any hazards such as downed power lines, spilled fuel, weapons, and an unstable vehicle. If the scene is not safe, you can either make it safe by removing the hazard, if possible, or retreat from the scene until it is made safe by the fire department, police department, power company, or other resource.

Once the scene is determined to be safe, you can approach the victim. As you are walking into the scene, inspect for any clues as to whether the victim is injured or ill. For example, if you note a ladder next to a person lying on the ground, you would assume the victim is injured from a fall. This is referred to as the *mechanism of injury*. If a person is found sitting in a chair in a restaurant, you would assume the victim is ill. Also, determine the number of people who are injured or ill at the scene. At the scene of an auto crash, you want to look inside and outside the cars for possible victims. Be suspicious, especially at a crash scene, that more than one person is injured.

Once you have determined the number of victims, you can then have a bystander contact the necessary resources. You may request emergency medical services, the fire department, the police department, or power company. You may request more than one ambulance if you find several people who are injured or ill.

Establishing Rapport and Control

Learning Objective 2 Describe how to establish rapport with the victim.

People who are injured are often frightened, anxious, angry, or in shock. To establish rapport with the victim and get control of the situation, you need to use the three Cs:

- Competence
- Confidence
- Compassion

Begin by observing any clues at the scene that may help you in assessment, such as damage to a vehicle, the victim's position, pills or food near the victim, or environmental temperature.

Next, approach the victim, ask for the victim's name, and say something like, "I'm [your name], and I'm trained in first aid care. I'd like to help you. Is that all right?" Tell the victim your level of care and what you'd like to do. Through this groundwork, you obtain the victim's consent.

Throughout the assessment and care, continue to call the victim by name, maintain eye contact, speak calmly and deliberately, and give orders quietly. People under stress or in medical shock process information more slowly, so speak distinctly and allow time for the victim or bystanders to respond.

> Learning Objective **3** Explain how to control the scene.

To establish control, do the following:

- Move smoothly and deliberately.

- Position yourself at a comfortable level in relation to the victim. Stay where the victim can see you without twisting his or her neck.

- Keep your eye level above that of the victim.

- Conduct your survey in an unhurried, systematic way.

- Emotions escalate quickly in tense situations, so keep your voice calm and quiet.

- If there is more than one victim, determine which victim(s) needs the most immediate care. **Triage**, a system of sorting victims into categories by treatment priority, is described in Chapter 28.

> **PROGRESS CHECK**
>
> 1. To establish scene control, use the three Cs—competence, confidence, and _____ . *(control/charisma/compassion)*
> 2. An important part of introducing yourself to the victim is obtaining _____ . *(the victim's name/consent for treatment/ a history of what happened)*

> 3. To maintain control, keep your voice _____ . *(calm and deliberate/powerful and authoritative/loud and demanding)*
> 4. Position yourself with your eye level _____ that of the victim. *(above/even with/below)*

3.2 Conducting the Primary Survey

> Learning Objective **4** Describe and conduct a primary survey.

The major goal of the primary survey is to check for life-threatening problems to the airway, breathing, and circulation. Unless you find a life-threatening situation that needs to be treated immediately, you should be able to complete the primary survey in approximately 60 seconds. Figure 3–1 on page 36 illustrates the order of the primary and secondary surveys. Start with the following three steps:

1. If the victim is conscious, ask, "What happened?" The response will provide information about the airway status, the adequacy of breathing, mental status, and mechanism of injury or nature of the illness (see Figure 3–2) on page 36.

2. Ask, "Where do you hurt?" The response will identify the most likely points of injury.

3. Visually scan the victim for general appearance, pale skin, **cyanosis** (blueness from lack of oxygen), and sweating.

These steps provide a quick assessment of the victim's overall condition. The rest of the primary survey consists of evaluating the **ABCDs**—airway, breathing, circulation (pulse and bleeding), and disability (nervous system disability, or altered responsiveness).

Always suspect a possible spinal injury in the victim who is unresponsive or who has an altered mental status. Do nothing that could aggravate possible spinal injury.

---

triage A system of sorting victims into categories by treatment priority

cyanosis Bluish discoloration from lack of oxygen

ABCDs Airway, breathing, circulation (hemorrhage), and disability

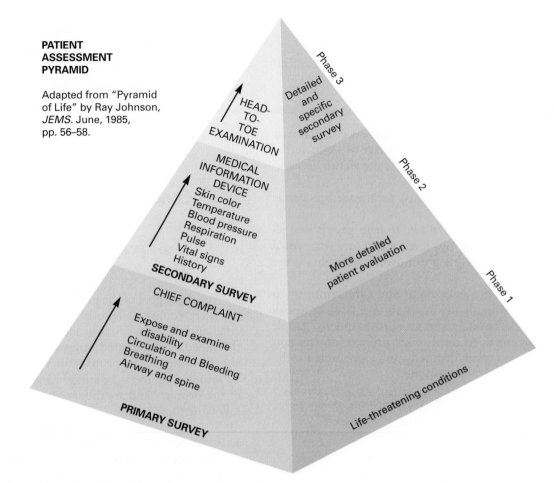

PATIENT ASSESSMENT PYRAMID

Adapted from "Pyramid of Life" by Ray Johnson, *JEMS*. June, 1985, pp. 56–58.

FIGURE 3–1. Remember the order of the primary and secondary surveys.

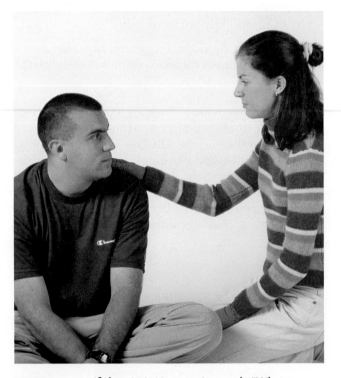

FIGURE 3–2. If the victim is conscious, ask, "What happened?" and "Where do you hurt?"

Airway and Spine Stabilization

Determine whether the airway is open. If the victim is conscious and talking without difficulty, the airway is open. If the airway is not open, use either the head-tilt/chin-lift maneuver or the modified jaw thrust maneuver to open it (see Chapter 4). Use the modified jaw thrust maneuver if a spine injury is suspected. If you suspect the victim has any possibility of a spinal injury, establish manual in-line spinal stabilization by bringing the victim's head and neck into a neutral in-line position. Have someone at the scene hold the victim's head so that the nose is in line with the navel (belly button) and the neck is not bent forward or backward. Instruct the victim not to move his or her head or neck.

According to the 2005 American Heart Association Guidelines for CPR and ECC, suspect possible spine injury if the victim

- is involved in any type of crash
- falls greater than the height of the victim
- complains of pain to his neck or back
- complains of tingling, numbness, or unusual sensation in his extremities

FIGURE 3–3. If the victim has an altered mental status, establish an airway, then check for adequate breathing by looking, listening, and feeling. Assure an adequate open airway by the head-tilt/chin-lift method.

FIGURE 3–4. If you suspect a spine injury, use a modified jaw thrust to open the victim's airway.

- appears to be intoxicated
- has an altered mental status
- is older than 65 years of age
- has an injury to the head or neck

Breathing

A responsive person who is alert and talking with ease is typically breathing adequately. To determine whether a victim with an altered mental status is breathing

- *Look* for chest rise and fall.
- *Listen* for sounds of air movement at the mouth and nose.
- *Feel* on your cheek for air passing in and out of the mouth or nose.

If the victim is not breathing spontaneously or not breathing adequately, begin artificial breathing immediately (see Chapter 4); continue until the victim is breathing spontaneously or until you are relieved by trained emergency personnel (see Figures 3–3 through 3–5).

If the victim is breathing adequately, continue with the primary survey.

Circulation

To assess for circulation, check the **radial pulse** (at the wrist on the thumb side) (see Figure 3–6 on page 38). If the victim is unconscious or you can't find the radial pulse, check the **carotid pulse** (in the groove of the neck) (see Figure 3–7 on page 38).

ASSESSING RESPIRATION

Observe the person for 10 to 15 seconds. If the person is breathing, keep the airway open and check for pulses. Absence of respiration calls for rescue breathing.

LOOK   for chest movement.
LISTEN for sounds of air movement.
FEEL   For any exhalation of warm air on your cheek.

After opening the airway, observe the victim's chest for rise and fall.

FIGURE 3–5. Assessing respiration

radial pulse The pulse at the wrist on the thumb side

carotid pulse The pulse at the groove on either side of the neck

FIGURE 3–6. Palpate (feel) the radial pulse at the wrist.

PALPATING CAROTID PULSE

FIGURE 3–7. Palpate the carotid pulse at either side of the neck.

If the patient is pulseless, not breathing, and unresponsive (shows no sign of life), begin cardiopulmonary resuscitation (CPR) immediately (see Chapter 5). If an automated external defibrillator (AED) becomes available, immediately attach the device and follow the prompts. Continue CPR until circulation resumes or you are relieved by trained emergency personnel.

If the victim is breathing and has a pulse, continue by checking for serious or profuse bleeding. Inspect for pools of blood or blood-soaked clothing.

If you find major bleeding—blood that is spurting or flowing freely—control it by direct pressure. Spurting or steady flow bleeding is the only kind of bleeding that should be treated during the primary survey.

Disability

The final step of the primary survey is to determine disability. Injuries to the brain generally result in an altered mental status or unresponsiveness, which usually indicates decreased oxygen to the brain or brain injury. There are four general levels of responsiveness:

- **Alert**—The victim's eyes are open.

- **Response to verbal stimuli**—The victim opens his or her eyes to verbal commands to do so.

- **Response to pain**—The victim appears to be asleep and does not respond when spoken to, but winces, grimaces, or jerks away when pinched.

- **Unresponsive**—The victim appears to be asleep and does not respond in any way when pinched.

If the victim has an altered mental status, he or she should be placed in a lateral recumbent position to protect the airway. If a spine injury is suspected, keep the victim in a supine position, maintaining the head and neck in a neutral in-line position. If the victim has a possible spine injury and has a possible compromise to the airway due to blood, secretions, or vomitus, or if you need to leave the victim to seek help, place the victim in the modified HAINES position.

The neuro exam, which is not strictly part of the primary survey, allows you to assess for disability in greater detail. The neuro exam is described in the next section.

PROGRESS CHECK

1. The major goal of the primary survey is to check for _____ . *(breathing/ heartbeat/life-threatening problems)*

2. You can determine both the level of consciousness and the adequacy of ventilation by _____ . *(watching for chest movement/checking the pulse/asking if the victim is okay)*

3. To conduct the primary survey, check the _____ . *(pulse/breathing/ABCDs)*

4. Unless you find life-threatening problems, you should be able to complete the primary survey in _____ . *(1 minute/2 minutes/5 minutes)*

5. The only kind of bleeding you should try to control during the primary survey is _____ . *(major bleeding/bleeding from a chest wound/bleeding from the head)*

3.3 Conducting the Neuro Exam

Learning Objective 5 Know how to conduct a neuro exam.

A neuro exam checks

- Mental status
- Motor function (such as voluntary movement)
- Sensory function (what the victim can feel)

To conduct the neuro exam, follow these steps:

1. Talk to the victim. A person who can't answer general questions such as "What time is it?" is disoriented. If the victim is an infant or young child, estimate alertness by observing voluntary movements and interest in surroundings.

2. Note the victim's speech. Vagueness, slurring of speech, or garbled speech indicates a decreasing mental status or possible brain injury.

3. If the victim can't speak, determine whether he or she can understand by assessing his or her response to a simple command, such as "Squeeze my hand" (see Figure 3–8).

4. If the victim has an altered mental status, determine how easily the victim can be aroused. If the victim doesn't respond to your voice, try a pain stimulus such as a pinch to the muscle at the base of the neck.

If you suspect a spinal injury, tell the victim to lie very still; stabilize the spine as well as you can, by keeping the head and neck in a neutral in-line position, and activate the EMS system (see Chapter 13).

FIGURE 3–8. Test whether the victim can understand you by stating, "Squeeze my hand" and waiting for a response.

PROGRESS CHECK

1. A neuro exam checks both motor and _____ function. *(visual/ sensory/psychological)*

2. Slurring of speech, garbled speech, or vagueness in answering questions indicates deteriorating _____ . *(mental status/motor control/ speech ability)*

3. If a victim can't speak, give a simple _____ to assess mental status. *(stimulus/test/command)*

4. Determine how easily victims can be aroused from an altered mental status by using either verbal or _____ stimuli. *(touch/ painful/sound)*

3.4 Chief Complaint and Vital Signs

Determining the Chief Complaint

Learning Objective 6 Explain how to determine the chief complaint.

Until now, you've concentrated on **signs**—things you can observe yourself (such as a leg deformed by fracture). Now you'll ask specific questions aimed at discovering the **symptoms**—what the victim feels and describes to you (such as abdominal pain) (see Figures 3–9 and 3–10).

Ask, "Tell me where you hurt." The answer is the *chief complaint.* Most chief complaints are characterized by pain or abnormal structure or function and can be pinpointed using observations made by the victim.

Even if injury is obvious, it's important to ask. For example, a victim of a car accident may have an obvious fracture to the leg, but if the chief complaint is "I can't breathe," you may discover an unsuspected chest injury.

Assessing Vital Signs

Learning Objective 7 Understand the significance of vital signs (pulse, respiration, and relative skin temperature).

signs Things you can observe about the victim, such as bleeding

symptoms Things the victim describes to you, such as abdominal pain

FIGURE 3–9. A victim exhibiting a sign, such as a deformed wrist.

FIGURE 3–11. Palpate the radial pulse at the wrist on the thumb side.

FIGURE 3–12. If the victim is unconscious or a radial pulse can't be felt, palpate the carotid pulse in the neck.

FIGURE 3–10. A victim describing a symptom, such as stomach pain.

Vital signs should be taken repeatedly at 5-minute intervals. Changes in vital signs reflect both changes in the victim's condition and the effectiveness of your first aid care.

Use your senses—sight, hearing, and touch—to determine pulse, respiration, and the temperature and color of the victim's skin.

PULSE

The pulse is the pressure wave generated when the heart beats; it reflects the rhythm, rate, and relative strength of the heart. You can take the pulse at any point where an artery crosses over a bone or lies near the skin, but the best place in a conscious victim is at the wrist (see Figure 3–11). If the victim is unconscious, take the pulse at the carotid artery (in the groove of the neck) (see Figure 3–12).

When you take the pulse, note its

- Rate—Normal heart rate range 60 to 100 beats per minute for an adult, 80 to 150 for a child, and 120 to 160 for a newborn.
- Strength—A normal pulse is full and strong.
- Rhythm—A normal pulse is regular.

To take the pulse, have the victim lie or sit down; use the tips of two fingers and assess the pulse gently by touch. Count the number of beats for 15 seconds, then multiply by four to determine the number of beats per minute. If the pulse is irregular, take it for a full minute. Write down the pulse immediately after taking it; don't rely on your memory.

Respiration (Breathing)

One respiration consists of one inhalation and one exhalation. Normal respirations are easy and spontaneous, without pain or effort. The normal range is 12 to 20 breaths per minute for an adult, 15 to 30 for a child, and 30 to 50 for a newborn. Place your hand on the victim's chest and feel for chest movement (see Figure 3–13). Do not tell the victim you are assessing the respirations since

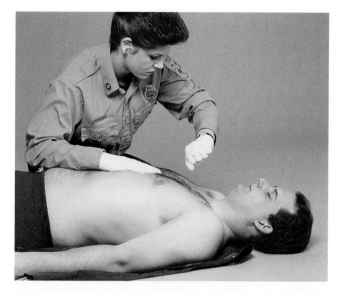

FIGURE 3–13. Measure respirations by placing your hand on the victim's chest or abdomen. Count the number of times the chest or abdomen rises in 30 seconds. Then multiply that number by two.

this may alter the rate. The chest should move up with each breath.

Cardinal signs of respiratory distress (see Figure 3–14) include flaring of the nostrils, use of accessory muscles in the neck, chest, and abdomen, fast breathing, increased heart rate, pale and cool skin, sweating, and decreasing mental status.

Temperature and Skin Color

Assess relative skin temperature (see Figure 3–15 on page 42) by placing the back of your hand against the skin of the victim's forehead neck or abdomen. Normal skin is fairly dry, as well as normal in temperature.

Hot skin temperature can be caused by fever, heat stroke, or a hot environment. Low skin temperature can be caused by shock, spinal injury, heat exhaustion, or exposure to cold.

Skin color can tell you a lot about a victim.

- Paleness (white tone) may be caused by shock, poor circulation, or heart attack.

- Redness may be caused by high blood pressure, spinal cord injury, alcohol abuse, sunburn, heat stroke, fever, or infectious disease.

- Blueness (cyanosis) may be caused by suffocation, lack of oxygen, heart attack, or poisoning. Cyanosis is always a serious problem. It usually appears first in the fingertips and around the mouth.

SIGNS AND SYMPTOMS OF RESPIRATORY DISTRESS

Wheezing, coughing, gurgling, high-pitched shrills, or other unusual noises

Dizziness, fainting, restlessness, anxiety, confusion, combativeness

Unable to speak in full sentences without catching breath

Bluish coloring

Flaring nostrils

Straining abdominal muscles

FIGURE 3–14. Look, listen, and feel for signs of respiratory distress.

FIGURE 3–15. For relative skin temperature, touch the victim's skin with the back of your hand.

FIGURE 3–16. Medic Alert bracelet

Capillary refill is one method of checking circulation. This procedure is performed by squeezing one of the victim's fingernails or toenails. When the nail is squeezed, the tissue under the nail turns white. When the pressure is released, color returns to the tissue. By measuring the time it takes for color to return under the nail, you are obtaining capillary refill. Two seconds or less is considered within normal limits for infants, children, and adult males. Females have an upper limit for normal refill of less than 3 seconds, and the upper limit for geriatrics (aged 65 years or older) is 4 seconds. A cold environment or various disease states could alter the capillary refill times. Capillary refill is most accurate in young children. If refill time is delayed, suspect shock or decreased blood flow to that extremity. Measure capillary refill time by counting "One one-thousand, two two-thousand," and so on.

Looking for Medical Information Devices

While taking vital signs, inspect for medical identification devices, such as a Medic Alert tag, necklace, or bracelet (see Figure 3–16). These medical information devices list the victim's medical problem and/or medications and an emergency 24-hour number you can call for more information.

Medical identification tags are often worn by people with hidden medical conditions, such as heart problems, diabetes, epilepsy, or allergies, or by those on special medications such as Coumadin, a drug that lengthens the time for blood clotting.

PROGRESS CHECK

1. The chief complaint is the victim's assessment of where he or she _____ . *(is injured/ is compromised/hurts)*

2. You can rely on your _____ to assess vital signs; you do not need specialized equipment. *(intuition/senses/wristwatch)*

3. Take the pulse of an unconscious victim at the _____ artery. *(carotid/brachial/radial)*

4. Take the pulse of a conscious victim at the _____ artery. *(carotid/brachial/radial)*

5. Use the back of your hand to check the victim's relative _____ . *(respiration/pulse/ temperature)*

3.5 Taking a History

Learning Objective 8 Explain how to take a history.

When taking a history:

- Assess the scene. The placement of the victim and objects at the scene can give clues about the injury.

- Ask questions. If the situation is urgent, ask yes-no questions ("Have you eaten today?"); if the situation is less urgent, ask open-ended questions ("Tell me about your last meal"). Whenever possible, ask open-ended questions, because you don't want to suggest answers to the victim.

- If the victim is unresponsive, seems confused, or is a child, get a history by talking to friends or family members.

An easy-to-remember mnemonic used to collect a history is SAMPLE. To collect a SAMPLE history, determine the following:

S   What are the *signs* and *symptoms* the victim is complaining of?

A   What is the victim *allergic* to?

M   What *medications* does the victim take, both prescription and over-the-counter?

P   What is the *pertinent past* medical history of the victim?

L   When was the *last time* the victim had something to eat or drink?

E   What were the *events* prior to the incident?

PROGRESS CHECK

1. When possible, ask the victim _____ questions. *(yes-no/open-ended)*

2. The sample history should be taken _____ the primary survey. *(before/after/during)*

3.6   Conducting a Secondary Survey

Learning Objective **9** Understand the sequence and practical application of a secondary survey.

In essence, a secondary survey is a closer look at the victim once life-threatening conditions are controlled and vital signs are recorded. During the secondary survey you conduct a full-body head-to-toe assessment by inspection and with your hands, checking for swelling, depression, deformity, bleeding, and other problems. Figure 3–17 illustrates the order of examination.

Explain to the victim what you are doing, and keep talking calmly throughout the survey. Keep the victim's head and neck in alignment, and don't move the victim unnecessarily if you suspect spinal injuries.

During the survey, use the following approach:

- *Look for* deformities, wounds, bleeding, discoloration, penetration, openings in the neck, and unusual chest movement.

- *Listen for* unusual breathing sounds, gurgling sounds, or **crepitus** (a sandpaperlike noise made by broken bone ends rubbing against each other).

- *Feel for* unusual masses, swelling, hardness, softness, mushiness, muscle spasms, pulsations, tenderness, deformities, and temperature.

- *Smell for* unusual odors on the victim's breath, body, or clothing.

The mnemonic DOTS can be used to assess signs or symptoms of injury:

D   Deformity

O   Open wounds

T   Tenderness

S   Swelling

Make every effort to protect the victim's privacy, but cut away any clothing that interferes with your ability to examine the victim properly.

When you finish the secondary survey, care for any injuries you find as time allows. The extent of the secondary survey and the first aid care you give will depend on how quickly the EMS system arrives on the scene.

THE SECONDARY SURVEY

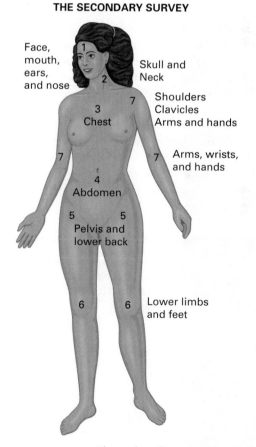

FIGURE 3–17. The order of examination in the secondary survey.

---

crepitus A sandpaperlike grating sound made by the ends of broken bones as they rub together

Face, Mouth, Ears, Nose

Figures 3–18 through 3–24 illustrate the survey of facial features. Check the following:

- Deformities, open wounds, tenderness, swelling
- Forehead, eye orbits, and facial structures for abnormalities
- Ears and nose for blood or clear fluid and injury
- Eyes for pupil size and reactivity to light
- Eyes for the ability to track a moving object smoothly and evenly in all four quadrants
- Mouth for lacerations, unusual breath odor, and teeth alignment

Skull and Neck

Figures 3–25 and 3–26 illustrate the survey of skull and neck. Check the following:

- Deformities, open wounds, tenderness, swelling
- Scalp for depressions and bruises
- Trachea for position (it should be in the middle of the neck)
- Neck for depressions, bruises, wounds, pain, and tenderness

The victim should be able to swallow without discomfort, and the voice should not be hoarse.

FIGURE 3–18. Run your fingers over the forehead, orbits of the eyes, and facial structure.

FIGURE 3–21 and FIGURE 3–22. Check the eyes for reactive pupils and possible damage.

FIGURE 3–19. Check the nose and ears for blood or clear fluid (cerebrospinal fluid).

FIGURE 3–20. Gently check the nose for any possible injury.

FIGURE 3–23 and FIGURE 3–24. Check the mouth for lacerations or obstructions. Is any unusual breath odor present? Check the face for symmetry and the teeth for alignment.

FIGURE 3–25. Gently palpate the skull for any depressions, deformities, open wounds, tenderness, and other abnormalities.

FIGURE 3–27. Apply light compression to the rib cage to discover any rib cage damage. At the same time, visually inspect the chest for deformities, wounds, and equal chest expansion (symmetry).

FIGURE 3–26. Gently palpate the neck to check for any deformities.

FIGURE 3–28. Gently press on the sternum for possible chest injury.

FIGURE 3–29. Inspect the abdomen then palpate each quadrant for tenderness and rigidity.

Chest

Figures 3–27 and 3–28 illustrate the inspection of the chest. Check for the following:

- Deformities, open wounds, tenderness, swelling

- Soft-tissue injuries, such as cuts, bruises, indentations, impaled objects, or open chest wounds

- Signs of fractures

- Respiratory distress and symmetry of chest rise and fall

- Pain, tenderness, or instability over the ribs

Abdomen

To survey the abdomen, place the victim in a supine position, keep the victim warm (shivering makes the abdominal muscles tense), and use a gentle touch (see Figure 3–29).

- Inspect and palpate for deformities, open wounds, tenderness, rigidity (hard and contracted abdominal muscles) and swelling.

- Look for protrusions, soft-tissue wounds, lumps, swelling, or bruising.

- Palpate the four quadrants separately with the pads of your fingers for hardening or abdominal masses. If you suspect injury, feel that quadrant last.

- Ask about pain.

Pelvic Region

Injury in the pelvic region can cause extreme pain and excessive bleeding, so be gentle. Examination can also be very embarrassing, so talk to the victim and explain what you are doing. If the victim is complaining of pain to the pelvis do not palpate it. (see Figures 3–30 and 3–31 on page 46).

- Inspect and palpate for deformities, open wounds, tenderness, and swelling.

- Put your hands on each side of the hips and compress inward. Check for tenderness, crepitus, and instability.

- Look for loss of bladder control, bleeding, or erection of the penis (a sign of central nervous system injury).

- Check the strength of the femoral pulse.

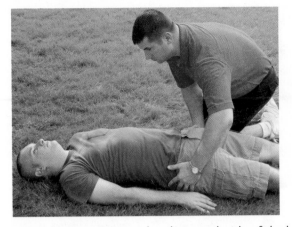

FIGURE 3–30. Put your hands on each side of the hips and compress inward, checking for tenderness, crepitus, and instability.

FIGURE 3–32. Check the back for point tenderness and deformity. Keep the head and neck in alignment, and be very careful not to move the victim.

- Feel for protrusions, depressions, and abnormal movement. Check for tenderness in the calves.

- Check each foot for a pulse (on top of the foot on the big toe side), sensation (by light touch and a pinch to each foot), motor function (by asking the victim to move his or her toes), and warmth.

Upper Extremities

- Inspect and palpate for deformities, open wounds, tenderness, and swelling (see Figures 3–37 through 3–39).

- Check for equal grip strength in both hands.

- Assess for motor function by asking the victim to squeeze your finger or wiggle his or her fingers.

- Assess for sensation by light touch and by a pinch to each hand.

FIGURE 3–31. Push down on the anterior of the iliac crest.

Back

If spine injury is suspected, *do not move the victim.* Without moving the victim, slip your hand beneath the back and feel for possible deformities, pain or tenderness, and bleeding (see Figure 3–32). Check for strength and sensation in all extremities.

Lower Extremities

Figures 3–33 through 3–36 illustrate the survey of the lower extremities.

- Inspect and palpate for deformities, open wounds, tenderness, and swelling.

- Check for abnormal position of the legs (a leg that is turned away, shortened, or rotated).

PROGRESS CHECK

1. During the secondary survey, conduct a full-body assessment _____ . *(from head-to-toe/from toe-to-head)*

2. Never move the victim unnecessarily until you are sure _____ . *(emergency personnel are on the way/there are no spinal injuries/the victim is not in pain)*

3. During the secondary survey, keep the head and neck _____ . *(aligned/immobile/comfortable)*

FIGURE 3–33. Check the upper leg for pain and deformity.

FIGURE 3–34. Palpate the knees and the patella (kneecap) for any pain or deformity.

FIGURE 3–35. Palpate the lower legs; the tibia, ankles, and feet.

FIGURE 3–36. Check each foot for a pulse, sensation, motor function, and temperature.

FIGURE 3–37. Palpate the clavicles for deformities, tenderness, or swelling.

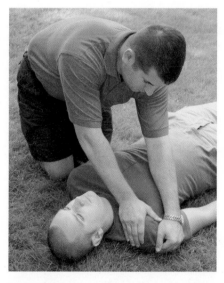

FIGURE 3–38. Palpate the complete shoulder girdle for deformities and tenderness.

FIGURE 3–39. Palpate each arm for deformities, open wounds, tenderness, and swelling. Assess the pulse and motor and sensory function.

Summary

- To begin, establish rapport with the victim by introducing yourself and explaining that you are there to help. Obtain consent to treat before assessing the victim.

- During the primary survey, check for and treat life-threatening injuries involving the airway, breathing, and circulation.

- The only bleeding you should try to control during the primary survey is spurting or steady flow hemorrhage.

- The brief neurologic examination lets you check mental status, motor function, and sensory function.

- The chief complaint—the answer you receive when you ask the victim where it hurts or what the problem is—points you to the most likely area of injury.

- Use your senses—look, listen, and feel—to assess the vital signs, including pulse, respiration, temperature, and skin color.

- When taking a history, ask open-ended questions when possible and remember the SAMPLE mnemonic.

- The secondary survey is a full-body assessment, during which you check for less-obvious injuries and medical problems. Depending on the time you have before emergency personnel arrive, you should provide care for the problems you find during the secondary survey.

Key Terms

Make sure you understand the following key terms:

triage	carotid pulse
cyanosis	signs
ABCDs	symptoms
radial pulse	crepitus

Critical Thinking Exercise

You are attending a high school football game when suddenly you note some unusual activity in the stands behind you. As you turn to see what the commotion is about, you hear someone yell "this man needs medical help." As you approach him, you note he is slumped between the bleacher seats, is not moving, and has a bluish complexion. You note vomitus coming from the mouth and nose.

1. What is your first immediate action to protect yourself?

2. How will you determine his level of responsiveness?

3. What assessment should be conducted first?

4. How would you manage the airway?

Chapter 3 Self-Test

Student:_____ Date:_____

Course:_____ Section #:_____

Part 1   True/False

If you believe the statement is true, circle the T. If you believe the statement is false, circle the F.

T F **1.** Serious internal injuries are usually very obvious to the First Aider.

T F **2.** It is important for a First Aider to know how an accident took place.

T F **3.** A normal pulse is full and strong.

T F **4.** The "B" in the ABCDs stands for "broken bones."

T F **5.** The number-one first aid priority in every first aid situation is establishing an open airway.

T F **6.** In a secondary survey, begin at the head and work down the body.

T F **7.** The normal breathing rate in the average adult is about 25 breaths per minute.

T F **8.** The normal resting pulse rate in an adult is 60 to 100 beats per minute.

Part 2   Multiple Choice

For each item, circle the correct answer or the phrase that best completes the statement.

1. In order of priority, which are the three primary first aid measures?
   a. maintain breathing, stop bleeding, manage shock
   b. open the airway, maintain breathing, maintain circulation
   c. prevent shock, stop bleeding, maintain breathing
   d. stop bleeding, prevent shock, avoid infection

2. What should you look for during the secondary survey?
   a. blood in the hair
   b. abdominal spasms and tenderness
   c. paralysis of the extremities
   d. all of the above

3. If you suspect a spinal injury during the course of a secondary survey, what should you do first?
   a. stop the survey and call for assistance
   b. stabilize the head
   c. continue the survey to find other problems
   d. stop the survey completely

4. How long should the First Aider spend on the primary survey?
   a. 10 to 12 minutes
   b. 5 to 10 minutes
   c. 2 to 3 minutes
   d. 1 minute or less

5. Medic Alert tags are worn to
   a. identify allergies
   b. warn of hidden medical conditions, such as diabetes
   c. provide pertinent information about a victim's special medical needs
   d. all of the above

6. The primary survey is conducted in the following order:
   a. check for bleeding, breathing, and pulse
   b. check for airway, breathing, pulse, and bleeding
   c. check for pulse, breathing, and bleeding
   d. check for bleeding, airway, breathing, pulse

7. The most common temperature taken by First Aiders in the field is the
   a. oral temperature
   b. relative skin temperature
   c. rectal temperature
   d. axillary temperature

8. The secondary survey is
   a. a repetition of the primary survey, to detect anything you missed the first time
   b. a full-body assessment, head to toe
   c. an assessment of the extremities
   d. a check for internal injuries

9. Vital signs should be taken
   a. during the primary survey
   b. after all fractures are immobilized
   c. during the secondary survey
   d. only after the primary and secondary survey

10. The artery in the neck where First Aiders most commonly take a pulse on an unconscious victim is called the
   a. cranial
   b. subclavian
   c. brachial
   d. carotid

Part 3   Matching

A young boy falls out of a tree onto a rock pile below. You are the first person to reach the boy, who is unconscious. Rearrange the items in the list below in the correct order under the headings "Primary Survey" and "Secondary Survey."

Primary Survey

1. _____
2. _____
3. _____
4. _____

Secondary Survey

5. _____
6. _____
7. _____
8. _____
9. _____
10. _____
11. _____
12. _____

A. Check the head for lacerations.

B. Check clavicles and arms for fractures.

C. Conduct a neuro exam.

D. Check for an open airway.

E. Check for adequate breathing.

F. Check the chest for movement on both sides and for fractures.

G. Check for a pulse.

H. Check the back for abnormalities.

I. Check the pelvis for fractures.

J. Check for any severely bleeding injuries.

K. Check the legs, ankles, and feet.

L. Check the abdomen for tenderness, spasms, or rigidity.

Part 4   What Would You Do If?

You are in a mall where an elderly woman has fallen. She says, "I'm dizzy," and she can't get up. Her lips are bluish and she is breathing in shallow gasps. When you ask her what day it is, she says, "I'm having a heart attack, aren't I?"

Which are signs and which are symptoms? How would you pursue a victim assessment? When would you decide to phone for an ambulance?

4

Basic Life Support: Artificial Ventilation

Learning Objectives

When you have mastered the material in this chapter, you will be able to

1 Describe the signs of respiratory distress

2 Explain proper victim assessment for breathing problems

3 Describe how to open the airway of a victim who does not have spinal injury

4 Describe how to open the airway of a victim you suspect has spinal injury

5 Understand the "look, listen, and feel" assessment method of determining breathlessness

6 Explain how to restore breathing through artificial ventilation

7 Adapt ventilation-support procedures to infants and children

8 Identify an obstructed airway

9 Use techniques for dislodging foreign objects that are obstructing the airway of a conscious person

10 Use the technique for dislodging foreign objects that are obstructing the airway of an unconscious person

On the Scene

On February 14, 2006, 58-year-old Richard Quail and his wife joined two other couples at a local steak house to celebrate Valentine's Day. When one woman told about a surprise party her children had planned and executed, all six laughed heartily. When the laughter died down, the others noticed that Richard had a panic-stricken look on his face. His wife put her hand on his arm and asked, hesitantly, "Are you all right?" Richard clutched the table edge with both hands and shook his head briskly; suddenly, clutching his throat as if he were choking, he struggled to his feet, knocking his chair over backward.

Both men at the table leaped toward him; "He's choking!" cried Stan Mortensen. While Stan ran toward the hostess to call for an ambulance, Judith Larsen approached from the next table. Standing behind Richard, she wrapped her arms around his waist. Positioning her fist, thumb side in, just above his navel, she powerfully thrust inward and upward. Still Richard clutched at his throat. After two more powerful thrusts, Richard expelled a large piece of steak, then started coughing. As Judith helped him to a chair, he began to vomit.

By the time EMTs arrived, Richard was shaken, but breathing normally.

he first priority in any emergency is to establish and maintain an adequate airway. Simply stated, your ability to do so can spell the difference between life and death.

In some instances, airway obstruction itself may be the emergency—a child may choke on a toy with small pieces, or a business executive at a banquet may choke on a piece of steak. In other cases, the injury process may cause a victim to stop breathing.

By understanding the physiological process of breathing and the methods of care, as outlined in this chapter, you can quickly initiate and maintain an airway adequate enough to save most victims until emergency help arrives.

4.1 Respiratory Distress

Breathing emergencies can be caused by a variety of accidents or medical disorders. The most common type of breathing emergency is **respiratory distress**. Respiratory distress can be caused by injury, asthma, hyperventilation, and anaphylactic shock. It represents the beginning of a life-threatening emergency.

The most common causes of **respiratory arrest** are electric shock, drowning, suffocation, toxic gas inhalation, head and chest injuries, heart problems, stroke, drug overdose, and allergic reactions. *Respiratory arrest is a true medical emergency.*

Signs and Symptoms

> Learning Objective 1 Describe the signs of respiratory distress.

The signs and symptoms of respiratory distress (see Figure 4-1) include the following:

- Abnormal breathing patterns (difficulty catching the breath, gasping for air, or slow or rapid breathing)
- Unusual breathing noises, such as wheezing, snoring, crowing, or gurgling
- Dizziness
- Pain in the chest
- Tingling in the hands and/or feet
- Clammy skin
- Abnormal skin color—paleness, flushed skin (redness), or cyanosis

> **respiratory distress** An abnormal condition where breathing is labored, noisy, irregular, or unusually fast or slow, or a combination of these
>
> **respiratory arrest** Total cessation of breathing or respiratory effort

Cyanosis (late sign)

Diminishing of speech

Is trachea in the midline? Or does it deviate to one side?

Retraction of neck muscles

Barrel chest?

Deformed chest in a trauma victim?

Does chest move symmetrically during respiration?

Any bulging or flailing during expiration?

Progressive restlessness, anxiety, confusion

Straining of facial and neck muscles

Flaring of nostrils

Presence of audible, noisy respirations indicating partial or progressive obstruction of the upper airway

Trachial tugging

Retraction of intercostal muscles

Use of abdominal muscles during exhalation; labored use of accessory muscles of respiration

FIGURE 4–1. Signs and symptoms of respiratory distress

Basic Life Support

When oxygen is cut off to the lungs—hence, to the brain and heart—the heart continues to pump, and oxygen stored in the lungs and blood will continue to circulate for a short time. Gradually, the heart stops beating, resulting in cardiac arrest.

The body's cells have a residual oxygen supply that keeps them alive for a short time even after breathing and heartbeat stop. The brain cells are the first to die, usually within 4 to 6 minutes after being deprived of oxygenated blood.

Basic life support describes the first aid procedures necessary to sustain life in an emergency situation. The first steps in basic life support are assessing the victim, opening the airway, and providing rescue breathing.

PROGRESS CHECK

1. A victim of respiratory distress may have skin that is either pale, flushed, or _____ . *(dry/hot/bluish)*

2. Basic life support describes the procedures needed to _____ in an emergency. *(summon help/sustain life/reverse damage)*

3. Brain cells begin to die within _____ minutes after being deprived of oxygenated blood. *(2 to 3/4 to 6/8 to 10)*

 4.2 ## Victim Assessment

Learning Objective **2** Explain proper victim assessment for breathing problems.

Your assessment of the victim is crucial. Assessment consists of four steps:

1. Determining unresponsiveness
2. Activating the EMS system
3. Positioning the victim and opening the airway
4. Observing for signs of life and determining breathlessness

Determining Unresponsiveness

To determine responsiveness in an adult or child, tap the victim gently on the shoulder and ask loudly, "Are you okay?" You are not looking for an answer as much as you are any kind of response—fluttering eyelids, muscle movement, turning to the sound, and so on. If there is no response, the victim is unresponsive. In an infant, gently tap the shoulder or flick the soles of the foot.

Activating the EMS System

When you have two or more people at an emergency, send one to call 9-1-1 while you begin care. If you are alone, you will either call first or care first:

- *Call first:* If you are alone and are treating an unresponsive victim who you believe may have a cardiac-related condition, activate EMS. If you have an Automated External Defibrillator, retrieve this before returning to the patient.

- *Care first:* If you are alone and treating an unresponsive victim who you believe to be suffering from a respiratory problem such as choking or drowning, perform five cycles of CPR (about 2 minutes). Then active EMS.

Positioning the Victim and Opening the Airway

Ideally, the victim should be lying on his or her back on a firm, flat surface. Place the victim's arms alongside his or her body, and kneel at the victim's side. If you have to move the victim, roll the victim as a unit so that head, shoulders, and torso move without twisting; maintain neutral alignment of the head and neck.

The most important part of rescue breathing is opening the airway. If the victim is unconscious, the tongue can relax, fall back, and block the airway; the epiglottis can also relax and block the throat. Sometimes, the victim's efforts to breathe can create negative pressure that draws the tongue or the epiglottis, or both, into the airway. In these cases, opening the airway may be all that is needed to restore breathing.

If you see liquids (such as vomitus) in the mouth, wrap your index and middle fingers in cloth and sweep the liquid out. If you can see solid foreign objects (such as broken teeth), quickly hook them out with your index finger.

You will use the head-tilt/chin-lift maneuver to open the patient's airway. We will also discuss the jawthrust maneuver. This will be used only if it is part of your training program.

---

basic life support   A term that describes the first aid procedures necessary to sustain life in an emergency situation

HEAD-TILT/CHIN-LIFT MANEUVER

Learning Objective **3** Describe how to open the airway of a victim who does not have spinal injury.

If you do *not* suspect cervical spine injury

1. Place the tips of the fingers of one hand underneath the lower jaw on the bony part near the chin; put your other hand on the victim's forehead and apply firm, backward pressure (see Figure 4-2).

2. Bring the chin forward, supporting the jaw and tilting the head backward; be careful not to compress the soft tissues underneath the chin. Maintain pressure on the victim's forehead to keep the head tilted backward.

3. Lift the chin so the teeth are nearly brought together; use your thumb to keep the mouth slightly open. Leave dentures in place if they are secure in the mouth. You will be able to form a better seal for ventilation with the dentures in place.

Take special precautions with children. Extending a child's head and neck too far can cause the trachea to collapse. Never tilt an infant's head beyond neutral position; in older children, tilt it only slightly beyond a sniffing position (the nose tilted slightly upward). Placing a folded towel under the shoulders may adjust the position enough.

Note: The most efficient method of opening the airway is the head-tilt/chin-lift maneuver. Use this technique unless instructed in the jawthrust maneuver and allowed by your level of certification.

JAW-THRUST MANEUVER

Learning Objective **4** Describe how to open the airway of a victim you suspect has spinal injury.

If the head-tilt/chin-lift position is unsuccessful or *if you suspect spine injury*

1. Facing the top of the victim's head, place your elbows on the surface on which the victim is lying, your hands at the sides of the victim's head.

2. Grasp the jawbone on both sides where it angles up toward the victim's ears (see Figure 4-3). Move the jaw forward and upward.

3. Retract the lower lip with your thumb if the lips close.

After you have displaced the jawbone forward, support the head carefully *without* tilting it backward or moving it side to side. **If at any time you have difficulty ventilating the patient, use the head-tilt/chin-lift maneuver.**

Determining Breathlessness

Learning Objective **5** Understand the "look, listen, and feel" assessment method of determining breathlessness.

With the airway open, check to see whether the victim is breathing. Place your ear close to the victim's mouth and nose for no more than 10 seconds, and:

- *Look* for the chest to rise and fall

- *Listen* for sounds of air movement at the mouth and nose

- *Feel* for the breath against your cheek

FIGURE 4-2. Head-tilt/chin-lift maneuver

FIGURE 4-3. Jaw-thrust maneuver

FIGURE 4-4. The recovery position

If the victim is breathing, maintain an open airway, and place the victim in the recovery position (see Figure 4-4). This position helps both conscious and unconscious victims maintain an open airway. If you suspect trauma or cervical spine injury, do not move the victim.

To place the victim in the recovery position, roll her or him onto one side, moving head, shoulders, and torso simultaneously without twisting. Then flex one leg at the knee. Place the bottom arm behind the back. Flex the top arm, placing the hand under the cheek. Continue with your primary survey as described in Chapter 3.

Inadequate breathing (breathing too slowly or shallowly to support life) may also be found. If you encounter this situation (e.g., four to six gasping, shallow breaths per minute) the victim will likely cease breathing soon. Place the victim supine and provide ventilations in between and in conjunction with the victim's attempts at breathing.

If the victim is not breathing, prepare to perform rescue breathing.

PROGRESS CHECK

1. The crucial first step in basic life support is _____ . *(opening the airway/assessing the victim/activating the EMS system)*

2. Tap the victim on the shoulder and ask if he or she is okay to determine _____ . *(unresponsiveness/breathlessness/arrest)*

3. Before you open the airway, the victim should be in a _____ position. *(prone/supine)*

4. During the head-tilt/chin-lift maneuver, maintain backward pressure on the victim's _____ . *(chin/forehead)*

5. In the jaw-thrust maneuver, you bring the victim's _____ forward instead of tilting the head backward. *(jaw/head)*

6. To assess for breathlessness, _____ for the chest to rise and fall. *(feel/look)*

7. To assess for breathlessness, _____ for air escaping during exhalation. *(listen/feel)*

8. To assess for breathlessness, _____ for breath against your cheek. *(feel/listen)*

4.3 Rescue Breathing

Learning Objective **6** Explain how to restore breathing through artificial ventilation.

If you determine that the victim is not breathing, keep the victim in a supine position and begin providing rescue breathing. Use a barrier device, such as a face shield or pocket face mask, when providing ventilations to prevent transmissional disease. Mouth to mouth ventilation will be described because you may choose to do this (e.g. on a family member) in the absence of a barrier device.

Mouth-to-Mouth Ventilation

Mouth-to-mouth ventilation is the simplest, quickest, and most effective way to perform rescue breathing, and it is preferred whenever possible. Figures 4-5 through 4-9 on page 56 illustrate mouth-to-barrier ventilation.

Before starting, make sure the victim is properly positioned and the airway is open, as described earlier. Then proceed as follows.

1. Use the thumb and finger of the hand tilting the victim's forehead to pinch the nostrils closed. If you used the jaw-thrust maneuver, continue to hold the

inadequate breathing Breathing that is too slow or shallow to support life

FIGURE 4-5. Open the airway using the head-tilt/chin-lift maneuver.

FIGURE 4-6. Check for breathing and other signs of life for no longer than 10 seconds.

FIGURE 4-7. In artificial ventilation, give two initial breaths. Allow deflation between breaths.

FIGURE 4-8. Observe the chest fall and feel the exhaled breath from the mask.

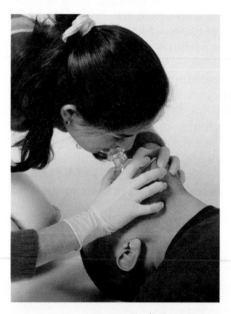

FIGURE 4-9. Once you determine that the victim has a pulse, continue mouth-to-mouth ventilation at the rate of one breath every 5–6 seconds.

lower lip down with your thumb and forefinger, and press your cheek against the victim's nostrils to seal them off.

2. Open your mouth wide, take in a breath, and cover the victim's entire mouth with yours, forming an airtight seal. Provide a steady, even breath over one second into the victim's mouth until you see the chest rise. Then remove your mouth and watch for

the chest to fall; feel for the victim's breath against your cheek. While your head is turned away, take in another breath.

3. Again cover the victim's mouth with yours, forming an airtight seal, and blow a second breath into the victim's mouth until you see the chest rise. Again remove your mouth and watch for the chest to fall.

4. If you don't see the chest rise and fall on the first attempt, reposition the airway and try again. (The most common cause of difficulty with ventilation is improper positioning of the head and chin.) If the second try also fails, assume the airway is blocked by a foreign object. Follow directions at the end of this chapter under Obstructed Airway Emergencies (see pages 60–64).

5. After the first two breaths, check the victim for a pulse. Using your fingertips, check the carotid pulse (located in the groove of the neck alongside the Adam's apple) on the side closest to you. The carotid pulse is easy to locate and easy to feel and is the last pulse to stop. Check for no more than 10 seconds (if the victim is hypothermic, check for 30 seconds). If there is no pulse, immediately start external chest compressions as described in Chapter 5. If the victim has a pulse, continue ventilation, giving one slow, full breath every 5 seconds, or approximately 12 per minute. Continue rescue breathing until the victim begins breathing spontaneously or until you are relieved by emergency personnel.

Note: Breaths that are given too rapidly or excessively will cause air to enter the stomach instead of the lungs. This can cause vomiting and passing of stomach contents into the lungs.

Mouth-to-Mouth Ventilation and Disease Transmission

Mouth-to-mouth ventilation is an effective method of ventilating a nonbreathing victim. You may, however, have concerns about contact with a communicable disease. If you're worried about disease transmission, keep these two things in mind:

- You are statistically more likely to perform ventilations or CPR on a family member or friend than on a stranger.

- Your concerns about disease transmission can be easily addressed by carrying a small (keychain- or pocket-sized) barrier device. Many school or office emergency kits also have barrier devices available.

Mouth-to-Barrier Ventilation

There are two kinds of clear plastic barrier devices that can be used in mouth-to-mouth ventilation to protect you from transmission of infectious diseases during rescue breathing.

1. The **face shield** covers the victim's mouth; in some face shields, a short airway extends into the victim's mouth to hold down the tongue. You breathe through the face shield to deliver ventilations;

because the face shield covers only the mouth, you must still pinch the victim's nose closed.

2. The **face mask** covers the victim's nose and mouth, creating an airtight seal; you deliver ventilations through a one-way valve so that the victim's exhaled breath does not enter your mouth. The American Heart Association recommends use of the face mask instead of the face shield, because it is more effective in creating an airtight seal. Figures 4-5 to 4-9 depict the use of a face mask.

To use a barrier device:

1. Extend the victim's neck and lift the chin.

2. Place the barrier device over the victim's mouth, or mouth and nose (depending on the type of device.)

3. Create an airtight seal.

4. If using a face shield, pinch the nostrils closed.

5. Deliver breaths smoothly and evenly over one second with enough force to make the chest rise.

Mouth-to-Nose Ventilation

Use mouth-to-nose ventilation when:

- You can't open the victim's mouth

- The victim's mouth is so large that you can't seal it off with your mouth

- The victim has no teeth, which interferes with the formation of a good seal

- The victim has mouth injuries

Proceed as follows.

1. With one hand, tilt the victim's forehead back. With your other hand, lift the lower jaw forward and seal the lips. If you used the jaw-thrust maneuver to open the airway, keep the jaw in place with your hand and seal the victim's mouth with your cheek.

2. Take a breath, then place your mouth over the victim's nostrils, forming a tight seal (see Figure 4-10). Blow air slowly and evenly through the victim's nose.

3. If you can, hold the victim's mouth open during exhalation; the victim will exhale more fully, emptying the lungs, if the mouth is open.

Continue rescue breathing as described for mouth-to-mouth ventilation.

> **face shield** A barrier device that covers a victim's mouth
>
> **face mask** A barrier device that covers a victim's mouth and nose

Mouth-to-Stoma Ventilation

A **stoma** is a small, permanent surgical opening in the neck through which the surgical patient breathes. Figure 4-11 illustrates how a neck breather's airway has been changed by surgery. Proceed with rescue breathing as follows.

1. Remove anything covering the stoma, such as a tie, scarf, or jewelry; clear the stoma of any foreign matter.

FIGURE 4–10. Mouth-to-nose ventilation

2. You don't have to perform a head tilt on a victim with a stoma—simply use one hand to pinch the victim's nose and close the victim's mouth. Pinch off the nose between your third and fourth finger, and seal the lips with the palm of your hand.

3. Take a deep breath, then breathe directly into the stoma, forming a seal around the stoma with your mouth. If there is a tracheostomy tube in the stoma, breathe through the tube.

Continue rescue breathing as described for mouth-to-mouth ventilation. Look, listen, and feel for breaths at the victim's stoma.

GASTRIC DISTENTION

During artificial ventilation, it is common for air to get into the esophagus and from there, into the stomach. **Gastric distention** (inflation of the stomach with air) occurs most often in children and in airway-obstructed victims when you have breathed too forcefully. To help prevent gastric distention:

> **stoma** A surgical opening in the neck
>
> **gastric distention** Inflation of the stomach with air

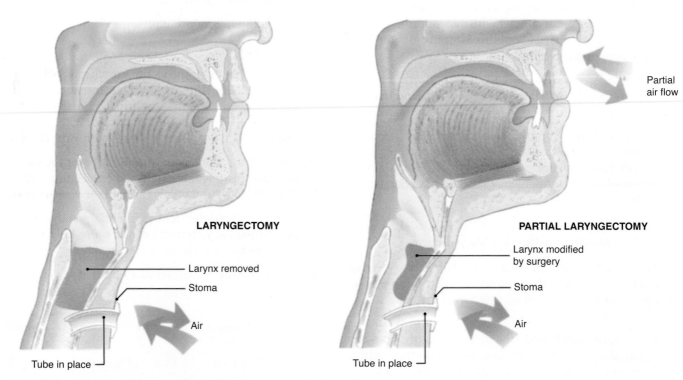

FIGURE 4–11. The neck breather's airway has been changed by surgery.

- Blow only hard enough to make the chest rise.

- Deliver steady breaths over 1 second with a volume of air that makes the chest rise.

- Make sure the airway is open.

Do not press on the abdomen to relieve gastric distention. Such pressure could force stomach contents back up into the mouth and down the trachea, causing **aspiration** (breathing foreign matter into the lungs), which interferes with ventilation.

VENTILATING INFANTS AND CHILDREN

> Learning Objective **7** Adapt ventilation-support procedures to infants and children.

If the victim is an infant (birth-to-1 year) or a child (1 year-to-about 12 years):

- Position the child on his or her back.

- Tilt the head only to a neutral position in an infant (see Figure 4-12); support the head and neck in one hand to maintain a neutral position. Tilt the head only to a sniffing position (the nose tilted slightly upward) in a child. The throat is much more pliable in an infant or child, and tilting the head back too far can actually obstruct the airway.

- With your mouth, cover both the nose and mouth of an infant with a tight seal (see Figure 4-13). Use your mouth to cover the mouth of a child.

- Deliver a slow breath of air over 1 second—just enough to make the chest rise. Be careful not to overinflate or blow too hard; gastric distention is much more common among infants and children.

- Turn your head to the side and watch for the chest to fall; listen for the child's breath, and feel for exhaled air against your cheek. With your head turned to the side, breathe in another deep breath of air.

- If the first breath did not go in (as indicated by the rise of the child's chest), reposition the airway and deliver a second breath. If the second breath does not go in, treat for an obstructed airway as described at the end of this chapter.

- If the second breath goes in, check for a pulse on the inside upper arm. (An infant's or child's neck is too thick and short to easily find the carotid pulse.) Check for no more than 10 seconds. If there is no pulse, start external chest compressions immediately, as described in Chapter 5.

- If there is a pulse, continue rescue breathing. Breathe once every 3 seconds. For both infants and children deliver the breath slowly (over 1 second.) Check the pulse about every 2 minutes (40 breaths) thereafter.

FIGURE 4–12. Head-tilt/chin-lift maneuver for an infant

FIGURE 4–13. Using the mouth to seal the mouth and nose of an infant

PROGRESS CHECK

1. The most effective form of artificial ventilation is _____ . *(mouth-to-mouth/mouth-to-barrier/mouth-to-nose)*

2. Deliver two full, slow rescue breaths, each one lasting about _____ second(s). *(1/3/4)*

3. Perform rescue breathing at the rate of about _____ breaths per minute. *(10/12/14)*

aspiration Breathing foreign matter into the lungs

4. The most common cause of ventilation difficulty is _____ . *(insufficient air/ obstructed airway/improper positioning of the head and chin)*

5. If the victim is an infant or child, ventilations should be faster and more _____ .*(shallow/forceful)*

4.4 Obstructed Airway Emergencies

Learning Objective **8** Identify an obstructed airway.

The most common cause of respiratory emergency is upper-airway obstruction—a foreign object blocking the nose, back of the mouth, or area around the larynx. The most common upper-airway obstruction in an unconscious victim is the tongue; the upper airway can also be blocked by food, small objects, or fluids, including saliva, mucus, blood, or vomitus.

Lower-airway obstruction can be caused either by a foreign object or by bronchospasms.

An obstruction can be partial or complete. If there is only partial obstruction, the victim will be able to cough; there may be a snoring sound as the victim breathes. If there is fairly good air exchange, encourage the victim to cough and expel the foreign object. Monitor the victim carefully, watching for the following signs of reduced air passage:

■ A weak, ineffective cough

■ A high-pitched wheeze during inhalation

■ Increased strain during breathing

■ Clutching at the throat

■ Slight cyanosis

Signs of complete airway obstruction are

■ Inability to speak, groan, cough, or cry out (the victim of a heart attack or other emergency will be able to at least whisper)

■ Absence of breath sounds

■ Labored use of muscles required in breathing—flared nostrils, strained neck and facial muscles

■ Progressive restlessness, anxiety, and confusion

■ Unresponsiveness

If you suspect airway obstruction as the cause of the victim's condition, you should attempt to clear the obstruction for about 2 minutes before stopping to activate EMS. You should be prepared to give first aid care in any case of complete airway obstruction.

First Aid for a Conscious Victim (Adult or Child)

Learning Objective **9** Use techniques for dislodging foreign objects that are obstructing the airway of a conscious person.

Victims who are conscious will usually be standing and often panicked because they are unable to breathe (see Figure 4-14). Assure the victim that you are trained to help. There are two techniques that will be used for the conscious adult and child patient: the back blow and the abdominal thrust (sometimes called the Heimlich Maneuver).

To care for a conscious victim who is unable to speak and has poor or no air exchange:

1. Stand to the side or slightly behind the victim. Place one arm across the victim's chest to provide support. Lean the victim forward.

2. With the heel of the other hand firmly strike the victim between the shoulder blades five times in rapid succession.

3. If the back blows do not dislodge the obstruction, provide five abdominal thrusts. Do this by standing behind the victim and wrapping your arms around the victim's abdomen. Make a fist with one hand and place the thumb-side in position between umbilicus (belly button) and the lower ribs (see Figure 4-15). The fist and lower arms should not come in contact with the ribs at all. Place your other hand over the fist.

4. Provide five inward and upward thrusts (see Figures 4-16 and 4-17).

FIGURE 4–14. The universal sign of choking. Ask the victim, "Are you choking?"

FIGURE 4–15. Position the fist, thumb side in, for the abdominal thrust.

FIGURE 4–16. Administering the abdominal thrust on a standing victim

FIGURE 4–17. Administering the abdominal thrust on a sitting victim

5. If the item is not dislodged, continue with five back blows and five abdominal thrusts until the victim can speak or becomes unconscious.

If you are alone and choking, you can perform abdominal thrusts on yourself by leaning forward and pressing your abdomen against a chair back or other similar object (Figure 4-18). The function of abdominal thrusts is illustrated in Figure 4-19. The administration of abdominal thrusts on a child is illustrated in Figure 4-20.

If the Victim Becomes or Is Unconscious

Learning Objective **10** Use the technique for dislodging foreign objects that are obstructing the airway of an unconscious person.

There are two ways will find an unresponsive victim who is choking. One will be to come upon a victim who is unresponsive and without signs of life. When you attempt to ventilate the victim you are unable to do so, even after repositioning the airway. You will then assume that the victim has airway obstruction.

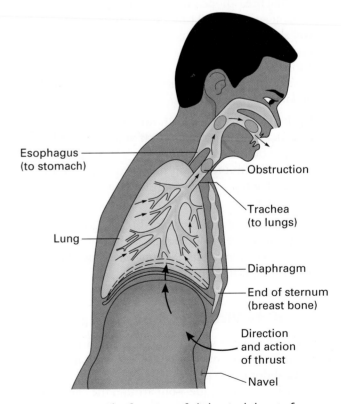

FIGURE 4–19. The function of abdominal thrusts for a complete airway obstruction victim

Esophagus (to stomach)

Obstruction

Trachea (to lungs)

Lung

Diaphragm

End of sternum (breast bone)

Direction and action of thrust

Navel

FIGURE 4–18. Self-administering an abdominal thrust

FIGURE 4–20. Abdominal thrusts on a child

The second way you will find an unconscious victim is when you have been performing obstructed airway maneuvers on a conscious victim who then becomes unresponsive. In either case you follow the same techniques which include chest thrusts, looking for the dislodged item in the mouth, and attempt to ventilate.

If you are unable to ventilate an unconscious victim:

1. Reposition the head. Tilt the head back a bit farther and attempt to ventilate. It is common for first aiders to not tilt the head back far enough the first time.

2. Provide 30 chest compressions. Place the heel of one hand at the center of the chest. This position is over the breastbone (sternum) between the nipples. Push at a rate of 100 times per minute. In the adult you should push approximately 1½ inch to 2 inches in depth, For a child you will compress about 1 to 1½ inches.
   Note: This technique is the same as performing CPR and will be discussed in greater detail in Chapter 5.

3. Look in the victim's mouth for any signs of the obstruction being dislodged. If you see something, scoop it out using your finger in a "hooking" motion. Do not force any objects deeper into the airway. Do not attempt to dislodge anything you cannot see.

4. Attempt rescue breaths. If the breaths go in, check the pulse. If breaths do not go in, continue cycles of 30 chest compressions, looking for dislodged items and attempts to ventilate.

If the Victim Is Obese or Pregnant

Obese or pregnant victims of choking pose a special concern. You may not able to get your arms around the victim's abdomen to perform a thrust. In this case perform the same technique—but around the chest rather than the abdomen. This is called a chest thrust. To perform the thrust on a conscious victim:

1. Stand behind the victim with your arms directly under the victim's armpits; wrap your arms around the victim's chest.

2. Position the thumb side of your fist on the middle of the breastbone. Be sure you are on the breastbone, not the ribs.

3. Grap your fist firmly with your other hand and thrust backward sharply.

4. Alternate chest thrusts with back blows for the conscious victim.

5. For the unresponsive victim, you will perform 30 compressions as described earlier in this chapter.

Figures 4-21 to 4-23 illustrate the technique used with an obese victim.

If the Victim Is an Infant

Do not use abdominal thrusts on an infant—there is significant risk of injuring the abdominal organs. Instead, do a combination of back blows and chest thrusts (see below). Never do a finger sweep in a conscious infant; perform a finger sweep in an unconscious infant only if you can see the foreign object.

Perform the following procedure only if the obstruction is a foreign body. If obstruction is caused by swelling from infection or disease, the infant should be transported immediately to a medical facility. An infant who is conscious but having difficulty breathing should also be transported.

1. Straddle the infant over one arm with his or her face down and lower than the trunk at about a 60 degree angle. Cradle the infant's head and neck in your hand, and rest your forearm on your thigh for support.

FIGURE 4–21. Ask the victim, "Are you choking?"

FIGURE 4-22. Position the thumb side of your fist at the midline of victim's sternum (breast bone).

FIGURE 4-24. Back blows for an infant

FIGURE 4-23. Seize your fist firmly with your other hand and thrust backward sharply.

FIGURE 4-25. Locating the finger position for chest thrusts in an infant

2. Using the heel of your other hand, deliver as many as five back blows rapidly and forcefully between the shoulder blades (see Figure 4-24).

3. While supporting the infant's head, sandwich her or his body between your hands, then turn onto the back, keeping the head lower than the trunk. Lay the infant on your thigh or over your lap.

4. Position the middle and ring fingers of your other hand on the lower third of the infant's sternum, approximately one finger's breadth below an imaginary line drawn between the nipples (see Figure 4-25). Deliver as many as five quick chest thrusts, thrusting straight back.

5. Repeat the cycle of back blows and chest thrusts until the object is expelled or the infant becomes unconscious.

6. If the infant is or becomes unconscious, use a gentle tongue-jaw lift to open the mouth. If you can see the obstructing object, sweep it out with your little finger. Attempt rescue breathing. If the infant's chest does not rise and fall, perform back blows and chest thrusts as described above. Continue the sequence of delivering five back blows, delivering five chest thrusts, checking for the object, removing the object if you can see it, and delivering one rescue breath.

TABLE 4–1	**Summary of Airway Procedures**		
	Adult (12 and older)	**Child (1 to approx 12 years)**	**Infant (birth to 1 year)**
Airway	Head-tilt/chin lift	Head-tilt/chin lift	Head-tilt/chin lift (do not hyperextend)
Initial breaths	Two breaths (1 second per breath)—each enough to make the chest rise	Two breaths (1 second per breath)—each enough to make the chest rise	Two breaths (1 second per breath)—each enough to make the chest rise
Rescue breathing	10–12/min, or every 5 seconds	About 20/min, or every three seconds	About 20/min, or every three seconds
Check for pulse and other signs of life (no longer than 10 seconds)	Carotid (neck)	Carotid (neck)	Brachial (upper arm)
Obstructed airway maneuvers	Back blows and abdominal thrusts	Back blows and abdominal thrusts	Back blows and chest thrusts

PROGRESS CHECK

1. The most reliable sign of complete airway obstruction is _____ . *(cyanosis/ a snoring sound during breathing/ complete inability to speak)*

2. The abdominal thrust is delivered just below the _____ . *(sternum/diaphragm/ rib cage)*

3. During the abdominal thrust, your thumb should be positioned slightly above the _____ . *(xiphoid process/ diaphragm/navel)*

4. If the victim with an obstructed airway is unconscious, the victim should be positioned on the _____ . *(back/side/stomach)*

5. If the victim with an obstructed airway is a conscious infant, you should first do _____ . *(back blows/chest thrusts/ a finger sweep)*

6. If the victim with an obstructed airway is an unconscious infant, you should first do _____ . *(back blows/chest thrusts/ a finger sweep)*

Summary

- Basic life support is a term that describes the first aid procedures necessary to sustain life in an emergency situation.

- The crucial first step of basic life support is assessment—you should perform proper assessment *before* you open the airway, do rescue breathing, or perform chest compressions.

- Open the airway with the head-tilt/chin-lift maneuver if you do not suspect spine injuries; if you suspect spine injuries, use the jaw-thrust maneuver.

- Assess for breathlessness by looking for the rise and fall of the chest, listening for air escaping, and feeling for breath against your cheek.

- For adult victims, activate the EMS system immediately—before you begin any rescue procedures—when acting alone.

- Infant and child (less than 8 years old) victims should receive 1 minute of first aid care before activating the EMS system when acting alone.

- If the victim is an infant or small child, seal *both* the mouth and the nose with your mouth, deliver breaths more often, and use less force.

- Perform the Heimlich maneuver only if there is a complete obstruction of the airway, signaled by the victim's inability to speak, groan, cough, or cry out.

Key Terms

Make sure you understand the following key terms:

basic life support   face mask
respiratory distress   stoma
respiratory arrest   gastric distention
inadequate breathing   aspiration
face shield

Critical Thinking Exercise

You are walking around a stack of books at the library when you hear a woman crying, saying, "I think he's dead." You see an older man on the floor of the library. As you move to the man's side you ask what happened. "He's a volunteer here," the woman says. "I just came around the corner and found him there."

You find the patient unresponsive and open his airway. You note a single, gasping breath in your 10-second check for breathing. It is very shallow. The man has a slow pulse.

1. Is this patient breathing adequately? Why or why not?

2. What would you do to treat this patient?

3. 9-1-1 must be activated. How would you do this?

4 Chapter 4 Self-Test

Student:_____ Date: _____

Course:_____ Section #:_____

Part 1   True/False

If you believe the statement is true, circle the T. If you believe the statement is false, circle the F.

T   F   **1.** If a choking person is unable to speak, you should assume the emergency is life threatening.

T   F   **2.** When resuscitating infants or small children, use more frequent, less powerful puffs of air into the mouth and nose simultaneously.

T   F   **3.** To check the effectiveness of artificial ventilation, you should watch to make sure the stomach is bulging.

T   F   **4.** If you suspect the heart has stopped beating, do not attempt artificial respiration.

T   F   **5.** An adult victim should be given one breath every 8 to 9 seconds.

T   F   **6.** You should do artificial ventilation for only as long as 30 minutes; after that, it is no good if the victim has not responded.

T   F   **7.** Barrier devices help prevent disease transmission from victim to rescuer.

Part 2   Multiple Choice

For each item, circle the correct answer or the phrase that best completes the statement.

1. The purpose of artificial ventilation is to
a. prevent the tongue from being swallowed
b. provide a method of air exchange
c. clear an upper-airway obstruction
d. clear a lower-airway obstruction

2. Which of the following combination of techniques is appropriate for an infant with a complete obstruction?
a. head-tilt/chin-lift, abdominal thrusts
b. back blows, abdominal thrusts
c. back blows, chest thrusts
d. no action, observe until EMS arrives

3. You can tell you are performing mouth-to-mouth or mouth-to-mask ventilation correctly if you can
a. see the victim's chest rise and fall
b. feel resistance as you blow air in
c. feel air escaping from the victim's mouth as he or she exhales
d. all of the above

4. When you are giving mouth-to-mouth resuscitation, you should
a. hold the victim's nostrils closed while breathing into the mouth
b. avoid touching the nostrils unless cardiopulmonary resuscitation is being given at the same time
c. pinch the nostrils as you lift your mouth from the victim's mouth
d. keep the nostrils open

5. Without oxygen, brain cells die
a. within 1 to 2 minutes
b. within 4 to 6 minutes
c. within 6 to 8 minutes
d. after 10 minutes

6. The preferable method of opening the airway is the
a. jaw thrust
b. neck-lift/jaw-thrust
c. head-tilt/jaw-thrust
d. head-tilt/chin-lift

7. The artificial ventilation rate for an infant is
a. once every 3 seconds
b. once every second
c. once every 5 seconds
d. about ten breaths per minute

8. The most common source of upper-airway obstruction in an unconscious person is
a. fluid
b. food
c. the tongue
d. swelling

9. The most reliable indication of a blocked airway in a conscious person is
a. the inability to talk
b. a compression accident
c. partially digested food in the mouth
d. cherry-red skin

67

The three major ways you can recognize adequate breathing are to

Look for _____ .
Listen for _____ .
Feel for _____ .

Part 4   What Would You Do If?

You are eating at a restaurant. Suddenly a man at the next table stands up, knocks over his chair, and places both hands over his throat. He looks alarmed, and his mouth is open. What is the probable cause of this emergency situation? What emergency care would you give in this situation? What would you do if the victim still was not breathing after you provided this first aid care?

Part 5   Skills Review

The following photographs show the stages for administering mouth-to-mouth ventilation. Number the photographs from 1 to 4 to show the correct order of the mouth-to-mouth sequence.

5

Basic Life Support: Cardiopulmonary Resuscitation

Learning Objectives

When you have mastered the material in this chapter, you will be able to

1 Identify the signs and symptoms of cardiac arrest

2 List the sequence of basic life support

3 Describe how to assess a victim for breathlessness

4 Describe how to assess a victim for pulselessness

5 Demonstrate proper hand placement for chest compressions

6 Describe how to deliver effective chest compressions

7 Explain the procedures for performing one-rescuer CPR

8 Know when to terminate CPR

9 Explain the procedures for performing two-rescuer CPR

10 Explain how to adapt CPR techniques to infants and children

11 Discuss the most common mistakes made when performing rescue breathing and chest compressions

12 Know when to withhold CPR

Sixty-one-year-old Eileen Sanders paused on the asphalt track behind the community recreation center. She had felt fine when she started briskly walking a few minutes earlier, but now she felt waves of nausea. As she headed toward a bench at the side of the track, she found it difficult to catch her breath; just before she reached the bench she collapsed, a squeezing pain in her chest suffocating her.

Just behind Eileen, two employees from the recreation center were taking a break by running a few laps. They rushed for Eileen. Thirty-year-old Madison White tapped Eileen's shoulders and shouted at her. No response. Her skin was pale, cool, and beaded with perspiration; when Madison didn't get a response, she sent her companion back to the office to call an ambulance.

Madison rolled Eileen onto her back, used the head-tilt/chin-lift maneuver to open her airway, and placed her cheek close to Eileen's face. There was no breath. Madison delivered two breaths by mouth-to-barrier resuscitation using a face shield from her keychain and felt for a pulse. There was none.

As EMTs ran across the lawn toward them, Madison was alternating between rescue breaths and chest compressions. The EMTs relieved her, performing two-rescuer CPR as a squad from the fire department arrived. Because of Madison's early action, Eileen's heart continued to circulate oxygenated blood, which preserved her life until emergency personnel could apply a defibrillator and shock her heart back into a normal heartbeat. Surgeons later performed bypass surgery to prevent another heart attack.

Heart attacks and associated heart disease are America's number-one killer: Cardiovascular disease takes the lives of almost 650,000 Americans each year. It attacks not only the elderly, but people in their thirties and forties.

Most people who die of a heart attack do so before they ever reach a hospital. Estimates are that many could be saved if immediate, efficient cardiopulmonary resuscitation (CPR), as outlined in this chapter, were provided quickly after the attack.

5.1 Cardiopulmonary Resuscitation

Learning Objective 1 Identify the signs and symptoms of cardiac arrest.

Cardiac arrest is a condition in which the heart has stopped beating. This may be due to the heart muscle not getting the blood—and therefore the oxygen and nutrients it needs—or it could be due to a sudden and serious heart rhythm abnormality.

Cardiac arrest may be a sudden event or preceded by signs and symptoms of a heart attack, including:

- Chest pain, heaviness, or tightness that radiates to the neck, shoulders, jaws, and arms
- Nausea or vomiting
- Cool, pale, moist skin
- Weak or irregular pulses
- Breathing difficulties

When a victim is in cardiac arrest you will find her or him totally unresponsive and without breathing activity. The victim will not move, gasp, breathe, or cough. The carotid pulse will be absent. In this case you should perform cardiopulmonary resuscitation (CPR), which consists of:

- Opening and maintaining the airway
- Providing artificial ventilation through rescue breathing
- Providing artificial circulation through chest compressions

After about 4 minutes without a pulse, chances of survival drop dramatically. CPR helps improve chances of survival by oxygenating and circulating blood until defibrillation and advanced cardiac life support can be provided by emergency personnel. Research shows that the keys to survival of a cardiac arrest victim are:

- Early access to the victim by rescuers or First Aiders trained in CPR
- Early notification of the EMS system
- Early defibrillation
- Early advanced cardiac life support by paramedics and/or physicians

Defibrillation is the application of electricity to the chest of a victim whose heart has stopped. When the heart stops, normal efficient heartbeats are replaced by chaotic, disorganized attempts at beating. Defibrillation, by literally "shocking" the heart, eliminates the disorganized electrical activity and allows normal beating to resume. Defibrillation is covered in Section 5.5. CPR skills are technical and may deteriorate over time. After your certification you should practice quarterly and renew your training every 1–2 years.

PROGRESS CHECK

1. In cardiac arrest, the heart stops because it is not getting the _____ it needs. *(electrical stimulation/rest/oxygen)*

2. CPR consists of opening the airway, providing rescue breathing, and providing _____ . *(chest compressions/defibrillation/intrathoracic massage)*

3. The key objectives of CPR are to _____ and circulate the blood. *(provide rescue breathing/defibrillate/oxygenate)*

4. After about _____ minutes, a victim's chances of survival drop dramatically. *(1/3/4/6)*

5. A key to survival in cardiac arrest is _____ CPR. *(early/effective/prolonged)*

5.2 Basic Life Support Sequence

Learning Objective 2 List the sequence of basic life support.

CPR is only one facet of *basic life support,* a term used to describe the first aid procedures necessary to sustain

---

cardiac arrest A condition in which the heart stops beating

defibrillation The application of electricity to the chest of a victim whose heart has stopped life in an emergency situation. The major steps in the basic life support sequence (illustrated in Figures 5-1 through 5-9) are:

- Determine responsiveness
- Activate the EMS system
- Open the airway
- Determine breathlessness
- Provide rescue breathing
- Determine pulselessness
- Deliver chest compressions
- Defibrillation where available

Determining Responsiveness

To determine responsiveness, tap the victim gently on the shoulder and ask loudly, "Are you okay?" You are not looking for an answer as much as you are any kind of response—fluttering eyelids, muscle movement, turning to the sound, and so on. If there is no response, the victim is unresponsive.

Activating the EMS System

If the victim is unresponsive, and you suspect a cardiac problem, activate the EMS system immediately. If possible, send a reliable person to call 9-1-1. This allows you to stay with the patient. The person who calls dispatch

FIGURE 5–1. Assess responsiveness.

FIGURE 5–2. Send someone to activate the Emergency Medical Services system.

FIGURE 5–3. Position the victim on a hard, flat surface.

FIGURE 5–4. Open the airway with the head-tilt/chin-lift maneuver.

FIGURE 5–5. Determine breathlessness and other signs of life.

FIGURE 5–6. Perform artificial ventilation. Give two breaths. Each should be one second and sufficient to cause the chest to rise.

FIGURE 5-7. Clear an obstructed airway if necessary.

FIGURE 5-8. Determine pulselessness by palpating the carotid artery and look for other signs of circulation.

FIGURE 5-9. Bare the chest (if necessary), landmark properly, and perform chest compressions.

should give the location of the emergency, the telephone number he or she is calling from, what happened, the number of victims involved (if more than one), what first aid care is being given to the victim, and any other requested information.

Opening the Airway

If the victim is unconscious, the tongue can relax, fall back, and block the airway. Sometimes, efforts to breathe can create negative pressure that draws the tongue into the airway. In these cases, opening the airway may be all that is needed to restore breathing.

Use the techniques described in Chapter 4 to open the airway.

Determining Breathlessness

> Learning Objective **3** Describe how to assess a victim for breathlessness.

With the airway open, check to see if the victim is breathing. Place your ear close to the victim's mouth and nose for no more than 10 seconds, and

- *Look* for the chest to rise and fall
- *Listen* for air escaping during exhalation
- *Feel* for the breath against your cheek
- *Observe* for signs of life such as movement or coughing.

If the victim is breathing, maintain an open airway and continue with your primary survey as described in

Chapter 3. If the victim is not breathing, prepare to perform rescue breathing.

Providing Rescue Breathing

If the victim is not breathing, provide rescue breathing as described in Chapter 4. Because mouth-to-mouth resuscitation is the most effective method, use it whenever possible. Begin by delivering two breaths of 1 second each; blow with just enough pressure to make the chest rise.

If the victim's chest does not rise and fall with each ventilation, there may be an airway obstruction. Take the necessary steps to remove the obstruction, as described in Chapter 4.

Determining Pulselessness

> Learning Objective **4** Describe how to assess a victim for pulselessness.

After you have given the first two breaths of rescue breathing, take the victim's pulse at the carotid artery to determine whether the victim's heart is beating (see Figure 5-10):

1. Maintain the head tilt with one hand on the victim's forehead, and place the first two fingers of your other hand on the victim's **larynx** (voice box).

2. Slide your fingers slightly toward you, into the groove alongside the larynx, to locate the carotid artery.

> **larynx** The voice box

FIGURE 5–10. After you have completed ventilation, check the carotid pulse. Palpate the thyroid cartilage in the midline with your index and middle fingers. Slide your fingers laterally to the groove between the trachea and the sternocleidomastoid muscle, and gently feel for the carotid pulse. If you feel no pulse, begin compressions.

3. Exert only gentle pressure to avoid compressing the carotid artery, and feel for a pulse for as long as 10 seconds.

4. While checking for the pulse, also be alert for other signs of life—including movements, breathing, gasping, or coughing—that could indicate a pulse is present.

If you do not feel a pulse at the carotid artery, you can assume that the patient is pulseless—the carotid pulse is one of the last to cease when the heart stops beating.

If you are not sure if there is a carotid pulse, but there are no other signs of life and breathing is absent, begin compressions.

PROGRESS CHECK

1. The first step in the basic life support sequence is to determine _____ . *(responsiveness/breathlessness/pulselessness)*

2. If you determine that the victim is unresponsive, you should immediately _____ . *(open the airway/start CPR/activate the EMS system)*

3. Before you can determine whether the victim is breathing, you need to _____ . *(open the airway/provide two rescue breaths/start CPR)*

4. Before you can determine whether the heart is beating, you need to _____ . *(position the victim/provide two rescue breaths/start CPR)*

5.3 Chest Compressions

If the victim's heart is not beating, as evidenced by a lack of carotid pulse or other signs of life, the next step in the basic life support sequence is to provide chest compressions—rhythmic compressions over the lower half of the sternum that keep the patient's blood circulating.

Chest compressions work on two principles to help circulate the blood: First, they increase pressure in the chest cavity, causing the heart to pump; and second, they provide direct compression to the heart itself. Paired with rescue breathing, chest compressions provide some circulation of oxygenated blood until breathing and circulation can be permanently restored by defibrillation and advanced cardiac life support.

For external chest compressions, the victim must be supine (lying on the back) on a firm, flat surface. The victim's head should not be elevated above the position of the heart. The victim's clothing doesn't hinder your ability to provide effective chest compressions, but it might keep you from properly positioning your hands; if necessary, pull clothing away.

Kneel next to one of the victim's shoulders; your knees should be spaced about as wide apart as your shoulders.

Positioning Your Hands

Learning Objective **5** Demonstrate proper hand placement for chest compressions.

The following steps refer to *adult* patients only.

Proper hand placement on the victim's chest (see Figures 5-11 and 5-12) is essential to avoid causing

LOCATION OF XIPHOID

COMPRESSION

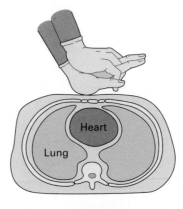

RELEASE

Posterior movement of xiphoid process may lacerate liver. Lowest point of pressure on sternum must be at xiphisternal junction or slightly above.

FIGURE 5–11. Proper hand placement for adult CPR

internal injury from chest compressions. Your hands *must* be above the **xiphoid process** (the lower tip of the sternum). To position your hands, place the heel of one hand in the center of the chest at the level of the nipples. Place the heel of your other hand on top of the first hand with the fingers of both hands pointing away from you. Interlock your fingers and extend them, keeping them off the victim's chest (Figures 5-13 and 5-14 on page 76). If your hands are weak or arthritic, you can grasp the wrist of your first hand with the other hand (Figure 5-15 on page 76).

Delivering Chest Compressions

Learning Objective **6** Describe how to deliver effective chest compressions.

To deliver chest compressions (see Figure 5-16 on page 76), proceed as follows:

1. With your hands properly placed, straighten your arms, lock your elbows, and position your shoulders directly over your hands. Your nose, shoulders, and navel should be aligned approximately vertically. In this position, each thrust you give will be straight down onto the victim's sternum.

2. Press straight down, using the weight of your upper body to compress the adult victim's sternum approximately 1½ to 2 inches, which will force blood from the heart. (You may have to compress the chest more in an obese or very muscular person and less in a very thin or small person.)

3. Release the pressure completely to allow blood to flow back into the heart. You should allow the chest to return to its normal position after every compression.

4. Keep your hands on the victim's chest at all times during chest compression—do not lift them or switch their position. Chest compressions should be smooth and rhythmic; there should be no jerking, jabbing, or starting-stopping movements with each compression.

5. Deliver chest compressions at the rate of about 100 per minute.

xiphoid process The lower tip of the sternum

Too far right:
May fracture ribs and cause lacerations to lung and liver.

Too far left:
May fracture ribs and cause lacerations to lung and heart.

Too high:
May crack sternum.

Too low:
May break off xiphoid process and lacerate the liver.

FIGURE 5–12. Improper positioning of the hands during CPR can damage the rib cage and underlying organs.

FIGURE 5–13. Place heel of hand on the center of the chest between the nipples.

FIGURE 5–14. Interlace fingers.

FIGURE 5–15. Alternative hand placement for CPR

FIGURE 5–16. Perform chest compressions fast and deep.

Performing One-Rescuer Adult CPR

Learning Objective 7 Explain the procedures for performing one-rescuer CPR.

If you are alone, determine unresponsiveness, activate the EMS system, open the airway, determine breathlessness, perform rescue breathing, and determine pulselessness as described above (see Figures 5-17 through 5-19). To perform CPR

1. Position your hands properly on the victim's chest as described above.

2. Deliver 30 chest compressions at the rate of about 100 per minute. Count aloud to keep track of the compressions.

3. Remove your hands from the victim's chest, open the airway, and deliver two rescue breaths of approximately 1 second each. Turn your head to the side while you inhale, and allow the victim's chest to deflate after each breath.

4. Position your hands on the victim's chest again, and deliver 30 more compressions at the rate of approximately 100 per minute.

FIGURE 5–17. Establish breathlessness with the look–listen–feel method, activate the EMS system, open the airway, establish breathlessness with the look–listen–feel method and perform 2 slow, full breaths.

FIGURE 5–18. Establish pulselessness by checking the carotid artery in the neck.

FIGURE 5–19. Place your hands in the center of the chest between the nipples. Compress 1½ to 2 inches on an adult at the rate of about 100 compressions per minute.

5. Repeat this cycle, performing five complete cycles of 30 compressions and 2 rescue breaths.

6. After five complete cycles (about 2 minutes), check again for circulation and breathing. If there is still no pulse, resume CPR. If there is a pulse but the victim is not breathing, perform rescue breathing at the rate of 10 to 12 breaths per minute but *do not* resume chest compressions. Continue to assess the victim every few minutes to determine whether breathing and pulse have returned.

New CPR guidelines indicate that CPR must:

■ Be fast and deep

■ Not be interrupted unless absolutely necessary

Terminating CPR

Learning Objective **8** Know when to terminate CPR.

You must continue performing CPR until the victim is breathing and has a pulse or until one of the following occurs:

■ Breathing and heartbeat start again spontaneously (this is unusual; most cases of cardiac arrest require defibrillation and advanced life support procedures)

■ Another trained rescuer, a physician, or an individual or team directed by a physician assumes responsibility for basic life support

■ A physician tells you to stop

■ The victim is transferred to an appropriate medical care facility

■ You are exhausted and unable to continue life support

■ Conditions (such as a fire, noxious fumes, or an unstable building) make it unsafe for you to continue

■ The victim is declared dead by a physician

Performing Two-Rescuer Adult CPR

Learning Objective **9** Explain the procedures for performing two-rescuer CPR.

If another person trained in CPR is at the scene, one of you should be positioned at the victim's side, the other at the head. Two-rescuer CPR is the preferred method because it results in more effective resuscitation and is less exhausting for the rescuers.

The First Aider at the victim's side should deliver thirty chest compressions, as described above, then pause while the First Aider at the victim's head delivers two breaths.

In two-rescuer CPR, the First Aider at the victim's side should not remove his or her hands from the victim's chest. The First Aider at the victim's head should maintain an open airway throughout resuscitation and should monitor the carotid pulse.

When the First Aider delivering chest compressions gets tired, the two First Aiders should rapidly switch positions, then resume resuscitation. Figures 5-20 through 5-26 illustrate two-rescuer CPR.

FIGURE 5–20. After establishing breathlessness, one rescuer gives two breaths while the other rescuer bares the chest (if necessary) and gets into position to perform chest compressions.

FIGURE 5–21. After establishing pulselessness, one rescuer begins chest compressions.

FIGURE 5–22. CPR continues at a ratio of 30 compressions to two ventilations. During the ventilations, the rescuer performing the compressions pauses.

FIGURE 5–23. Stop CPR to assess the carotid pulse after two minutes, and every two minutes thereafter.

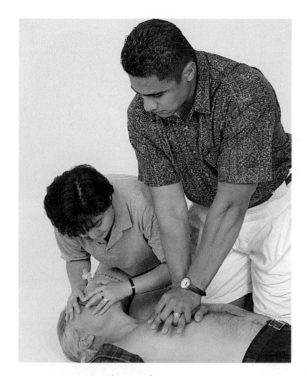

FIGURE 5–24. The tired compressor requests a switch.

FIGURE 5–26. Completing the change: If no pulse is found, the rescuers continue CPR.

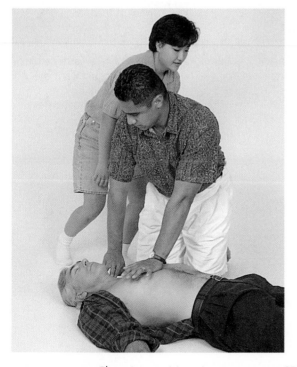

FIGURE 5–25. Changing positions in two-rescuer CPR: The rescuer ventilating delivers two breaths as usual, then positions herself to provide compressions. The rescuer performing the compressions quickly moves to the victim's head and checks the carotid pulse and breathing for no more than 10 seconds. The other rescuer readies for compression.

Performing CPR on Infants and Children

Learning Objective **10** Explain how to adapt CPR techniques to infants and children.

Because children are more likely to have a respiratory problem, it is recommended that, if you are alone, you *perform CPR for 2 minutes before activating the EMS system.* As with adults, you should never perform rescue breathing or deliver chest compressions unless you have determined breathlessness and/or pulselessness. (See Figures 5-27 through 5-35 on page 80 for illustrations.)

In an infant or child, unresponsiveness is characterized by the following signs and symptoms:

- No brachial or carotid pulse
- No chest movements
- Blue or pale skin
- No response to gentle shaking or tapping (tap, but do not shake, an infant)

In infants under 1 year of age, determine pulselessness at the pulse on the inner side of the upper arm (the brachial pulse). To perform CPR:

1. Determine proper placement of your fingers on the infant's chest by placing your index finger in the center of the chest just below the level of the nipples.

2. Place your other hand on the infant's forehead or under the infant's shoulders for support. Lift your

FIGURE 5–27. Determine unresponsiveness in the infant by shouting. Do not shake an infant. You may also try flicking the soles of the baby's feet.

FIGURE 5–28. Gently open the airway using the head-tilt/chin-lift maneuver. Do not tilt the head back very far.

FIGURE 5–29. Establish breathlessness by the look–listen–feel method.

FIGURE 5–30. Infant mouth-to-mouth and nose ventilation: The rescuer covers the baby's mouth and nose with a good seal, then gives two ventilations.

FIGURE 5–31. Check the infant for pulselessness by palpating the brachial artery.

FIGURE 5–32. Perform cardiac compressions in an infant by placing two fingers on the center of the chest just below the nipple line.

FIGURE 5–33. The lower sternum is depressed ½ to 1 inch at a minimum compression rate of 100 per minute.

FIGURE 5–34. Perform CPR, then activate the EMS system. Provide two breaths after performing 30 compressions. Each breath should be over 1 second and be just enough to make the chest rise.

FIGURE 5–35. Performing infant CPR while carrying the baby

FIGURE 5–36. The technique for CPR differs for adults, children, and infants.

index finger off the infant's chest, and use your middle and ring fingers to deliver chest compressions.

3. Depress the infant's sternum ½ inch to 1 inch—a third to a half the depth of the chest—at the rate of at least 100 compressions per minute.

4. Deliver 30 compressions, then two rescue breaths. Continue in cycles of 30 compressions to two slow breaths; do five cycles, then check the infant's pulse to determine whether the heart has started beating.

In children who have not reached puberty (usually 1–12 years of age) determine pulselessness at the carotid artery. To perform CPR:

1. Deliver compressions to the lower half of the sternum.

2. Use the heel of only one hand to depress the sternum; place your second hand on the child's forehead. Never place your second hand on top of the first one.

3. Depress the sternum 1 to 1½ inches.

4. Deliver 30 compressions, then two slow rescue breaths. Continue in cycles of 30 to two.

You will perform compressions at the rate of 100/min. for infants, children, and adults. Remember to minimize any interruptions in CPR. See Figure 5-36 and Table 5-1 for a comparison of techniques for adults, children, and infants.

PROGRESS CHECK

1. You must properly position your _____ during chest compressions, or you can injure the victim. *(shoulders/hands/knees)*

2. The xiphoid process is the tip of the _____ . *(rib/clavicle/sternum)*

3. During chest compressions, keep your shoulders straight and your elbows _____ . *(bent/locked/aligned)*

4. After every two rescue breaths, deliver _____ chest compressions. *(10/20/30)*

TABLE 5–1	**CPR for Adults, Children, and Infants**		
	Adult	**Child (Aged 1–8)**	**Infant**
Hand Placement	Two hands on the center of the chest at the nipple level.	One hand on the center of the chest at the nipple level.	Two fingers on the center of the chest just below the nipple line.
Compression	1½–2"	1–1½"	½–1"
Breaths	Until chest rises (1 second per breath)	Until chest rises (1 second per breath)	Until chest rises (1 second per breath)
Cycle	30 compressions 2 breaths	30 compressions 2 breaths	30 compressions 2 breaths
Rate of Compression	30 compressions in about 22 seconds	30 compressions in about 22 seconds	30 compressions in about 22 seconds

5. Once you start CPR, you must continue it until breathing and pulse return, someone else takes over, or _____ . *(you are told to stop/you are too tired to continue/you injure the victim)*

6. During two-rescuer CPR, the First Aider at the victim's side should never _____ . *(lift hands off the chest/deliver rescue breaths)*

7. If delivering chest compressions to an infant, use _____ . *(two fingers/one hand/both hands)*

5.4 Mistakes, Complications, and When to Withhold

Some theories in CPR have changed over the years. It is now believed that compressions should be delivered "fast and hard" as required by Red Cross and AHA guidelines. To this end, first aiders should switch between compressions and ventilations (when two first aiders are available) to prevent fatigue and assure adequate CPR. Interruptions in CPR should be kept to a minimum.

Many first aiders also worry about performing CPR on patients who may actually have a pulse. If a patient is not breathing and has no other signs of life (coughing, gasping, movement) and you are not sure about the pulse, perform CPR. It is unlikely that the patient has a pulse. This is better than withholding CPR from a patient who needs it.

Mistakes in Performing CPR

Learning Objective **11** Discuss the most common mistakes made when performing rescue breathing and chest compressions.

The most common ventilation mistakes are:

- Failing to tip the head back far enough in adults
- Failing to maintain an adequate head tilt
- Failing to maintain an adequate seal over the mouth and/or nose, letting air escape
- Not giving slow, full breaths
- Failing to watch and listen for exhalation

Common chest compression mistakes are:

- Bending the elbows
- Not having the shoulders directly over the hands

- Placing the hands on the victim's chest improperly
- Letting the fingers touch the victim's chest during compressions
- Not compressing fast enough
- Not compressing deep enough
- Jerky rather than smooth compressions
- Lifting or moving the hands between compressions

Complications Caused by CPR

Even properly performed, CPR can cause the following complications:

- Fracture of the ribs or sternum
- Separation of rib cartilage (common in the elderly)
- Pneumothorax
- Hemothorax
- Bruising of the lung
- Lacerations of the liver

Even if it causes complications, *effective CPR is necessary;* the alternative is death.

Withholding CPR

Learning Objective **12** Know when to withhold CPR.

You are legally required to begin CPR on any victim who needs it—unless there is a legal or medical reason to withhold it:

- There is rigor mortis or other signs of death.
- The victim is decapitated.
- The victim has wounds that will certainly cause death.

PROGRESS CHECK

1. To be effective in CPR, you must _____ the head far enough. *(lift/tilt/turn)*

2. If you think you might be injuring a victim during CPR, you should _____ . *(continue CPR/stop CPR/assess the injury)*

3. If you are on duty, you are legally required to begin CPR on any victim who needs it unless the victim _____ . *(does not give consent/cannot be properly positioned/has obviously fatal wounds)*

5.5 Defibrillation

Defibrillation is done by automated external defibrillators (AEDs), medical devices that deliver a controlled shock through pads or electrodes placed in specific locations on the victim's chest. AEDs are made so that they can be used easily and safely by members of the public. You may have noticed defibrillators on the walls of public areas like shopping malls, airports—even your school. Defibrillation is the only definitive care for cardiac arrest.

The heart beats because electrical impulses stimulate the heart muscle to compress in an organized fashion. When the electrical activity becomes random and disorganized ventricular fibrillation occurs and the heartbeat and pulse stop. **Ventricular fibrillation** is a chaotic, unorganized beating effort of the heart that is incapable of producing a pulse or circulation. This abnormal rhythm can be corrected by early defibrillation. Defibrillation is designed to literally shock the heart into the proper organized rhythm, which will restore the heartbeat.

The AED is not only able, but also extremely accurate, in identifying heart rhythms. You will never have to interpret or identify the rhythm. The AED will also provide prompts that will guide you through the defibrillation process.

Successful defibrillation has been performed in public places by those who have had no formal training. To provide defibrillation:

1. Perform basic life support procedures including activation of the EMS system, two initial ventilations and pulse check (see Figure 5-37). *Only apply an AED to victims who DO NOT have a pulse.*

2. If the patient collapses in your presence or within a few minutes of your arrival, apply the defibrillator. If you believe the patient has been down longer than a few minutes, many physicians recommend 5 cycles of 30:2 CPR (2 minutes) prior to defibrillation.

3. Turn the AED on. The device will provide instructions as explained next (see Figures 5-38 through 5-42).

4. Apply the electrodes to the victim's chest as indicated in the drawings on the electrode face.

5. Push the "analyze" button. Be sure no one is touching or moving the victim (i.e., the victim is "clear").

6. If the AED detects ventricular fibrillation, it will charge and advise you to push the shock button. After making sure you and others are not touching the victim, push the shock button. A shock will be delivered.

7. Follow the voice prompts of the AED. Generally the defibrillator will instruct you to stop CPR every 2 minutes so that the rhythm can be analyzed to determine if another shock is indicated.

Some AEDs are fully automated and do not require you to push any buttons at all. Simply turning the device on and applying the electrodes will begin the process. At this point, simply follow the instructions provided by the device.

PROGRESS CHECK

1. Ventricular fibrillation is an _____ beating effort of the heart. *(accelerated/unorganized/ordinary)*

2. If you are alone with a victim in cardiac arrest and you have an AED available, you should perform _____ first. *(CPR/defibrillation/a neuro exam)*

3. Before analyzing or shocking a victim with an AED you should _____ the victim. *(roll/clear/ventilate)*

FIGURE 5–37. Check for pulse and other signs of heartbeat.

---

ventricular fibrillation A chaotic, unorganized beating effort of the heart that is incapable of producing a pulse or circulation

FIGURE 5–38. Turn on defibrillator. Follow prompts given by unit.

FIGURE 5–39. Attach pads to chest. The pads show proper placement.

FIGURE 5–40. Be sure no one is touching the victim or the cables and press analyze.

FIGURE 5–41. If directed by the AED, be sure everyone is clear of the victim and press the "shock" button.

FIGURE 5–42. Perform CPR for 2 minutes. The AED will prompt you to stop CPR so it can analyze the rhythm. Follow further prompts from the AED.

Summary

- Cardiac arrest occurs when the heart stops beating.

- Cardiopulmonary resuscitation consists of opening and maintaining the airway, providing rescue breathing, and providing chest compressions.

- The key objectives of CPR are to oxygenate and circulate the blood of a cardiac arrest victim until advanced cardiac life support can be given.

- Defibrillation is the most effective method of restoring a heartbeat to a pulseless victim.

- The sequence of basic life support is to determine responsiveness, activate the EMS system, open the airway, determine breathlessness, provide rescue breathing, determine pulselessness, and provide chest compressions.

- Determine pulselessness after performing rescue breathing by checking the carotid artery in the neck and noting absence of movement, breathing, gasping, or coughing.

- Chest compressions consist of smooth, regular, rhythmic applications of pressure over the lower half of the sternum.

- Keys to effective CPR are fast, deep compressions.

- Once you start CPR, you should continue it until breathing and pulse start again spontaneously, another trained person takes over, a physician tells you to stop, the victim is transported, you become too exhausted to continue, conditions make it unsafe for you to continue, or a physician declares the victim dead.

- In one-rescuer CPR, the First Aider delivers both rescue breaths and chest compressions; in two-rescuer CPR, one First Aider delivers rescue breaths and monitors the carotid pulse while the other performs chest compressions.

- You need to modify your technique if you are performing CPR on an infant or child under the age of 12; children over the age of 12 are treated as adults.

- Even though properly performed CPR can cause complications, such as rib or sternum fracture, you should still perform it—the alternative is death.

- You are legally required to provide CPR to someone who needs it unless the person is obviously dead or the person has injuries that will certainly cause death.

Key Terms

Make sure you understand the following key terms:

cardiac arrest
defibrillation
larynx
xiphoid process
ventricular fibrillation

Critical Thinking Exercise

While delivering meals for the local Meals on Wheels, you come to the house of Mr. and Mrs. Ellington. They are a very pleasant older couple you have met on several occasions. You come to the door where you are met by Mrs. Ellington. She looks concerned. "It is good to see you. I can't seem to wake up Ted. He never sleeps this late."

Your accept her offer to come in and observe that everything seems safe. You find Mr. Ellington in bed unresponsive. He is not breathing and has no pulse. You find that he has a long history of heart problems. Mrs. Ellington seems too worried and confused to call 9-1-1.

1. Since Mrs. Ellington is too upset to call 9-1-1, would you do this yourself or perform CPR first?

2. Can you perform CPR on the bed? Why or why not?

3. List the steps you would follow to perform CPR on Mr. Ellington.

5 Chapter 5 Self-Test

Student: _____ Date: _____

Course: _____ Section #: _____

Part 1   True/False

If you believe the statement is true, circle the T. If you believe the statement is false, circle the F.

T   F   **1.** Chest compressions on an adult man should depress the sternum 4 to 5 inches.

T   F   **2.** The best way to find out if a person has stopped breathing is to check the carotid pulse.

T   F   **3.** You should start chest compressions as soon as you find out the victim is not breathing.

T   F   **4.** For adult CPR, proper hand placement on the chest is two finger widths above the xiphoid process.

T   F   **5.** When performing one-rescuer CPR, deliver compressions at the rate of 60 per minute.

T   F   **6.** The compression rate for infants is 100 per minute.

T   F   **7.** Determine heartbeat in an infant by palpating the brachial pulse.

Part 2   Multiple Choice

For each item, circle the correct answer or the phrase that best completes the statement.

1. The correct hand position for administering CPR to an infant is
   a. two fingers above the substernal notch
   b. at the base of the sternum
   c. in the lower third of the sternum
   d. two fingers placed just below an imaginary line drawn between the nipples

2. After each chest compression, your hands should
   a. come completely off the chest
   b. apply a small amount of pressure on the chest
   c. rest on the chest in the normal CPR position
   d. none of the above

3. If you are alone and giving CPR, you should give _____ compression(s) after each _____ ventilations.
   a. 30/2
   b. 15/2
   c. 1/2
   d. 1/4

4. Basic life support consists of
   a. recognizing cardiac arrest and providing artificial ventilation and circulation
   b. checking for breathing and applying rescue breathing
   c. checking for heartbeat and applying artificial circulation
   d. checking for heartbeat and applying rescue breathing

5. CPR must begin when a need for it is recognized and must continue until all of the following occur *except*
   a. the victim is declared dead by the First Aider
   b. the victim is resuscitated
   c. the rescuer can no longer go on
   d. a qualified medical person takes over

6. To check the carotid pulse for circulation
   a. use your thumb
   b. take the pulse on the opposite side of the trachea so that you can feel air exchange in the trachea
   c. check the pulse with your fingertips after you give two full rescue breaths
   d. none of the above

7. You should periodically stop and check to see whether the heartbeat has returned by
   a. checking the pupils
   b. checking the pulse
   c. listening for a heartbeat with a stethoscope
   d. never stop CPR unless the victim is obviously revived

Part 3 What Would You Do If?

You are eating at a restaurant with your family when a middle-aged man at another table clutches at his chest and collapses on the floor. You hear the commotion and run to his table. You ask, "Is he choking?" No one can tell you. People are crowded around the body, the man's wife is shaking him and screaming, but no one is in charge. What signs and symptoms would tell you that the man is suffering a heart attack? What first aid step would you perform first? Identify the steps you would perform under each category:

A–Airway

B–Breathing

C–Circulation

D–Disability

6

Bleeding and Shock

Learning Objectives

When you have mastered the material in this chapter, you will be able to

1 Describe and demonstrate how to control external bleeding with direct pressure

2 Describe and demonstrate how to control external bleeding with pressure points

3 Describe and demonstrate how to control external bleeding with air splints

4 Describe and demonstrate how to control external bleeding with tourniquets

5 Identify the most common signs and symptoms of internal bleeding

6 Describe and demonstrate the general procedures for controlling internal bleeding

7 Understand the basic pathophysiology of shock

8 Understand the factors that may influence the severity of shock

9 Recognize the various types of shock

10 Identify the signs and symptoms of shock

11 Describe and demonstrate the management of shock

12 Identify the signs and symptoms of anaphylactic shock

13 Describe the management of anaphylactic shock

On the Scene

Fourteen-year-old Jessica Franklin rounded the curb on her new mountain bike, slid in an area of loose gravel, and flipped up over the handlebars of the bike. A large, jagged laceration on her leg caused by one of the gear handles began bleeding profusely.

Bart Billings, passing on his way to a job interview, stopped to provide aid. His rapid primary assessment showed that the bleeding leg was the only serious injury; he shouted to a woman standing on a neighboring lawn to call 9–1–1.

Because he didn't have gloves, Bart quickly removed his clean shirt, folded it over a number of times, and used it as a thick pad to prevent contact with Jessica's blood. He then elevated the leg, propping it on his knee, and applied direct pressure to the laceration. When it looked like the bleeding might still be profuse enough to soak through all the layers of his shirt, Bart used his free hand to apply pressure on the femoral artery. Bart maintained both direct pressure and pressure on the artery and monitored Jessica for signs of shock until EMTs arrived 4 minutes later.

he life processes depend on an adequate and uninterrupted supply of blood. The loss of 2 pints of blood in an adult is usually serious; the loss of 3 pints of blood can be fatal if it occurs over the course of a few hours. Bleeding in certain parts of the body—such as from the large blood vessels in the neck—can prove fatal within just a few minutes.

The loss of blood causes a state of physical shock that results because there is insufficient blood flowing through the body to provide tissues with nutrients and oxygen. All the body processes are affected by shock. If the conditions causing shock are not reversed, the victim will die.

This chapter discusses the various ways to control bleeding and outlines the first aid care that should be given a victim in shock.

FIGURE 6–1. Bleeding from the unconscious victim's mouth or nose can be a serious threat to the airway and respiration. Be sure to establish an open airway and position the patient to allow for drainage of blood.

6.1 Bleeding and Its Effects

The severity of bleeding depends on

- How fast the blood is flowing from the vessel
- The size of the vessel
- Whether the vessel is a vein or an artery
- Whether the bleeding is internal or external
- Where the bleeding originated
- The victim's age and weight
- The victim's general physical condition
- Whether the bleeding is a threat to the airway and respiration

Bleeding starts a specific chain of events in the body that is designed to compensate for the loss of fluid and for the potential loss of oxygen that circulates to the heart, brain, lungs, and other organs.

Simply, the body starts to manufacture extra red blood cells; excess fluid is reabsorbed into the bloodstream; platelets collect at the wound site to promote clotting; and white blood cells collect to help control infection.

If the bleeding becomes uncontrolled, the body can't compensate quickly enough to maintain the necessary volume of blood, and the bleeding becomes a life-threatening emergency (see Figure 6-1). Uncontrolled bleeding can lead to moderate shock (loss of 15 percent of blood volume), or severe shock (loss of greater than 30 percent of blood volume).

The severity of bleeding depends on its source: artery, vein, or capillary (see Table 6-1 and Figure 6-2). Figure 6-3 on page 92 illustrates four stages of hemorrhage.

TABLE 6–1	Sources of Bleeding and Their Effects		
Source	**Color**	**Speed**	**Effect**
Artery	Bright red	Rapid (spurting or pulsating)	Under high pressure, most difficult to control
Vein	Dark red	Steady flow	Difficult to control; large veins may suck in air
Capillary	Medium red	Slow, even ooze or steady drip	Often clots spontaneously, usually causes little blood loss

PROGRESS CHECK

1. When bleeding is uncontrolled, the body can't compensate quickly enough, and _____ results. *(cardiac arrest/ heart failure/shock)*

2. A loss of _____ pints of blood can be fatal if it occurs over a period of a few hours. *(1/2/3)*

3. Blood from an artery is _____ . *(red/bright red/dark red)*

4. Blood from a vein is _____ . *(red/bright red/dark red)*

5. Blood from a capillary is _____ . *(red/dark red/medium red)*

6. The most difficult bleeding to control comes from _____ . *(arteries/veins/capillaries)*

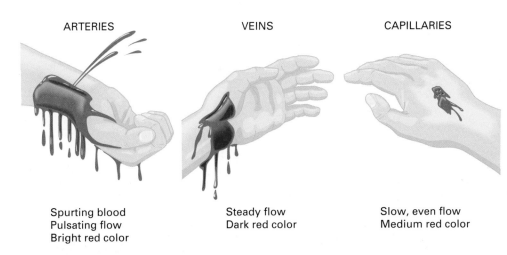

ARTERIES

Spurting blood
Pulsating flow
Bright red color

VEINS

Steady flow
Dark red color

CAPILLARIES

Slow, even flow
Medium red color

FIGURE 6–2. Bleeding sources and characteristics

A **hemophiliac** (sometimes called a *bleeder*) is a person whose blood will not clot because of congenital abnormalities in the clotting mechanisms. Even a slight wound that cuts a blood vessel can cause a hemophiliac to bleed to death. When treating a victim who is a hemophiliac, in addition to providing aggressive care, you must activate the EMS system immediately for rapid transport to a hospital even though the wound would be considered minor in other victims.

6.2 Control of Bleeding

When confronted with a bleeding victim, follow these steps:

1. Stop the bleeding.

2. Determine the cause and source of the bleeding and the general condition of the victim (see Figure 6-4 on page 93); expose the wound to determine where the blood is coming from.

3. Place the victim in a position in which he or she will be least affected by the loss of blood.

4. Maintain an open airway.

After bleeding is controlled, take measures to prevent or control shock, take vital signs every 5 minutes and repeat victim assessment every 15 minutes, and stay alert for the complications of blood loss.

Taking Infection-Control Precautions

Whenever you help a victim who is bleeding or losing other body fluids, take the following precautions to protect yourself against transmission of infectious disease (see Chapter 1):

- Place a barrier between you and the victim's blood. If you can, wear protective gloves; if not, use plastic wrap, aluminum foil, extra gauze bandages, or a clean, thick, folded cloth. As a last resort, use the victim's own hand.

- Avoid touching your mouth, nose, or eyes or handling food while providing first aid care.

- As soon as you finish treating the victim, wash your hands thoroughly with soap and hot water or an antiseptic cleanser, even if you wore gloves. Use a fingernail brush to clean thoroughly under your fingernails.

- Wash all items that have the victim's blood or body fluids on them in hot, soapy water. Rinse well.

Applying Direct Pressure and Elevation

> **Learning Objective 1** Describe and demonstrate how to control external bleeding with direct pressure.

The best method of controlling bleeding—and the one you should try first—is applying pressure directly to the wound (see Figures 6-5 through 6-10, page 93):

1. Place a sterile dressing over the wound so that it is covered completely. If you do not have a sterile dressing, use the cleanest available material (such as a handkerchief, sanitary napkin, or bed sheet).

> **hemophiliac** A person whose blood will not clot because of congenital abnormalities in the clotting mechanism

THE CLASSES OF HEMORRHAGE

CLASS 1	CLASS 2	CLASS 3	CLASS 4
Up to 15% blood loss	Up to 25% blood loss	Up to 30% blood loss	More than 30% blood loss

HOW THE BODY RESPONDS

The body compensates for blood loss by constricting blood vessels (vasoconstriction) in an effort to maintain blood pressure and delivery of oxygen to all organs of the body.	• Vasoconstriction continues to maintain adequate blood pressure, but with some difficulty now. • Blood flow is shunted to vital organs, with decreased flow to intestines, kidneys, and skin.	• Compensatory mechanisms become overtaxed. Vaso-constriction, for example, can no longer sustain blood pressure, which now begins to fall. • Cardiac output and tissue perfusion continue to decrease, becoming potentially life threatening. (Even at this stage, however, the patient can still recover with prompt treatment.)	• Compensatory vasoconstriction now becomes a complicating factor in itself, further impairing tissue perfusion and cellular oxygenation.

EFFECT ON PATIENT	EFFECT ON PATIENT	EFFECT ON PATIENT	EFFECT ON PATIENT
• Victim remains alert. • Blood pressure stays within normal limits. • Pulse stays within normal limits or increases slightly; pulse quality remains strong. • Respiratory rate and depth, skin color and temperature all remain normal.	• Victim may become confused and restless. • Skin turns pale, cool, and dry because of shunting of blood to vital organs. • Diastolic pressure may rise or fall. It's more likely to rise (because of vasoconstriction) or stay the same in otherwise healthy patients with no underlying cardio-vascular problems. • Pulse pressure (difference between systolic and diastolic pressures) narrows. • Sympathetic responses also cause rapid heart rate (over 100 beats per minute). Pulse quality weakens. • Respiratory rate increases because of sympathetic stimulation. • Delayed capillary refill.	• Victim becomes more confused, restless, and anxious. • Classic signs of shock appear—rapid heart rate, decreased blood pressure, rapid respiration and cool, clammy extremities.	• Victim becomes lethargic, drowsy, or stuporous. • Signs of shock become more pronounced. Blood pressure continues to fall. • Lack of blood flow to the brain and other vital organs ultimately leads to organ failure and death.

*The average adult has 5 liters (1 liter = approximately 1 quart) of circulating blood; 15% is 750 ml (or about 3 cups). With internal bleeding 750 ml will occupy enough space in a limb to cause swelling and pain. With bleeding into the body cavities, however, the blood will spread throughout the cavity, causing little, if any initial discomfort.

FIGURE 6–3. The four classes of hemorrhage are based on the amount of blood lost.

FIGURE 6–4. Detecting and controlling severe bleeding are parts of the primary survey.

FIGURE 6–5. Bleeding from a lacerated wound on the forearm

FIGURE 6–6. Control bleeding with a combination of direct pressure and elevation. If dressings are unavailable, use a gloved hand or other clean material, such as a shirt, towel, or pillowcase.

FIGURE 6–7. If bleeding soaks through the dressing, do not remove it.

FIGURE 6–8. Add a new dressing on top of the original. Continue with direct pressure and elevation. After bleeding is under control, bandage the dressing in place.

FIGURE 6–9. In cases of profuse bleeding, do not waste time hunting for a dressing. Immediately apply direct pressure to the bleeding vessel.

FIGURE 6–10. Bandage the wound.

2. Press firmly over the dressing with your fingertips directly to the site of bleeding. Keep the pressure firm and constant for at least 10 minutes. Wounds on the scalp, face, and hands will bleed more profusely because those areas are so richly supplied with blood.

3. Elevate the bleeding part above heart level unless you suspect a fracture, dislocation, impaled object, or spinal injury. *Note that elevation alone is not effective in controlling bleeding—it must be used along with direct pressure.*

4. You can use a cold pack over the wound as you apply direct pressure and elevation; cold can reduce blood flow to the area. Make sure you place a layer of gauze or other thin material under the cold pack anywhere it might contact the victim's skin.

5. Check the dressing every few minutes. If it soaks through with blood, do not remove it—simply place another dressing on top of it and continue to apply or reapply pressure.

6. *Never apply direct pressure to a wound if there is an object embedded in the wound or if a bone is protruding from the wound.* In these cases, use a doughnut-shaped pad over the wound, then apply pressure to the pad. To make a doughnut-shaped pad, loop a cravat or other narrow bandage around your four fingers several times, then wind the remainder of the bandage in and out around the ring until the entire bandage is wound into the pad.

Leave the dressing in place for at least 10 minutes *after* the bleeding has stopped. Taking it off earlier can disturb the clot and cause the bleeding to start again.

If necessary, you can increase the pressure on the dressing with a pressure bandage, air splint, or blood pressure cuff.

Using a Pressure Bandage

A pressure bandage is used to create pressure over a dressing (see Figure 6-11). To use a pressure bandage:

1. Cover the wound completely with a thick dressing; make sure all edges of the wound are covered.

2. Holding the dressing in place, wrap the pressure bandage around the dressing tightly enough to exert moderate pressure.

3. Periodically check the distal pulses, and frequently check for mottled skin or blanched nails, signs that the pressure bandage is too tight.

Using Indirect Pressure

Learning Objective **2** Describe and demonstrate how to control external bleeding with pressure points.

If direct pressure and elevation don't control the bleeding, bleeding from an artery or vein can be controlled by using your thumb or finger to apply pressure on a **pressure point**—a place where the artery is close to a bony structure and also near the skin surface. Pressure

pressure point A place where an artery is close to the skin surface and lies over a bone

FIGURE 6–11. Applying a pressure bandage

points can be difficult to locate and use, but pressure applied at these points can be effective in controlling the flow of blood to the injury site (see Figures 6-12 and 6-13).

Never substitute indirect pressure for direct pressure—both should be used simultaneously. Hold the pressure point only as long as necessary to stop the bleeding; reapply indirect pressure if bleeding recurs.

Major arterial pressure (pulse) points (see Figure 6-14 on page 96) include the maxillary, temporal, brachial, radial and ulnar, femoral, posterior tibial, and dorsalis pedis arteries. See Table 6-2 on page 96 for the locations of these pressure points.

Use pressure points with caution, because indirect pressure can cause damage from inadequate blood flow. Never use indirect pressure if you suspect that the bone below the artery might be injured.

The most commonly used pressure points are the brachial and the femoral.

BRACHIAL ARTERY

Pressure on the brachial artery is used to control severe bleeding from a wound on the arm. The pressure point is located in a groove on the inside of the arm between the armpit and the elbow. To apply pressure:

1. Grasp the middle of the victim's arm with the thumb on the outside of the arm and the fingers on the inside.

2. Press the fingers toward the thumb.

3. Use the flat, inside surface of the fingers, not the fingertips. This inward pressure collapses the artery by pressing it against the humerus.

FIGURE 6–12. Apply pressure to the brachial artery pressure point to control bleeding in the arm.

FIGURE 6–13. Apply pressure to the femoral artery pressure point to control bleeding in the leg.

Arterial pulse points are places where an artery lies close to the skin or passes over a bony prominence. When an artery is so located, it can be palpated, or felt with gentle fingertip pressure. Since most body parts are supplied by more than one artery, the use of arterial pressure points alone rarely controls hemorrhage. However, compression of arterial pulse points *in addition to direct pressure* can sometimes help to control severe bleeding. Major arterial pulse points include:

- **Carotid arteries** are located on each side of the neck next to the larynx. These two arteries supply blood to the head. *Do not exert pressure on the carotid pressure points.*

- **Maxillary arteries** supply much of the blood to the face. One can be palpated on each side of the face on the inner surface of the lower jaw.

- **Temporal arteries** supply part of the blood supply to the scalp. One can be palpated on each side of the face just above the upper portion of the ear.

- **Brachial arteries**, located on the inner arms just above the elbows, supply blood to the arms.

- **Radial** and **ulnar arteries**, located in the wrist, also supply blood to the arms and hands.

- **Femoral arteries**, which pass through the groin, supply blood to the legs.

- **Posterior tibial artery**, which passes through the ankle, and the **dorsalis pedis artery**, on the front surface of the foot, can determine circulation to the feet.

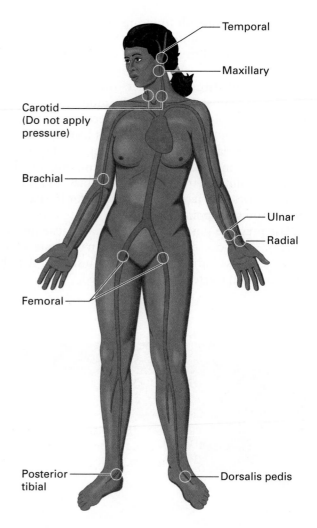

FIGURE 6–14. Arterial pulse points

TABLE 6–2	**Major Arterial Pressure Points and Their Locations**	
Pressure Point	**Location**	**Controls Blood Flow to**
Maxillary	Each side of the face, on the inner surface of the lower jaw	Face
Temporal	Each side of the face, just above the ear	Scalp
Brachial	Inner arm, just above the elbow	Arms
Radial and ulnar	Wrist	Arms and hands
Femoral	Each side of the groin	Legs
Posterior tibial	Inner side of ankle behind the ankle bone (medial malleolous)	Foot
Dorsalis pedis	On top of the foot on big toe side	Foot

FEMORAL ARTERY

Pressure on the femoral artery is used to control severe bleeding from a wound to the leg. The pressure point is located on the front center part of the crease in the groin area. This is where the artery crosses the pelvic basin on the way into the lower extremity. To apply pressure:

1. Place the victim flat on his or her back, if possible.

2. Kneeling on the side opposite the wounded limb, place the heel of one hand directly on the pressure point, and lean forward to apply pressure to collapse the artery.

3. If bleeding is not controlled, it may be necessary to press directly over the artery with the flat surface of the fingertips and apply additional pressure on the fingertips with the heel of the other hand.

Using an Air Splint

Learning Objective **3** Describe and demonstrate how to control external bleeding with air splints.

An air splint (see Figure 6-15) can be used to create a pressure bandage and control bleeding in an extremity. Using an air splint has one additional benefit: It frees your hands so you can manage other injuries. Use an air splint as follows:

1. Cover the wound with a thick, sterile dressing.

2. Slip the splint over the dressing, taking care not to shift or remove the dressing.

3. Inflate the splint. Take care not to overinflate—you should be able to depress the surface of the splint at least half an inch with your fingertips.

FIGURE 6–15. Air splints can be used to apply pressure and control bleeding from an extremity.

4. Check distal pulses often if they are not covered by the splint; check frequently for mottled skin or blanched nails, signs that the splint is too tight.

Never deflate an air splint unless directed to by EMS personnel.

Using a Tourniquet

Learning Objective **4** Describe and demonstrate how to control external bleeding with tourniquets.

A tourniquet should be used *only as a last resort*, after all other methods of controlling life-threatening bleeding have failed. It can be used only on an extremity; using a. tourniquet may lead to amputation of the extremity below the tourniquet. As a general rule, consider a tourniquet only under either of these conditions:

- A large artery has been severed and the bleeding cannot be controlled by direct pressure, elevation, cold application, or pressure points.

- A limb has been partially or totally severed, and bleeding is uncontrollable.

- A mass casualty incident where several patients are injured and you are unable to spend the time applying pressure to a bleeding wound.

You can improvise a tourniquet from a strap, belt, suspender, handkerchief, towel, necktie, cloth, folded triangular bandage, or other suitable material that is at least 3 inches wide. *Never* use wire, cord, or anything else that could cut into the flesh. *Never* use a clamp or hemostat on a blood vessel.

To apply a tourniquet (see Figure 6-16), follow these steps:

1. Hold the appropriate pressure point to control bleeding temporarily, then place the tourniquet between the heart and the wound, leaving at least 2 inches of uninjured flesh between the tourniquet and the wound.

2. Put a thick pad over the tissue that will be compressed.

3. Wrap the tourniquet material tightly around the limb twice, then tie it in a half-knot on the upper surface of the limb.

4. Place a short stick or other similar object at the half-knot, then tie a square knot.

5. Twist the stick to tighten the tourniquet *only* until the bleeding stops. Secure the stick in place with the

1. Apply pad

2. Tighten tourniquet

3. Fix in place

4. Record time

FIGURE 6–16. Apply a tourniquet as a last resort.

ends of the tourniquet or another strip of cloth. Leave the tourniquet uncovered.

6. Write a note detailing the location of the tourniquet, the time it was applied, and the vital signs at the time you applied it. Pin the note to the victim's clothing. Then write *T* or *T/K* on the victim's forehead with lipstick or marker and write the time the tourniquet was applied.

Never loosen or remove a tourniquet except under the direction of a physician.

Using a Blood Pressure Cuff

In some cases, you can use a blood pressure cuff to control bleeding (see Figure 6-17). If you use a cuff,

- Secure it well so the Velcro does not pop open.

- Inflate it to a pressure that causes the bleeding to stop, usually 10 to 20 mm Hg above the systolic blood pressure.

- Never deflate the cuff unless a physician orders you to do so.

A blood pressure cuff can safely remain inflated for as long as 30 minutes.

PROGRESS CHECK

1. Direct pressure is pressure applied directly to the _____ . *(artery/pressure point/wound)*

2. If a dressing soaks through with blood, you should _____ . *(remove it/remove and replace it/leave it in place and put another one over it)*

3. In addition to direct pressure, _____ the limb and apply cold packs. *(elevate/compress/splint)*

4. Indirect pressure is applied at _____ . *(wound sites/pressure points/joints)*

5. The pressure point that controls bleeding to the arms is the _____ . *(femoral/temporal/brachial)*

6. The femoral pressure point is located in the _____ . *(neck/inner arm/groin)*

7. Material used for a tourniquet should be at least _____ inches wide. *(2/3/4)*

8. Release a tourniquet only when _____ . *(bleeding has stopped/EMTs arrive/a physician is present)*

FIGURE 6–17. A blood pressure cuff can be used to apply pressure and control bleeding in an extremity.

 ## 6.3 Internal Bleeding

Internal bleeding generally results from blunt or penetrating trauma or certain fractures (such as a pelvic fracture). Though not visible, internal bleeding can be very serious—even fatal—because a large amount of blood can be lost and shock can develop rapidly (see Figure 6-18).

You should suspect internal bleeding based on signs and symptoms as well as the mechanism of injury.

Signs and Symptoms

Learning Objective **5** Identify the most common signs and symptoms of internal bleeding.

The signs and symptoms of internal bleeding are similar to those of shock: restlessness and anxiety; cool, clammy skin; weak, rapid pulse; rapid breathing; and, ultimately, a drop in blood pressure. There may be additional signs and symptoms, depending on the source of the bleeding (see Table 6-3). Internal bleeding may not cause signs or symptoms for hours or days; realize that internal bleeding may be occurring even if there are no signs or symptoms.

First Aid Care

Learning Objective **6** Describe and demonstrate the general procedures for controlling internal bleeding.

The highest priorities in terms of treatment are internal bleeding into the chest cavity, the abdominal cavity, the pelvic cavity, and around the femur when fractured.

The most common cause of internal bleeding due to trauma is a fracture, and the most severe fracture-related blood loss occurs in fractures of the pelvis and femur.

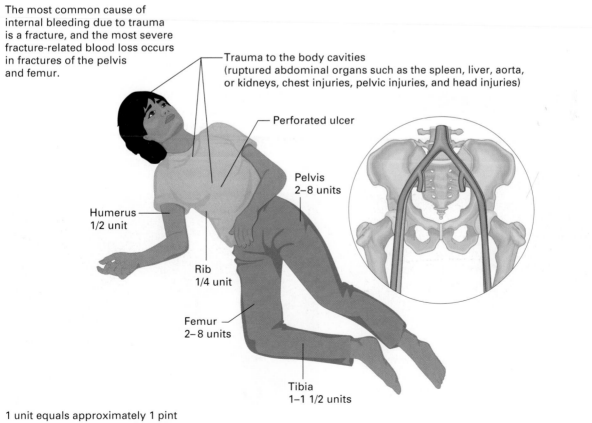

Trauma to the body cavities (ruptured abdominal organs such as the spleen, liver, aorta, or kidneys, chest injuries, pelvic injuries, and head injuries)

Perforated ulcer

Pelvis
2–8 units

Humerus
1/2 unit

Rib
1/4 unit

Femur
2–8 units

Tibia
1–1 1/2 units

1 unit equals approximately 1 pint

FIGURE 6–18. Internal bleeding

TABLE 6-3	Common Causes of Internal Bleeding and Their Signs and Symptoms
Common Causes	**Signs and Symptoms**
Blunt and penetrating trauma	Bruising; pain, tenderness, swelling, or discoloration at the site of injury; in blunt trauma to the head, bleeding from the mouth and blood or bloody fluid in the nose or ears; in blunt trauma to the abdomen, bleeding from the rectum or nonmenstrual bleeding from the vagina; open wounds to head, chest, abdomen, pelvis, or extremities
Fractured ribs or sternum	Coughing up of bright red, frothy blood; shallow, rapid respiration
Bleeding ulcer or ingestion of a sharp object	Vomiting of bright red blood or dark brown partly digested blood that resembles coffee grounds
Intestinal disease, parasites, blunt trauma to the abdomen	Black, tarry stools; rigidity of the abdomen; spasms of abdominal muscles
Blockage of urethra or pelvic fracture	Blood in the urine or urine that is smoky colored

For victims of internal bleeding, activate the EMS system; then:

1. Secure and maintain an open airway, and monitor the ABCDs.

2. Check for fractures; splint if appropriate.

3. Keep the victim quiet. Position and treat the victim for shock by elevating the feet only 8 to 12 inches and covering him or her to maintain body heat. (Do not elevate the feet if you suspect leg or spine injuries.) If the victim starts to vomit, place in the coma position.

4. Monitor vital signs every 5 minutes until emergency personnel arrive.

PROGRESS CHECK

1. Internal bleeding is extremely serious because it can cause _____ . *(extremity damage/brain damage/shock)*

2. If internal bleeding is present the heart rate will be _____ . *(decreased/normal/increased)*

3. The most common cause of internal bleeding is _____ . *(blunt and penetrating trauma/perforated ulcer/skull fracture)*

4. The signs and symptoms of internal bleeding are much like those of _____ . *(external bleeding/cardiopulmonary disease/shock)*

5. Basic treatment of internal bleeding involves _____, opening the airway, and positioning the victim to prevent shock. *(applying pressure/activating the EMS system/ elevating the affected part)*

6.4 Nosebleed

Nosebleeds are a relatively common source of bleeding that can result from injury, disease, activity, temperature extremes, or other causes. Severe, uncontrolled nosebleeds can cause enough blood loss to cause shock.

If you suspect the nosebleed was caused by a fractured skull, *do not try to stop the flow of blood*; to do so will increase pressure on the brain. Cover the opening of the nose *loosely* with a dry, sterile dressing to absorb the blood, activate the EMS system, and treat the victim for skull fracture, as outlined in Chapter 13.

If you suspect a nosebleed is caused by something *other* than a fractured skull:

1. Keep the victim quiet and in a sitting position, leaning forward to prevent aspiration of blood (see Figure 6-19). Never have the victim tilt his or her head back.

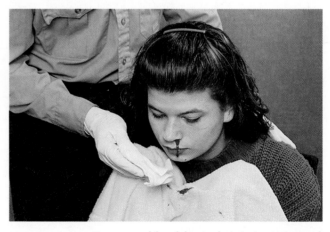

FIGURE 6–19. For a nosebleed, keep the victim quiet and leaning forward in a sitting position.

FIGURE 6–20. Apply pressure by pinching the nostrils and, if necessary, apply cold compresses to the nose and face.

2. If you do not suspect nasal fracture, pinch the nostrils together (see Figure 6-20).

3. Apply cold compresses to the bridge of the nose.

4. If the bleeding does not stop, call 9-1-1 to activate EMS.

PROGRESS CHECK

1. To control nosebleed, keep the victim _____ . *(sitting up/lying down/ in a position of comfort)*

2. Unless you suspect nasal fracture, pinch the nostrils together, then apply _____ . *(pressure/cold compresses/indirect pressure)*

3. If you suspect _____, do not try to stop a nosebleed. *(heart attack/elevated blood pressure/skull fracture)*

6.5 Shock

Shock is defined as an inadequate delivery of blood to the cells. Left untreated, shock is fatal. Unless you recognize and treat shock immediately, the victim can die.

The Causes of Shock

Learning Objective **7** Understand the basic pathophysiology of shock.

Shock is a progressive process that can be either gradual or rapid in onset; throughout the development of shock,

the victim's condition constantly changes. Figures 6-21 and 6-22 illustrate the continuous cycle of traumatic shock.

Learning Objective **8** Understand the factors that may influence the severity of shock

Basically, shock is the inadequate delivery of oxygen and nutrients to the cells. This is also known as inadequate tissue perfusion. **Perfusion** refers to the circulation of oxygen-rich blood through organs and tissues. The cells most sensitive to a lack of oxygen are those in the heart, brain, and lungs.

There are four basic causes of shock: (see Table 6-4, page 103.)

1. Fluid is lost from the circulatory system (generally a result of bleeding, burns, or dehydration). See Figure 6-23, page 103.

2. The heart fails to pump the blood effectively.

3. The blood vessels dilate, causing blood to pool in extremities and non-vital areas.

4. The body's supply of oxygen is inadequate.

Factors influencing the severity of shock include age (infants and the elderly are at most risk), multiple injuries, pre-existing medical conditions, pregnancy, physical condition, and amount of blood loss. Shock often progresses rapidly in children and the elderly.

The Types of Shock

Learning Objective **9** Recognize the various types of shock.

Shock is progressive and occurs in three stages: **compensatory**, **progressive (decompensatory)**, and **irreversible shock** (see Table 6-5 and Figure 6-24, page 104).

---

shock Inadequate tissue perfusion.

perfusion Circulation of oxygen-rich blood to cells.

compensatory shock The first stage of shock, in which the body attempts to overcome the decrease in tissue perfusion.

progressive (decompensatory) shock The second stage of shock, in which the compensatory mechanisms have failed, the blood pressure begins to decrease, and the organs are beginning to suffer from the lack of perfusion

irreversible shock The final stage of shock, in which body organs start to die

TRAUMA OF ANY KIND

Depressed circulation due to blood loss externally, and pooling of blood in large internal vessels.

Tissues and organs receive inadequate supply of blood.

Rapid heart rate and weak pulse from blood loss.

Blood vessels in extremities constrict to conserve blood, causing *cold, clammy skin.*

Low levels of oxygen and nutrient supplies to body tissues cause a decrease in body temperature.

Decrease in waste elimination from lungs and kidneys.

Low levels of oxygen to breathing control centers of the brain make respiration rapid and shallow.

Nervous system reaction results in profuse sweating.

Muscles in the blood vessel walls relax, and blood pressure drops.

Leaking capillaries lead to loss of vital blood plasma, causing circulatory depression and thirst.

Unconsciousness and death may result.

FIGURE 6–21. Continuous cycle of traumatic shock

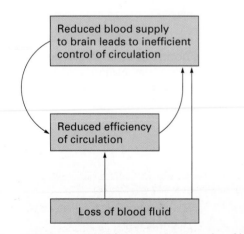

Reduced blood supply to brain leads to inefficient control of circulation

Reduced efficiency of circulation

Loss of blood fluid

FIGURE 6–22. The progressive circle of hermorrhagic shock

Shock in a child can present a somewhat different picture—generally, it develops early with little evidence and progresses extremely rapidly. A child may show no signs or symptoms at all, or only very subtle ones, then suddenly exhibit the dramatic signs of progressive shock. For this reason, *always begin first aid care of a child very early.* Never wait to see if symptoms develop.

Pregnant patients will lose large amounts of blood before signs and symptoms of shock become evident.

Signs and Symptoms of Shock

Learning Objective **10** Identify the signs and symptoms of shock.

Figure 6-25 on page 105 illustrates the signs and symptoms of shock. Signs of shock in a dark-skinned victim may be more subtle (see Figure 6-26 on page 105).

A healthy person with dark skin will usually have a red undertone and show a healthy pink color in the nail beds, lips, mucous membranes of the mouth, and tongue. However, a dark-skinned victim suffering from a lack of oxygen does not exhibit marked skin color changes. Rather, the skin around the nose and mouth will have a grayish cast, the mucous membranes of the mouth and tongue may be blue (cyanotic), and the lips and nail beds will have a blue tinge. If shock is due to bleeding, the mucous membranes in the mouth and tongue will not look blue but will have a pale, graying, waxy pallor. Other landmarks include the tips of the

TABLE 6—4	Types of Shock

Type	Description and Cause
Hemorrhagic	Loss of blood, usually from multiple trauma and severe burns; there is not enough blood in the system to provide adequate circulation to all parts (see Figures 6-22 and 6-23).
Neurogenic	Spinal or head injury resulting in loss of nerve control; blood vessels dilate, and there is not enough blood to fill them.
Psychogenic	Something psychological affects the victim; blood drains from the head and pools in the abdomen, causing fainting.
Cardiogenic	The cardiac muscle does not pump effectively enough to circulate blood, usually because of injury, heart attack, or heart disease.
Metabolic	Insulin shock, diabetic coma, vomiting, diarrhea, or some other condition causes loss of fluids and change in biochemical balance.
Septic	Toxins from severe infection cause dilation of blood vessels, pooling of blood in the small capillaries, and bacterial invasion of blood vessels.
Anaphylactic	Severe allergic reaction occurs, usually to insect sting, food, or medicine.

HEMORRHAGIC SHOCK

Watch for shock in all trauma patients. They can lose fluids not only externally through bleeding, vomiting, or burns, but also internally through crush injuries and organ punctures.

FIGURE 6–23. Loss of body fluids can be external and internal.

ears, which may be red during fever. The palms of the hands and soles of the feet will appear more pale.

Management of Shock

Learning Objective 11 Describe and demonstrate the management of shock.

Activate the EMS system immediately; then:

1. Secure an open airway. Give extra attention to any victim whose airway is obviously compromised.

2. Place the victim on his or her back *unless* the victim has an object impaled in the back of the body, difficulty breathing, or heart attack symptoms. In these cases, position the victim in a half-sitting position to make breathing easier. A victim who is obviously pregnant should be placed on her left side or supine with her right hip elevated. Any victim who has a suspected spinal injury should be placed in a supine position with the head and neck maintained in a neutral in-line position.

3. Control any obvious bleeding.

4. Elevate the legs *no more than* 8 to 12 inches above heart level. Never tilt the entire body so that the feet are elevated and the head is lower than the body—doing so can impair breathing. *Never elevate the legs of a person with leg injuries* (marked by deformity or swelling).

TABLE 6-5	Signs and Symptoms of the Three Stages of Shock	
Stage	**What Happens**	**Signs and Symptoms**
Compensatory	The body tries to use its normal defense mechanisms to maintain normal function.	Minimal–normal blood pressure; increased pulse; cool, clammy skin; dull, pale skin; weakness, anxious, restlessness
Progressive	Body shunts blood away from the extremities and abdomen to the heart, brain, and lungs.	Extremely pale skin; dropping blood pressure; profuse sweating; extreme thirst; nausea and/or vomiting; dizziness; altered levels of consciousness
Irreversible	Blood is shunted from the liver and kidneys to the heart and brain; organs die; blood pools away from vital organs; death occurs.	Dull, lusterless eyes; dilated pupils; shallow, irregular breathing; loss of consciousness

RECOGNIZING THE STAGES OF SHOCK

Shock is inadequate perfusion of bodily tissues. It is not a disease in itself but occurs secondary to trauma or illness. Shock may develop when serious injury causes significant blood loss, pump (heart) damage, spinal cord injury, or pulmonary injury, or when serious illness causes peripheral vasodilation or severe dehydration. Remember — in order for blood to circulate properly there must be adequate blood volume, a good working pump, and an intact vascular system.

When the cells of the body are not adequately oxygenated and/or nourished, a sequence of events may occur that, if left uncorrected, will result in death. The body will set in motion a series of complex mechanisms in an attempt to achieve homeostasis and compensate for shock. If the state of shock is severe or prolonged, it may become irreversible. If this occurs, no intervention will save the victim. Recognizing the signs and symptoms of each stage of shock will help you classify the victim's condition according to its severity so you can intervene appropriately.

COMPENSATORY STAGE

- Restlessness, anxiety, irritability, apprehension
- Slightly increased heart rate
- Pale and cool skin in hemorrhagic shock, warm and flushed skin in septic, anaphylactic, and neurogenic shock
- Slightly increased respiratory rate
- Slightly decreased body temperature (except fever in septic shock)

PROGRESSIVE (UNCOMPENSATED) STAGE

- Listlessness, apathy, confusion, slowed speech
- Rapid heart rate
- Weak, thready pulse
- Decreased blood pressure
- Cold, clammy, cyanotic skin
- Rapid breathing
- Severely decreased body temperature
- Confusion and incoherent, slurred speech, possibly unconsciousness
- Dilated pupils, slow to react
- Slow, shallow, irregular respirations

MAY LEAD TO PROGRESSIVE STAGE

IF APPROPRIATE EMERGENCY CARE IS NOT GIVEN

IRREVERSIBLE SHOCK AND DEATH

FIGURE 6–24. The stages of shock

Restlessness, anxiety, and a feeling of impending doom may precede any other signs.

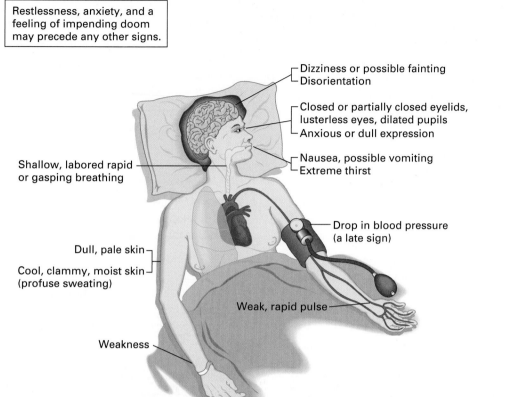

Dizziness or possible fainting
Disorientation

Closed or partially closed eyelids, lusterless eyes, dilated pupils
Anxious or dull expression

Nausea, possible vomiting
Extreme thirst

Shallow, labored rapid or gasping breathing

Drop in blood pressure (a late sign)

Dull, pale skin
Cool, clammy, moist skin (profuse sweating)

Weak, rapid pulse

Weakness

FIGURE 6–25. Signs and symptoms of shock

Skin around mouth may be grayish.

Tongue may be blue.

Lips may be blue.

Nail beds may be blue.

Mucous membranes of mouth may be blue or have a pale, grayish, waxy pallor.

FIGURE 6–26. Look for more subtle signs of shock in a dark-skinned person.

5. Splint any fractures; this can reduce shock by controlling bleeding and relieving pain.

6. Keep the victim warm by conserving body heat, but *do not overheat.*

7. Keep the victim quiet and still; shock is aggravated by rough and/or excessive handling.

8. Give the victim nothing by mouth because of the possible need for surgery, possible injury to the digestive system, and possible vomiting. If the victim complains of intense thirst, moisten his or her lips with a wet towel.

9. Monitor vital signs and mental status at 5-minute intervals until emergency personnel arrive.

Preventing Shock

Never wait for the signs or symptoms of shock to develop; it is much better to prevent shock. Any victim of injury or illness can develop shock; you can prevent shock by:

- Making sure the victim is breathing adequately; if necessary, provide rescue breathing
- Controlling any bleeding
- Loosening restrictive clothing
- Reassuring the victim and staying calm and in control yourself
- Splinting and immobilizing fractures
- Taking measures to relieve pain (properly dressing, bandaging, splinting, and positioning the victim)
- Positioning the victim supine with feet elevated no more than 8–12 inches, if the victim is alert or responding appropriately; if the victim is in an altered mental state, on his or her side
- Keeping the victim warm without overheating

Figures 6-27 through 6-33 illustrate body positioning and care for preventing shock.

FIGURE 6–27. Normally, the lower extremities should be elevated. Gravity will reduce the blood flow in the elevated extremities and may improve the blood supply to the heart. If the victim has leg fractures, the legs should not be elevated unless they are well splinted.

FIGURE 6-28. Maintain body heat.

FIGURE 6–29. If shock is due to a heart attack or heart failure and there are breathing difficulties, the victim may be more comfortable with the head and shoulders raised—that is, in a semisitting position.

FIGURE 6–30. If the victim is unconscious, he or she should be placed on his or her side in the recovery position.

FIGURE 6–31. If circumstances require it, the individual should be left in the position found.

FIGURES 6–32 and 6–33. Along with proper positioning to prevent shock, it is also important to assure adequate breathing, control bleeding, immobilize fractures, maintain body heat, and reassure the victim.

6.6 Anaphylactic Shock

Anaphylactic shock is a severe allergic reaction caused by misdirected immune response to an allergen—usually to insect stings, foods, medicines, or other allergens or antigens. Anaphylactic shock is a dire medical emergency (see Figure 6-34). (See the section on insect stings in Chapter 23.) An allergen or antigen is usually a protein that is viewed as a foreign substance by the body. As a rule, anaphylactic reactions occur more frequently and rapidly if the antigen is injected.

Anaphylactic shock is a severe allergic reaction of the body to sensitization by a foreign protein, such as insect sting; foods; medicine; ingested, inhaled, or injected substances. It can occur in minutes or even seconds following contact with the substance to which the victim is allergic. This is a grave medical emergency.

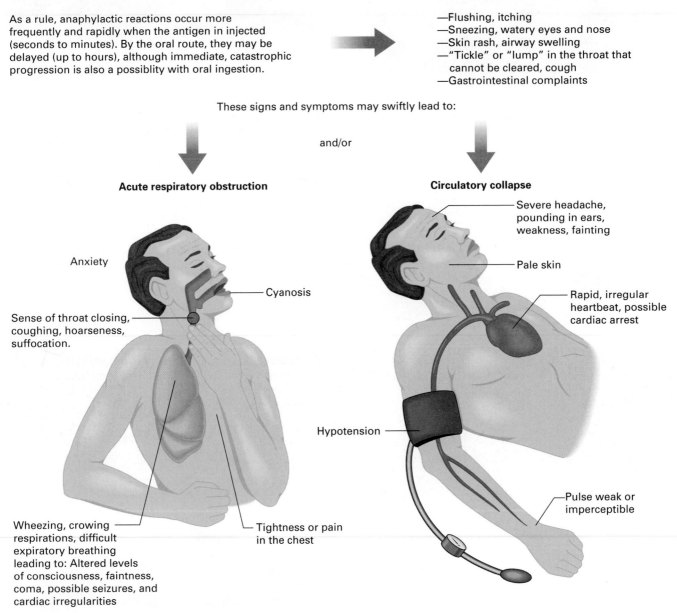

Rapidity of onset

As a rule, anaphylactic reactions occur more frequently and rapidly when the antigen in injected (seconds to minutes). By the oral route, they may be delayed (up to hours), although immediate, catastrophic progression is also a possiblity with oral ingestion.

Common early symptoms and signs

—Flushing, itching
—Sneezing, watery eyes and nose
—Skin rash, airway swelling
—"Tickle" or "lump" in the throat that cannot be cleared, cough
—Gastrointestinal complaints

These signs and symptoms may swiftly lead to:

and/or

Acute respiratory obstruction

Anxiety

Sense of throat closing, coughing, hoarseness, suffocation.

Cyanosis

Wheezing, crowing respirations, difficult expiratory breathing leading to: Altered levels of consciousness, faintness, coma, possible seizures, and cardiac irregularities

Tightness or pain in the chest

Circulatory collapse

Severe headache, pounding in ears, weakness, fainting

Pale skin

Rapid, irregular heartbeat, possible cardiac arrest

Hypotension

Pulse weak or imperceptible

FIGURE 6–34. Anaphylactic shock

Untreated, victims can die—often within a few minutes of contacting the allergen or antigen.

Of those who die from anaphylactic shock, more than two-thirds die because they cannot breathe (because of swollen air passages) and approximately one-fourth die from shock (because not enough blood is circulating through the body due to loss of fluid and an increase in the size of the blood vessels).

Signs and Symptoms

Learning Objective **12** Identify the signs and symptoms of anaphylactic shock.

The initial signs and symptoms of anaphylactic shock can occur in any combination, affecting the skin, heart and blood vessels, respiratory tract, gastrointestinal tract, and central nervous system.

Skin

- Itching and burning, with flushing
- Cyanosis around the lips
- Raised, hivelike patches with severe itching
- Swelling of the face, tongue, hands, feet
- Redness or flushed, pale or mottled face

Heart and Blood Vessels

- Weak, rapid pulse
- Low blood pressure
- Dizziness or lightheadedness

Respiratory Tract

- A painful, squeezing sensation in the chest
- Difficulty in breathing
- Coughing
- Wheezing

Gastrointestinal Tract

- Nausea
- Vomiting
- Abdominal cramps
- Diarrhea

Central Nervous System

- Restlessness
- Faintness
- Convulsions
- Altered mental status (occurs very early in anaphylactic shock)

These initial signs and symptoms progress rapidly to either acute airway obstruction, respiratory failure or circulatory collapse, then death.

Management of Anaphylactic Shock

Learning Objective **13** Describe the management of anaphylactic shock.

Activate the EMS system immediately; the victim will need rapid transport for life-saving treatment. While emergency personnel are en route, proceed as follows:

1. Secure an open airway.

2. If indicated, begin rescue breathing or CPR.

3. If the victim has an epinephrine autoinjector, help the victim use it *if allowed by local protocol.*

PROGRESS CHECK

1. As a rule, anaphylactic shock occurs most rapidly if the antigen is _____ . *(swallowed/inhaled/injected)*

2. Initial signs and symptoms may lead swiftly to _____ or circulatory collapse. *(loss of consciousness/respiratory failure/ irregular heartbeat)*

3. To manage anaphylactic shock, activate the EMS system, then immediately _____ . *(start CPR/secure an open airway/start rescue breathing)*

Summary

- The sudden loss of 3 pints of blood in an adult can be fatal.
- Severity of bleeding depends on how fast the blood is flowing, whether it is flowing from an artery or a vein, where the bleeding originated, and whether the blood is flowing freely externally or into a body cavity.
- Bleeding from an artery is more difficult to control than bleeding from a vein or capillary; arterial blood is bright red and spurts or pulsates out.
- You can control bleeding with direct pressure, elevation, pressure points and the use of splints.
- The use of a tourniquet to control bleeding should be a last resort only, when all other methods have failed or in a mass casualty incident.

- Internal bleeding can be a serious cause of shock, and usually requires surgical intervention.
- Shock occurs when the cells do not receive an adequate amount of oxygenated blood.
- Shock is a progressive condition that occurs in three stages; left untreated, it causes death.
- Shock in a child develops early and progresses extremely rapidly; never wait for signs and symptoms to occur before beginning treatment.

Key Terms

Make sure you understand the following key terms:

hemorrhage
hemophiliac
pressure point
shock
perfusion
compensatory shock
progressive (decompensatory) shock
irreversible shock

Critical Thinking Exercise

You are out working in the yard when you hear your neighbor screaming for help. She runs out onto the front porch with a dish towel soaked in blood wrapped around her right wrist. She tells you she was moving her glass-top coffee table when the glass cracked and sliced into her wrist. You remove the towel to inspect the injury and note bright red blood spurting from the wound.

1. Would you consider the bleeding to be severe?

2. How would you manage the bleeding?

3. If you fail to control the bleeding, what steps would you take next?

4. What signs and symptoms would heighten your suspicion that the patient is going into shock?

6 Chapter 6 Self-Test

Student: _____ Date: _____

Course: _____ Section #: _____

Part 1   True/False

If you believe the statement is true, circle the T. If you believe the statement is false, circle the F.

T **(F)** **1.** Indirect pressure is a good substitute for direct pressure.

(T) F **2.** Pressure on the arterial pulse points may help slow bleeding when direct pressure is inadequate.

T **(F)** **3.** Blood from a vein flows in spurts with each heartbeat.

T **(F)** **4.** Bleeding from capillaries rarely clots spontaneously.

(T) F **5.** A victim with internal bleeding can develop life-threatening shock before the bleeding is apparent.

(T) F **6.** A completely severed artery can sometimes constrict and seal itself off.

(T) F **7.** Internal bleeding usually results from blunt trauma or fractures.

(T) F **8.** Normally, the lower extremities should be elevated to treat for shock.

T **(F)** **9.** During shock, the oxygen supply is decreased because the heart needs less oxygen.

(T) F **10.** Losing fluid from the circulatory system is one of the primary causes of shock.

T **(F)** **11.** Give a shock victim fluids if he or she is conscious.

T **(F)** **12.** If a victim is unconscious, place her or him in a semisitting position.

Part 2   Multiple Choice

For each item, circle the correct answer or the phrase that best completes the statement.

1. Which of the following is the best method for controlling severe bleeding and should be applied first?
   a. elevation
   b. pressure point
   c. direct pressure
   d. tourniquet

2. List the four methods of controlling bleeding in order of preference: (1) elevation; (2) direct pressure at the wound; (3) indirect pressure (pressure points); (4) tourniquet.
   a. 2,1,3,4
   b. 2,3,1,4
   c. 1,2,3,4
   d. 3,2,1,4

3. Uncontrolled bleeding of the lower arm may be controlled by applying pressure to the
   a. femoral artery
   b. temporal artery
   c. radial artery
   d. brachial artery

4. When a dressing becomes saturated with blood, you should
   a. remove it and apply a new dressing
   b. apply a tourniquet
   c. leave the dressing in place and apply an additional dressing on top of it
   d. tie the knot on the bandage tighter

5. What condition may cause a person to bleed to death from a minor wound?
   a. anemia
   b. leukemia
   c. hypochondria
   d. hemophilia

6. Do *not* try to stop a nosebleed if you suspect
   a. a broken nose
   b. a fractured skull
   c. a fractured jaw
   d. high blood pressure

111

7. A victim with a nosebleed should
   a. lean forward and then pinch the nostrils to apply pressure *(circled)*
   b. blow the nose until the bleeding stops
   c. tilt the head back or lie flat while applying pressure to the bridge of the nose
   d. lean forward, pack the nostrils, and apply heat

8. Perfusion is
   a. the process of blood clotting
   b. the manufacture of red blood cells
   c. another word for transfusion
   d. delivery of blood to an organ *(circled)*

9. Which of the following characterizes arterial bleeding?
   a. dark red color and spurting flow
   b. bright red color and spurting flow *(underlined)*
   c. dark red color and steady flow
   d. bright red color and steady flow

10. What is a pressure point?
   a. a point where the blood pressure drops low enough to stop bleeding
   b. a place where an artery is protected on all sides by bone and muscle
   c. a place where an artery is close to the skin surface and over a bone *(circled)*
   d. a point where an artery is near the wound

11. Use a tourniquet only if
   a. there is severe hemorrhage
   b. bleeding cannot be controlled by direct pressure
   c. bleeding cannot be controlled by pressure at the appropriate pressure points

   d. all other methods of controlling life-threatening hemorrhage have failed *(circled)*

12. Anaphylactic shock should be considered
   a. a true medical emergency *(circled)*
   b. an emergency only in a sensitized person
   c. an emergency only if the person has been stung on the face or hand
   d. a nonemergency situation

13. Which of the following shock processes occurs first?
   a. the brain loses its ability to function
   b. vital organs and the brain do not receive enough blood *(circled)*
   c. blood rushes to the brain and vital organs, thus depriving other body cells of nutrients
   d. internal organs and brain cells begin to die

14. Which of the following is *not* a means of preventing shock?
   a. keep the victim's body temperature above normal *(circled)*
   b. reassure the victim
   c. loosen constrictive clothing
   d. control hemorrhage

15. Which of the following is *not* a type of shock?
   a. hypothermic *(underlined)*
   b. neurogenic
   c. septic
   d. cardiogenic

16. A person may be in anaphylactic shock from
   a. seeing a bloody accident
   b. eating berries *(marked)*
   c. injuring the head
   d. a severe illness

Part 3   Matching

1. Tourniquets should be used only for severe, life-threatening bleeding that cannot be controlled by any other means. Order the following procedures for proper application of a tourniquet:

_____5_____ Secure the stick in place.

_____3_____ Wrap the tourniquet around the limb twice and tie in a half-knot on the limb's upper surface.

_____7_____ Do not cover a tourniquet.

_____6_____ Twist the stick to tighten the tourniquet only until bleeding stops.

_____2_____ Place the tourniquet between the heart and the wound.

_____1_____ Activate the EMS system.

_____4_____ Place a short stick at the half-knot and tie a square knot.

_____8_____ Make a written note of the location and time the tourniquet was applied.

2. Match each type of shock with the correct cause:

Type		Definition
1. __B__	Septic	**A.** Spinal or head injury results in loss of nerve control and integrity of blood vessels.
2. __D__	Hemorrhagic	
3. __F__	Cardiogenic	**B.** Toxins cause pooling of blood in the extremities.
4. __A__	Neurogenic	
5. __C__	Anaphylactic	**C.** Allergic reaction of the body.
6. __E__	Psychogenic	**D.** Loss of blood.
		E. Something psychological affects the victim; blood drains from the head and pools in the abdomen.
		F. The heart does not pump efficiently.

Part 4 What Would You Do If?

1. You arrive at the scene of an auto/bicycle accident and find a teenager who has a large laceration on the lower leg and is bleeding profusely.

2. Your neighbor is stung by a bee and has flushed, itching skin, watery eyes, tightness in the chest, and feels as if his throat is closing.

7

Soft-Tissue Injuries

Learning Objectives

When you have mastered the material in this chapter, you will be able to

1 List the types of closed soft-tissue injuries

2 Describe the first aid care of a victim with a closed soft-tissue injury

3 List the types of open soft-tissue injuries

4 Discuss the threat of infection for a victim of human bites

5 Describe the first aid care of a victim with an open soft-tissue injury

6 Discuss first aid care considerations for a victim with a penetrating chest injury

7 Discuss first aid care considerations for a victim with an open wound to the abdomen

8 Describe the special concerns and cautions necessary in the first aid care of wounds containing impaled objects

9 Outline the special concerns and cautions necessary in the first aid care of clamping injuries

On the Scene

wenty-two-year-old Clay Millett slipped in the mud at a construction site where he was working. During the fall, a large Phillips screwdriver Clay was using plunged into his abdomen, just to the right side of his navel.

Kent Hansen, working nearby, ran to the aid of his co-worker, who was bent over, screaming. Kent rolled Clay over onto his back and helped him lie down; a surprisingly small amount of blood oozed into Clay's clothing around the impaled screwdriver.

Kent sent the supervisor to call for emergency help, elevated Clay's feet by propping them on a toolbox, and took off his own jacket, draping it over Clay's chest and shoulders to help him stay warm. Kent stabilized the impaled screwdriver by spreading out the fingers of one hand and holding his hand still against Clay's abdomen, preventing the screwdriver from moving. When EMTs arrived, they stabilized the screwdriver with dressings, then transported Clay to the hospital, where the screwdriver could be surgically removed and internal injuries repaired.

oft tissues are the layers of skin, fat, and muscles that protect underlying structures and organs. While a soft-tissue injury is often an obvious and dramatic one, it is seldom the most serious type of injury—unless it compromises the airway or causes massive hemorrhage. Because of these possibilities, it is important that you conduct a thorough secondary survey to rule out other, more serious injuries or life-threatening conditions before you take time to treat soft-tissue injuries.

An injury to the skin and underlying musculature is commonly referred to as a **wound**. More specifically, a wound is an injury, caused by trauma, that disrupts the normal continuity of the tissue, organ, or bone affected. Wounds may be generally classified as closed or open, single or multiple.

This chapter outlines the care of both closed and open wounds—including penetrating injuries—and details the treatment of victims wounded with impaled objects.

7.1 Closed Injuries

> Learning Objective 1 List the types of closed soft-tissue injuries.

In a closed injury, such as a bruise, soft tissues beneath the skin are damaged, but the skin is not broken.

Types of closed injuries include contusions (bruises), hematomas, and crush injuries.

Contusion

In a **contusion** (see Figure 7-1), the **epidermis** (outer layer of the skin) remains intact; in the **dermis** (underlying layer of skin), however, cells are damaged and blood vessels are torn.

Contusions are characterized by local pain and swelling. If small blood vessels beneath the skin have been broken, the area will gradually turn black and blue as blood and fluid leak into the damaged tissue.

Hematoma

If large vessels have been torn beneath a bruised area, a **hematoma**—a collection of blood beneath the skin—develops. Hematomas are characterized by a lump with bluish discoloration. Blood from a deep bruise can actually separate tissue and pool in a pocket. The victim can lose 1 or more liters of blood from a large hematoma.

FIGURE 7–1. Contusions are injuries that cause bleeding beneath the skin but do not break the skin.

Crush Injuries

The force of a sudden blow or blunt trauma can cause a crush injury. With a crush injury, underlying layers of skin sustain severe damage; the internal layers of skin can actually rupture. A crush injury is especially treacherous because the resulting internal injuries can cause few, if any, external signs. Although the injury site may be painful, swollen, or deformed, there is usually little or no external bleeding.

The victim of a crush injury can look fine at first, but his or her condition may quickly deteriorate, resulting in deep shock and/or death. For this reason, always suspect hidden internal damage in victims with crush injuries.

First Aid Care

> Learning Objective 2 Describe the first aid care of a victim with a closed soft-tissue injury.

Small bruises generally require no treatment. Larger bruises and crush injuries, however, can cause serious internal injury and blood loss. Treat them as follows:

1. If you suspect internal bleeding or the victim shows the signs and symptoms of shock, treat for shock as outlined in Chapter 6.

> **wound** An injury to the skin and underlying musculature that disrupts the normal continuity of the affected tissue, organ, or bone
>
> **contusion** A bruise
>
> **epidermis** The outermost layer of the skin
>
> **dermis** The second layer of skin, which contains the hair follicles, sweat glands, oil glands, and nerves
>
> **hematoma** A collection of blood beneath the skin

2. Apply ice or cold compresses to help relieve pain and reduce swelling. Never apply ice directly to the skin, and do not apply ice for more than 20 minutes at a time.

3. Splint painful, swollen, or deformed extremities to help control pain and swelling and prevent further injury. If large bruised areas are present, assess carefully for fracture, especially if any swelling or deformity is present (see Chapter 11).

PROGRESS CHECK

1. A contusion is a _____ . *(closed fracture/bruise/laceration)*

2. A hematoma is _____ under the skin. *(blood/swelling/ecchymosis)*

3. Crushing injuries don't break the skin but can cause internal injury severe enough to cause _____ . *(hemorrhage/fracture/shock)*

4. Apply _____ to reduce the pain and swelling associated with closed injuries. *(cold compresses/manual pressure/splints)*

7.2 Open Injuries

Learning Objective **3** List the types of open soft-tissue injuries.

In an open wound, the skin is broken and the victim is susceptible to external bleeding and wound contamination. Remember: The wound itself may be only part of the victim's injury—an open wound may be only the surface evidence of a more serious injury, such as a fracture. Figure 7-2 illustrates the classifications of open wounds.

Abrasion

An **abrasion** is a superficial wound caused by rubbing, scraping, or shearing (see Figure 7-3). Part of the skin layer—usually the epidermis and part of the dermis—is

---

abrasion A superficial wound caused by rubbing, scraping, or shearing

---

CLASSIFICATION OF OPEN WOUNDS

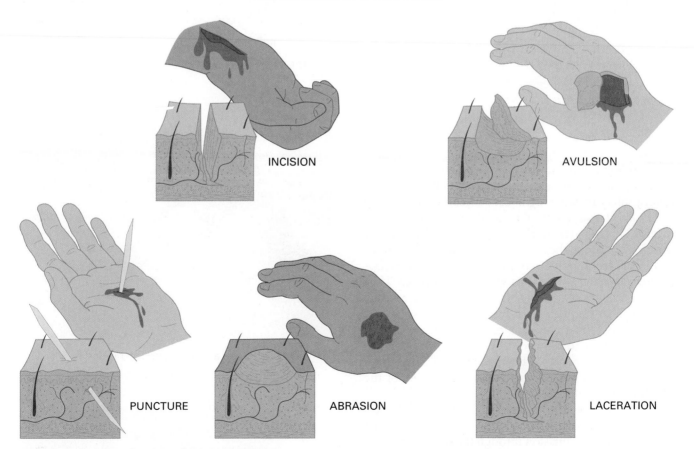

INCISION

AVULSION

PUNCTURE

ABRASION

LACERATION

FIGURE 7–2. Classification of open wounds

FIGURE 7–3. An abrasion is an open wound caused by rubbing and scraping off layers of skin.

FIGURE 7–4. Incisions and lacerations

FIGURE 7–5. Laceration of the forehead and scalp

FIGURE 7–6. Deep abrasions and lacerations

lost. All abrasions, regardless of size, are extremely painful because of the nerve endings involved.

Blood may ooze from the abrasion, but bleeding is usually not severe. Abrasions can pose a threat if large areas of skin are involved (as can happen in a motorcycle accident when the rider is thrown against the road). The most serious threat from abrasions is that of contamination and infection.

Laceration

A **laceration** is a break in the skin of varying depth. Lacerations can be either linear (regular) or irregular, and can occur either in isolation or together with other types of soft-tissue injury (see Figures 7-4 through 7-6). Lacerations can cause significant bleeding if the sharp object also cuts the wall of a blood vessel, especially an artery. This is particularly true in areas where major arteries lie close to the skin surface, such as in the wrist.

Linear lacerations, also known as *incisions*, are characterized by sharp, even cuts with smooth edges. They are caused by a sharp, cutting object, such as a knife, razor blade, or broken glass. Linear lacerations tend to bleed freely. The greatest dangers with linear lacerations are severe (often profuse) bleeding and damage to tendons and nerves. They usually heal better than irregular lacerations, though, because the edges of the wound are smooth and straight.

A stellate (irregular) laceration is a tear caused by a sharp, uneven instrument (such as a broken bottle) that produces a ragged incision through the skin surface and underlying tissues.

> **laceration** A break in the skin; lacerations can have either smooth or rough edges and can be of varying depth.

Avulsion

An **avulsion** is the tearing loose of a flap of skin, which may either remain hanging or be torn off altogether; scarring is often extensive. Avulsions usually bleed profusely; in some cases, however, blood vessels might seal themselves and retreat into surrounding tissue, limiting the amount of blood loss.

If the avulsed tissue is still attached by a flap of skin and is folded back, circulation to the flap can be severely compromised. The seriousness of an avulsion depends on how disrupted circulation is to the flap.

The most commonly avulsed skin on the body is that on the fingers and toes, hands, forearms, legs, feet, ears, nose, and penis (see Figures 7-7 and 7-8). Avulsions commonly occur in automobile accidents and industrial settings.

Penetrating and Puncture Wounds

A puncture wound is caused by the penetration of a sharp object (such as a nail) through the skin and underlying structures. The opening in the skin may appear very small, resulting in little external bleeding, but the puncture wound may be extremely deep—causing severe internal bleeding and posing a serious threat of infection (see Figure 7-9).

Internal organs may also be damaged by punctures. In some cases, the object that causes the injury remains embedded in the wound.

Gunshot wounds may cause both entrance and exit wounds. The entrance wound is usually much smaller than the exit wound, which is generally two to three times larger and tends to bleed heavily. Many victims have multiple gunshot wounds; you should look carefully for additional wounds, especially in regions where they may be disguised, such as those covered by hair or bulky clothing.

Knife and stab wounds are dangerous—often fatal. Because knife wounds are easy to see, First Aiders too frequently concentrate only on the superficial skin wound and fail to consider the damage to underlying organs. Remember—the superficial skin wound is almost never fatal. The fatalities all relate to the injured organs that lie beneath the skin wound.

Amputations

The ripping, tearing force of industrial and automobile accidents can be great enough to tear away limbs from the body; amputations can also involve other body parts (see Figures 7-10 through 7-12).

Because blood vessels are elastic, they tend to spasm and retract into surrounding tissue in cases of complete amputation; therefore, complete amputations may cause relatively limited bleeding. In partial or degloving amputations, however, lacerated arteries continue to bleed profusely, and blood loss can be massive.

> **avulsion** The tearing loose of a flap of skin, which may either remain hanging or be torn off altogether

FIGURE 7–7. Forearm avulsion

FIGURE 7–8. Avulsion of the finger

FIGURE 7–9. Puncture wound of the foot

FIGURE 7–10. Finger amputation

FIGURE 7–11. Finger amputation

FIGURE 7–12. Toe amputation

FIGURE 7–13. Dog bites

FIGURE 7–14. Dog bite

FIGURE 7–15. Horse bite

New techniques in microreconstructive surgery make it possible to save many amputated limbs or digits, so care of the amputated part has become almost as crucial as care of the victim. See pages 124–125 in this chapter for more information on care of amputated parts.

Bites

Learning Objective **4** Discuss the threat of infection for a victim of human bites.

More than two million domestic animal bites and more than two thousand snakebites occur in the United States each year. The number of human bites is not recorded, but would likely be significant if known.

Nine out of ten animal bites are inflicted by dogs; complications can include infection, cellulitis, and tetanus. The worst dog bites are those that leave puncture wounds and those that occur in areas with few blood vessels (see Figures 7-13 through 7-15).

A bite wound is actually a combination of a penetrating injury and a crush injury. A bite wound can involve soft tissues, internal organs, and bones, and may include rupturing of tissues or organs. The power of a dog's jaws can cause a severe crush injury; a large breed can bite with the estimated force of 400 pounds per square inch. Figure 7-16 details first aid care for dog bites.

The most difficult bite to manage is a human bite because of the high infection rate associated with it. The human mouth harbors millions of bacteria in a greater variety than found in the mouths of animals, and massive contamination may result from a bite.

First Aid Care

Learning Objective **5** Describe the first aid care of a victim with an open soft-tissue injury.

Always take measures to avoid contact with body substances when caring for a victim of a soft-tissue injury, because there is a high chance of contact with the victim's blood, body fluids, mucous membranes, traumatic wounds, or sores. Use protective gloves. If

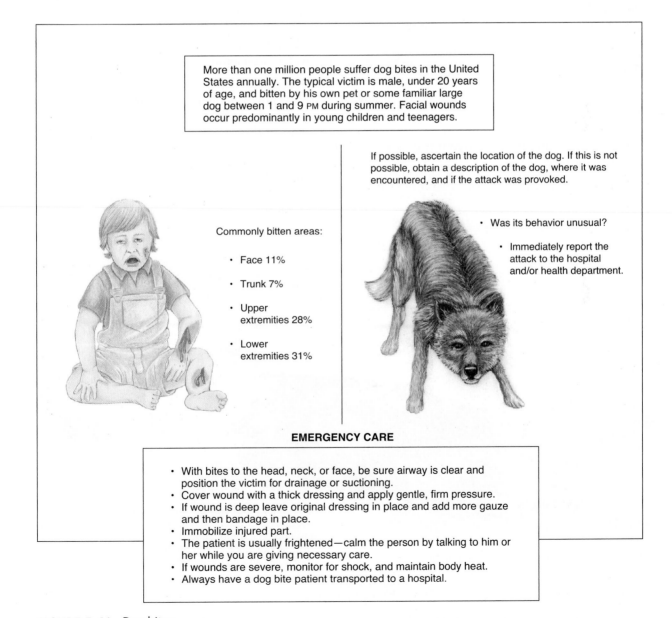

More than one million people suffer dog bites in the United States annually. The typical victim is male, under 20 years of age, and bitten by his own pet or some familiar large dog between 1 and 9 PM during summer. Facial wounds occur predominantly in young children and teenagers.

If possible, ascertain the location of the dog. If this is not possible, obtain a description of the dog, where it was encountered, and if the attack was provoked.

Commonly bitten areas:

- Face 11%
- Trunk 7%
- Upper extremities 28%
- Lower extremities 31%

- Was its behavior unusual?
- Immediately report the attack to the hospital and/or health department.

EMERGENCY CARE

- With bites to the head, neck, or face, be sure airway is clear and position the victim for drainage or suctioning.
- Cover wound with a thick dressing and apply gentle, firm pressure.
- If wound is deep leave original dressing in place and add more gauze and then bandage in place.
- Immobilize injured part.
- The patient is usually frightened—calm the person by talking to him or her while you are giving necessary care.
- If wounds are severe, monitor for shock, and maintain body heat.
- Always have a dog bite patient transported to a hospital.

FIGURE 7–16. Dog bites

there is a chance of spraying or spattering blood, protect your face and clothes. After caring for the victim, dispose of the gloves and wash your hands thoroughly with soap and hot water.

Before you begin to treat the injury itself, maintain an airway and provide artificial ventilation if necessary. Treat soft-tissue injuries as follows (see Figure 7-17):

1. Expose the wound so you can see it clearly; if necessary, cut the victim's clothing from around the wound.

2. Control bleeding with direct pressure, using your gloved hand and a dry, sterile compression bandage, if possible. (See Chapter 6 for guidelines on controlling bleeding.)

3. Prevent further contamination by keeping the wound as clean as possible. Avoid touching the wound with anything that is not clean. Leave the cleaning of the wound to medical personnel.

4. Apply a dry, sterile dressing to the wound and bandage it securely in place. (See Chapter 10.)

In general, you should activate the EMS system if any of the following are true:

- The wound has spurted blood, even if you have controlled the bleeding.
- The wound is deeper than the outer layer of skin.
- There is uncontrolled bleeding.

- There is embedded debris, an embedded object, or extensive contamination.
- The wound involves nerves, muscles, or tendons.
- The wound involves the mouth, tongue, face, genitals, or any area where a scar would be disfiguring.
- The wound is a human or animal bite.

Cleaning Wounds and Preventing Infection

In *most* cases, you should not try to clean a wound yourself. Let an EMT or personnel at the emergency room take care of cleaning wounds, especially those that are large, have embedded debris, are extremely dirty, may require stitches, or are life-threatening.

For a *shallow* wound

- Wash the area around the wound with soap and water (see Figure 7-18).
- Irrigate the wound with clean tap water; the water must flow at moderate pressure and be clean enough to drink. *Never scrub the wound—you can damage the wounded tissues.*
- Gently pat the wound dry with sterile gauze and apply antibiotic ointment (such as Neosporin).
- Cover the wound with a sterile, nonstick dressing, and bandage in place.

Control Bleeding

Prevent further contamination: all open wounds will already be contaminated, but a dressing and bandage will prevent further contamination.

Do not remove an impaled object: it may be cut if necessary to move the victim but should remain in place until the victim receives hospital care. The object should be stabilized with bulky dressings.

Immobilize the part and keep the victim quiet.

Do not try to replace protruding organs: that is, protruding eyeballs or protruding intestines should be covered as they are and no attempt should be made to replace them in their normal positions within the body cavity. The covering for intestines should be kept moist.

Preserve avulsed parts: torn off parts should be saved, and flaps of skin may be folded back to their normal position before bandaging.

FIGURE 7–17. First aid care for open wounds

FIGURE 7–18. Clean the area around a shallow wound using separate small strokes and by wiping away from the edges.

Never apply hydrogen peroxide, isopropyl alcohol, Merthiolate, Mercurochrome, or iodine to a wound—these can injure the tissues and delay healing.

Do not close a wound with adhesive tape, Steri-strips, or butterfly strips—these increase the risk of infection.

Removing Slivers

Left embedded in the skin, slivers almost always cause infection, so it is important to remove them. If a sliver is deeply embedded and you cannot see one end of it, take the victim to a physician for removal of the sliver.

If you can see the end of the sliver, use tweezers to remove it. Grasp the sliver firmly and pull at the same angle at which the sliver penetrated the skin. Pull slowly and firmly, and make sure you remove all of the sliver. If you pull too quickly or at the wrong angle, you may break off the sliver and leave part of it behind.

If you can see the end of the sliver but can't grasp it with tweezers, use a sterilized needle to gently bring it to the surface; then remove it with tweezers, as described above.

Once you have removed the sliver, clean the area with soap and water, apply antibiotic ointment, and apply an adhesive strip to discourage infection.

Removing a Fishhook

You can safely remove a fishhook if the point *but not the barb* has penetrated the skin. To remove the hook, apply ice to the skin temporarily to numb it, then back the fishhook out. Wash the wound with soap and water, apply antibiotic ointment, and apply an adhesive strip.

If the barb has penetrated the skin, gently tape the fishhook to the skin so it won't move—movement causes pain and increases injury—and wait for a physician to remove the hook.

PROGRESS CHECK

1. The greatest threat from an abrasion is _____ . *(infection/pain/blood loss)*

2. Linear lacerations heal better than stellate lacerations because _____ . *(there is less blood loss/the edges are smooth/infection is less likely)*

3. The most dangerous dog bites are those in areas with few _____ . *(nerve endings/blood vessels/underlying tissues)*

4. The greatest danger with an avulsion is compromised _____ in the flap. *(sensation/circulation/pain reception)*

5. The most serious bites are _____ bites. *(snake/dog/human)*

6. Blood loss from an amputation may actually be slight, because the elastic blood vessels may _____ . *(be crushed/retract into surrounding tissue/shut down)*

7.3 Special Treatment Considerations

The preceding first aid guidelines apply to most soft-tissue injuries, but you must be aware of special considerations in the case of chest or abdominal injuries, impaled objects, amputations, and clamping injuries.

Chest Injuries

Learning Objective **6** Discuss first aid care considerations for a victim with a penetrating chest injury.

In the case of penetrating chest injuries, activate the EMS system, then put an **occlusive** (airtight) dressing over the open wound and tape it on three sides.

occlusive Waterproof and airtight

You can use household plastic wrap or another occlusive object (one that air will not pass through). One corner should be left untaped enough to flutter as the victim breathes.

For more information on the first aid care of chest injuries, see Chapter 9.

Abdominal Injuries

> Learning Objective 7 Discuss first aid care considerations for a victim with an open wound to the abdomen.

If organs protrude through an open abdominal wound, activate the EMS system; then:

1. Do not touch abdominal organs or try to replace them in the abdomen.

2. Cover protruding abdominal organs with a clean, moist, sterile dressing. Use sterile gauze compresses if available, and moisten them with clear water. *Never use absorbent cotton or any material that clings or shreds when wet, such as paper towels or toilet tissue.*

3. Cover the moist dressing with an occlusive material, such as plastic wrap, to retain moisture and warmth.

4. Gently wrap the dressing in place with a bandage or clean sheet (see Chapter 9).

Impaled Objects

> Learning Objective 8 Describe the special concerns and cautions necessary in the first aid care of wounds containing impaled objects.

Never remove an impaled object unless it penetrates the cheek or interferes with chest compressions. To treat:

1. Remove the victim's clothing if necessary to expose the wound; cut it away without disturbing the impaled object.

2. Manually secure the impaled object to prevent any motion. Moving the impaled object even slightly can increase bleeding and cause damage to underlying tissues, such as muscles, nerves, blood vessels, bones, and organs.

3. Control bleeding with direct pressure, but do not exert any pressure on the impaled object or on the edges of the skin around the cutting edge of the object.

4. Stabilize the impaled object with bulky dressings and bandage in place. The impaled object itself must be completely surrounded by bulky dressings—the objective in packing dressings around the object and

taping them securely in place is to reduce motion to a minimum.

5. Calm and reassure the victim as you monitor for shock.

6. Keep the victim at rest.

7. Do not attempt to cut off, break off, or shorten an impaled object unless transportation is not possible with it in place. If the object must be cut off, stabilize it securely before cutting. Remember—any motion of the impaled object is transmitted to the victim and can cause additional tissue damage and shock. This step should be done by EMS personnel if possible.

8. Activate the EMS system immediately.

An object impaled in the cheek should be removed in the field when you are more than 1 hour away from medical help (*follow local protocol*); profuse bleeding into the mouth and throat can impair breathing.

To remove an object impaled in the cheek

1. Feel inside the victim's mouth to determine whether the object has penetrated completely.

2. Remove the object by pulling it back out the way it entered.

3. Control bleeding on the cheek and dress the wound.

4. If the object penetrated completely, pack the inside of the cheek (between the cheek wall and the teeth) with sterile gauze to control bleeding.

5. Activate the EMS system.

If you encounter too much resistance in trying to remove the object from the cheek, maintain the airway and activate the EMS system immediately. Stabilize the penetrating object while waiting for emergency personnel.

Amputations

A concern in the first aid care of amputations is the appropriate treatment of the amputated part: The way you handle an amputated part can help determine whether it can be reattached later by a surgeon.

Generally, you should not waste time searching for amputated parts or neglect victim care while you look for amputated parts. If you can find the amputated parts quickly or if someone you assign can find them, proceed as follows:

1. If possible, rinse the amputated part with clean water, but *do not scrub*. Wrap the part in a dry sterile gauze dressing secured in place with a self-adherent roller bandage.

2. Place the wrapped part in a plastic bag, in accordance with local protocol.

3. Place the wrapped and bagged part in a cooler or any other available container so that it is on top of a cold pack or a sealed bag of ice (do not use dry ice). The part should be kept as cool as possible, without freezing. Do not cover the part with ice or immerse it in any kind of liquid.

4. When EMTs arrive, give them the amputated part so it can be transported with the victim.

An important consideration in amputation is to preserve as much as possible of the original length of the limb. Even if a limb has been severely mangled and will eventually require amputation, the flap of skin holding the limb together may be used by the surgeon to cover the end of the stump, preserving a significant amount of limb length. In addition, the strands of soft tissue connecting the limb might contain nerves or blood vessels that, with proper surgical management, might allow the limb to survive.

Clamping Injuries

> Learning Objective **9** Outline the special concerns and cautions necessary in the first aid care of clamping injuries.

Most clamping injuries involve the hand—more specifically a finger, which can be strangled when it is stuck into a hole and cannot be pulled out. The longer the tissue remains in the clamping object, the harder it will be to remove, because swelling becomes more severe by the minute.

To treat a clamping injury:

1. Remove the clamping object as quickly as possible. If you cannot remove the clamping object, apply a lubricant, such as green soap, and slowly but firmly wiggle the body part until it is loose.

2. If possible, elevate the affected extremity while you remove the clamping object.

3. If you are unable to loosen the body part or remove the clamping object, activate the EMS system.

PROGRESS CHECK

1. To treat a chest injury, cover the wound with an occlusive dressing and tape it on _____ sides. *(two/three/all)*

2. Cover protruding abdominal contents with a dressing, then _____ material. *(occlusive/porous/adherent)*

3. The goal in treating a wound with an impaled object is to prevent _____ as much as possible. *(bleeding/pain/motion)*

4. If you find an amputated part, wrap it in gauze, then keep it _____ . *(moist and cool/dry and cool/dry and room temperature)*

5. In cases of a clamping injury, activate the EMS system if _____ . *(the wound bleeds/ you cannot remove the clamping object/there is severe pain)*

Summary

- Closed wounds are those in which the tissue beneath the skin is damaged, but the skin is not broken; examples are bruises and hematomas.

- Open wounds are those in which the skin is broken; examples are abrasions, incisions, lacerations, punctures, avulsions, bites, and amputations.

- The most serious threat from an abrasion is infection; blood loss is usually minimal.

- Lacerations with smooth edges heal better than those with ragged edges.

- The biggest threat from an avulsion is lack of circulation to the flap; make sure the flap is not bent back.

- If you can find an amputated part, your proper care of it can dramatically improve the odds of the surgeon's successfully reattaching it.

- Even if a limb is severely mangled, you should never complete an amputation; nerves and blood vessels in even small strands of tissue may enable the surgeon to reattach the limb completely.

Key Terms

Make sure you understand the following key terms:

wound	abrasion
contusion	laceration
epidermis	avulsion
dermis	occlusive
hematoma	

Critical Thinking Exercise

You are doing an internship at a local manufacturing company. As you walk down a hallway near one of the shops, you hear a commotion. A man working a band saw has cut off a finger and left a second finger dangling by a thread.

1. Would you expect severe bleeding from the stump where the finger was cut off? Why or why not?

2. The second finger has been cut through the bone and is only attached by tissue. Should you complete the amputation? Why or why not?

3. The finger was found by a coworker. How would you direct her to handle the amputated finger?

7 Chapter 7 Self-Test

Student: _____   Date: _____

Course: _____   Section #: _____

Part 1   True/False

If you believe the statement is true, circle the T. If you believe the statement is false, circle the F.

T F   **1.** Always thoroughly clean a wound before dressing and bandaging it.

T F   **2.** Avulsed parts or flaps of skin should not be folded back into place; this causes more contamination.

T F   **3.** Nine out of ten animal bites are inflicted by dogs.

T F   **4.** Do not attempt to remove objects embedded in a wound.

T F   **5.** Proper handling of a severed body part may allow it to be reattached successfully.

T F   **6.** Always break or cut off an impaled object before the victim is transported.

T F   **7.** Objects impaled in the neck should be removed.

T F   **8.** Objects impaled in the cheek should rarely be removed.

T F   **9.** Be patient with clamping injuries of the finger—the longer a finger is stuck, the easier it will be to remove.

Part 2   Multiple Choice

For each item, circle the correct answer or the phrase that best completes the statement.

1. What type of wound has as its greatest danger severe bleeding and cut tendons and nerves?

 a. an incision
 b. a laceration
 c. a contusion
 d. a puncture

2. An open wound characterized by jagged skin edges and free bleeding is

 a. a laceration
 b. an incision
 c. a contusion
 d. a puncture

3. What type of wound has the greatest danger of infection?

 a. an incision
 b. a laceration
 c. a contusion
 d. a puncture

4. When a puncture wound is caused by an impaled object

 a. remove the object and cover the wound with a sterile dressing
 b. stabilize the object with a bulky dressing
 c. apply slight pressure on the object to control bleeding
 d. always shorten the object so it will be easier to move the victim

5. A serious injury in which large flaps of skin and tissues are torn loose or pulled off is called an

 a. abrasion
 b. amputation
 c. avulsion
 d. incision

6. Proper handling of a severed part includes

 a. cleaning it with an antiseptic solution
 b. wrapping it in gauze or a clean towel
 c. freezing the part as quickly as possible
 d. applying a tourniquet to the severed part to preserve fluids

7. Most clamping injuries involve

 a. the hands
 b. the feet
 c. the arms
 d. the legs

8. Gunshot wounds generally

 a. have no exit wounds
 b. have a smaller exit wound than entrance wound
 c. have identical-sized entrance and exit wounds
 d. have a larger exit wound than entrance wound

1. A patron at a local gas station is stabbed in the chest with a large screwdriver. When you arrive, the victim is unconscious and the screwdriver is still in place.

2. You hear a gunshot in your apartment building. On investigation, you find a middle-aged man with a gunshot wound to the upper thigh of his right leg. His wife tells you he was cleaning the gun when it accidentally discharged.

8

Injuries to the Face, Eye, and Throat

On the Scene

Thirteen-year-old Melissa Gentry was jumping on the trampoline with three friends when she slammed into her friend's knee, knocking out her front tooth. Hearing Melissa's cries, Carrie Scofield looked out the kitchen window as Melissa's tooth bounced across the surface of the trampoline and Melissa clapped her hands across her mouth. Carrie called out through the window, telling the girls not to touch the tooth, and poured a cup of cold milk before running out to the backyard.

Carrie picked up the tooth by the crown, carefully avoiding touching the root, and dropped the tooth into the cup of cold milk. She handed the cup to her daughter. Katy, and instructed her to hold it.

Carrie led Melissa into the house, asked Melissa to rinse out her mouth gently with cool water, then asked her to bite down on a rolled piece of gauze to help control the bleeding. She quickly called Melissa's mother, who took Melissa and the tooth—still soaking in the cold milk—to the dentist. The tooth was successfully implanted within the hour.

The specialized structures of the face, prone to injury because of their location, can be permanently and irreversibly damaged. Injuries to the face are quite common: Approximately 75 percent of all victims involved in motor vehicle accidents sustain at least minor facial trauma.

While some injuries to the face are minor, many face and throat injuries are life threatening because they compromise the upper airway, impairing the victim's ability to breathe. In addition, many injuries of the face and throat stem from impacts strong enough to cause spinal damage or skull fracture. Because the neck also contains major blood vessels, injuries to the neck or throat can cause severe, life-threatening bleeding.

In addition to facial injuries, more than 1.5 million eye injuries occur each year in the United States; proper assessment and treatment can be instrumental in saving the victim's eyesight.

This chapter outlines the proper assessment and first aid care of victims with eye injuries as well as injuries to the face, jaw, and throat.

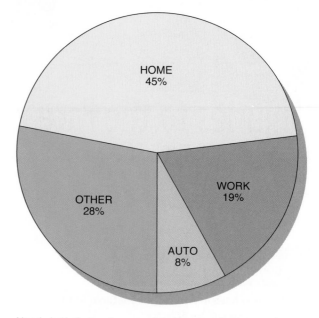

Nearly half of all serious eye injuries occur in or around the home. Most could be prevented by wearing safety glasses while doing chores.

FIGURE 8–1. Eye injuries

8.1 Injuries to the Eye

> Learning Objective 1 Describe how to assess eye injuries.

Few true eye (**ocular**) emergencies occur, but when they do, they tend to be urgent. The eyes are easily damaged by injury; eye injuries account for approximately 10 percent of all injuries. An injury to the eye can involve the bone and soft tissues surrounding the eye, but can also injure the eyeball itself; in some cases, the eyeball may be penetrated.

Injury to the eye probably causes greater anxiety to the victim than any other type of injury. Because of the potential for permanent damage, never assume that an eye injury is minor; all eye injuries should receive medical attention immediately.

Nearly half of all serious eye injuries occur in or around the home (see Figure 8-1).

Assessment

Ask the victim when the accident or pain occurred, what the victim first noticed, and how the eyes were affected. Then examine the eyes separately and together with a small penlight to evaluate the following:

- See if the eye sockets (**orbits**) show signs of bruising (ecchymosis), swelling, laceration, or tenderness.
- Check the lids for bruising, swelling, and laceration.
- Look for redness, pus, and foreign bodies in the linings of the eyelids (**conjunctivae**).

- Determine whether the eyeballs (**globes**) are red, abnormally colored, or lacerated.
- Check the pupils for size, shape, equality, and reaction to light; they should be black, round, equal in size, and they should react to light (get smaller when light is shined on them).
- Check eye movements in all directions for abnormal gaze, paralysis of gaze, or pain on movement.

Suspect significant damage if the victim has loss of vision that does not improve when he or she blinks, loses part of the field of vision, has severe pain in the eye, has double vision, or is unusually sensitive to light.

If the victim is unconscious, gently close the eyes and cover them with moist dressings. An unconscious person loses normal reflexes such as blinking that help protect the eyes.

Basic First Aid Care for Eye Injuries

> Learning Objective 2 Describe general first aid care procedures for eye injuries.

ocular Having to do with the eye

orbit The bony socket that holds the eyeball

conjunctivae The transparent mucous membrane lining the eyelids and covering the outer surface of the eyeball

globe The eyeball

In general, care for soft tissue injuries around the eye as you would any other soft tissue injury; however, *never put direct pressure on the eyeball, even if you do not think it is injured.* Regardless of the eye injury, these basic rules apply:

- Do not irrigate an injured eye except in the case of a chemical burn or if there is a foreign object in the eye.

- Do not put salves or medicine in an injured eye.

- Do not remove blood or blood clots from the eye.

- Do not try to force the eyelid open unless you have to wash out chemicals or a foreign object.

- Have the victim lie down and keep quiet.

- Limit use of the uninjured eye; it is usually best to patch it along with the injured eye.

- Give the victim nothing by mouth in case general anesthesia is required at the hospital.

- Every victim with an eye injury must be evaluated by a physician.

Foreign Objects in the Eye

Foreign objects—such as particles of dirt, sand, cinders, coal dust, or fine pieces of metal—can be blown or driven into the eye and lodged there (see Figure 8-2). If they are not removed, they can cause significant damage, including inflammation, infection, and scratches of the cornea. You should always consider foreign objects in the eye to be hazardous, especially if they contain iron or copper.

The pain caused by foreign objects in the eye is usually severe, and the eye generally produces tears immediately in an attempt to flush out the irritants. The victim may not be able to open the eye, especially since light causes further irritation.

Never let a victim with foreign objects in the eye rub the eye. If tears do not flush out the foreign objects, ask the victim to blink several times; this will often remove loose objects. You should try to remove only those objects in the transparent mucous membrane lining the eyelids and covering the outer surface of the eyeball; never try to remove an object from the cornea.

FIRST AID CARE

> Learning Objective **3** Describe first aid care for foreign objects in the eye.

If blinking does not remove the object:

1. Flush the eye gently with clean water, holding the eyelids apart with your fingers (see Figure 8-3).

2. Remove an object lodged under the upper eyelid by drawing the upper lid down over the lower lid; as the upper lid returns to its normal position, the undersurfaces will be drawn over the lashes of the lower lid, removing the foreign object.

3. If the foreign object remains in the eye, grasp the eyelashes of the upper lid and turn the lid up over a cotton swab or similar object. Carefully remove the foreign object from the eyelid with the corner of a piece of sterile gauze (see Figure 8-4, page 132).

4. If the foreign object is lodged under the lower lid, pull down the lower lid, exposing the lid's inner surface, and remove the foreign object with the corner of a piece of sterile gauze or cotton swab.

5. If the object becomes lodged in the eyeball, do not disturb it; place a bandage compress over both eyes and activate the EMS system (see Figure 8-5, page 132).

Injuries to the Eye Sockets

Injury to the face may result in the fracture of one or several of the bones of the skull that form the eye sockets (orbits) (see Figure 8-6, page 132). Whenever an eye

FIGURE 8-2. Foreign object lodged in the eye

FIGURE 8-3. Flushing foreign objects from the eye

FIGURE 8–4. To remove particles from the white of the eye, pull down the lower eyelid while the victim looks up or pull up the upper lid as the victim looks down.

FIGURE 8–5. If a foreign object becomes lodged in an eye, bandage both eyes to minimize motion.

FIGURE 8–6. Eye socket injury

socket has been fractured, assume there is also head injury. Signs and symptoms of fracture to the eye sockets include:

- Double vision
- Markedly decreased vision
- Loss of feeling above the eyebrow, over the cheek, or in the upper lip due to nerve damage
- Nasal discharge, which may be profuse
- Paralysis of upward gaze (the victim's eyes will not be able to follow your finger upward)

Injury to the face commonly causes a black eye ("shiner"), in which the delicate blood vessels around the eye rupture and result in bruising. Blows to the eye range in severity, depending on the force and the angle. The actual bleeding associated with a black eye is usually insignificant, but remember that a black eye may hide a more serious injury, such as a fracture to the eye socket or damage to the eyeball. Generally, a victim of a black eye should seek medical attention to rule out associated injury.

Any victim of any eye injury should seek medical attention if there is bruising (a black eye), pain, or impaired/reduced vision.

FIRST AID CARE

> Learning Objective **4** Describe first aid care for injury to the eye sockets.

Fractures of the eye sockets require hospitalization and possible surgery. Activate the EMS system; then:

1. If the eyeball has *not* been injured, place ice packs over the injured eye for 15 minutes to reduce swelling. Keep the victim in a sitting position until emergency personnel arrive, and *do not exert pressure on the eyeball.*

2. If you suspect injury to the eyeball, avoid using ice packs. Keep the victim in a supine position until emergency personnel arrive.

Injuries to the Eyelids

Lid injuries include black eyes (ecchymosis), burns, and lacerations (see Figure 8-7). Because the eyelid is richly supplied with blood vessels, lacerations to the lid can cause profuse bleeding.

Anything that cuts the lid can also cause damage to the eyeball, so assess the injury carefully.

FIRST AID CARE

> Learning Objective **5** Describe first aid care for eyelid injuries.

In general, first aid care consists of controlling bleeding and protecting the injured tissue and underlying

FIGURE 8–7. Eyelid injury

structures. *Never try to remove anything that is embedded in the eyeball.* Activate the EMS system; then:

1. Control eyelid bleeding with light pressure from a light dressing; use no pressure at all if the eyeball itself is injured.

2. Cover the lid with moistened sterile gauze to keep the wound from drying. If the eyelid skin is torn off the eyelid, preserve it so it can be transported with the victim for later grafting.

3. If the eyeball is not injured, cover the injured lid with cold compresses to reduce swelling.

4. Cover the uninjured eye with a bandage to decrease movement of the injured eye.

Injuries to the Eyeball

Injuries to the eyeball include bruising, cuts, damage caused by foreign objects, and abrasions. Deep lacerations can cut the cornea, causing the contents of the eyeball to spill out; severe blunt trauma or projectile injury can rupture the eyeball.

Some injuries to the eyeball—such as lacerations or embedded objects—are immediately apparent. Other signs and symptoms of injury to the globe include

- A pear-shaped or irregularly shaped eyeball
- Blood in the front chamber of the eye

FIRST AID CARE

> Learning Objective **6** Describe first aid care for injuries to the eyeball.

Injuries to the eyeball are best treated in the emergency room, where specialized equipment is available. Activate the EMS system; then take these steps:

1. Apply light patches to both eyes. Do not use a patch or any kind of pressure if you suspect a ruptured eyeball, because pressure can force eye contents out.

2. Keep the victim lying on his or her back until emergency personnel arrive.

Chemical Burns of the Eye

Chemical burns of the eye (see Figure 8-8) represent a dire emergency: Permanent damage to the eye can occur within seconds of the injury, and the first 10 minutes following injury often determine the final outcome.

Alkalies—such as ammonia, drain cleaner, cement, and plaster—cause more damage to the eye than acids because they continue to burn and penetrate more deeply. Common acids include battery acid, hydrochloric acid, and nitric acid. Regardless of the substance, though,

FIGURE 8–8. Chemical burn of the eye

FIGURE 8–9. Chemical burns of the eye should be irrigated continuously for 30 to 60 minutes.

burning and tissue damage will continue as long as any substance is left in the eye, even if that substance is diluted.

The signs and symptoms of chemical burns include

- Irritated, swollen eyelids
- Redness or red streaks across the surface of the eye
- Blurred or diminished vision
- Excruciating pain in the eyes
- Irritated, burned skin around the eyes

FIRST AID CARE

> Learning Objective 7 Describe first aid care for chemical burns of the eye.

Activate the EMS system, then follow these steps:

1. Holding the eyelids open, continuously and gently irrigate the eye with running water for at least 30 to 60 minutes, beginning as soon as you encounter the victim (see Figures 8-9 and 8-10). *Do not try to neutralize the chemical*; use only water. Eye wash systems (Figure 8-10) are sometimes available at work sites. When possible, use warm water. Never use any chemical antidote, including diluted vinegar, baking soda (sodium bicarbonate), or alcohol. Never use eye drops.

2. Pour the water from the inside corner of the eye across the eyeball to the outside edge; take care not to contaminate the uninjured eye. Ask the victim to roll the eyeball, which helps wash out the eye.

3. Remove or flush out contact lenses; left in, they will trap chemicals between the contact lens and the cornea. (See "Removing Contact Lenses" later in this chapter.)

4. Remove any solid particles from the surface of the eye with a moistened cotton swab.

FIGURE 8–10. If possible, irrigate chemical burns of the eye in an eye wash system.

5. Continue irrigation until emergency personnel arrive.

6. If the arrival of emergency personnel is delayed and you have rinsed the eye with running water for at least 60 seconds, loosely bandage both eyes with cold, wet dressings until emergency help arrives.

Following irrigation, avoid contaminating your own eyes by washing your hands thoroughly and using a nail brush to clean under your fingernails.

Light Burns of the Eye

Looking at a source of ultraviolet light can burn the eyes, resulting in severe pain between 1 and 6 hours after exposure. One of the most common sources of light burns to the eyes is sunlight reflected off snow; other causes include tanning lamps and arc welders.

A victim of light burns to the eye should be seen by an ophthalmologist, who can determine how extensive the burns are and prescribe necessary treatment or medication. In the meantime:

1. Move the victim *out of the sunlight.* If possible, the victim should be in a dark room, away from sources of light.

2. Cover both eyes with gauze pads that have been moistened with cold water.

3. Discourage the victim from rubbing his or her eyes; rubbing will further inflame injured tissues.

Impaled Objects in the Eye and Extruded Eyeball

A sharp object that penetrates the eyeball may come back out, or it may become impaled or embedded in the eyeball. Objects impaled or embedded should be removed only by a physician. First aid care consists of stabilizing the object to prevent accidental movement or removal until the victim receives medical attention (see Figures 8-11 through 8-14).

During a serious injury, the eyeball may be forced out of the socket, or **extruded** (see Figure 8-15 on page 136). Never attempt to replace the eye in the socket.

FIRST AID CARE

> Learning Objective **8** Describe first aid care for a victim with an object impaled in the eye.

> Learning Objective **9** Describe first aid care for an eyeball that is forced out of the socket.

Activate the EMS system; then follow these steps:

1. With the victim lying on his or her back, stabilize the head with sandbags or large pads.

FIGURE 8–12. Place padding around the object.

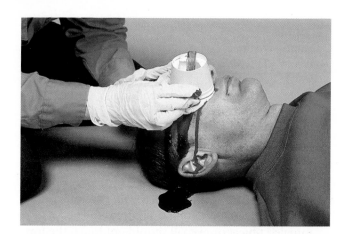

FIGURE 8–13. Stabilize the impaled object with a cup or other object.

FIGURE 8–14. Bandage the cup in place.

FIGURE 8–11. Object impaled in the eye

> **extruded** Forced out of position; an extruded eyeball has been forced out of the socket.

FIGURE 8–15. Eyeball forced out of the socket

2. Gently cover an eyeball that has been forced out of the socket with a clean, moist dressing—such as sterile gauze that has been moistened with clean water—to help keep the eyeball moist. Or, encircle the eye and the impaled object with a gauze dressing or other suitable material, such as soft, sterile cloth. Never apply pressure. Cut a hole in a single bulky dressing to accommodate an impaled object.

3. Place a metal shield, paper cup, or cone over the impaled object or extruded eyeball. Do not use a styrofoam cup, because it can crumble. The impaled object or eyeball should not touch the top or sides of the cup.

4. Hold the cup and dressing in place with a self-adhering bandage compress or roller bandage that covers both eyes; do not wrap the bandage over the cup, because pressure from the bandage can push the cup down onto the impaled object or extruded eyeball. If the victim is unconscious, close the uninjured eye before bandaging to prevent drying of tissues.

5. Cover the uninjured eye to prevent movement of the injured eye.

6. Treat for shock: give the victim nothing by mouth.

Removing Contact Lenses

> Learning Objective **10** Describe how to remove contact lenses.

An estimated 18 million Americans wear contact lenses of some type, some in only one eye; some, especially the elderly, wear both contact lenses and eyeglasses. Therefore, don't dismiss the possibility of contact lenses just because the victim is wearing eyeglasses.

To detect lenses, shine a penlight or flashlight into the eye: A soft lens will show up as a shadow on the outer portion of the eye; a hard lens will show up as a shadow over the iris.

When determining whether to remove contact lenses, follow local protocol. Generally, you should remove contact lenses if there is a chemical burn to the eye or if transport will be delayed; generally, you should not remove contact lenses if the eyeball has any injury other than a chemical burn.

After you remove contact lenses, store them in clean containers marked L and R (for the left and right contact). If possible, store the contact lenses in saline or water.

Removing Hard Contact Lenses

About the size of a shirt button, a hard lens fits over the cornea. To remove a hard lens (see Figure 8-16)

1. Separate the eyelids; manipulate them to position the lens over the cornea.

2. Place your thumbs gently on the top and bottom eyelids, and gently press the eyelids down and forward to the edges of the lens.

FIGURE 8–16. Removing a hard corneal contact lens

3. Press the lower eyelid slightly harder, and move it under the bottom edge of the lens.

4. Moving the eyelids toward each other, slide the lens out between them.

Removing Soft Contact Lenses

A soft lens is slightly larger than a dime and covers all of the cornea and some of the white of the eye (the **sclera**). To remove a soft lens (see Figure 8-17)

1. With your middle fingertip on the lower lid, pull the lid down. With the other hand, pull the upper lid up.

2. Place your index fingertip on the lower edge of the lens, then slide the lens down to the white of the eye.

3. Compress the lens gently between your thumb and index finger, allowing air to get underneath it, and remove it from the eye.

If the lens has dehydrated on the eye, run sterile saline across the eye surface, slide the lens off the cornea, and pinch the lens up to remove it.

FIGURE 8–17. Removing a soft (flexible) contact lens

8.2 Injuries to the Face

Learning Objective **11** Describe general first aid care for injuries to the face.

In victims with trauma to the face, mouth, and jaw, you should suspect spinal injuries of the neck and back. Victims of significant facial trauma may also have fractures of the jaw and damage to or loss of teeth (see Figures 8-18 through 8-22, page 138).

To give first aid to a person with a facial injury

1. Establish an airway. Inspect the mouth for small fragments of teeth or broken dentures, bits of bone, pieces of flesh, or fragments of foreign objects on which the victim might choke. Remove them as thoroughly as possible. Pull the tongue forward to open the airway. If you have trouble grasping the tongue, open the throat by pulling the chin forward or grasping the angle of the jaw and pressing it forward.

2. Completely immobilize the neck to prevent aggravation of possible spinal neck injuries (cervical spine injuries).

3. Control bleeding—several major arteries run through the face, and they can bleed profusely and rapidly enough to cause death. Apply extremely gentle pressure if you suspect that bones under the wound may be fractured or shattered.

sclera The white of the eye

FIGURE 8–18. Injury to the face

FIGURE 8–20. Injury to the mouth

FIGURE 8–19. Injury to the face

FIGURE 8–21. Injury to the chin and jaw

FIGURE 8–22. Injury to the chin

4. If nerves, tendons, or blood vessels have been exposed, cover them with a moist, sterile dressing.

5. Make sure you inspect both the outside *and* the inside of the cheek; if the face is injured, the teeth may cut the tissue inside the cheek. To control bleeding inside the cheek, place a rolled gauze bandage between the teeth and the cheek, securing it to the outside of the victim's mouth with a piece of tape so the bandage doesn't get swallowed. To control bleeding on the cheek, cover with a gauze bandage and apply direct pressure; remember not to use force if the teeth or bones beneath the cheek are broken.

Learning Objective **12** Describe first aid care for injuries to the mouth and jaw.

Examine the mouth for broken or missing teeth. If a tooth has been lost, try to find it; a surgeon can reimplant a tooth within 2 hours and can use bone fragments to reconstruct the jaw. For treatment procedures, see Section 8.3 on pages 143 to 145.

If dentures are in and unbroken, leave them in place—they can help support the structures of the mouth. If dentures are broken, remove them.

Fractures of the Face and Jaw

Fractures of the face and jaw (maxillofacial fractures) may be simple, such as undisplaced nasal fractures, or extensive, involving severe lacerations, bony fractures, and nerve damage (see Figure 8-23 on page 140). Spinal injury, tearing or rupture of an eyeball, and facial burns often accompany facial fracture.

SIGNS AND SYMPTOMS

The signs and symptoms of facial fracture include

- Distortion of facial features
- Numbness or pain
- Severe bruising and swelling
- Bleeding from the nose and mouth
- Limited jaw motion
- Teeth not meeting normally
- Double vision, when bone around the eye is fractured
- Irregularities in the facial bones that can be felt before swelling occurs
- Distance between the eyes appears too wide

The signs and symptoms of upper jaw (**maxilla**) fracture include

- Movement of the upper jaw
- Nosebleed
- Black eyes
- Numbness of the upper lip or cheek
- Eyes that appear unlevel

The signs and symptoms of lower jaw (**mandible**) fracture (see Figure 8-24 on page 141) include

- The mouth is usually open (some victims may be unable to open the mouth)
- Saliva mixed with blood flowing from the corners of the mouth

- Drooling (pain prevents the victim from swallowing)
- Painful and difficult speech
- Missing, loosened, or uneven teeth (even if teeth are not missing, the victim will complain that teeth do not "fit together right")
- Pain around the ears

FIRST AID CARE

Learning Objective **13** Describe first aid care for fractures of the face and lower jaw.

The first priority in caring for a victim of face or jaw fracture is establishing and maintaining the airway, which can be compromised by blood, swelling, or structural defects. Activate the EMS system; then follow these steps:

1. Clear the airway; remove any debris from the mouth.

2. Immobilize the neck if you suspect spinal injuries, then position the victim to allow for drainage.

3. Control bleeding; place bandages carefully to allow for vomiting and drainage of blood.

4. If you suspect lower jaw fracture, carefully immobilize the lower jaw with a cervical collar or cravats. Monitor for vomiting.

5. If you suspect a fracture of the nose, control nosebleed as described in Chapter 6. Apply an ice pack to the nose for as long as 20 minutes to reduce swelling and relieve pain. *Never try to straighten the nose.*

OBJECTS IMPALED IN THE CHEEK

The only time you should try to remove an impaled object is when it is impaled in the cheek, has penetrated all the way through the cheek, and is loose—threatening to obstruct the airway. To remove, activate the EMS system; then follow these steps:

1. Pull or push the object out of the cheek in the same direction in which it entered the cheek. Never pull the object through to the inside of the mouth.

2. Pack dressing material between the victim's teeth and the wound; leave some of the dressing outside the mouth and tape it there to prevent the victim from swallowing the dressing (see Figure 8-25 on page 141).

3. Dress and bandage the outside of the wound to control bleeding.

maxilla The upper jaw
mandible The lower jaw

COMMON FRACTURES OF THE FACE AND JAW

Facial fractures often result from impact injuries to the face. The main danger of facial fractures is airway problems. Bone fragments and blood may obstruct the airway. Common signs of a fractured jaw may include irregularity of bite, loss of teeth, bleeding in the mouth, deformity and/or loose bone segments, increased salivation, and the inability to swallow or talk.

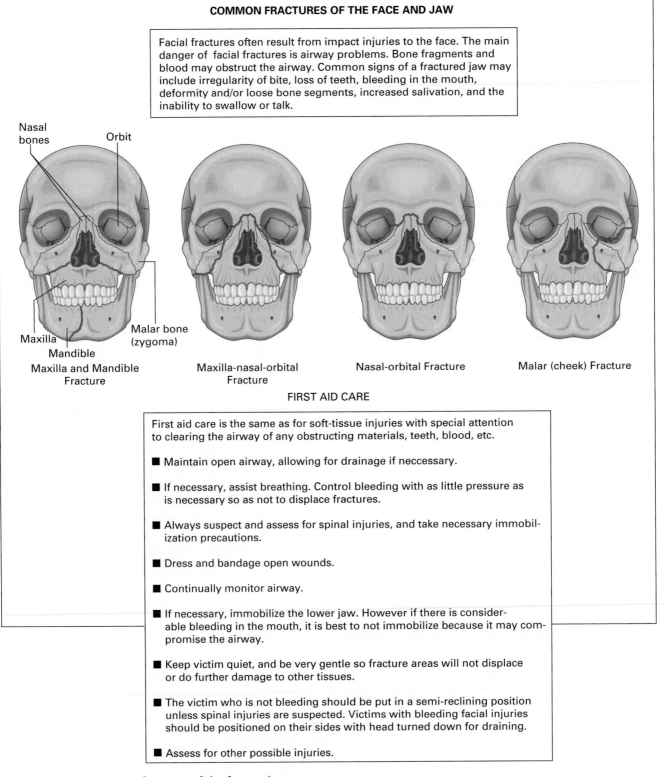

Nasal bones
Orbit
Maxilla
Mandible
Malar bone (zygoma)

Maxilla and Mandible Fracture

Maxilla-nasal-orbital Fracture

Nasal-orbital Fracture

Malar (cheek) Fracture

FIRST AID CARE

First aid care is the same as for soft-tissue injuries with special attention to clearing the airway of any obstructing materials, teeth, blood, etc.

■ Maintain open airway, allowing for drainage if neccessary.

■ If necessary, assist breathing. Control bleeding with as little pressure as is necessary so as not to displace fractures.

■ Always suspect and assess for spinal injuries, and take necessary immobilization precautions.

■ Dress and bandage open wounds.

■ Continually monitor airway.

■ If necessary, immobilize the lower jaw. However if there is considerable bleeding in the mouth, it is best to not immobilize because it may compromise the airway.

■ Keep victim quiet, and be very gentle so fracture areas will not displace or do further damage to other tissues.

■ The victim who is not bleeding should be put in a semi-reclining position unless spinal injuries are suspected. Victims with bleeding facial injuries should be positioned on their sides with head turned down for draining.

■ Assess for other possible injuries.

FIGURE 8–23. Common fractures of the face and jaw

FIGURE 8–24. Soft-tissue injuries and fracture of the lower jaw

FIGURE 8–25. Impaled objects in the cheek may be removed. Dress outside of wound and put dressing on inside of wound between cheek and teeth. Hold dressing in place if necessary.

FIGURE 8–26. Nose injury

FIGURE 8–27. Nose injury

INJURIES OF THE NOSE

Learning Objective 14 Describe first aid care for injuries of the nose.

Injuries to the nose are generally caused by blunt trauma, such as a blow to the nose by a fist. Care for soft-tissue injuries of the nose (see Figures 8-26 and 8-27) as you would other soft-tissue injuries. Take special care to maintain an open airway, and position the victim so that blood does not drain into the throat. Blood that drains into the throat can interfere with breathing and can cause the victim to vomit. Generally, the best position is to have the victim sit, leaning slightly forward.

If the nose is bleeding, pinch the nostrils together; if bleeding is not controlled, place an ice pack on the bridge of the nose or apply pressure on the upper lip just below the nose. For guidelines on nosebleed, see Chapter 6.

Generally, a victim of nosebleed doesn't require medical attention if no other injury is present and if the bleeding stops. An exception is when the nosebleed is *posterior*, meaning that it occurs in the back of the throat. Bleeding from posterior nosebleeds is usually extremely heavy.

Foreign objects in the nose usually occur among small children. If part of the object is protruding and you can easily grasp it, pull it out. Do not probe into the nostril to try to remove an object; you could push it farther in, blocking breathing and making removal more difficult. Try to make the victim sneeze by tickling the opposite nostril; sneezing may dislodge the object. You can also ask the victim to blow the nose gently while you compress the opposite nostril. If the object is not dislodged, reassure and calm the child and parent, then activate the EMS system. Special lighting and instruments available at the hospital minimize the risk of removal.

Nasal fractures are the most common type of facial fracture because of the delicate structure of the nose; the most common signs and symptoms are swelling and deformity. To treat, apply ice compresses to reduce swelling, then activate the EMS system. *Never try to straighten a crooked nose.*

Injuries of the Ear

Learning Objective 15 Describe first aid care for injuries of the ear.

Cuts and lacerations of the ear are common (see Figures 8-28 and 8-29), but are rarely life threatening. Pierced earrings commonly catch and tear, causing injury. Occasionally, a section of the ear may be severed. Treat as you would other soft tissue injuries; exert direct pressure to control bleeding. Save any parts that are torn off; wrap them in moistened gauze and save for transport with the victim.

When dressing an injured ear, place part of the dressing between the ear and the side of the head. As a general rule, don't probe into the ear.

Never pack the ear to stop bleeding from the ear canal. Clear or bloody fluid draining from the ear can indicate skull fracture. Place a loose, clean dressing across the opening of the ear to absorb blood, but do not exert pressure to stop the bleeding.

Foreign objects in the external ear are a common problem among children; most common are small, hard objects such as beans and peanuts. If you can see the object and it is at the opening of the ear canal, gently remove the object with tweezers. Otherwise, do not stick anything in the ear to try to remove the object; instead, the victim should be taken to the hospital, where good lighting and appropriate equipment are available. *Never irrigate the ear in an attempt to dislodge a foreign object;* liquid will cause many objects (such as beans) to swell, making removal more difficult.

If the victim has an insect in the ear, never insert anything sharp into the ear canal in an attempt to kill the insect. Most insects are attracted to light: gently pull down on the earlobe to straighten the ear canal and shine a flashlight into the ear to lure the insect out. If the eardrum is intact and the ear canal is not injured, you can also drown the insect by placing a few drops of vegetable oil or light mineral oil into the ear canal; never use motor oil. Once the insect stops moving, carefully and gently irrigate the opening of the ear canal with warm water to remove the insect. If that is unsuccessful and you are certain there is no injury to the ear canal or eardrum, you can use a bulb syringe to gently suction out the insect's body.

The inner ear may also be injured by blunt force, a blow to the head, rapid changes in pressure, or explosions. A direct blow to the head may also rupture the eardrum. The victim might lose hearing in the affected ear or might have problems keeping balance. Do not try to care for internal ear injuries; victims need professional care.

Injuries of the Throat

The throat can be injured by any crushing blow; common causes include hanging (accidental or intentional), impact with a steering wheel, or running or riding into a stretched wire or clothesline (see Figure 8-30 and 8-31). If the throat is cut, bleeding from a major artery or vein can occur, and air bubbles may enter the blood vessels.

SIGNS AND SYMPTOMS

Besides obvious lacerations, swelling, or bruising, signs and symptoms of an injured throat include (see Figure 8-32 on page 144):

FIGURE 8–28. Injury to the ear

FIGURE 8–29. Injury to the ear

FIGURE 8–30. Injury to the throat

FIGURE 8–31. Injury to the throat

- Displacement of the trachea to one side
- Difficulty speaking
- Grating sounds during speaking or breathing as air escapes from an injured voice box
- Loss of the voice
- Airway obstruction that is not obviously due to other sources (such obstruction is caused by swelling of the throat)

FIRST AID CARE

> Learning Objective 16 Describe first aid care for injuries of the throat.

Maintaining an airway is extremely important in throat injuries, because blood clots when it is exposed to air and clots can threaten the airway. Activate the EMS system; then follow these steps:

1. Open the airway; if necessary, give rescue breathing.

2. Keep the victim lying down to lessen the chance of air entering the blood vessels. Position the victim on the left side with the body tilted downward at a 15-degree angle.

3. Control bleeding with slight to moderate pressure and bulky dressings. If you think the blood is coming from a vein, apply pressure above and below the site to prevent air from entering the bloodstream. Monitor pressure carefully—too much pressure will block the flow of blood to the brain. Never apply pressure to both sides of the neck at the same time.

4. Treat for shock.

PROGRESS CHECK

1. The priority in treating injuries to the face is to _____ . *(maintain the airway/prevent shock/control bleeding)*

2. _____ often accompanies trauma to the mouth and jaw. *(Severe bleeding/Spinal injury/Severe pain)*

8.3 Dental Emergencies

> Learning Objective 17 Describe first aid care for common dental injuries.

Dental emergencies are rarely life threatening but can be extremely painful and can cause the victim considerable anxiety. Rapid first aid care dramatically improves the outcome and can make it possible for a dentist to make permanent repairs. A victim with any kind of dental emergency should be referred to a dentist or oral surgeon for treatment as quickly as possible; many injuries can be repaired only within a relatively narrow window of time.

If you don't suspect a head, neck, or back injury, place the victim in a sitting position, leaning slightly forward. This position allows blood to drain and helps maintain an open airway. If the victim cannot sit, position the victim on the side so that blood can drain from the mouth.

If an injury to the mouth involves the tongue, apply a dressing to the tongue and use direct pressure to control bleeding. If the lip is penetrated, place a piece of rolled-up gauze between the lip and the gum, and a second gauze dressing on the outer lip; use direct pressure to control bleeding. If you are not able to control bleeding quickly, seek immediate medical attention, because the airway can be compromised by uncontrolled bleeding in the mouth.

Toothache

Most commonly, a toothache is caused by tooth decay. Though pain may be limited to the affected tooth, it may also radiate to other teeth, the opposite side of the jaw, or even to the eye, ear, or neck. In most cases, a decayed tooth will be sensitive to heat, cold, and sometimes sweets. Any person with a toothache should receive attention from a dentist immediately.

Until a victim can be seen by a dentist, identify the affected tooth by tapping the teeth gently, one at a time, with a spoon handle. To help relieve pain:

1. Ask the victim to rinse the mouth with warm water; the water should not be too hot or too cold.

2. Using dental floss, remove any seeds or particles of food that might be caught between the teeth (pressure can cause pain).

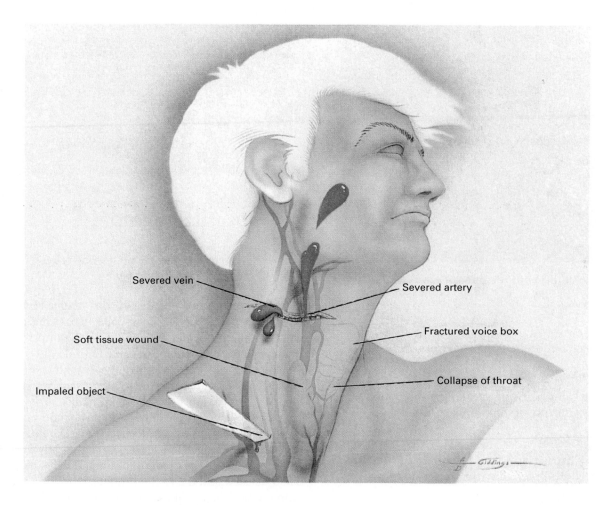

Severed vein

Severed artery

Soft tissue wound

Fractured voice box

Impaled object

Collapse of throat

BLUNT OR CRUSHING INJURY

- Loss of voice.
- Severe airway obstruction even though the mouth and nose are clean and no foreign body is present.
- Deformity, bruises, or depressions in the neck.
- Swelling in the neck and sometimes face and chest. When the swollen areas are touched there are crackling sensations under the skin due to air leakage in the soft tissues.
- If one of the above signs is present, it is an extreme emergency, and the victim needs to be transported to a medical facility immediately.
- Calm and reassure the victim, encouraging him to breathe slowly.
- Administer artificial ventilation as needed.
- Be alert for possible injuries to the spine of the neck, and take appropriate immobilization measures.
- Activate the EMS system immediately.

OPEN INJURIES

- Serious open wounds of the neck can cause profuse bleeding.
- If an artery has been severed and there is bright red spurting blood, apply direct pressure with a sterile (if possible) bulky dressing. If blood soaks through the dressing, do not remove it — just add another dressing on the first one. Maintain firm pressure with your hand until you arrive at the hospital. CAUTION: Pressure dressing around the neck can compromise the airway.
- Do not apply pressure over the airway or on both sides of the neck at the same time.
- If necessary, apply pressure to the carotid pressure point. Do not apply pressure on both carotid arteries at the same time. If there is an impaled object, stabilize in place with bulky dressings. Do not remove.
- Keep victim lying on his or her back with legs elevated, and activate the EMS system immediately.
- If a large vein (profuse, steady flow of dark red to maroon-colored blood) is severed, attempt to control bleeding using direct pressure with a bulky dressing. If bleeding is controlled, cover with an occlusive dressing.
- If bleeding is not immediately controlled, apply pressure above and below the point of bleeding. It is imperative that air not be allowed to be sucked into the vein (air embolism) and be carried into the circulatory system. This can be rapidly fatal. This is more likely to occur if the victim is sitting or standing.
- Cover wound with an airtight dressing or plastic wrap, and tape all edges snugly to form an airtight seal over the severed vein.
- Position the victim on his side.
- Activate the EMS system. Administer artifical ventilation as needed.
- Monitor airway.

FIGURE 8–32. Common neck and throat injuries

3. Use a cotton swab soaked with oil of cloves on the tooth to help relieve the pain; avoid touching the gums, lips, or other surfaces of the mouth.

4. Give the victim an over-the-counter pain reliever, such as aspirin, acetaminophen, or ibuprofen.

Loose Tooth

Any injury to the face can carry enough impact to loosen one or more teeth. To check for a loose tooth, grasp the tooth gently with your fingers and apply slight pressure on both sides of the tooth. The slightest movement indicates that the tooth has been loosened from its socket. To prevent further injury, have the victim bite down firmly, but not too hard, on a piece of gauze. The pressure should be enough to keep the tooth in the socket, but not enough to further loosen it. *Never pull out a loose tooth.*

Broken Tooth

The most common teeth to be broken are the top front teeth; in addition to being broken when the victim suffers head or facial injury, they are often broken in falls, fights, motor vehicle accidents, and sporting events. A broken tooth can be extremely painful, because the nerve may be exposed; immediate dental care is essential. Until the victim can be treated by a dentist:

1. Use a clean cloth and water to gently clean blood, dirt, and other debris away from the broken teeth; if there are still tooth fragments in the mouth, remove them to prevent choking.

2. If the jaw is not fractured, have the victim gently rinse the mouth with warm water to thoroughly clean it. If you suspect that the jaw is fractured, stabilize the jaw by wrapping a bandage under the chin and over the top of the head; do not have the victim rinse the mouth with water.

3. Apply an ice pack or cold compress to the victim's face over the broken teeth to relieve pain and reduce swelling.

Knocked-Out Tooth

An estimated 2 million people have teeth knocked out every year in the United States; as many as 90 percent of those teeth could be saved with proper first aid and *rapid* treatment by a dentist. The ligament fibers necessary for successful reimplantation begin to die soon after the injury, so time is of the essence; a tooth can usually be successfully reimplanted if it is inserted back into the socket within 30 minutes. The odds of a successful implantation decrease 1 percent for every minute that the tooth remains out of the socket. Keeping the tooth moist until it is placed in the socket dramatically increases the odds of success.

A top priority in the case of a knocked-out tooth is finding the tooth and handling it properly. *Never touch the root of the tooth*; handle it only by the crown so you don't damage the ligament fibers necessary for reimplantation. Do not rinse the tooth unless you are reinserting it into the socket. To treat the victim and the tooth properly:

1. Have the victim rinse his or her mouth gently with warm water to wash out blood, dirt, and debris.

2. Place a rolled sterile gauze pad against the socket and have the victim bite firmly on it to help control bleeding.

3. Handling the tooth gently and by the crown only, immerse it in the solution found in the commercial Save-a-Tooth™ kit. Called Hank's Solution, it is a balanced-pH cell-culture medium that helps restore the ligament fibers on the tooth. While it is most effective in the 6 to 12 hours after the injury occurs, it has been approved by the FDA for use as long as 24 hours after the injury. These kits are available over the counter in drugstores.

4. If you don't have access to a commercial kit, immerse the tooth in either saliva or cold milk (which contains a concentration of calcium and magnesium) in a closed container. Ideally, whole milk is best. Never use reconstituted powdered milk or milk byproducts, such as yogurt or cottage cheese; these contain substances that will damage the ligaments. *Do not place the tooth in alcohol or mouthwash*; in an emergency, you can use water. Make sure the container will not dry or crush the outside of the tooth.

Saliva is the perfect solution for protecting a tooth, but it is not a good idea to ask an injured person to hold the tooth in his or her mouth—an injured person may become anxious, confused, or upset and may swallow the tooth. If there is nothing else available, ask a family member to hold the tooth *gently* in his or her mouth while the victim is being taken to a dentist or oral surgeon.

PROGRESS CHECK

1. A knocked-out tooth can almost always be reimplanted if the procedure is done within _____ . *(30 minutes/1 hour/24 hours)*

2. To protect a knocked-out tooth, always handle it by _____ . *(the root/the crown)*

3. To increase the odds of successful reimplantation, keep a knocked-out tooth _____ . *(wet/dry/cold/warm)*

4. To transport a knocked-out tooth, immerse it in _____ . *(water/mouthwash/milk)*

Summary

- Use a small penlight or other light to examine the eyes; examine them both separately and together.

- Never try to remove a foreign object that is lodged in the eye.

- All victims of eye injury must be evaluated by a physician.

- Bleeding from the eyelids can be profuse; never apply pressure to the eyelid if you think the eyeball itself might be injured.

- In chemical burns of the eye, irrigate the affected eye for at least 30 minutes or until emergency personnel arrive.

- Remove contact lenses if there has been a chemical burn to the eye or if transport will be lengthy or delayed.

- The amount of force necessary to injure the face will usually also cause spinal injury.

- The top priority in treating victims with injury or fracture of the face or jaw is maintaining the airway.

- Rapid first aid care of a dental injury dramatically improves long-term outcome.

Key Terms

Make sure you understand the following key terms:

ocular	extruded
orbit	sclera
conjunctiva	maxilla
globe	mandible

Critical Thinking Exercise

You are peacefully riding your bicycle down a neighborhood road. Suddenly that peace is shattered by screams of pain and cries for help. You immediately come to a stop and quickly scan the home the screaming is coming from. An open garage door reveals an older man bending forward and covering his eyes with his hands. He is still yelling for help.

1. What immediate action would you first take?

2. What clues to the situation would you quickly look for as you enter the garage?

3. What assessment should be conducted?

4. What first aid would you render?

8 Chapter 8 Self-Test

Student:_____ Date: _____

Course: _____ Section #:_____

If you believe the statement is true, circle the T. If you believe the statement is false, circle the F.

T   F   **1.** Both eyes should be bandaged if a foreign object is lodged in just one eye.

T   F   **2.** It is always best to try gently to remove an object lodged in the eyeball.

T   F   **3.** A chemical burn of the eye should be irrigated for approximately 5 minutes.

T   F   **4.** Never force the eyelids open in an attempt to irrigate a chemical burn.

T   F   **5.** Never use cold compresses on injuries to the globe.

T   F   **6.** If the eyelids do not cover the eyeball in a lid injury, use a light, moist dressing to prevent drying.

T   F   **7.** Do not try to remove contact lenses, especially in a chemical burn.

T   F   **8.** Do not remove blood or blood clots from the eye.

T   F   **9.** A victim of trauma to the mouth and face should have the head and neck immobilized.

T   F   **10.** If you find a missing tooth, scrub it thoroughly and pack it in ice.

T   F   **11.** Never apply ice or cold packs to a suspected nasal fracture.

T   F   **12.** A knocked-out tooth should be immersed in cold water.

Part 2   Multiple Choice

For each item, circle the correct answer or the phrase that best completes the statement.

1. The first priority in treating a chemical burn to the eye is to
   a. irrigate the eye with clean water
   b. irrigate the eye with a chemical antidote
   c. instruct the victim to close the eye
   d. apply a cold compress to the affected eye

2. If a victim has a foreign object embedded in the eyeball
   a. remove the object, then dress and bandage the eye
   b. place a loose dressing over the object
   c. prepare a thick pressure dressing and secure a protective cone over the impaled object, leaving the uninjured eye unbandaged
   d. prepare a thick dressing and secure a protective cone over the impaled object, bandaging the uninjured eye also

3. If an eyeball is knocked out of the socket, which of the following should you not do?
   a. leave the eyeball out of the socket
   b. cover the eyeball with a cup and thick dressing
   c. cover both eyes with a thick dressing
   d. gently replace the eyeball in the socket, then cover with a dressing

4. Eyelid injuries should be
   a. irrigated with cool water
   b. covered with a compress and roller band
   c. treated with antibiotic salve
   d. covered with a light dressing

5. For all chemical burns of the eye
   a. irrigate with water and vinegar solution
   b. have the victim blink repeatedly and wash the eyes
   c. irrigate continuously for at least 30 minutes
   d. irrigate with baking soda

6. A whole tooth can sometimes be reimplanted; the key to successful reimplanting is to keep the dislodged tooth
   a. in an airtight bag
   b. moist
   c. warm
   d. covered with baking soda

7. When a victim sustains a possible facial fracture
   a. keep the victim supine with head and neck immobilized
   b. check all possible eye movements
   c. use ice packs over the area
   d. flush the area with clean water

8. The most important aim of emergency care of jaw fractures is to
   a. find teeth that have been knocked out
   b. apply wraps to keep the lower jaw stable
   c. ensure an airway
   d. pack the area in ice to control swelling

Part 3   Matching

Match the first aid care procedure in the right-hand column with the injury in the left-hand column.

Injury

1. _____ Foreign body in the eye
2. _____ Injury to the eye sockets
3. _____ Lid injuries
4. _____ Eyeball injuries
5. _____ Chemical burns
6. _____ Object impaled in the eye

First Aid Care

A. Position a cup or cone over the injured eye, then bandage.
B. Check all possible eye movements.
C. Cover eyes with a sterile, moist dressing.
D. Cover the eyes with a light dressing (moist if necessary).
E. Flush the eyes with clean water.
F. Irrigate continuously for at least 30 minutes.

Part 4   What Would You Do If?

1. You are at a construction site where a carpenter is cutting some lumber with a power rip saw. A fragment of wood flies into the carpenter's eye.

2. You are at the scene of a motorcycle accident. The victim was not wearing a helmet and has abrasions and lacerations around the mouth and lower jaw.

9

Injuries to the Chest, Abdomen, and Genitalia

On the Scene

Fifty-one-year-old Thomas Meservy was celebrating the arrival of warm weather by playing a spirited game of football with his three sons and five grandsons. As a group struggled to gain control of the football, Thomas took a strong elbow thrust to the heart.

Thomas fell to his knees, holding his hands over a painful area on the right side of his chest. As the group gathered around him, he whispered that it hurt him to move, cough, or even breathe deeply. Examining him more closely, his son Keith saw that there was slight deformity, and felt a grating sensation when he gently palpated the chest.

Keith suspected from the pain, deformity, and grating sound that his father had broken several ribs. Keith sent his brother in the house to call 9-1-1 and get a pillow. Keith instructed Thomas to hold the pillow against his painful side for support, then draped a coat around his shoulders to help keep him warm. When emergency personnel arrived, they were able to stabilize the ribs before transporting Thomas to the hospital.

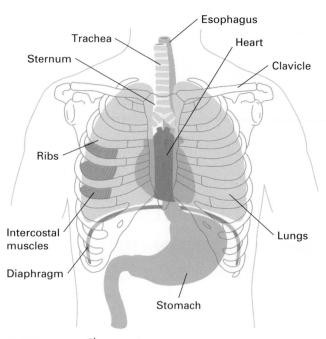

FIGURE 9–1. Chest cavity

hest injury is the second leading cause of death from trauma—second only to head injury. *All* chest injuries should be considered life threatening until proven otherwise, and you should always assume cardiac and lung damage until they are ruled out. Victims of chest injury can look relatively fine, but can deteriorate suddenly and rapidly.

Injuries to the abdomen can result in severe bleeding from rupture or laceration of abdominal organs. Many injuries to the abdomen require surgical repair. You should suspect abdominal organ injury in any victim with evidence of blunt or penetrating injury to the abdominal cavity.

This chapter outlines the first aid care procedures for victims with injuries to the chest, abdomen, and genitalia.

9.1 Chest Injuries

> Learning Objective 1 Identify the three main types of chest injury.

There are two general categories of chest injury: closed and open. In closed (blunt) chest injuries, the skin remains intact. Although the skin is not injured, serious underlying damage can occur, especially lacerations to or rupture of the heart, lungs, and large vessels.

In open (penetrating) chest injury, the skin is broken, either by a penetrating object or the end of a broken rib. Severe internal damage can occur, especially if a bullet mushrooms, tumbles, or fragments or if a knife damages the tissues and organs along the path of penetration. Figure 9-1 illustrates the chest cavity.

Remember: The most dramatic or alarming chest injuries may not be the most life-threatening ones. Types of chest injury include:

- Blunt trauma (caused by a forceful blow to the chest)

- Penetrating injury (an object penetrates the chest wall)

- Compression injury (the chest cavity is compressed rapidly, usually during an automobile accident)

General Signs and Symptoms of Chest Injury

> Learning objective 2 Identify the general signs and symptoms of chest injury.

Whether the injury is open or closed, certain signs and symptoms will occur in major chest trauma, many of them simultaneously (see Figure 9-2):

- Pale, cool, clammy skin

- Cyanosis (bluish coloring of the fingernails, fingertips, lips, or skin)

- **Dyspnea** (shortness of breath or difficulty breathing)

- Rapid breathing (more than 20 breaths per minute)

- **Tracheal deviation**

- Pain during breathing

- Distended neck veins

- Pain at the injury site, or pain near an injury that is made worse by breathing

- Coughing up of blood (**hemoptysis**), usually bright red and frothy

- Failure of the chest to expand normally during inhalation

- Shock

- Rapid, weak pulse (more than 100 beats per minute)

- Open wounds to the chest

- Bruising or deformity to chest wall

- Changing mental status, including confusion, agitation, restlessness, and irrational behavior

Two important signs of chest injury are an increase in the respiratory rate and a change in the normal

> **dyspnea** Shortness of breath or difficulty in breathing
>
> **tracheal deviation** Displacement of the trachea to one side or the other
>
> **hemoptysis** Coughing up of blood

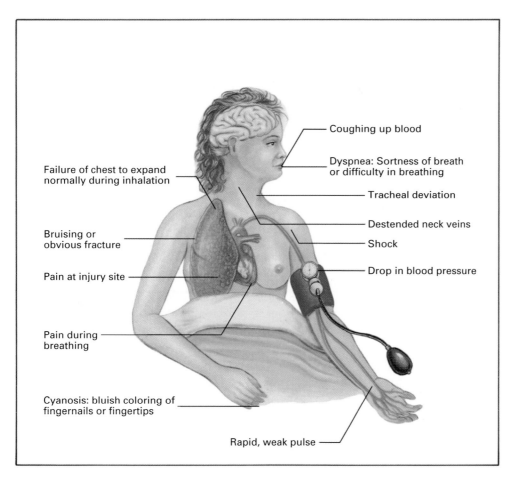

Coughing up blood

Dyspnea: Sortness of breath or difficulty in breathing

Tracheal deviation

Destended neck veins

Shock

Drop in blood pressure

Failure of chest to expand normally during inhalation

Bruising or obvious fracture

Pain at injury site

Pain during breathing

Cyanosis: bluish coloring of fingernails or fingertips

Rapid, weak pulse

FIGURE 9–2. Signs and symptoms of chest injury

breathing pattern. If an adult victim breathes more than 20 times in a minute, experiences pain when breathing, or finds it difficult to take a deep breath, there is probably chest injury. Another important sign of chest injury is evidence of injury to the chest such as bruising or open wounds.

General First Aid Care Principles for Chest Injuries

Learning Objective **3** Describe and demonstrate the first aid care principles for chest injuries.

Activate the EMS system immediately; then follow these steps:

1. Your first priority is to open the airway if necessary; ensure adequate ventilation. If breathing is inadequate, provide rescue breathing.

2. Place an occlusive dressing over any open wounds to the chest (described later in this chapter); control external bleeding.

3. Never try to remove an impaled object; stabilize it to prevent movement until the victim can receive medical help.

4. If there is an object impaled in the chest:

- Cut away clothing to expose the wound.
- Dress the wound around the impaled object to control bleeding and control a sucking chest wound.
- Stabilize the impaled object with rolls of self-adhering bandages or bulky dressings.
- Tape bandages in place to stabilize the impaled object.

PROGRESS CHECK

1. One of the two most important signs of chest injury is a change in _____. *(skin color/ normal breathing pattern)*

2. One of the two most important signs of chest injury is the _____ rate. *(respiratory/heart)*

3. The first priority in caring for a victim of chest injury is to _____ . *(control bleeding/ ensure adequate ventilation/prevent further injury)*

4. You should _____ an impaled object in the chest. *(remove/stabilize, then remove/immobilize and leave in place)*

Specific Chest Injuries

Flail Chest

> Learning Objective **4** Recognize flail chest and demonstrate the appropriate first aid care for it.

Flail chest occurs when the chest wall becomes unstable because two or more adjacent ribs are fractured in two or more places. It can affect the front, back, or sides of the rib cage (see Figure 9-3). Because it usually involves bruising of the lung tissues and inadequate oxygenation, flail chest is a life-threatening injury.

Most often, multiple ribs are fractured in multiple places; the segment of chest wall over them becomes free-floating. When the victim inhales, the area does not expand but moves inward; when the victim exhales, the flail section protrudes—a pattern called **paradoxical movement**.

Signs and symptoms of flail chest include:

- Difficulty breathing
- Paradoxical chest wall movement accompanied by severe pain
- Bruising to the injured area
- Signs of shock
- Victim's attempt to support the chest wall with arms and hands
- Pale, cool, clammy skin
- Cyanosis

- Nasal flaring and neck muscle use
- Increased breathing rate

If the heart has been severely compressed, there may be bluish discoloration of the head, neck, shoulders, lips, and tongue; bulging neck veins; bulging, bloodshot eyes; and obvious deformity of the chest.

To check for flail chest, inspect the chest for paradoxical movement and palpate for an unstable area on the chest.

FIRST AID CARE

Immediately activate the EMS system; then:

1. Maintain an open airway and administer artificial ventilation if the breathing is inadequate.

2. Use *gentle* palpation to locate the edges of the flail section; stabilize with a pad of dressings or a pillow (see Figure 9-4). Secure with wide tape. Do not ever place anything completely around the chest.

3. Position the victim with the flail segment against an external support in a semisitting position or lying in a supine position with the segment splinted with the arm; monitor vital signs and care for shock.

> **flail chest** Instability of a section of chest wall
>
> **paradoxical movement** A condition in which the injured area of the chest moves opposite the rest of the chest during breathing

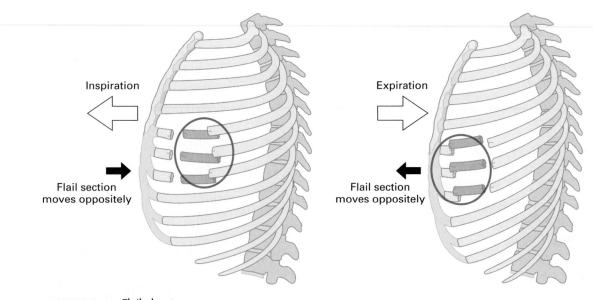

Inspiration

Flail section moves oppositely

Expiration

Flail section moves oppositely

FIGURE 9–3. Flail chest

FIGURE 9–4. Stabilize flail chest by applying a pillow or bulky dressing.

Compression Injuries and Traumatic Asphyxia

Learning Objective **5** Recognize compression injuries of the chest and demonstrate appropriate first aid care for them.

A life-threatening emergency, severe and sudden compression of a victim's chest (such as when a person is thrown against a steering wheel) causes a rapid increase in pressure inside the chest. Most serious, the sternum exerts sudden and severe pressure on the heart, causing it to be bruised.

Traumatic asphyxia occurs from a sudden compression of the chest wall, causing blood to stop flowing or to flow backward in the vessels.

Signs and symptoms include

- Pale, cool, clammy skin
- Weak pulses
- Increased heart rate
- Increased breathing rate
- Distended neck veins
- Bloodshot, protruding eyes
- Cyanotic tongue and lips
- Coughing or vomiting blood
- Swollen, cyanotic appearance of the head, neck, and shoulders

FIRST AID CARE

Activate the EMS system immediately; then:

1. Maintain an open airway and administer artificial ventilation if breathing is inadequate.

2. Control any bleeding that results from the trauma.

3. Monitor the victim closely; position the victim in a supine position.

Broken Ribs

Learning Objective **6** Recognize broken ribs and demonstrate appropriate first aid care for them.

Although broken ribs themselves are not life threatening, they can cause injuries that *are*, such as injury to the heart, lungs, or great blood vessels.

The most common symptom of rib fracture is pain; it usually hurts the victim to move, cough, or breathe deeply (see Figure 9-5). Other signs and symptoms (see Figure 9-6 on page 154) can include

- Severe pain at the fracture site
- Grating sound upon palpation (**crepitus**)
- Chest deformity
- Shallow, rapid breathing
- Bruising or lacerations at the suspected fracture site
- Frothy blood at the nose or mouth (indicating lung laceration)

FIGURE 9–5. Typical "guarded" position of victim with rib fracture

traumatic asphyxia Sudden compression of the chest wall that forces blood to flow the wrong way.

crepitus A sandpaperlike grating sound made by the ends of a broken bone as they rub together

Pain at fracture site.
Pain on moving, coughing, or breathing deeply.
Shallow breathing.
Chest deformity.
Bruising or lacerations.
Grating sound upon palpation.
Crackling sensation near site.
Frothy blood at nose or mouth (lung puncture).

FIGURE 9–6. The most common symptom of rib fracture is severe pain. Other signs and symptoms may not be present.

FIRST AID CARE

The top priority in first aid care is making sure the victim can breathe adequately by splinting the chest as needed. Activate the EMS system, then give the victim a pillow or blanket to hold against the chest for support (see Figure 9-7). If the victim can't hold a pillow, do the following:

1. Use a sling and swathe to utilize the victim's arm as a splint and support; the forearm of the injured side positioned across the chest (see Figures 9-8 and 9-9).

2. Position the victim in a supine position.

3. Monitor the victim's ABCDs, watching for signs of internal bleeding that could lead to shock.

Do not do this:

- Wrap anything completely around the chest
- Tape the ribs

Hemothorax, Tension Pneumothorax, Open Pneumothorax, and Pneumothorax

Learning Objective 7 Recognize hemothorax, tension pneumothorax, open pneumothorax, and pneumothorax, and demonstrate appropriate first aid care for each.

In three conditions—**tension pneumothorax**, open pneumothorax, and **pneumothorax** (see Figure 9-10)—air enters the space between the lung and the outer pleural lining, causing pressure to be placed against the lungs and/or heart that can interfere with breathing and circulation. Blood enters the space in a **hemothorax**. All four are life threatening (see Table 9-1 on page 156). For each condition, activate the EMS system immediately; *tension pneumothorax is one of the few emergencies in which*

hemothorax An accumulation of blood in the chest cavity

tension pneumothorax A situation in which air enters the pleural space through a one-way defect in the lung, resulting in a progressive increase in pressure in the pleural cavity that causes the lung to collapse and that impairs circulation

pneumothorax A condition in which air from a lung or from the outside fills the chest cavity, but does not fill the lung

FIGURE 9–7. Place a pad between arm and chest.

FIGURE 9–8. Supporting with a sling

FIGURE 9–9. Immobilizing the arm and sling with a swathe, a bandage that stabilizes the sling

seconds count. Figures 9-12 through 9-15 on page 157 illustrate first aid care of a victim with possible pneumothorax.

PROGRESS CHECK

1. In flail chest, the chest wall _____ when the victim exhales. *(collapses/moves/protrudes)*

2. Flail chest most often occurs when multiple _____ are fractured. *(bones/ribs/joints)*

3. To check for flail chest, have the victim lie on his or her back and check for _____ as the victim breathes. *(crepitus/pain/paradoxical motion)*

4. Traumatic asphyxia occurs from sudden _____ of the chest wall. *(compression/collapse/penetration)*

5. The most common symptom of rib fracture is _____ . *(deformity/pain/bruising)*

6. The greatest priority in treating rib fracture is to splint the chest so the victim _____ . *(can breathe adequately/is not in pain/will not be further injured by broken bone ends)*

7. In treating a rib fracture, you should use _____ . *(tape/continuous strapping/a sling and swathe)*

8. In a hemothorax, _____ enters the chest cavity. *(air/blood/pressure)*

9. To help prevent tension pneumothorax, you should always leave one corner of a chest bandage _____ . *(over the wound/untaped/at least 2 inches beyond the wound)*

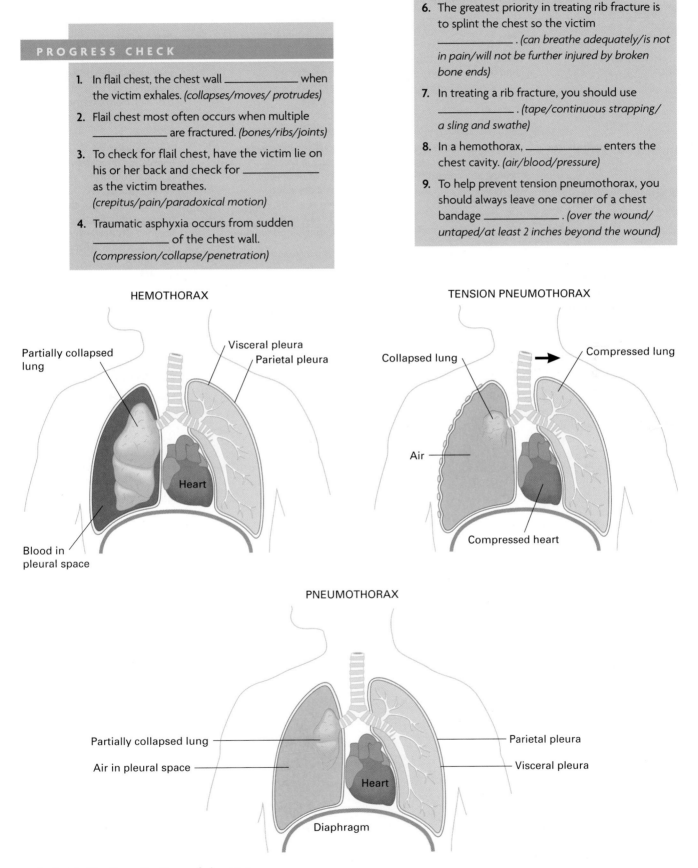

FIGURE 9–10. Complications of chest injury

	TABLE 9–1	Life-Threatening Conditions of the Chest Cavity	
Condition	Cause	Signs and Symptoms	First Aid Care
Hemothorax	Blood fills the chest cavity, compressing the lung	• Shock • Rapid heartbeat • Rapid breathing • Weak pulse • Hemoptysis • Frothy or bloody sputum	Administer artificial ventilation if breathing is inadequate; control bleeding from external wounds; treat for shock
Tension pneumothorax	Air builds up in the chest cavity, completely collapsing the lung and compressing the heart	• Obvious and increasing difficulty in breathing • Bulging of neck veins • Tracheal deviation • Uneven chest movements • Rapid heart rate • Decreasing blood pressure	Administer artificial ventilation if breathing is inadequate; if the chest is bandaged, leave one corner of the bandage untaped, creating a flutter valve (see Figure 9-11); treat for shock
Open pneumothorax (sucking chest wound)	Open chest wound allows air into the chest cavity	• Moist sucking or bubbling sound as air passes in and out of the wound	Apply an occlusive dressing over the wound to create a flutter valve, leaving one corner untaped; administer artificial ventilation if breathing is inadequate
Pneumothorax	Air enters the chest cavity and compresses the lung	• Sudden, sharp chest pain • Difficulty in breathing	Maintain open airway; administer artificial ventilation if breathing is inadequate; apply occlusive dressing to any open chest wounds and leave one corner untaped

On inspiration, dressing seals wound, preventing air entry

Collapsed lung

Expiration allows trapped air to escape through untaped section of dressing

FIGURE 9–11. Creating a flutter valve to relieve tension pneumothorax

FIGURE 9–12. Sucking chest wound and possible pneumothorax

FIGURE 9–13. Tape dressing in place.

FIGURE 9–14. Position occlusive covering, which should contact the chest wall directly

FIGURE 9–15. Position victim to ease breathing.

9.3 Abdominal Injuries

> Lerining Objective **8** Describe the differences between open and closed abdominal wounds.

A wide range of trauma, from motor vehicle accidents to shootings, affect the organs of the abdomen; because the abdominal cavity contains not only vital organs but a rich supply of blood vessels, abdominal injuries are life threatening and demand prompt and proper treatment. Figure 9-16 on page 158 illustrates injuries to the abdomen, chest, and pelvic cavity.

If a victim has suffered abdominal trauma, also suspect that he or she has also suffered chest trauma until proven otherwise.

An open wound that penetrates the abdominal cavity is extremely dangerous because of possible damage to internal organs. The stomach or intestine may be perforated, internal bleeding may occur, and infection may develop. Bacteria may be introduced into the peritoneal cavity from the outside or from a perforated intestine.

In closed abdominal wounds, the abdomen is damaged by a severe blow or crushing injury, but the skin remains unbroken (blunt trauma). Such wounds may be extremely dangerous—they can cause serious injury to the internal organs, internal bleeding, and shock.

Assessment of Abdominal Injuries

> Learning Objective **9** Describe the assessment of a victim with abdominal injury.

Injury to heart or major cardiopulmonary vessels

Sternal fracture

Sternal separation

Torn blood vessels (hemothorax)

Rib fracture

Perforation of pleura and/or lung (sucking chest wound or pneumothorax)

Puncture wound (by missile)

The organs most frequently damaged by penetrating abdominal trauma are the liver, small intestine and colon.

Vertebral dislocation (any level)

Remember, with gunshot and stab wounds there may be an entry and an exit wound. Bullets and stab wounds can cause injuries to multiple organs and bullets can be deflected internally causing damage in areas not anticipated.

Lacerated and punctured kidneys

Transected ureter and urethra

Ruptured bladder

FIGURE 9–16. Injuries to the chest, abdomen, and pelvic cavity

To assess a victim for abdominal injury:

1. Have the victim lie supine with knees flexed and supported; remove or loosen clothing over the abdomen.

2. Inspect for lacerations, open wounds, bruising, impaled objects, or protruding abdominal organs.

3. Gently palpate all four quadrants for guarding, rigidity, pain, and tenderness.

Signs and Symptoms of Abdominal Injuries

Learning Objective **10** Describe the common signs and symptoms of abdominal injuries.

The amount of blood you can see is not necessarily indicative of the severity of injury: Deep underlying damage may occur with only little external hemorrhage. Abdominal injuries may cause any of several signs and symptoms (see Figure 9-17):

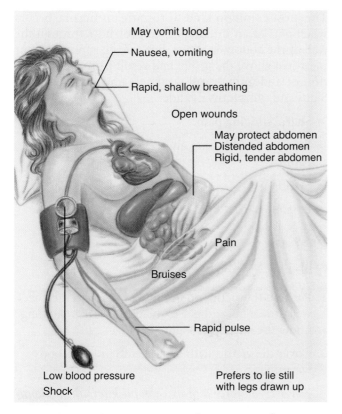

FIGURE 9–17. Common signs and symptoms of abdominal injuries

- Distended or irregularly shaped abdomen

- Bruising of the abdomen flank or back

- Tenderness (pain on palpation)

- Pain, ranging from mild discomfort to intense, intolerable pain

- Pain other than at the injury site

- Pain radiating to either shoulder

- "Guarding" (voluntary contraction of the abdominal muscles)

- Fetal position or lying with legs drawn up toward the chest and abdomen (see Figure 9-18)

- Weak peripheral pulses

- Abdominal cramping

- A rigid, boardlike, stiff or hard abdomen on palpation (abdominal rigidity)

- Nausea and/or vomiting; the victim may vomit blood

- Rapid, shallow breathing

- Rapid pulse

- Open wounds and penetrations

- Organs protruding through open wounds

FIGURE 9–18. Victims with abdominal injuries often lie with their legs drawn up in the fetal position.

- Blood in the urine

- Extreme weakness

- Thirst

- Low blood pressure

General First Aid Care

Learning Objective **11** Describe general first aid care for abdominal injuries.

As with all injured victims, top priorities are airway, breathing, and circulation. Activate the EMS system; then follow these steps:

1. Take measures to prevent shock; keep the victim warm, but do not overheat.

2. Control bleeding and dress all open wounds with a dry, sterile dressing. If organs are protruding, follow the guidelines under "Abdominal Evisceration," on page 160.

3. If any object has penetrated or impaled the victim
   - Cut clothing away from the object.
   - Dress the wounds around the object to control bleeding.
   - Stabilize the object with bulky dressings.
   - Bandage the object in place to prevent movement.

4. Position the victim for greatest comfort; victims may want to lie on the back with the knees flexed. If possible, elevate the feet.

5. Be alert for vomiting; position the victim for adequate drainage. Constantly monitor vital signs and abdominal condition.

6. Do not give the victim anything by mouth.

Abdominal Evisceration

Learning Objective **12** Demonstrate appropriate first aid care for abdominal eviscerations.

If abdominal contents are protruding through a wound (**evisceration**), immediately activate the EMS system; then:

1. Cover protruding abdominal organs with a clean dressing moistened with sterile water if possible or clear water that is clean enough to drink. Never use absorbent cotton or any material that clings or disintegrates when wet, such as paper towels or toilet tissue.

2. Cover the moist dressing with an occlusive material, such as clean plastic wrap, to retain moisture and warmth. Gently wrap the dressing in place with a bandage or clean sheet. Keep the bandage and dressing loose enough so that they do not exert pressure on the abdominal organs or cause injury.

3. Prevent shock, and constantly monitor the victim's vital signs.

Never touch abdominal organs or try to replace them in the abdominal cavity. See Figures 9-19 through 9-23.

Rupture or Hernia

Learning Objective **13** Describe appropriate first aid care for rupture, or hernia.

The most common kind of rupture, or **hernia**, occurs when part of an internal organ protrudes through the wall of the abdomen. Most, but not all, ruptures occur in or just above the groin, and result from a combination of abdominal wall weakness and muscle strain. Signs and symptoms include

- Sharp, stinging pain
- Feeling of something giving way at the site of the rupture
- Swelling
- Possible nausea and vomiting

FIRST AID CARE

Activate the EMS system; then:

1. Position the victim on his or her back with the knees well drawn up, and place a blanket or other padding under the knees (see Figure 9-24).

2. Cover the victim with a blanket to preserve body warmth.

Never try to force a protrusion back into the abdominal cavity.

---

evisceration The protrusion of abdominal contents through a laceration or other wound

hernia Protrusion of an internal organ through the abdominal wall or into another body cavity

---

FIGURE 9–19. Abdominal evisceration—an open wound resulting in protrusion of an organ, usually the intestines

FIGURE 9–20. Cut away clothing from wound and support knees in a flexed position.

FIGURE 9–21. Place dressing over wound. Do not attempt to replace intestines within abdomen.

FIGURE 9–22. Moisten dressing with clean water. (Note that under ideal conditions you will premoisten the dressing before application.)

FIGURE 9–23. Gently and loosely tape the dressing in place, then apply an occlusive material such as plastic wrap. Tape loosely over dressing to keep dressing moist.

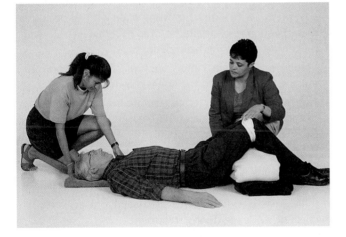

FIGURE 9–24. First aid care for a rupture or hernia

9.4   Injuries to the Genitalia

In treating injuries to the genitalia, act in a calm, professional way; protect victims from onlookers and help protect their privacy by using sheets, towels, or other material as a drape over the genital area.

PROGRESS CHECK

1. The amount of _____ does not necessarily indicate how serious abdominal injury is. *(pain/external blood/deformity)*

2. Most abdominal injury victims are most comfortable on their back with the _____ . *(feet elevated/head elevated/knees drawn up)*

3. If abdominal organs protrude through a wound, you should _____ them. *(cover/replace/remove)*

Male Genitalia

Learning Objective **14** Describe appropriate first aid care for injuries to the male genitalia.

Although injuries to the external male genitalia— lacerations, avulsions, abrasions, penetrations, and contusions—are excruciatingly painful, they are not necessarily life threatening. However, the amount of pain involved and the nature of the injury can cause great concern to the victim.

To treat, activate the EMS system; then:

1. Wrap the penis or scrotum in a soft, sterile dressing moistened with sterile or clean water. If there is external bleeding, control it with direct pressure.

2. If there is a penetrating or impaled object, do not remove it; stabilize it with a bulky dressing to prevent movement.

3. If part of the penis or scrotum is caught in a zipper, cut off the zipper fastener and separate the teeth; if a long section of skin is caught, cut the zipper out of the pants to make the victim more comfortable.

4. Apply an ice bag or cold compresses to relieve pain and reduce swelling.

5. If there are avulsed parts, wrap in sterile gauze moistened with clean water and send them with the victim.

Female Genitalia

Learning Objective **15** Describe appropriate first aid care for injuries to the female genitalia.

Injuries to the external female genitalia are rare but can occur with straddle injuries, sexual assault, blows to the perineum, or abortion attempts; following childbirth; or when foreign objects are inserted into the vagina. Because the area is richly supplied with blood vessels and nerves, the injury can cause extreme pain and considerable bleeding.

To treat, activate the EMS system; then:

1. Control bleeding with direct pressure.

2. Dress the wounds, keeping the dressing in place with a diaper-type bandage. Stabilize any impaled objects or foreign bodies.

3. Use ice packs or cold compresses to relieve pain and reduce swelling.

If the woman was a victim of sexual assault, preserve the chain of evidence:

- Do not allow her to bathe or douche.

- Do not allow her to wash her hair or clean under her fingernails.

- If possible, do not clean wounds.

- Handle her clothing as little as possible.

- Put all items of clothing and other items in separate bags; if there is blood on any object, do not use plastic bags.

PROGRESS CHECK

1. In both male and female victims with injuries to the genitalia, apply _____ to relieve pain and reduce swelling. *(direct pressure/an ice bag/sterile gauze)*

2. Always try to _____ avulsed skin. *(preserve/finish detaching/clean)*

3. If a woman was the victim of sexual assault, try to _____ . *(comfort her/find the assailant/preserve the chain of evidence)*

Summary

- All injuries to the chest are life threatening.

- Two of the most important signs of chest injury are the respiratory rate and any change in the normal breathing pattern.

- The first priority in treating chest injuries is to ensure the airway is open and ventilation is adequate.

- Flail chest usually occurs when multiple ribs are fractured in multiple places, resulting in a section of chest that is unstable.

- Broken ribs are rarely life threatening, but they can cause injuries that *are*; stabilize them with a sling and swathe.

- In a hemothorax, blood fills the chest cavity (pleural cavity) and compresses the lungs, interfering with respiration.

- Tension pneumothorax, in which air pressure collapses the lung and compresses the heart, is one of the few emergencies in which seconds count.

- To prevent a pneumothorax from worsening, cover any open chest wound with an occlusive material; leave one corner untaped so air can escape on expiration.

- Never try to remove a penetrating or impaled object from the chest or abdomen; stabilize the object to prevent movement.

- The amount of blood is not necessarily indicative of the severity of abdominal injury; severe internal damage can result from blunt, closed trauma.

- Never touch abdominal organs that protrude through a wound, and never try to replace them in the abdomen; cover them with a moist dressing, then with an occlusive material such as clean plastic wrap to retain warmth and prevent the dressings from drying.

- Victims of abdominal injury are typically more comfortable on the back with the knees drawn up.

- Few injuries to the external genitalia are life threatening, but the amount of pain and the nature of the injury can cause the victim great concern.

- In injuries to the genitalia, control bleeding, dress wounds, and apply ice packs or cold compresses to relieve pain and reduce swelling.

- If a woman is a victim of sexual assault, preserve the chain of evidence during treatment.

Key Terms

Make sure you understand the following key terms:

dyspnea	crepitus
tracheal deviation	hemothorax
hemoptysis	tension pneumothorax
flail chest	pneumothorax
paradoxical movement	evisceration
traumatic asphyxia	hernia

Critical Thinking Exercise

You are attending a local concert at the park when suddenly a crowd develops and someone begins to scream for help. As you approach the crowd, you notice a male who is approximately 19 years of age with what appears to be a stab wound to the right side of his chest just above the nipple. He is having difficulty breathing.

1. How would you immediately manage the stab wound?

2. What signs and symptoms would indicate a severe chest injury?

3. What additional first aid would you provide to the patient?

9 Chapter 9 Self-Test

Student: _____   Date: _____

Course: _____   Section #: _____

Part 1   True/False

If you believe the statement is true, circle the T. If you believe the statement is false, circle the F.

T   F   **1.** Traumatic asphyxia occurs from sudden compression of the chest wall.

T   F   **2.** Flail chest most often occurs when two or more adjacent ribs are broken in two or more places.

T   F   **3.** In paradoxical movement, the injured chest wall moves in and the uninjured chest wall moves out.

T   F   **4.** Stabilize a flail chest with pads or a pillow.

T   F   **5.** Position a flail chest victim so the flail segment is not against any external support.

T   F   **6.** Do not tape the ribs or use continuous strapping on a flail chest victim.

T   F   **7.** Common signs and symptoms of abdominal injury include slow, shallow breathing and rapid pulse.

T   F   **8.** Do not remove penetrating or impaled objects from the abdomen.

T   F   **9.** Most hernias occur in or just below the groin.

T   F   **10.** A dull, pulsating pain is the most common symptom of a hernia.

T   F   **11.** Bleeding from an injury to the genitalia should always be controlled at the femoral pressure point.

Part 2   Multiple Choice

For each item, circle the correct answer or the phrase that best completes the statement.

1. In what position should you place a victim with broken ribs?

  a. semisitting or supine
  b. upright
  c. semiprone, injured side down
  d. flat on the back

2. Which of the following is *not* likely a sign of a chest injury?

  a. coughing blood
  b. shock
  c. strong, bounding pulse
  d. distended neck veins

3. The leakage of blood into the chest cavity from lacerated vessels or from the lung, causing the lung to compress, is called

  a. pneumothorax
  b. flail chest
  c. traumatic asphyxia
  d. hemothorax

4. Paradoxical movement occurs when

  a. compression injuries cause gasping breaths interspersed with extremely shallow breathing
  b. a compressed lung lacks oxygen
  c. air remains in the chest cavity outside the lungs
  d. the motion of the injured chest area is opposite the motion of the remainder of the chest

5. The two general categories of chest wounds are

  a. open and closed
  b. simple and compound
  c. fracture and puncture
  d. lung related and heart related

6. Pneumothorax occurs when

  a. air enters the chest cavity but does not enter the lung from a wound site
  b. the descending aorta is lacerated
  c. blood fills up the chest cavity
  d. three or more ribs break and the chest wall that lies over the break area collapses

7. Which of the following is *not* appropriate care for abdominal injuries?

   a. carefully remove impaled objects
   b. do not give the victim anything by mouth
   c. work to prevent shock
   d. have the victim lie on the back with knees flexed

8. Eviscerated organs should be

   a. replaced within the abdomen
   b. covered with a dry dressing
   c. covered with a moist sterile dressing and an occlusive dressing
   d. rinsed thoroughly with copious amounts of water

9. The most common form of rupture or hernia occurs when

   a. a portion of an internal organ protrudes through the abdominal wall
   b. a portion of a thoracic organ protrudes through the thoracic wall
   c. veins or arteries become weak and bulge or rupture
   d. any of the above

Part 3   Matching

Match the definitions in the left column with the conditions in the right column.

1. _____ Air enters the chest cavity through a sucking wound
2. _____ Blood leaks into the chest cavity and compresses the lung
3. _____ Air pressure collapses the lung and compresses the heart
4. _____ Sudden compression of the chest wall disturbs ventilation and blood flow

A. Traumatic asphyxia
B. Hemothorax
C. Tension pneumothorax
D. Open pneumothorax

Part 4   What Would You Do If?

1. A victim has been stabbed in the chest with a large kitchen knife. When you arrive, the knife has been removed. When the victim breathes, a bubbling is produced at the wound site.

2. You are at a construction site where a worker has fallen on some reinforcisng rods. He is lying on his back and has an obvious abdominal evisceration.

3. You are at the home of a victim who has been lifting and moving heavy boxes. He complains of nausea and sharp, stinging pain just above the groin. There is swelling and protrusion in the area of pain.

10

Dressing and Bandaging

Learning Objectives

When you have mastered the material in this chapter, you will be able to

1 Identify the various types of dressings

2 Identify the various types of bandages

3 Demonstrate how to apply triangular bandages to different parts of the body

4 Demonstrate how to apply cravat bandages to different parts of the body

5 Demonstrate how to apply roller bandages to different parts of the body

6 Describe the basic principles of dressing and bandaging wounds

7 Demonstrate how to apply a pressure dressing

8 Demonstrate how to use a sling

On the Scene

Keaton Shaw was playing with some friends in a shallow creek that ran behind their group of houses. Suddenly a sharp pain shot through his foot; he yanked it out of the water and discovered that he had stepped on a sharp object lodged in the sandy creek bottom, cutting the bottom of his foot.

Keaton's brother ran a little more than a block to get their mother while Keaton sat on the bank of the creek, resting his foot on a large boulder. Elizabeth Shaw, carrying the family's first aid kit to the site, quickly ascertained that the wound was not large or deep enough to require stitches, and knew that Keaton was up to date on his tetanus shots. The wound had bled enough to wash out any contaminants, and Elizabeth knew her priority was to dress and bandage it to keep it dry and prevent infection.

She gently applied a light coating of antibiotic cream to the laceration. Tearing open a 2-inch-square gauze pad and holding it carefully by the corners, she placed it on top of the cut, completely covering it. She then used a self-adhering roller bandage, wrapping it snugly around Keaton's foot to hold the dressing in place. Finally, she slipped a clean sock on the injured foot, helped Keaton put on his sandals, and helped him walk home.

Once bleeding from a wound has been controlled, the wound should be dressed and bandaged. All open wounds need some kind of covering to prevent infection and control bleeding. Proper wound care also enhances healing, adds to the comfort of the victim, and promotes more rapid recovery. Improper wound care can delay healing, cause infection, cause severe discomfort to the victim, and—in rare cases—result in the loss of a limb.

The basic purposes of dressings and bandages are to

- Control bleeding
- Prevent further contamination and injury
- Keep the wound dry
- Immobilize the wound site

This chapter outlines the principles of dressing and bandaging and includes a discussion of specific types of dressings and bandages that can be used in wound care.

10.1 Dressings

Learning Objective 1 Identify the various types of dressings.

A **dressing** is a sterile covering for a wound that covers and touches the surface of the wound. All open wounds need to be covered to prevent infection; dressings can also control bleeding, absorb blood and fluids, and prevent further injury to the wound. A dressing should be:

- **Sterile**, meaning that any microorganisms and spores on the dressing have been killed
- **Aseptic**, meaning it is free of bacteria
- Held in place with a bandage tightly enough to control bleeding, but not so tightly that it stops blood circulation
- Larger than the wound, so that it extends beyond all the edges of the wound
- Soft, thick, and compressible so that it provides even pressure over the entire surface of the wound

Most dressings are also porous, which allows air to circulate to the wound to promote healing.

Large or deep wounds should always be cleaned and treated at a medical facility to reduce the risk of infection; don't try to clean these wounds yourself. A medical professional can determine whether a tetanus shot is needed. Once you have provided basic first aid care by controlling bleeding, make sure a victim with a large or deep wound sees a medical professional.

The ideal dressing is layered, free of lint, consists of coarse mesh gauze to allow air to circulate to the wound, is bulky enough to immobilize tissues and protect the wound, and is soft, thick, and pliable. A dressing is always placed against the wound, and the dressing is held in place with a bandage; the bandage is never placed directly against the wound.

There are several types of commercial dressings (see Figures 10-1 through 10-4):

- **Occlusive**—plastic wrap or other dressing that forms an airtight seal, usually used for chest or abdominal wounds.
- **Compress**—a thick, bulky, usually sterile dressing intended to stop or control bleeding.
- **Trauma**—a 5-by-36-inch piece of thick, sterile, absorbent dressing that can be used to cover a larger area in cases of more serious or widespread injury (also called a *universal* dressing).
- **Adhesive strips**—a combination of a sterile dressing and a bandage, individually packaged and used for small wounds (often called a Band-Aid®). These may come in special shapes for wounds on fingertips or knuckles. Butterfly bandages help hold together the edges of wounds.
- **Adhesive tape**—Often used to hold the edges of wounds together, it comes in rolls of various widths. It is generally not applied directly to the wound, but is most often used to secure small dressings or roller bands in place. Adhesive tape must be applied directly to the skin; if it is applied only to gauze, bandages, or other fabric, it will slip.

Gauze Pads

Gauze is used several ways in dressings; plain gauze can be used in place of a bandage compress to cover large wounds. Plain gauze in various-sized pads, designed for smaller wounds, is sterilized and sold commercially in individually wrapped packages. Make sure you don't touch the part of the gauze that will contact the wound.

The most popular sizes of sterile **gauze pads** are 2-by-2s, 4-by-4s, and 4-by-8s. In cases of major multiple trauma, nonsterile bulk packages of 4-by-4 dressings are often used.

---

dressing A sterile covering for a wound

sterile Free of all microorganisms and spores

aseptic Free of bacteria

occlusive Waterproof and airtight

gauze pads Commercially manufactured, individually wrapped sterile pads made of gauze

FIGURE 10–1. Sterile gauze pads

FIGURE 10–2. Nonelastic, self-adhering dressing and roller bandages

FIGURE 10–3. Multitrauma dressing

FIGURE 10–4. Burn dressings

Some gauze pads are penetrated with ointment or have a plasticlike coating to prevent them from sticking to the wound. You can improvise by applying a small amount of antibiotic ointment, such as Neosporin, to the gauze pad before placing it against the wound. Be careful to hold the gauze pad by its corner and touch it only with ointment to avoid contaminating it.

Special Pads

Large, thickly layered bulky pads, some with waterproof outer surfaces, are available in several sizes for quick application to an arm or leg or to a large area of the trunk. They are used where bulk is required to stop profuse bleeding and to stabilize impaled objects. Such **special pads** are also referred to as multitrauma dressings, trauma packs, general-purpose dressings, burn pads, or ABD dressings.

You can use individually wrapped sanitary napkins in place of special pads when necessary; however, even individually wrapped sanitary napkins are not sterile and can introduce infection to the wound.

Bandage Compresses

A bandage compress (see Figure 10-5 on page 170) is a special dressing designed to cover open wounds and to help control heavy bleeding. It consists of a pad made of several thicknesses of gauze attached to the middle of a strip of bandaging material that can simply be secured by tying, and usually comes in a sterile package. The pad sizes range from 1 to 4 inches. Unless otherwise specified, all bandage compresses and all gauze dressings should be covered with open triangular, cravat, or roller bandages.

> **special pads** Large, thickly layered bulky pads used to control bleeding and stabilize impaled objects

FIGURE 10–5. Already prepared bandage compresses are available in individual packages.

Applying a Sterile Dressing

Gauze pads and other sterile dressings are generally packaged individually and remain sterile until the package is opened. To help prevent the risk of infection:

- Wear protective gloves whenever possible.

- Avoid touching the surface of the wound.

- Use a dressing that is large enough to cover all the edges of the wound.

- Hold the dressing carefully by the corner; do not touch the part of the dressing that will come into contact with the wound.

- Place the dressing directly on top of the wound; do not slide or shift it into place after it touches the skin.

- Cover the dressing with a bandage that is tight enough to hold the dressing securely in place without impairing circulation.

To apply an adhesive strip, remove the wrapping and, holding it by the protective strips, pull back on the strips without removing them. Without touching the pad, place it directly on the wound; carefully pull away the protective strips, then press down the ends and edges of the adhesive strip.

PROGRESS CHECK

1. A sterile dressing is one on which there are no _____ . (bacteria/microorganisms/viruses)

2. An aseptic dressing is free of _____ . (bacteria/microorganisms/viruses)

3. Use petroleum gauze when you don't want the dressing to _____ . (get wet/shred/stick to the wound)

---

4. An occlusive dressing is _____ . (dry/moist/airtight)

5. A compress dressing is used to _____ . (control bleeding/prevent infection/absorb fluids oozing from the wound)

6. A 9×36-inch piece of thick, absorbent material is called a _____ dressing. (occlusive/universal/compress)

10.2 Bandages

Learning Objective 2 Identify the various types of bandages.

The most common kind of bandage is the adhesive strip, such as a Band-Aid®. There are many other types and sizes of bandages, though. A **bandage**

- Holds a dressing in place over a wound

- Creates pressure that controls bleeding

- Helps keep the edges of the wound closed

- Secures a splint to an injured part of the body

- Provides support for an injured part of the body

- Helps prevent or reduce swelling

Properly applied, bandages promote healing, prevent severe complications, and help the victim stay comfortable. Never place a bandage directly on the wound; use it only to cover a dressing. The bandage should be clean, but does not need to be sterile.

Bandages should be properly applied and well secured. If a bandage gets loose, wounds may bleed or become infected, and broken bones can further displace. Make sure you don't leave loose ends on a bandage, since they can catch on objects and cause further injury.

The two most common mistakes in bandaging are bandaging too loosely and bandaging too tightly. Bandages should be firm enough to hold the dressing in place, but not so tight that they restrict circulation. Most bandages gradually stretch, so check to make sure it is still holding the dressing in place. You should immediately loosen any bandage that is too tight. Never cover the fingers or the toes with a bandage unless they are injured; doing so prevents you from being able to tell if you have applied a bandage too tightly. The following are signs that a bandage is too tight:

- The skin around the bandage becomes pale or bluish in color (cyanotic).

bandage Material used to hold a dressing in place

- There is a bluish tinge to the nearest fingernails or toenails.

- The victim complains of pain, usually only a few minutes after you apply the bandage.

- The skin beyond the bandage (distal) is bold.

- The skin beyond the bandage (distal) is tingling or numb.

- You cannot feel the pulse beyond the bandage (distal), or it is very weak.

- Capillary refill is absent or diminished in the fingernails or toenails beyond the bandage (when you press on the nail, the nailbed does not immediately turn pink again).

- The victim cannot move his or her fingers or toes.

When tying a bandage, square knots are best—they don't slip, hold well, and are easy to untie. If you think a knot might cause the victim discomfort, place a pad between the knot and the body.

Triangular and Cravat Bandages

Learning Objective **3** Demonstrate how to apply triangular bandages to different parts of the body.

Learning Objective **4** Demonstrate how to apply cravat bandages to different parts of the body.

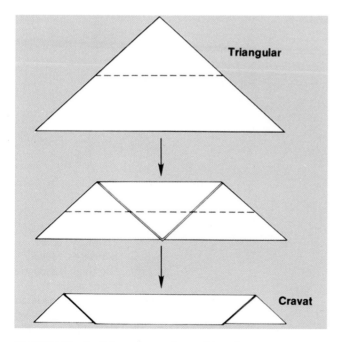

FIGURE 10–6. Triangular and cravat bandages

A standard **triangular bandage** (see Figure 10-6) is made from a piece of unbleached cotton cloth—most commonly preshrunk cotton muslin—that is cut diagonally from a square that is 36 to 40 inches. A triangular bandage is easy to apply and can be applied so the part over the dressing will not be soiled. When applied correctly, a triangular bandage can be used on most parts of the body. Folded, a triangular bandage becomes a **cravat**.

A triangular bandage is most commonly used to

- Support fractures and dislocations

- Apply splints

- Form slings

- Make improvised tourniquets

In an emergency, you can make a triangular bandage from a clean handkerchief, a cotton towel, or a clean piece of shirt. If a regular-sized bandage is too short, tie a second bandage to one end.

Roller Bandages

Learning Objective **5** Demonstrate how to apply roller bandages to different parts of the body.

Roller bandages are made from gauze-like material; they come in a variety of widths, and the different widths can be used for different parts of the body. (For example, a 1-inch bandage is used for fingers; a 2-inch for hands, wrists, and feet; a 3-inch for arms and elbows; and a 4- or 6-inch for legs, knees, and ankles.)

The most popular and easy-to-use roller bandage is a self-adhering (nonelastic), form-fitting **roller bandage**, which can be secured easily with several overlapping wraps and can then be cut and tied or taped in place (see Figures 10-7 through 10-15 on pages 172–173). Roller bandages come in a variety of widths and lengths, ranging from ½ inch to 12 inches wide and as long as 10 yards. Because they adhere to themselves, they are easy to use. Examples of commercial self-adhering roller bandages are Kerlix and Kling. Roller bandages can also be used as dressings.

Another type of roller bandage is the elastic bandage; while it is used to compress strains, sprains, and

triangular bandage Triangle-shaped piece of cloth used to apply splints and form slings

cravat A folded triangular bandage

roller bandage A form-fitting bandage designed to be wrapped around a wound site

FIGURE 10–7. Head and/or eye bandage. In case of eye injury, cover both eyes.

FIGURE 10–8. Head or ear bandage. Keep the bandage near the eyebrows and low at the back of the head.

FIGURE 10–9. Shoulder bandage. Begin at the lowest part of the arm and work toward the shoulder; wrap in a figure-8 across the chest, under the opposite arm, and across the back.

FIGURE 10–10. Elbow bandage. Use a figure-8 pattern, covering half to three-fourths of each previous layer.

FIGURE 10–11. Lower arm bandage. Make the bandage more secure by starting at the wrist and moving up to the wider part of the arm.

FIGURE 10–12. Thigh and ankle bandages. Make the thigh bandage more secure by starting at the knee and moving toward the wider part of the thigh.

FIGURE 10–13. Knee bandage. Keeping the knee slightly bent, start with two wraps around the kneecap, then use a figure-8 wrap, covering half to three-fourths of each previous layer.

FIGURE 10–14. Hand bandage. Begin by wrapping twice around the palm, then use a figure-8 pattern to wrap diagonally from palm to wrist and back.

2. Crisscross the bandage over itself as you circle until the complete wound area is covered. Do not cover the fingers or toes.

3. Fasten the bandage in place with tape, safety pins, or clips that come with the bandage. You can also tie a roller bandage. The easiest way is to split the tail of the bandage about 12 inches, then tie a knot to prevent the bandage from splitting further. Then simply wrap the ends in opposite directions and tie them together.

You can also use two gauze rolls, wrapping alternately around and across the wound, until it is wrapped completely.

Elastic roller bandages are applied in the same way and are used to control swelling, support an injured limb, or provide continuous pressure. Make sure the elastic roller bandage is not too tight; frequently check the color and warmth of skin beyond the bandage. Generally, elastic roller bandages are not used over open wounds.

FIGURE 10–15. Foot or ankle bandage. Use a figure-8 pattern to provide compression for an ankle. Begin with two wraps around the foot's instep, then use figure-8 turns to wrap diagonally from foot to ankle and back.

contusions, it is generally not recommended as a bandage to cover dressings because it is difficult to determine when the bandage is too tight.

To apply a roller bandage over a dressing:

1. Place the end of the roller bandage on the dressing, then wrap it around the body part in a circular fashion.

PROGRESS CHECK

1. Bandages are applied on top of a
_____ . (wound/dressing/splint)

2. A bandage should normally not contact a
_____ . (wound/dressing/splint)

3. Cold, numb, or tingling skin distal to a bandage indicates the bandage is _____ .
(too tight/too loose/controlling bleeding)

4. A folded triangular bandage is a _____
bandage. (roller/compress/cravat)

5. The easiest roller bandages to use are
   _____ . (gauze/elastic/self-adhering)

6. You should NOT use an elastic roller bandage
   over a _____ wound.
   (closed/open/puncture)

10.3 Principles of Dressing and Bandaging

Learning Objective 6 Describe the basic
principles of dressing and bandaging wounds.

It is very important that you dress a wound carefully.
Please follow these steps to ensure proper care:

- The dressing is opened carefully and handled so it
  does not get contaminated. Always wash your
  hands before dressing and bandaging a wound.

- The original dressing is not removed; if blood soaks
  through, add another dressing on top of the original.

- The dressing adequately covers the entire wound.

- Bandages are not placed directly against the wound.

- Wounds are bandaged snugly, but not too tightly.

- Bandages are not too loose; neither the dressing nor
  the bandage should shift or slip.

- There are no loose ends of cloth, gauze, or tape that
  could get caught; when possible, you should tie
  bandage ends in a square knot, then tuck them
  under. If the knot causes discomfort, place a gauze
  or cloth pad under it.

- The bandage covers all edges of the dressing.

- Tips of the fingers and toes are left exposed when
  arms and legs are bandaged so you can check for
  impaired circulation.

- A small bandage on an arm or leg is covered with
  a larger bandage to more evenly distribute the
  pressure and to avoid causing a pressure point.

- Start a bandage on an arm or leg at the end nearest
  the hand or foot, then work upward to prevent
  applying the bandage too tightly.

- The body part is bandaged in the position in which
  it is to remain; you can bandage over a joint, but
  don't try bending the joint after you apply the
  bandage.

- Ask the victim how the bandage feels; if it is too
  tight, loosen it and make it comfortable but snug.

- Never use a circular bandage around the neck; it
  could cause strangulation.

Improvising Dressings and Bandages

In some injury situations, you may not have access to
commercial dressings or bandages; in those cases, you
need to improvise—sometimes very quickly—to provide
proper care for a victim.

There are no hard-and-fast rules for dressing and
bandaging wounds; often, adaptability and creativity
are far more important than even the best-intentioned
rules. In dressing and bandaging, use the materials you
have on hand and the methods to which you can best
adapt, as long as you meet the following conditions:

- The materials you use are as clean as possible.

- Never touch the wound itself or the part of the
  dressing that touches the wound.

- Bleeding is controlled; generally, you should not
  bandage any wound with anything other than a
  pressure bandage until bleeding has stopped.

In an emergency, you can use the following for dressings, as long as they are clean:

- Handkerchief

- Washcloth or towel

- Sheet or pillowcase

- Cloth

- Sanitary napkin

A piece of plastic wrap can be used as an occlusive
dressing.

Never use elastic bandages, fluffy cotton, cotton
balls, paper towels, toilet tissue, or any other material
that could shred, disintegrate, or cling to the wound.
Cotton balls are especially dangerous, since cotton
fibers can contaminate the wound.

If you have time, you can partially sterilize an improvised dressing by ironing it with a hot iron for a few
minutes or by boiling it and letting it dry completely
before applying it to the wound.

To improvise a roller bandage, use a necktie or strips
of cloth torn from sheets or other clean fabric.

To improvise a sling for an arm, you can use a belt,
scarf, necktie, or other wide strip of fabric, or try one of
the following:

- Bend the elbow and place the victim's hand
  inside his or her buttoned shirt or jacket at the
  appropriate level.

- Bend the elbow, then loop a belt or necktie across
  the back of the neck and around the wrist, adjusting to the appropriate level.

- Pin the victim's sleeve to his or her shirt or jacket.

- Turn the lower edge of the victim's shirt or jacket
  up over the arm, and pin the upper part to the
  shoulder so it creates a sling of an appropriate level.

Applying Special Dressings and Bandages

PRESSURE DRESSINGS

Learning Objective **7** Demonstrate how to apply a pressure dressing.

Pressure dressings are those that are applied snugly enough to create pressure against the wound. Use a pressure dressing to control profuse bleeding.

1. Cover the wound with a bulky, sterile dressing.

2. Apply direct pressure with your hand over the dressing until bleeding stops.

3. Apply a firm roller bandage (preferably self-adhering) and monitor continuously for signs that the bandage is too tight. You can also use an air splint or a blood pressure cuff to hold a pressure dressing in place (see Chapter 6). Use an elastic roller bandage only in cases of difficult-to-control, profuse bleeding.

4. If blood soaks through the original dressing and bandage, do not remove them; leave them in place and apply another dressing and roller bandage over the originals.

SLINGS

Learning Objective **8** Demonstrate how to use a sling.

Slings are used to support injuries of the shoulder, arms, or ribs. If available, use a commercial triangular bandage as a sling; in an emergency, use one of the materials or methods described in the section on improvising dressings and bandages on page 174.

To tie a triangular sling that will support an injured arm (see Figure 10-16), follow these steps:

1. Place one end of the base of an open triangular bandage over the shoulder of the uninjured side.

2. Allow the bandage to hang down in front of the chest so its apex will be behind the elbow of the injured arm.

3. Bend the arm at the elbow with the hand slightly elevated (4 to 5 inches). When possible, the fingertips should be exposed so you can monitor for impaired circulation.

4. Bring the forearm across the chest and over the bandage.

5. Carry the lower end of the bandage over the shoulder of the injured side, and tie a square knot at the uninjured side of the neck; make sure the knot is at the *side* of the neck.

6. Twist the apex of the bandage and tuck it in or pin it at the elbow. Figures 10-17 through 10-30 on

1

2   3

FIGURE 10–16. Triangular bandage as an arm sling. Support the arm slightly away from the chest, with the wrist slightly higher than the elbow. Bring the lower point up and behind the neck; tie to secure.

pages 176–178 illustrate how to apply triangular bandages and cravats to the forehead or scalp, jaw or face, eye, ear, chest or back, shoulder, elbow, hand, hip, leg, knee, ankle, and foot.

PROGRESS CHECK

1. Material used for dressings should be as _____ as possible. *(strong/thick/clean)*

2. Generally, the only dressing you should bandage in place while a wound is still bleeding is a _____ dressing. *(compress/universal/pressure)*

3. If blood soaks through the original dressing, you should _____ . *(remove it/replace it with a new dressing/leave it in place and put a new dressing on top of it)*

4. Make sure the bandage covers the entire _____ . *(wound/dressing/extremity)*

5. All loose ends of the bandage should be _____ . *(tucked in/tied/cut off)*

6. If you bandage across a joint, bandage it in _____ . *(a straightened position/a bent position/the position in which it is to remain)*

FIGURE 10–17. Triangular bandage for forehead or scalp

FIGURE 10–18. Triangular bandage for chest or back

1   2

3   4

FIGURE 10–19. Triangular bandage for shoulder

1   2

3   4   5

FIGURE 10–20. Triangular bandage for hand

1   2   3

FIGURE 10–21. Triangular bandage for hip

FIGURE 10–22. Triangular bandage for foot

FIGURE 10–23. Cravat for head or ear

FIGURE 10–24. Cravat for jaw or cheek

FIGURE 10–25. Cravat for eye; if treating an injury to the eyeball or eye socket, both eyes must be covered to prevent movement of the injured eye.

FIGURE 10–26. Cravat for elbow

FIGURE 10–27. Cravat for knee

FIGURE 10–28. Cravat for leg

FIGURE 10–29. Cravat ankle wrap

FIGURE 10–30. Cravat pressure bandage—palm of hand

Summary

- A dressing is a sterile covering for a wound; the ideal dressing is layered and consists of coarse gauze.
- Never use as a dressing paper towels, toilet tissue, or other material that could shred or cling to the wound.
- A bandage holds a dressing in place and does not touch the wound.
- An airtight (occlusive) dressing can be improvised from plastic wrap or petroleum gauze.
- Signs that a bandage is too tight include paleness or bluish discoloration (cyanosis) of the skin around the bandage and cold, tingling, or numb skin beyond the bandage.
- Triangular, cravat, and roller bandages are special kinds of bandages.

Key Terms

Make sure you understand the following key terms:

dressing
sterile
aseptic
occlusive
gauze pads
special pads
bandage
triangular bandage
cravat
roller bandage

Critical Thinking Exercise

You are approaching your school campus in your car, trying to make it on time to your early morning class. Another student is just ahead of you on his motorcycle. As he enters the intersection on a green light, a motorist runs a red light and just misses the motorcycle. Swerving to avoid a collision, the helmeted motorcyclist lays the bike down, and skids along the roadway. As you come to a rapid stop, he lays on the pavement in front of your vehicle.

1. What immediate action would you take to protect yourself and the accident victim?

2. Would you allow anyone to move him?

3. How would you determine his level of responsiveness?

4. How would you assess the victim?

5. What first aid would you give at the scene?

Chapter 10 Self-Test

Student:_____ Date:_____

Course:_____ Section #:_____

Part 1   True/False

If you believe the statement is true, circle the T. If you believe the statement is false, circle the F.

T   F   **1.** A bandage should normally be placed directly on a wound.

T   F   **2.** Bandages should be applied firmly and fastened securely.

T   F   **3.** The most popular and adaptable bandage is the cravat.

T   F   **4.** A bandage compress is a special dressing for covering open wounds and controlling heavy bleeding.

T   F   **5.** Triangular bandages are made from cloth that is approximately 20 inches square.

T   F   **6.** You should always bandage a dressing in place before the bleeding has been controlled.

T   F   **7.** Do not attempt to bandage an area any larger than the wound site.

T   F   **8.** Cotton balls make an ideal dressing because of their absorbency.

T   F   **9.** If blood soaks through the original dressing, remove it and apply a new dressing.

T   F   **10.** Elastic roller bandages should not be used except in cases of profuse bleeding.

Part 2   Multiple Choice

For each item, circle the correct answer or the phrase that best completes the statement.

1. If the fingers or toes of an injured limb become cold, swollen, blue, or numb, you should
   a. immediately loosen the bandage
   b. elevate the affected limb
   c. cover the limb with a warm blanket
   d. treat the victim for shock

2. The primary reason elastic roller bandages are not recommended for use in first aid care is
   a. they are difficult to remove
   b. they tend to stretch after a period of time
   c. they may seriously constrict blood flow
   d. they do not absorb moisture

3. Which type of knot is most frequently used in bandaging?
   a. square knot
   b. slip knot
   c. half hitch
   d. claw hitch

4. Which of the following is an example of an airtight (occlusive) dressing?
   a. adhering roller gauze
   b. plastic wrap
   c. butterfly bandage
   d. gauze roller

5. Bandages should never
   a. be applied directly over the wound without a dressing
   b. be applied tightly enough to hinder circulation
   c. be applied loosely
   d. all of the above

6. Which of the following is *not* a principle of bandaging?
   a. when bandaging the arm, leave the fingers uncovered
   b. place the body part to be bandaged in the position in which it is to remain
   c. leave no loose ends that could get caught
   d. if in doubt, leave a bandage tied loosely

7. Which of the following is *not* a guideline for use of an arm sling?
   a. it should support the entire hand
   b. the knot should not be tied in the middle of the back of the neck
   c. bend the arm at the elbow and elevate the hand 4 to 5 inches
   d. the apex of the bandage should be behind the elbow of the injured arm

8. Which of the following is *not* a recognized type of wound dressing?
   a. bacteriostatic dressing
   b. aseptic dressing
   c. occlusive dressing
   d. dry sterile dressing

Match the type of wound dressing with its description.

1. _____ A dressing that may not be sterile
2. _____ A dressing that forms an airtight seal
3. _____ A sterile dressing
4. _____ Sterile gauze saturated with a substance
   to prevent the dressing from sticking to an open wound
5. _____ A dressing that is free of moisture
6. _____ A bulky, usually sterile dressing

A. Aseptic
B. Compress
C. Wet
D. Dry sterile
E. Specialized gauze pad
F. Occlusive

Part 4   What Would You Do If?

A pedestrian is hit by a car and sustains a large avulsion on the left thigh.

11

Musculoskeletal Injuries

Learning Objectives

When you have mastered the material in this chapter, you will be able to

1 Describe the common signs and symptoms of sprains, dislocations, strains, cramps, and contusions

2 Describe and demonstrate first aid care for a sprain

3 Describe and demonstrate first aid care for a dislocation

4 Describe and demonstrate first aid care for a strain

5 Describe and demonstrate first aid care for a cramp

6 Differentiate between an open and a closed injury to a bone (fracture)

7 Describe how to assess a painful, swollen, deformed extremity

8 Describe and demonstrate first aid care for a victim with a fracture

9 State the reasons for splinting

10 List the general rules of splinting

11 List the complications of splinting

On the Scene

Seventeen-year-old Michael Draper was camping at Lake Powell, Utah, with his best friend Calvin's family. He and Calvin were competing with each other to see who could jump feet first off the highest cliff into the deep water below. From the top of a 70-foot cliff, Michael got a running start and jumped off the rock ledge. Unfortunately, his body didn't enter the water at a 90-degree angle, and the force of the water on his back and torso caused his head to flex violently forward. Michael felt a pain in his neck, but was able to surface and swim to a nearby boat. Calvin's uncle, 27-year-old Lester Johnston helped Michael into the boat, stabilized his head and neck with an improvised towel roll, and held Michael still while another family member drove them 3 hours to the nearest hospital. By the time they reached the hospital, Michael's neck pain had ceased and he only complained of pain in his wrist. He asked Lester to forget about the hospital and simply drive him home, but Lester insisted that Michael see a physician immediately. The physician X-rayed Michael's neck and discovered a burst fracture of the seventh cervical vertebrae. Bone fragments came within 2 millimeters of his spinal cord. For the next four months, Michael wore a halo-type neck brace 24 hours a day.

As a First Aider, you could be placed in a situation just like Lester's. Your actions may determine what the future holds for those in your care. If Michael wasn't cared for properly, he would probably be in a wheelchair today. However, because of the prompt and appropriate actions of a First Aider, Michael leads a normal life and has no evidence of a traumatic injury.

njuries to muscles, joints, and bones are some of the most common situations encountered by First Aiders. These injuries can range from simple and not life-threatening ones (such as a broken finger or sprained ankle) to critical, life-threatening ones (such as a fracture of the femur or spine). Regardless of whether the injury is mild or severe, your ability to provide first aid care efficiently and quickly may prevent further painful and damaging injury and may even keep the victim from suffering permanent disability or death.

This chapter covers assessment skills and care guidelines for sprains, strains, and fractures, including splinting.

11.1 The Musculoskeletal System

The human musculoskeletal system is composed of 206 bones, 6 types of joints, and more than 600 muscles. The skeletal system itself has 4 major functions:

1. It gives shape or form to the body.

2. It supports the body, allowing it to stand erect.

3. It provides the basis for locomotion, or movement, by giving muscles a place to attach, and it contains joints (where bones are joined together by ligaments) that allow movement.

4. It forms protection for major body organs, such as the brain (skull), the heart and lungs (rib cage), pelvic organs, and the spinal cord (vertebrae).

Bones

Bones are made up of dense tissue that is richly supplied by nerves and blood vessels; some bones even manufacture red blood cells. When bones are broken, bleeding can be serious.

The bones of children are softer and more porous than those of adults, so they tend to break more easily. The bones of the elderly also tend to break more easily—as people age, their bones naturally lose mass and density.

Bones are classified by their size and shape: long bones (such as those of the thigh, lower leg, upper arm, and forearm); short bones (such as those of the hands and feet); flat bones (such as the ribs and the shoulder blade); and irregular bones (such as the vertebrae and the skull bones).

Joints

Joints are formed when the ends of two or more bones come together in a single place. If joints allow movement, the ends of the bone are held together by ligaments, tough and fibrous connective tissues. Some joints, such as the shoulder, allow a wide range of movement; others, such as the hip, allow a more limited range of movement. In some cases, the bone ends are fused and the joints don't move; a good example are the joints of the skull.

When a joint is forced beyond its normal range of motion, the ligament can tear, causing swelling, pain, and deformity. These kinds of injuries are especially serious when they involve weight-bearing joints, such as knees and ankles.

Muscle

Muscle is a special type of tissue that contracts, or shortens, when stimulated. All body movement results from muscles contracting and relaxing. An involuntary muscle is one that is not controlled by conscious thought. Examples of involuntary muscles are those of the heart and the digestive tract, such as the esophagus, stomach, and colon. The voluntary (skeletal) muscles are under conscious control. Voluntary muscles make up the arms, legs, upper back, and hips and cover the ribs and the abdomen. Skeletal muscles are attached to the bones either directly or by tendons (tough, fibrous, connective tissue). When a voluntary muscle is stimulated to contract, it shortens and pulls on a part of the skeletal system, causing movement.

Tendons

Tendons are highly specialized connective tissue. They allow for maximum strength because they are oriented in the direction of muscle pull. Tendons form a shiny white band that attaches to the muscles and, through a network of tiny fibers, connects with a bone. If sharp, sudden force is applied, the tendon may pull loose from the bone and may even pull a small piece of bone with it.

Ligaments

Ligaments connect bone to bone. When a ligament is injured, sections of it give way at different places along the entire ligament length. Skin lacerations are rarely involved. Ligaments are usually injured without any external tissue damage.

Most joints of the body have ligaments at the side farthest from the center plane of motion. More complex joints (like the knee) feature ligaments that are attached to the joint capsule. The ligament is often injured simultaneously with the joint; consequent internal bleeding causes early joint swelling.

11.2 Sprains, Dislocations, Strains, and Cramps

> Learning Objective **1** Describe the common signs and symptoms of sprains, dislocations, strains, cramps, and contusions.

A **sprain** is an injury to a joint in which ligaments are stretched and partially or completely torn, usually from the sudden twisting of the joint beyond its normal range of motion. It can be very difficult to tell the difference between a sprain and a fracture, because the signs and symptoms are similar. A **dislocation** is the separation of a bone end from a joint, leaving the bone end out of alignment with the joint. For the common signs and symptoms of dislocation, see Figure 11-1. A **strain** is a soft-tissue injury of the muscle. A **cramp** is an uncontrolled spasm of a muscle. A **contusion** is a bruise to muscle.

Sprains

The signs of a severe sprain are similar to those of a fracture. The most common signs and symptoms are

- Pain
- Swelling
- Deformity
- Discoloration of the skin
- Inability to use the affected part normally

The joints most often sprained are the thumb and fingers, knee, and ankle. Severe sprains may rupture ligaments or dislocate or fracture the bones that form the

> **sprain** An injury in which ligaments are stretched and partially or completely torn
>
> **dislocation** An injury in which the joint comes apart and stays apart; the bone ends are no longer in contact with each other
>
> **strain** An injury to a muscle that occurs when the muscle is stretched beyond its normal range of motion, causing the muscle to tear
>
> **cramp** Uncontrolled spasm of a muscle
>
> **contusion** A bruise to the tissue of a muscle

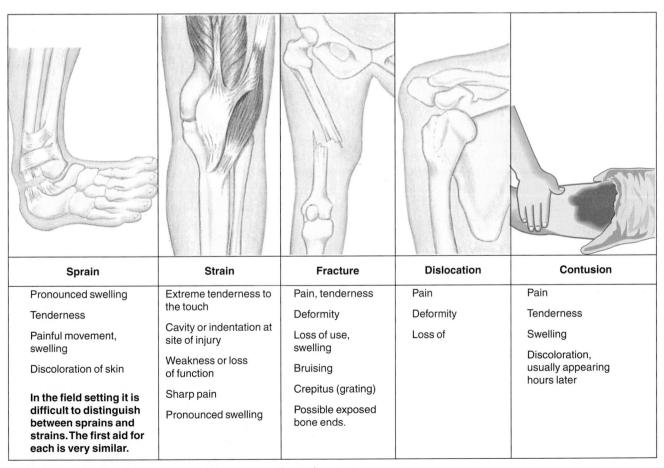

Sprain	Strain	Fracture	Dislocation	Contusion
Pronounced swelling	Extreme tenderness to the touch	Pain, tenderness	Pain	Pain
Tenderness		Deformity	Deformity	Tenderness
Painful movement, swelling	Cavity or indentation at site of injury	Loss of use, swelling	Loss of	Swelling
Discoloration of skin	Weakness or loss of function	Bruising		Discoloration, usually appearing hours later
In the field setting it is difficult to distinguish between sprains and strains. The first aid for each is very similar.	Sharp pain	Crepitus (grating)		
	Pronounced swelling	Possible exposed bone ends.		

FIGURE 11–1. Signs and symptoms of common orthopedic injuries

joint. It is critical to quickly apply cold to the sprain. Mild sprains, which only stretch ligament fibers, generally heal quickly (within a few days to a few weeks).

> Learning Objective **2** Describe and demonstrate first aid care for a sprain.

In most cases, it would be difficult to tell the differences between a fracture and a sprain without an X-ray, so you should care for a sprain as if it were a fracture, and immobilize it accordingly. The goal of first aid treatment is to prevent further injury to the ligament. To treat, do not allow the victim to use the sprained joint; provide care based on the acronym RICE:[1]

1. **R**est—Have the victim stay off the injured part completely and not use the joint at all. Splint the sprained joint to give it complete rest. Any movement increases blood circulation to the joint, which increases swelling.

2. **I**ce—Cold relieves pain and prevents or reduces swelling and inflammation. Immediately put cold packs, crushed ice, or cold towels on the injured area, or immerse it in ice water for 20 to 30 minutes at a time every 2 hours. *Don't stop applying cold too soon;* it should be continued for the first 24 to 48 hours. (Don't apply it any longer than 20 to 30 minutes at a time, or you could cause frostbite; always remove the cold pack when the skin becomes numb.) You can make an ice pack by putting crushed ice or ice cubes in a towel or a double plastic bag or a hot water bottle or ice bag; you can also use a bag of frozen corn or peas (refreeze it and use it later as an ice pack). If you use a commercially manufactured chemical cold pack, follow manufacturer's directions; in most cases, you will snap or squeeze the pack to activate it. Use each chemical cold pack only once, and take extra care not to rupture or puncture the bag—leaks can cause chemical burns. If needed, hold the cold pack in place with an elastic bandage, taking care not to wrap the bandage too tightly. Do not apply cold if the victim has Raynaud's syndrome, circulatory disease, an abnormal sensitivity to cold, or if the injured area is or has been frostbitten.

3. **C**ompression—To limit internal bleeding and compress fluid from the injury site, wrap a compression bandage (usually an elastic one) in an overlapping spiral that supports the entire injured area. Use a 2-inch-wide elastic bandage for injuries of the wrist and hand; a 3-inch-wide bandage for injuries of the

arm, elbow, or ankle; and a 4- to 6-inch-wide bandage for injuries of the leg, knee, or ankle. The victim should wear the bandage continuously for 18 to 24 hours, except when applying a cold pack. The bandage should exert even pressure without being too tight; fill any hollow areas with padding (such as a folded sock or washcloth) before you apply the bandage. Start several inches below the injured area, and wrap in upward, overlapping spirals, gradually wrapping more loosely above the injury. Leave the fingers and toes exposed so you can make sure the bandage is not too tight. Pale skin, pain, tingling, and numbness are signs that the bandage is too tight.

4. **E**levation—Limits circulation, reduces swelling, and encourages lymphatic drainage. Elevate the injured area to heart level or just above *if* you do not suspect fracture.

For maximum effect, start the RICE treatment within 10 minutes of the injury; follow up by activating the EMS system or transporting the victim to a medical facility.

Dislocations

A dislocation is a displacement or separation of a bone from its normal position at a joint, usually caused by severe force. The joint comes apart and stays apart, and the ends of the bones are no longer in contact. The joints most frequently dislocated are those of the hip, knee, ankle, shoulder, elbow, and finger.

Signs and symptoms of a dislocation are similar to those of a fracture. The principal symptoms are pain or a feeling of pressure over the involved joint and a loss of motion in the joint. The principal sign is deformity. If the dislocated bone end is pressing on a nerve, numbness or paralysis may occur below the dislocation; if it presses on a blood vessel, loss of pulse may occur below the dislocation.

> Learning Objective **3** Describe and demonstrate first aid care for a dislocation.

Immediately assess blood flow by assessing capillary refill and checking distal pulses, and assess nerve function by checking for loss of sensation, numbness, or paralysis. Absence of a pulse or diminished capillary refill means the extremity is not receiving enough blood; activate the EMS system *immediately.* Because dislocations are often accompanied by fractures, you should

1. Immobilize all dislocations *in the position found.* Splint above and below the dislocated joint with an appropriate splint that will keep the joint immobile. (See Figure 11-2 for an example.) *Do not try to*

---

[1]Alton L. Thygerson, "Muscle Injuries," *Emergency* (July 1985): 50–51; Susanna Levin, "Sprains Are a Pain," *Walking Magazine* (June/July 1987): 75.

FIGURE 11–2. Use of cravat with pad and sling to immobilize dislocated shoulder

straighten (**reduce**) *the dislocation.* Check the distal pulse and capillary refill again after you have applied the splint.

2. Use the RICE method.

3. Treat for shock; keep the victim warm and quiet and in the position most comfortable.

Strains

Often the result of overexertion, strains are a stretching and tearing of muscle fibers. They occur when muscles are stretched beyond their normal range or when cold or tight muscles are suddenly exerted. Neglected, they often recur. The lower back is a common area for strains. Strains are usually marked by rapid and pronounced swelling. Some victims may say they felt a burning or tearing sensation when the injury occurred.

Signs and symptoms of a strain are:

- Extreme pain
- Severe tenderness
- Pain or stiffness if the muscle is moved
- A bump or indentation that can be seen or felt
- Loss of function of the injured muscle

Learning Objective **4** Describe and demonstrate first aid care for a strain.

Assume that the injury may be a fracture, and immobilize accordingly; then

1. Place the victim in a comfortable position that takes pressure off the strained muscles.

2. Apply cold directly to the strained area, as described in step 2 of the RICE system.

3. Activate the EMS system or transport the victim to a medical facility.

Cramps

It's not known exactly what causes cramps—uncontrolled spasms of a muscle that cause severe pain and loss or restriction of movement—but they are associated with certain illnesses, can follow physical activity, are a sign of dehydration, may occur when a victim loses too many electrolytes (usually through heavy perspiration), and sometimes occur during sleep.

Learning Objective **5** Describe and demonstrate first aid care for a cramp.

Though it may seem natural to massage a cramp, massage can actually increase the pain and rarely helps relieve the cramping. Instead, treat a cramp as follows:

1. Have the victim gently stretch the cramping muscle; gradual lengthening of the muscle can relieve the cramp by lengthening the muscle fibers. Because cramps are extremely painful, the victim may need you to gently pull the affected area to stretch out the muscle. If the muscle is in the calf of the leg, standing on the affected leg will lengthen the muscle and relieve the cramp.

2. Apply steady, firm pressure to the cramping muscle with the heel of your hand.

3. Apply an ice pack over the cramped muscle.

4. Try using an acupressure point: pinch the upper lip hard to relieve cramping of a calf muscle.

5. If the cramp occurs during or after heavy physical activity, have the victim drink a commercial electrolyte drink or lightly salted water (¼ teaspoon of salt dissolved in a quart of water).

reduce To straighten

Muscle Contusions

A muscle contusion is a bruise to the muscle tissue that usually occurs from a direct blow to the muscle. The signs and symptoms are:

- Pain
- Tenderness
- Swelling
- Discoloration that usually occurs several hours after the injury

To care for a muscle contusion, use the RICE procedure.

PROGRESS CHECK

1. An injury in which ligaments are stretched and partially or completely torn is a _____ . (sprain/strain/dislocation)

2. A soft-tissue injury or muscle spasm around a joint is a _____ . (sprain/strain/dislocation)

3. You should care for sprains and dislocations as if they were _____ . (life threatening/fractures/strains)

4. Treat a cramp with _____ . (gentle massage/firm massage/stretching)

 ## Injuries to Bones

Learning Objective 6 Differentiate between an open and a closed injury to a bone (fracture).

A fracture is a crack or break in the continuity of a bone (see Figure 11-3). A bone or joint injury can be one of two kinds (see Figure 11-4):

- Closed (simple), in which the overlying skin is intact; no wound is nearby.
- Open (compound), in which the skin over the fracture site has been damaged or broken, either by the ends of the bone or by the blow that broke the bone; the bone might or might not protrude through the wound, and you might or might not be able to see the bone through the wound (see Figure 11-5 on page 190). The greatest threat in a compound fracture is to the soft tissue and organs that lie around the bone ends.

In assessing and treating injuries to the bones and joints, it is important to determine the mechanism of injury as well as the signs and symptoms of the injury itself (see Figures 11-6 through 11-8 on page 190).

Impacted Oblique Transverse

Comminuted Greenstick Spiral

FIGURE 11–3. Types of fractures

CLOSED
Skin is intact.

OPEN
Bone is protruding or has
protruded through the skin.

FIGURE 11–4. Closed and open fractures

Mechanisms of Injury

The force that injures a bone or joint may also cause injuries to the surrounding soft tissues (such as nerves and arteries), or even to body areas distant from the bone injury site. You can get a good idea of how much damage may have occurred by determining the mechanism of injury.

As you approach the accident scene and talk with the victim or bystanders, try to imagine the forces the victim's body was subjected to and the direction in which those forces propelled the body. The forces that may cause bone and joint injury (see Figure 11-9 on page 190) include the following.

DIRECT FORCE

The fracture from direct force, or a direct blow, occurs at the point of impact. For example, a victim in an automobile accident who is not wearing a seatbelt might be thrust forward, the knees hitting the dashboard; as a result, the patella (kneecap) is fractured.

INDIRECT FORCE

Indirect force affects one end of a limb, causing injury to the limb some distance away from the point of impact. In this case, the previous scenario might lead to a hip fracture or dislocation. Another example is a woman thrown from a horse may land on two outstretched hands. One arm sustains a fractured wrist, and the clavicle (collarbone) at the end of the other arm is fractured.

TWISTING FORCE

When a bone is fractured by twisting force, one part of the bone remains stationary while the rest of the bone twists. For example, a child running across a field may step into a hole. The foot is rammed snugly into the hole and stays stationary, while the rest of the lower leg twists

FIGURE 11–5. X-ray of a broken humerus

FIGURE 11–6
Closed fracture
of the humerus

FIGURE 11–7
Open fracture
of the fibula

FIGURE 11–8
Closed fracture;
observe the
deformity.

Direct force

Indirect force

Severe twisting
force

FIGURE 11–9. Different types of force can cause different types of injuries.

and is fractured. Bone and joint injuries from twisting force commonly occur in football or skiing accidents.

Signs and Symptoms

> Learning Objective 7   Describe how to assess a painful, swollen, deformed extremity.

With rare exceptions, fractures and other bone injuries are not life threatening. And although they are often the most obvious and dramatic injuries a victim suffers, fractures may not necessarily be the most serious. Therefore, it is important that you complete the primary survey and manage any life-threatening conditions *before* you look for the signs and symptoms of bone and joint injury (see Figure 11-10):

- Deformity, shortening, or angulation; deformity is not always obvious, but when the normal and the injured extremity are compared, there is a difference in the size, length, shape, or position of the injured one.

- Pain and tenderness, usually only at the site of injury.

- Increased skin temperature at the injury site.

- **Crepitus**, a grating noise that can be heard or sensation that can be felt as broken fragments of bone grind against each other. *Never move an injured area in an attempt to hear whether there is crepitus.*

- Rapid and immediate swelling, which is caused by bleeding.

- Discoloration or redness, followed by bruising 2 or 3 days later.

- Open wound, with or without exposed bone ends; it may be a puncture wound.

- Joint locked into position.

- Guarding (victim tries to hold the injured area in a comfortable position and avoids moving it).

- Possible loss of function; in some cases, the victim can use or move the bone with little or no pain, even when there is a fracture.

Children's bones are much more flexible than those of adults, and fractures are often incomplete (called *greenstick fractures*). Localized pain and swelling in a child often indicates fracture or possibly an injury to the growth plate, not a sprain.

First Aid Care

> Learning Objective 8   Describe and demonstrate first aid care for a victim with a fracture.

It is difficult to tell whether a bone is broken, so when in doubt, always treat the injury as a fracture. Fractures should be treated in priority order, as follows:

- Spinal fractures

- Fractures of the head and rib cage

- Pelvic fractures

- Fractures of the lower limbs

- Fractures of the upper limbs

Remember—if there was enough force to damage the pelvis or to cause severe head or facial injuries, assume there are also injuries to the spine.

The most important first aid care is immobilization of any suspected fracture or extensive soft-tissue injury. You should immobilize before you apply ice or elevate the injured part; doing so

- Minimizes damage to soft tissue, muscle, or bone sheathing that may become wedged between fracture fragments

> **crepitus** grating sound or sensation that occurs when the ends of a broken bone rub against each other

Bruising	Tenderness
Pain	Discoloration
Swelling	Exposed bone ends
Deformity	Disability

FIGURE 11–10. Signs and symptoms of fractures

■ Prevents a closed fracture from becoming an open one

■ Prevents more damage to surrounding nerves, blood vessels, and other tissues from the broken bone ends

■ Minimizes bleeding and swelling

■ Diminishes pain, which helps control shock

■ Prevents restriction of blood flow by bone ends compressing blood vessels

Any fracture of the spine is always a first priority for treatment; for guidelines in managing spine fractures, see Chapter 13. Treat a fracture as follows (see Figures 11-11 and 11-12):

1. Gently remove any clothes that cover the injured area. Cut clothing at the seams to avoid unnecessary movement of the injured area.

2. Support the injured part; gently remove clothing and jewelry around the injury site without moving the injured area.

3. Cover any open wounds with sterile dressings to control bleeding and prevent infection. Gently wipe away dirt and debris, and irrigate the exposed bone end with clean water.

4. Assess blood flow and nerve function; this step is essential, since the most serious complication of fracture is reduced blood flow and subsequent tissue death. Check the distal pulse of the suspected fracture site—the radial pulse of the wrist (on the thumb side of the wrist) for an arm fracture, the posterior tibial pulse (between the inside ankle bone and the Achilles tendon) for a leg fracture. *Lack of a pulse indicates a significant medical emergency*—tissues of the arms and legs can't survive for more than 2 to 3 hours without blood flow. Seek immediate medical attention. Gently manipulate the limb once in an attempt to restore circulation. Also check the capillary refill by pressing on the nailbeds. As you let go, the nails will turn from white to pink, if normal. To assess nerve function, gently squeeze the victim's fingers or toes; ask the victim to wiggle the fingers or toes if they are not injured. If the victim can't feel you squeeze the fingers or toes, there may be nerve or spinal damage.

5. If there is severe deformity or angulation, apply minimal **traction**—a firm, steady pull to bring the limb into more normal alignment—except for crushing injuries; immobilize joints above and below the fracture. When applying traction, grasp an arm with one hand on either side of the injury, and pull gently and steadily in line with the bone. For a fractured leg, position both your hands below the fracture and pull gently and steadily downward. *Do not attempt to push bone ends back underneath the skin, and avoid excessive pressure on the wound.* Remember that traction is not used to completely correct a deformity—something that can be done only in a hospital—but to *reduce* the amount of angulation. *As a general rule, never straighten a wrist, elbow, knee, or shoulder.* Except for the wrist and shoulder, make one attempt to straighten closed, angulated fractures *if no distal pulse is found.* If pain, resistance, or crepitus increases, stop. Wrap from the distal end of the splint to the proximal end; splint firmly enough to immobilize but not tightly enough to stop blood circulation. Follow specific guidelines for splinting listed in the next section.

6. Check distal pulses and capillary refill and sensation after the splint is in place to make sure circulation is still adequate.

7. Use the RICE procedure.

> **traction** gentle, steady pulling movement of a bone in alignment with its natural position

FIGURE 11–11 An open tibia fracture

FIGURE 11–12. Support and stabilize the limb above and below the injury, control bleeding, locate a distal pulse, and apply a splint. Brace the fracture with your hand under the fracture site.

1. In assessing for fracture, it is important to consider the _____ as well as the signs and symptoms. *(history/mechanism of injury/pain)*

2. Though fractures may be the most obvious and dramatic injuries suffered by a victim, they are often not the most _____ ones. *(life-threatening/easy-to-manage/painful)*

3. Before you try to identify fractures, you should complete _____ . *(artificial ventilation/chest compressions/the primary survey)*

4. The most important first aid care for suspected facture is _____ . *(control of bleeding/immobilization/replacing bone ends)*

5. _____ helps minimize damage to soft tissue, surrounding nerves, and blood vessels by broken bone ends. *(Immobilization/Splinting/Compression)*

6. If the forearm is fractured, you should also immobilize the _____ . *(upper arm/shoulder/wrist and elbow)*

7. You _____ try to straighten the wrist, elbow, knee, or shoulder. *(should/should not)*

11.4 Splinting

Learning Objective **9** State the reasons for splinting.

Any device used to immobilize (prevent movement of) a fracture or dislocation is a *splint*. A splint can be soft or rigid, commercially manufactured or improvised from virtually any object that can provide stability.

Splints are used to support and immobilize suspected fractures, dislocations, or severe sprains; to help control bleeding; to help control pain; and to prevent further damage to tissues from the movement of bone ends. Any victim with suspected fracture, dislocation, or severe sprain should be splinted before being moved.

Rules for Splinting

Learning Objective **10** List the general rules of splinting.

Regardless of where you apply the splint (see Figure 11-13), follow these general rules:

- Do not splint if it will cause more pain for the victim.

- Both before and after you apply the splint, assess the pulse and sensation below the injury. You should evaluate these signs every 15 minutes after applying the splint to make sure the splint is not impairing circulation.

- Immobilize the joints both above and below the injury.

- Splint an injury in the position you found it. If there is no distal pulse or movement, you may attempt to return the bone to its normal alignment by placing one hand above the injury and another below. Then pull with gentle traction while moving the injury back toward the correct anatomical position.

- Remove or cut away all clothing around the injury site with a pair of bandage scissors so you won't accidentally move the fractured bone ends and complicate the injury. Remove all jewelry around the fracture site.

- Cover all wounds, including open fractures, with sterile dressing before applying a splint (see Figure 11-14 on page 194), then gently bandage. Avoid excessive pressure on the wound.

- If there is a severe deformity or the distal extremity is cyanotic or lacks pulses, align the injured limb with gentle traction before splinting, following the guidelines above.

- Never intentionally replace protruding bone ends.

- Pad the splint to prevent pressure and discomfort to the victim.

- Apply the splint before trying to move the victim.

- When in doubt, splint the injury.

- If the victim shows signs of shock, maintain body temperature as needed, align the victim in the normal anatomical position and arrange for immediate transport without taking the time to apply a splint.

Types of Splints

There are three general types of splints:

RIGID SPLINTS

Rigid splints are commercially manufactured inflexible devices (see Figure 11-15 on page 194) made of wood, aluminum, wire, plastic, cardboard, or compressed wood fibers. Some are designed in specific shapes for arms and legs and are equipped with Velcro closures; others are pliable enough to be molded to fit any appendage. One of the most popular commercial

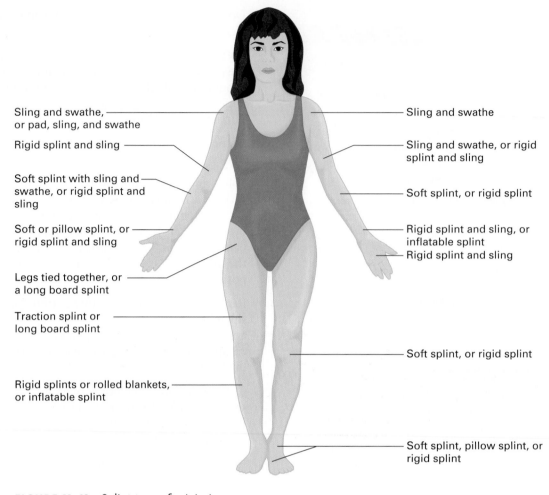

Sling and swathe, or pad, sling, and swathe

Rigid splint and sling

Soft splint with sling and swathe, or rigid splint and sling

Soft or pillow splint, or rigid splint and sling

Legs tied together, or a long board splint

Traction splint or long board splint

Rigid splints or rolled blankets, or inflatable splint

Sling and swathe

Sling and swathe, or rigid splint and sling

Soft splint, or rigid splint

Rigid splint and sling, or inflatable splint

Rigid splint and sling

Soft splint, or rigid splint

Soft splint, pillow splint, or rigid splint

FIGURE 11–13. Splint types for injuries

FIGURE 11–14. Splint immobilizes fractures and dislocations.

FIGURE 11–15. A set of commercial splints

FIGURE 11–16. SAM splint

FIGURE 11–17. You must know how to make emergency splints from whatever materials are available.

splints is the SAM splint (see Figure 11-16), a light-weight splint made of pliable aluminum sandwiched between layers of foam; it can be molded to fit any body part. Some commercial splints come with washable pads, but others must be padded before being applied. The splint must be long enough to extend both above and below the fracture.

TRACTION SPLINTS

Traction splints gently pull in the direction opposite the injury, alleviating pain, reducing blood loss, and minimizing further injury. Traction splints are not intended to reduce the fracture, but simply to immobilize the bone ends and prevent further injury. A traction splint should be used only for a broken thigh, and should be applied only by EMTs or those who have had special training in applying traction splints.

IMPROVISED SPLINTS

You may have access to a commercial splint, but it is much more likely that you will need to improvise at the scene. A splint can be improvised from a cardboard box, folded newspaper, cane, ironing board, pillow, rolled-up magazine, folded blanket, baseball bat, umbrella, broom handle, catcher's shin guard, or any other similar object (see Figure 11-17).

You can also use a *self-splint* (also called an *anatomical splint*) by tying or taping an injured part to an adjacent uninjured part; for example, splint a finger to a finger, a toe to a toe, a leg to the other leg, or an arm to the chest (see Figure 11-18). An effective improvised splint must be:

- Light in weight, but firm and rigid

- Long enough to extend past the joints and prevent movement on either side of the fracture

- As wide as the thickest part of the fractured limb

- Padded well so the inner surfaces are not in contact with the skin

FIGURE 11–18. Improvised self-splint

An ordinary bed pillow can be an effective improvised splint when wrapped around the area and secured with several cravats.

Hazards of Improper Splinting

Learning Objective 11 List the complications of splinting.

Improper splinting can:

- Compress the nerves, tissues, and blood vessels under the splint, aggravating the existing injury and causing new injury

- Delay the transport of a victim who has a life-threatening injury

- Reduce distal circulation, threatening the extremity

- Aggravate the bone or joint injury by allowing movement of the bone fragments or bone ends or by forcing bone ends beneath the skin surface

- Cause or aggravate damage to the tissues, nerves, blood vessels, or muscles as a result of excessive bone or joint movement

Special Considerations in Splinting

Never straighten a fracture or dislocation of the spine, elbow, wrist, hip, or knee—these joints are too close to blood vessels or nerves that could be permanently damaged. There are certain special techniques to remember when splinting long bones or joints or when using a traction splint.

SPLINTING A LONG BONE

Splint a long bone as follows:

1. Gently grasp the limb and apply gentle, steady pressure to stabilize the bone.

2. Assess the pulse and sensory function below the injury site. Look for **paresthesia** (a pricking or tingling sensation that indicates loss of circulation) or paralysis. If the injury involves an upper extremity, nerve function is intact if the victim can make a fist, undo the fist, spread the fingers, and make a hitchhiking sign with the thumb. If the injury involves a lower extremity, nerve function is intact if the victim can tighten the kneecap and move the foot up and down as if pumping an automobile accelerator.

3. If the limb is severely deformed, is cyanotic, or lacks distal pulses, align it by providing steady, gentle pressure along with traction (see Figure 11-19); if pain or crepitus increases, stop.

4. Measure the splint to make sure it is the right size. The splint should be long enough to immobilize the entire bone plus the joints above and below the fracture site (see Figure 11-20). If you are immobilizing the leg, ideally, the outside splint should be long enough to reach from the victim's armpit to below the heel; the inner splint should be long enough to reach from the groin to below the heel.

5. Apply the splint, immobilizing the bone and the joint both above and below the injury (see Figures 11-21 through 11-23).

6. Secure the entire injured extremity; you can use the straps or Velcro closures that come with commercial splints, or wrap roller bandages around improvised splints and secure them with cravats.

7. Immobilize the hand or foot in the normal position of function. Make sure you can still see and feel the hand or foot so you can assess pulse and sensation.

> **paresthesia** Pricking or tingling sensation that indicates loss of circulation

FIGURE 11–19. Applying traction

FIGURE 11–20. Cardboard splint of the lower arm

A pad is between the fractured arm and the body. A padded splint is tied to the outer arm.

The arm is supported by a wide cravat. The knot is to the side, not pressed against the neck.

A swathe binds the arm to the chest.

FIGURE 11–21. A fracture of the humerus immobilized by a splint

Splinting a Joint

Splint a joint as follows:

1. Stabilize the joint manually; one First Aider should apply firm but gentle stabilization while a second readies the splint.

2. Assess the pulse and sensory function below the injury site; check for paresthesia or paralysis.

3. Immobilize the site of the injury in the position you found it with a splint.

4. Immobilize the site of the injury with a splint.

5. Immobilize the bones both above and below the injured joint to help prevent accidental movement of the joint (see Figures 11-24 through 11-27 on pages 198–199).

6. After applying the splint, reassess pulse and sensation every few minutes throughout care.

FIGURE 11–22. Pillow splint for fractures of the forearm, wrist, and hand

> **PROGRESS CHECK**
>
> 1. You should not apply a split if it will cause more _____ for the victim. *(pain/disability/deformity)*
>
> 2. You should assess the victim's _____ both before and after you apply a splint. *(breathing/pulses/level of consciousness)*
>
> 3. You should immobilize _____ both above and below the injury. *(bones/ joints/ tissues)*

FIGURE 11–23. Fixation splint of the tibia/fibula, using padded boards

FIGURE 11–24. Some splints can be formed to the injured limb, but they should be well-padded, and secured with gauze rolls.

FIGURE 11–25. Fractured elbow immobilized with a board splint

FIGURE 11–26. Splint a dislocated or fractured elbow in the position found.

FIGURE 11–27. Immobilizing a fracture of the ankle and foot; always untie laces if a shoe is left on the foot.

Summary

- A sprain is an injury in which ligaments are stretched and partially or completely torn.

- A strain is a soft-tissue injury or muscle spasm around a joint.

- Use gentle stretching to care for a cramp; you can also apply ice or firm pressure to a cramping muscle.

- A dislocation is the displacement of a bone end from a joint.

- First aid care for sprains consists of the RICE treatment—rest, ice, compression, and elevation.

- You should always assume that strains and dislocations are features, and treat accordingly.

- Never try to straighten a dislocation; splint it in the position you found it.

- A fracture is a break in the continuity of a bone; fractures can be either open (in which the skin over the fracture site is broken) or closed (in which the skin over the fracture site is intact).

- Injuries to bones can be caused by direct force, indirect force, or twisting force.

- A fracture may often be the most obvious or dramatic injury the victim has, but few are life threatening;

therefore, it is critical that you complete the primary survey and manage life-threatening conditions before attempting to identify fractures.

- Fractures should be treated in priority order: spinal fractures, fractures of the head and rib cage, pelvic fractures, fractures of the lower limbs, and fractures of the upper limbs.

- The most important first aid care for fractures is immobilization; you should always immobilize before you apply ice or elevate the injured part.

- As a general rule, never straighten a wrist, elbow, knee, ankle, or shoulder.

- Always immobilize the joints just above and below a fractured bone; always immobilize the bones just above and below an injured joint.

- Always check pulses both before and after you splint.

- Any device used to immobilize a fracture or dislocation is a splint; splints are used to support, immobilize, and protect injured parts. You can use a rigid splint, traction splint, or improvised splint.

- Never try to straighten a dislocation; splint it in the position you found it.

- Improvised splints must be light in weight but firm and rigid; long enough to extend past the joints and prevent movement on either side of the fracture; as wide as the thickest part of the fractured limb; and padded well so the inner surfaces are not in contact with the victim's skin.
- Improper splinting can compress nerves, tissues, and blood vessels and can reduce circulation to the limb.

Key Terms

Make sure you understand the following key terms:

sprain
dislocation
strain
cramp
contusion
reduce
creptitus
traction
paresthesia

Critical Thinking Exercise

Summer has finally arrived. You join your friend for a great afternoon swimming at a favorite local spot, an old gravel pit that fills with water from the river nearby. Your friend Jeff dives in first, unaware that ledges of rock jut out from that side of the gravel pit. Shortly after plunging into the water, Jeff's head collides with a rock shelf. He comes to the surface and struggles to say that his legs are tingling and he can't move his arms very well. Blood flows from a gash in his scalp.

1. What is your first immediate action to protect Jeff's life?

2. How will you determine the extent of Jeff's injury?

3. How would you stabilize Jeff's head and neck so that no further spinal damage would occur?

Chapter 11 Self-Test

Student: _____ Date: _____

Course: _____ Section #: _____

Part 1   True/False

If you believe the statement is true, circle the T. If you believe the statement is false, circle the F.

T F **1.** It is usually impossible to tell the difference between a sprain and a closed fracture without an X-ray.

T F **2.** To test for fracture, ask the victim to try to move the injured part or walk on the injured leg.

T F **3.** In cases of suspected dislocation, correct the deformity before splinting it.

T F **4.** Permanent nerve damage can result from a splint that is too tight; you should carefully monitor for signs of discoloration and swelling.

T F **5.** Apply heat to a sprained joint for the first 24 hours.

T F **6.** A fracture is a crack or splinter in a bone that is not broken.

T F **7.** A closed fracture can become an open fracture through mishandling.

T F **8.** A splint should be placed directly against the skin without padding or dressings for maximum effectiveness.

T F **9.** A splint should not extend beyond the joints above and below the suspected fracture.

T F **10.** A fractured elbow should always be immobilized in the position in which it is found.

Part 2   Multiple Choice

For each item, circle the correct answer or the phrase that best completes the statement.

1. The primary objective in first aid care for a fracture is to
   a. set the bone
   b. immobilize the fracture
   c. push a protruding bone end back into its original position
   d. all of the above

2. In cases of fracture, the purpose of a splint is to
   a. reduce the chance of shock
   b. decrease pain
   c. prevent motion of the injured limb
   d. all of the above

3. What is a sign or symptom of a strain?
   a. immediate swelling
   b. inability to move
   c. sharp pain that lasts for prolonged periods
   d. a sudden burning sensation

4. An injury in which ligaments are partially torn is
   a. a sprain
   b. a strain

   c. tendinitis
   d. a dislocation

5. Displacement of a bone end from a joint with associated ligament damage is called a
   a. strain
   b. sprain
   c. dislocation
   d. fracture

6. To treat a bleeding open fracture
   a. wash the wound thoroughly with either disinfectant or clear running water
   b. control bleeding with pressure through a dressing
   c. if the bone is protruding, do not cover the wound
   d. replace bone fragments before covering the wound with a dressing

7. If you suspect a fracture of the upper arm, you should immobilize

    a. the elbow
    b. the upper arm
    c. the shoulder
    d. all of the above

8. The **I** in **RICE** stands for

    a. immobilize
    b. ice
    c. injury
    d. instant pain

Part 3   Matching

Match each of the four conditions with both its definition and its care.

1. _____ Strain
2. _____ Dislocation
3. _____ Sprain
4. _____ Fracture

A. Overstraining of muscles and/or tendons, causing muscles and tendons to stretch and/or rupture
B. Displacement of bone ends that form the joint
C. Crack or break in the continuity of the bone
D. Injury to ligaments around the joint, producing undue stretching or tearing of tissues
E. Make comfortable and apply cold
F. Control any bleeding and immobilize
G. Use rest, ice, compression, and elevation
H. Mobilize in the position found

Part 4   What Would You Do If?

1. At the scene of an automobile accident, you diagnose a young man as having a closed fracture of the forearm. You also suspect that he might have a spinal injury. What first aid would you administer if an ambulance will reach you within 10 minutes? How would you splint the fractures if no ambulance will respond and you will have to transport the victim in a medical facility?

12

Common Sport and Recreational Injuries

Learning Objectives

When you have mastered the material in this chapter, you will be able to

1 Describe and demonstrate first aid care of a fractured clavicle

2 Describe and demonstrate first aid care of a shoulder separation

3 Describe the usual mechanism of injury that causes a shoulder dislocation

4 Describe the usual mechanism of injury that causes a dislocated elbow

5 Describe the signs and symptoms of a fractured radial head

6 Define Colles's and Smith's fractures and describe the usual mechanism of injury for each

7 Describe the mechanisms of injury that cause fractures to the carpal and metacarpal bones, dislocations of the carpal bones, and fractured or dislocated fingers

8 Describe first aid care for injuries to the hip

9 Describe first aid care for injuries to the hamstring and knee ligaments

10 Describe the signs and symptoms of a dislocated kneecap (patella)

11 Describe the first aid care of an achilles tendon rupture

12 Describe the first aid care of sprains or fractures of the ankle and foot

On the Scene

Sixteen-year-old Shauna Randall was playing volleyball on a field behind the high school where two coaches had set up a series of nets. When a player from the opposing team spiked the ball just over the net, Shauna dived to reach it; instead, her outstretched hand slammed into the turf.

Coach Linda Ames ran to Shauna, who was complaining of pain in the shoulder and holding her elbow up into her side. Coach Ames sent another player into the gym to call for emergency help, then assessed Shauna. There was an obvious lump over the tip of Shauna's shoulder that was extremely painful to the touch; Coach Ames suspected a second- or third-degree separation of the acromioclavicular joint—more simply stated, shoulder separation.

Helping Shauna to her office, Coach Ames used both vertical and horizontal swathes and a sling to support Shauna's arm. When emergency personnel arrived, Coach Ames was holding a cold compress against the injured shoulder joint, to help control pain and swelling.

This chapter written by David O. Draper, Ed. D., A.T. C.

Because of the nature of sport and recreational activities, injuries are common; first aid on the scene can prevent additional pain and injury and can dramatically improve the victim's eventual outcome.

Each section in this chapter discusses the likely mechanisms of injury, the most likely signs and symptoms you will find during assessment, and the immediate first aid care you should give at the scene. All victims of the injuries described in this chapter need medical and/or surgical care; either activate the EMS system or transport the victim yourself to a medical facility after providing appropriate first aid care.

12.1 Injuries to the Shoulder, Elbow, Wrist, and Hand

Fractured Clavicle

The most frequently injured bone of the shoulder is the clavicle, or collarbone, it is more common in children than adults. A fractured clavicle occurs from blunt trauma, such as when two rugby players collide. The most common mechanism of injury is a fall—such as when a gymnast falls off the beam headfirst or a rider falls off a horse. As the athlete attempts to break the fall with the hand, the force goes up the arm, and the clavicle is actually pinched between the humerus and the sternum. The clavicle usually breaks in the middle third, which is its weakest point.

Because the clavicle lies directly over the blood vessels and nerves that supply the upper arm, it is important to immediately immobilize it so you prevent further injury to the tissues surrounding the break.

SIGNS AND SYMPTOMS

Signs and symptoms are similar to those of other fractures, as described in Chapter 11. Because the clavicle lies just under the skin, you might be able to see and feel a lump over the fracture sight; the lump will be tender, swollen, and deformed. The athlete generally feels pain in the shoulder that might radiate to the upper arm. He or she typically supports the arm and holds it near his or her chest.

FIRST AID CARE

> **Learning Objective 1** Describe and demonstrate first aid care of a fractured clavicle.

1. Don't move the victim until you have splinted the fracture with one of the following three methods:
   - *Sling and swathe*
   - *Figure-8 bandage* (see Figure 12–1) or *butterfly sling*, which provides slight traction on the fracture site, stabilizing the area and relieving some pain
   - *Improvised immobilization* using cravats tied together, a roller bandage, or elastic wrap

2. Gently apply an ice pack or cold compresses to the fracture site to alleviate pain.

3. Allow the victim to stay in the most comfortable position, usually sitting.

Shoulder Separation

A shoulder separation involves the **acromioclavicular joint**, the most freely movable joint in the body and the joint where the clavicle, scapula, and humerus meet.

> **acromioclavicular joint** The joint in the shoulder where the clavicle, scapula, and humerus join

FIGURE 12–1. A figure-8 bandage seen from the front and the back

Separation occurs when the bones of the shoulder come apart and stay apart. Three major ligaments support this joint, and the severity of the injury is measured by the number of ligaments damaged and the extent of the damage (see Figure 12–2). Because of its extreme range of motion, the shoulder is one of the most commonly dislocated joints, second only to the joints in the fingers.

The most common mechanism of injury in shoulder separation (see Figure 12–3) is falling directly on the tip of the shoulder—such as when a wrestler is thrown to the mat or a hurdler trips and lands shoulder-first on the track. A second mechanism of injury is falling on an outstretched hand. In either situation, the ligaments supporting the joint are stretched or torn.

FIGURE 12–3. Acromioclavicular joint separation—mechanism of injury is falling on the point of the shoulder.

(a)   1st Degree

(b)   2nd Degree

(c)   3rd Degree

FIGURE 12–2. The extent of damage in the three categories of sprains, which involve damage to the ligaments that support joints. (a) First-degree sprain with minimal disruption of tendons in the shoulder. (b) Second-degree sprain with significant tearing. (c) Third-degree sprain with complete tearing and loss of joint stability.

SIGNS AND SYMPTOMS

With a slight (first-degree) separation, there is little swelling or deformity over the joint. A second- or third-degree separation is marked by the following symptoms:

- An obvious and **palpable** lump over the tip of the shoulder; the lump is the tip of the clavicle that has dislodged from the scapula (see Figure 12–4 on page 206).

- Extreme pain at the site of the separation.

- *Guarding*—supporting of the injured arm by holding the elbow up. Almost all victims hold the upper arm away from the body (if the arm is fractured, the victim generally holds the arm against the body for support).

- The shoulder looks "squared" instead of rounded.

- The athlete can't touch the opposite shoulder with the hand of the injured arm.

FIRST AID CARE

> Learning Objective **2** Describe and demonstrate first aid care of a shoulder separation.

To care for a mild (first-degree) separation, immobilize the shoulder with a roller or elastic bandage and apply an ice pack or cold compress. If there is deformity,

palpable Able to be felt by the First Aider

FIGURE 12–4. Dislodged clavicle as a result of shoulder separation

suspect a second- or third-degree separation. To treat a second- or third-degree separation:

1. Immobilize the shoulder with both horizontal and vertical swathes and a sling.

2. Apply an ice pack or cold compress to the shoulder joint if the victim can tolerate it.

Dislocated Shoulder

> Learning Objective **3** Describe the usual mechanism of injury that causes a shoulder dislocation.

A shoulder dislocation is a more severe injury than a separation, because the dislocation involves the articulating surface of the shoulder (the glenohumeral joint). Many nerves and arteries pass through the area of the joint and can be involved in the injury.

The most common mechanism of injury causing shoulder dislocation is when the athlete's arm is held out from the side with the palm at shoulder height, then pulled backward; a classic example is a football player reaching out to tackle an oncoming opponent (see Figure 12–5). The force of the opposing player causes the head of the humerus to dislocate from its attachment on the scapula. Figure 12–6 illustrates a dislocated shoulder.

SIGNS AND SYMPTOMS

Signs and symptoms of a dislocated shoulder include:

- The usually rounded part of the shoulder is flattened.

- The injured arm appears longer than the opposite arm.

- The victim exhibits a guarding of the shoulder and an inability to lift the arm.

- You may be able to feel the head of the humerus in the victim's armpit.

FIRST AID CARE

1. Check for a pulse in the wrist and sensation in the hand; if either is missing, activate the EMS system immediately.

2. Immobilize the shoulder in the position found; *never attempt to straighten a dislocated shoulder.*

Dislocated Elbow

> Learning Objective **4** Describe the usual mechanism of injury that causes a dislocated elbow.

The elbow is a joint formed by the bone of the upper arm (humerus) and the two bones of the forearm (radius and ulna). Because all the blood vessels and nerves to the forearm and hand pass through the elbow, injuries to the elbow are potentially very serious. Remember that the elbow can be injured in either a straight or a bent position.

FIGURE 12–5. Mechanism of an anterior dislocation. The arm is forced into extension, abduction, and external rotation.

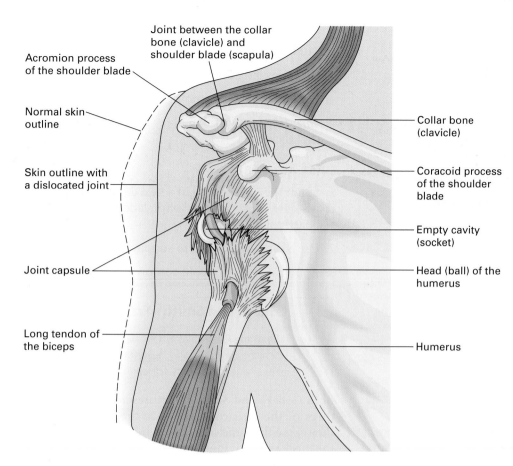

Joint between the collar
bone (clavicle) and
shoulder blade (scapula)

Acromion process
of the shoulder blade

Normal skin
outline

Skin outline with
a dislocated joint

Joint capsule

Long tendon of
the biceps

Collar bone
(clavicle)

Coracoid process
of the shoulder
blade

Empty cavity
(socket)

Head (ball) of the
humerus

Humerus

FIGURE 12–6. Dislocated
shoulder

Although not a common injury in sports and recreation, gymnasts and wrestlers occasionally suffer a dislocated elbow (see Figure 12–7) because their sport involves supporting their weight on their hands. A typical mechanism of injury is having one's wrestling opponent fall on the back of the arm that is supporting one's weight. Occasionally a gymnastics coach or spotter dislocates an elbow trying to catch an off-balance athlete.

A dislocated elbow is not the same as **tennis elbow**, an injury that causes inflammation on the outside bony protrusion of the elbow. Tennis elbow actually involves the tendons of the wrist, and results from quick snapping twists of the wrist in any activity, not just tennis. The tendon in the elbow is attached to the muscle that controls wrist and finger movement, so the tennis player experiences extreme pain when using either the wrist or the elbow.

Golfer's elbow is very similar to tennis elbow, except the injury and pain are on the inside of the elbow. The inflammation occurs in the tendon attached to the inner side of the elbow.

Humerus

Radius

Ulna

FIGURE 12–7. Dislocation of the elbow joint

tennis elbow Inflammation of the bony
protrusion of the elbow

golfer's elbow Inflammation in the tendon
attached to the inner side of the elbow

As with a dislocated shoulder, a dislocation of the elbow carries the risk of injuring the numerous nerves and blood vessels that pass through the elbow. Accompanying fractures are common.

SIGNS AND SYMPTOMS

The signs and symptoms of a dislocated elbow include:

- Gross deformity of the elbow
- A golf-ball-sized lump on the back of the elbow
- A shortened forearm on the injured side
- Inability to bend the elbow

FIRST AID CARE

1. Immobilize the injury in the position found; *never try to straighten a dislocated elbow.* If possible, use a ladder splint, Sam splint, or vacuum splint; do not use an air splint, because it forces the bones into the shape of the splint.

2. Apply an ice pack or cold compress.

Fracture of the Radial Head

The head of the radius is on the lateral side of the elbow; typically, it is fractured when a victim falls on an outstretched hand, such as when hiking or bicycling. Although the elbow itself usually doesn't hit the ground, energy travels from the ground to the hand, then up the arm, causing the humerus to compress the radial head.

SIGNS AND SYMPTOMS

> **Learning Objective 5** Describe the signs and symptoms of a fractured radial head.

The most common symptom of radial head fracture is pain while rotating the forearm. To assess, have the victim hold out the arm with the elbow slightly bent and the hand cupped. Then have the victim turn the palm down, as if pouring water from the palm. If that kind of rotation causes significant pain, suspect radial head fracture.

Other signs and symptoms include the following:

- Mild deformity, if any
- Slight swelling over the lateral side of the elbow
- Head of the radius painful to the touch
- Guarding (the victim will try to hold the elbow slightly bent)

FIRST AID CARE

1. Splint the injured arm in a flexed position; if possible, use a vacuum splint, ladder splint, or board splint.

2. Use a sling and swathe to support the injured arm.

3. Apply an ice bag or cold compress to the injury site.

Colles's and Smith's Fractures

> **Learning Objective 6** Define Colles's and Smith's fractures and describe the usual mechanism of injury for each.

Both Colles's and Smith's fractures are displaced fractures of the forearm just above the wrist. Although they cause the same signs and symptoms, they differ in the mechanism of injury.

- **Colles's fracture** (see Figure 12–8) occurs when the victim falls on the palm of the hand with the wrist extended.
- **Smith's fracture** occurs when the victim falls on the back of the hand with the wrist flexed.

Both injuries are most common in children and adolescents—usually from falls on the playground

> **Colles's fracture** A displaced fracture of the forearm caused when the victim falls on the palm of the hand with the wrist extended
>
> **Smith's fracture** A displaced fracture of the forearm caused when the victim falls on the back of the hand with the wrist flexed

FIGURE 12–8. Colles's fracture

or during in-line skating or skateboarding—because the growth plate just above the wrist does not fully mature until around the age of 18 and is more prone to fracture.

SIGNS AND SYMPTOMS

Both Colles's and Smith's fractures cause extreme pain and a classic "silver fork deformity"—a hollow or depression in the lower third of the forearm and a prominence and swelling at the wrist.

FIRST AID CARE

1. Splint the forearm; if possible, use a SAM splint, ladder splint, or vacuum splint. Immobilize both the wrist and the elbow, but leave the fingers exposed.

2. Because a number of blood vessels pass through the area, check circulation by monitoring the capillary refill in the fingernails.

3. Apply an ice pack or cold compress to the injury site to reduce swelling and pain.

Fracture and Dislocation of the Carpal Bones

> Learning Objective 7 Describe the mechanisms of injury that cause fractures to the carpal and metacarpal bones, dislocations of the carpal bones, and fractured or dislocated fingers.

In sports and recreation, carpal fracture and dislocation most commonly result from falling on an outstretched, extended hand. The most commonly fractured carpal bone—the navicular—has a limited blood supply and heals very poorly unless promptly and properly treated. Thus, you should never dismiss wrist injury as a simple sprain.

SIGNS AND SYMPTOMS

Both fracture and dislocation may cause swelling, deformity, and tenderness on the back of the wrist. In addition, navicular fracture causes pain and a throbbing sensation in the **anatomical snuffbox** (the area of the wrist through which the radial artery passes) (see Figure 12–9).

FIRST AID CARE

1. If there is no deformity, splint the wrist and hand with an air splint or other appropriate splint.

2. If there is deformity, splint the wrist and hand with a SAM splint, ladder splint, vacuum splint, or other splint that will conform to the shape of the deformity; do not use an air splint if there is deformity.

3. Use an ice pack or cold compress to reduce pain and swelling.

FIGURE 12–9. The "anatomical snuffbox." Tenderness on palpation is highly suggestive of a fractured navicular.

Metacarpal Fractures

Fractures of the metacarpal bones can occur to the base, neck, or shaft. A *boxer's fracture*, or compacted fracture, typically results from a mistimed punch with a closed fist. Other fractures occur from severe twisting or severe hyperextension, such as when a basketball player catches a finger in an opposing player's jersey (see Figure 12–10).

SIGNS AND SYMPTOMS

Typical signs and symptoms include:

- Pain in the hand (often so mild that the victim insists the injury is only a sprain)
- Swelling of the hand
- Possible twisting of the finger so the nailbed is turned to one side

FIRST AID CARE

1. If there is no gross deformity, splint the hand with a SAM splint, ladder splint, or vacuum splint. Keep the fingertips, exposed.

2. Assess for circulation by checking capillary refill every few minutes while you take the patient to a medical facility.

Fractured or Dislocated Fingers

Both fractures and dislocations of the fingers are common; the fingers are the most commonly broken bones in the body. Finger fractures and dislocations occur most often in football and gymnastics when the athlete lands on the hand in an awkward position or when the ball hits the tips of the fingers.

> **anatomical snuffbox** The area of the wrist through which the radial artery passes

FIGURE 12–10. Fracture due to hyperextension of a finger

SIGNS AND SYMPTOMS

Signs and symptoms of dislocated fingers are:

- Pain
- Swelling
- Inability to move the joint
- Appearance of a lump at the joint
- Possible loss of sensation and/or circulation
- Shortening of the finger

While dislocations and severe fractures are usually obvious, nondisplaced fractures can cause very little deformity; swelling may or may not occur. Whether or not the victim experiences deformity and swelling, pain is usually severe. The finger may hurt even when it is not being moved. Loss of function doesn't always occur; the victim might be able to move fingers that are broken.

FIRST AID CARE

1. Splint the fingers; if there is little deformity, splint the injured finger to an adjacent uninjured finger (see Figure 12–11).

2. *Never* try to reduce (straighten) a dislocated finger.

3. Apply an ice pack or cold compress to reduce pain and swelling.

Sprained Thumb (Gamekeeper's Thumb)

A potentially disabling injury to an individual is *gamekeeper's thumb*, a sprain to the ulnar collateral ligament. The unusual name for this injury is taken from injuries to the thumb that occurred while bird hunting. If a hunter wounded a bird, he would grab it by the head and wring its neck. Sometimes this awkward action caused the bird to hit and hyperextend the thumb, spraining the ligaments. This injury now

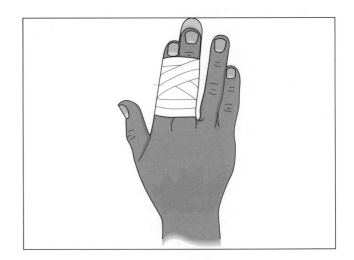

FIGURE 12–11. Finger splinted to an adjacent uninjured finger

occurs mainly in sporting events like football or basketball, when the athlete hyperextends the thumb while trying to catch an object. This injury is also fairly common to the recreational skier.

SIGNS AND SYMPTOMS

The thumb might appear swollen or discolored, depending on how much time has elapsed since the injury occurred. The thumb will be tender over the attachment of the ulnar collateral ligament on the inside of the thumb by the web space. A key sign is that the victim will not be able to apply much of a pinch grip between the affected thumb and the index finger.

FIRST AID CARE

1. An ice pack should be applied to the area to control swelling and pain.

2. The thumb should be immobilized or buddy taped to the index finger.

3. Refer to a physician.

In most cases, a physician will splint the thumb for 2 to 3 weeks. If the ability to pinch does not return after 2 to 3 weeks, the victim should see a physician that specializes in hand surgery. Sometimes the small muscles of the thumb block the ends of the ulnar collateral ligament from rejoining. Surgery might be needed to free the ends of the ligament and sew it back together. Otherwise, the ability to grip objects might be impaired indefinitely.

PROGRESS CHECK

1. If the arm on the injured side appears longer than the one on the other side, suspect _____ of the shoulder. *(fracture/dislocation/separation)*

2. In shoulder fracture or separation, there is generally a lump at the tip of the shoulder; with dislocation, the tip of the shoulder is typically _____. *(swollen/prominent/flattened)*

3. Use slight traction or pulling to immobilize all shoulder injuries other than _____. *(separation/dislocation/fracture)*

4. You should splint an elbow dislocation _____. *(with the arm straightened/ in the position found/with the elbow bent)*

5. Do not use a (n) _____ splint on a dislocated elbow. *(air/Sam/ladder)*

6. To assess fractured radial head, have the victim _____. *(bend the elbow/straighten the elbow/rotate the forearm)*

7. In all splints of the forearm, wrist, and/or hand, leave the _____ exposed. *(elbow/wrist/fingertips)*

8. The general first aid care procedure for all injuries to the shoulder, elbow, wrist, and hand is to _____. *(apply traction/ use a sling/immobilize, usually by splinting)*

12.2 Injuries to the Hip, Leg, Knee, Ankle, and Foot

Hip Pointer

A *hip pointer*, or bruising of the area over the iliac crest of the pelvis, results from blunt trauma—typically from two athletes colliding or an athlete landing on the hip while diving for a ball.

SIGNS AND SYMPTOMS

Signs and symptoms include:

- Inability to bear full weight on the injured side, causing limping

- Tenderness to the touch

- Red discoloration, later turning purple

FIRST AID CARE

> Learning Objective 8 Describe first aid care for injuries to the hip.

Because a fracture needs to be ruled out, the victim should be transported to a medical facility. To relieve pain and reduce swelling until a physician can evaluate the injury, apply an ice pack or cold compress held in place with a roller bandage.

Hip Dislocation

The ball-and-socket hip joint is extremely stable and requires a great deal of force to dislocate. A hip dislocation can occur from powerful direct force to the foot, knee, or thigh, or from a fall that impacts any of these areas. It may also occur if an athlete falls hard on the knee.

Signs and symptoms of hip dislocation are:

- Severe pain

- Obvious deformity

- Inability to flex the foot or toes

- Loss of motion

It is very difficult to differentiate between a hip dislocation and a hip fracture.

Hip Fracture

A fractured hip is most often caused by a fall. The fracture occurs at the top end of the femur (thigh bone), not in one of the bones of the pelvis.

Signs and symptoms of a hip fracture are:

- Severe pain in the groin
- The leg appears to be shortened
- The leg is rotated, with the toes pointing outward
- Inability to lift the leg

Ischial Tuberosity Fracture

During a sprint or other activity in which the hip is flexed and the leg extended—such as running, jumping, and hurdling—an athlete can suffer an **ischial tuberosity** fracture (an avulsion fracture of the hamstring attachment). This kind of injury is most common in children and adolescents because of the soft growth plate in the hip.

SIGNS AND SYMPTOMS

Ischial tuberosity fracture causes

- Pain in the buttocks where the ischial tuberosity attaches
- Swelling in the buttocks on the affected side
- A lump in the buttocks on the affected side

FIRST AID CARE

1. Use a roller bandage to support the affected buttocks.
2. Apply an ice pack or cold compress to relieve pain and reduce swelling.
3. Because this injury makes it extremely difficult to walk, provide crutches, a stretcher, or other way to transport the victim.

Hamstring Strain

An athlete who flexes the hip and extends the knee can also strain the hamstring (see Figure 12–12); unlike an ischial tuberosity fracture, hamstring strain occurs among people of all ages, not just the young.

There are varying degrees of injury; however, a common symptom is tenderness over the injured aspect of the muscle. The more severe the muscle tear, the greater the deformity and the greater the difficulty in bending the leg. Within a few days to a week, the area becomes discolored.

Treat as for ischial tuberosity fracture.

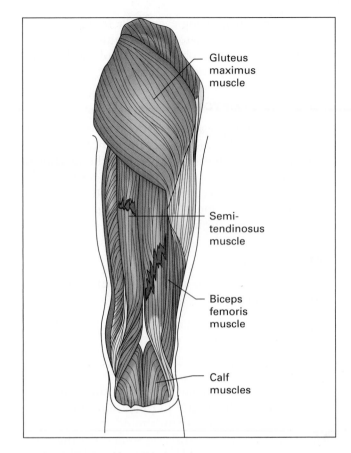

FIGURE 12–12. Hamstring strain

Sprained Knee Ligaments

Any external or internal force that causes the leg to go beyond the normal range of motion can tear a knee ligament (see Figure 12–13). These forces include hyperextension, twisting, and forces that either bow the legs or knock the knees. Depending on the ligament involved, surgical reconstruction may be necessary.

SIGNS AND SYMPTOMS

Signs and symptoms include pain and possible swelling. In some cases, there is an audible "pop" when the injury occurs.

FIRST AID CARE

> Learning Objective 9 Describe first aid care for injuries to the hamstring and knee ligaments.

1. Wrap the knee in the most comfortable position with a pillow splint, or immobilize the knee and the bones above or below it with a vacuum splint or padded splint.

> **ischial tuberosity** The spot where the top of the hamstring attaches

FIGURE 12–13. Valgus knee injury. If a valgus force is applied to the knee while the foot is fixed, a tear of the medialligamentous structures will occur. If the force is great enough, the anterior cruciate ligament may also be torn as well as the medial meniscus.

2. Apply an ice pack or cold compress to relieve pain and reduce swelling.

Dislocated Patella

Learning Objective **10** Describe the signs and symptoms of a dislocated kneecap (patella).

A twisting, hyperextension, or *knock-knee* force can dislocate the **patella** (kneecap), generally to the lateral side of the leg. For example, a tennis player who plants a foot, then twists to reach the ball might suffer this kind of injury. A kneecap that is dislocated can be clearly felt laterally.

SIGNS AND SYMPTOMS

Signs and symptoms include:

- An audible "pop" as the injury occurs
- Extreme pain
- Inability to straighten or extend the injured leg
- Severe swelling
- Lateral dislocation of the kneecap that can be palpated

FIRST AID CARE

A dislocated kneecap or knee needs immediate medical attention; if the injury is untreated for more than 8 hours, the athlete could lose his or her leg. The greatest concern during first aid is for the major artery that runs behind the knee joint: It can be compressed

by the patella, cutting off blood flow to the lower leg. To treat:

1. Check the ankle pulse. If it is absent, try once to straighten the knee. *Never try to straighten or extend the knee for any other reason.*

2. Splint the injured leg in the position in which it was found; use a pillow splint, Sam splint, or vacuum splint to immobilize the knee and the bones above and below it, taking care not to push against the patella.

3. Apply an ice pack or cold compress to relieve pain and reduce swelling.

Achilles Tendon Rupture

Learning Objective **11** Describe the first aid care of an achilles tendon rupture.

Most frequently seen in recreational athletes over thirty years old, achilles tendon rupture results from jumping and cutting maneuvers, such as those that typically occur in basketball and tennis.

SIGNS AND SYMPTOMS

The victim may hear an audible "pop" during the injury itself, and may feel as though he or she has been shot in the leg. A partial tear causes only pain and limited range of motion. If the tear is complete, the victim may also have extreme deformity; the tendon may roll up in a ball, or there may be a divot in the muscle.

patella The kneecap

FIGURE 12–14. Thompsen's test

FIGURE 12–15. Ankle sprain

Don't be fooled by this injury however, since complete achilles tendon ruptures might exhibit little deformity or pain. If you squeeze the victim's calf muscle and the foot does not flex (Thompsen's test), the tear is complete (see Figure 12–14). Surgery is often required to repair the torn tendon.

FIRST AID CARE

1. Splint the affected leg with a lower leg splint, with the foot slightly plantar flexed.

2. Apply an ice pack or cold compress to the area, and secure it with a roller bandage.

Ankle Sprains

> Learning Objective **12** Describe the first aid care of sprains or fractures of the ankle and foot.

Probably the most common injury that occurs in sports and recreation is a sprained ankle. The majority of the time, the foot rolls inward (see Figure 12–15)—such as when a basketball player comes down on another player's foot. As the ankle rolls beyond its normal range of motion, ligaments can be stretched or torn. Although rare, ankle sprains can also result from the foot rolled outward.

It is difficult to tell the difference between a fractured ankle and a sprained ankle. Some guidelines to determine whether the athlete needs an x-ray are:

- Ask if he or she can put weight on the foot. A sprain will cause some pain, but if the person can take four or more steps, the injury is probably a sprain.

- If hopping on the good foot causes too much pain to tolerate in the injured foot, the injury is probably a fracture.

- If swelling occurs on only one side of the ankle or foot, it is probably a sprain. If swelling occurs on both sides, it is probably a fracture.

- If the athlete got nauseated immediately following the injury, it is more likely a fracture.

- Press gently along the injured bones. It is most likely a fracture if the pain or tenderness occur on the back or tip of either of the ankle bones or the inside or outside of the middle foot.

SIGNS AND SYMPTOMS

Signs and symptoms include:

- Pain or tenderness over the ligaments that were stressed

- Swelling over the area of the ligaments that were stressed

- Difficulty walking or even standing, depending on the severity of the sprain

FIRST AID CARE

1. Immediately apply an ice pack to the area to help control swelling.

2. Apply compression with an elastic wrap or an air splint if there is no apparent deformity.

3. Elevate the limb.

4. Transport the victim to a medical facility to rule out a fracture.

Dislocated Ankle

Figure 12–16 shows a dislocated ankle that occurred in a soccer game. In this case, most, if not all, of the main ligaments that support the medial side of the ankle were torn. This injury needs to be treated with care, since pressure on arteries and nerves could lead to permanent damage. This injury needs to be splinted in the position in which it is found, and the victim should be rushed to a medical facility. Ice application will help to control swelling, muscle spasm, and pain.

FIGURE 12–16. Dislocated ankle

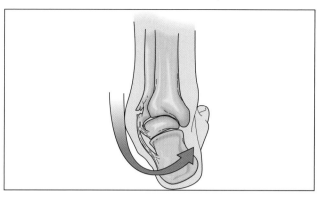

FIGURE 12–17. Fibula fracture

Fractured Tibia or Fibula

The bones of the lower leg—the tibia and fibula—can be fractured by a direct blow to the leg and by the forces that cause a sprained ankle. If the foot rolls outward, the tibia may fracture; if the foot rolls inward, the fibula may fracture (see Figure 12–17).

SIGNS AND SYMPTOMS

Signs and symptoms include:

- Swelling, almost always on both sides of the ankle (swelling is usually on one side only if the ankle is sprained instead of fractured)

- Possible deformity over the injured area

- Pain when the bottom of the foot is tapped

FIRST AID CARE

1. If there is no displacement or deformity, immobilize the leg with an air splint; otherwise, use a Sam splint, ladder splint, vacuum splint, or similar splint to immobilize the leg.

2. Apply an ice pack or cold compress to relieve pain and reduce swelling.

PROGRESS CHECK

1. An ischial tuberosity fracture causes pain in the _____ . (hip/leg/buttocks)

2. Care for torn knee ligament by splinting the leg in a _____ position. (straight/flexed/comfortable)

3. Splint a dislocated patella in _____ . (the position in which it was found/a straight position/a flexed position)

4. Achilles tendon rupture typically causes _____ if the tear is partial. (gross deformity/limited range of motion/paralysis)

5. The same force that causes sprained ankle can also cause fracture in the _____ . (foot/lower leg/knee)

Summary

- Because it can be difficult to distinguish between fractures and other injuries, victims of the sports injuries discussed in this chapter should always be evaluated by a physician.

- Applying a sling and swathe or an elastic bandage that supplies slight traction is appropriate for a fracture or separation of the shoulder; you should not apply pressure or traction if the shoulder is dislocated.

- Always splint a dislocated joint in the position found.

- Never use an air splint for an injury in which there is deformity, because the air splint forces the limb to conform to its shape. Instead, use a splint that will conform to the deformity.

- Apply ice packs or cold compresses to injuries involving fractures, strains, sprains, dislocations, and separations to relieve pain and reduce swelling. Use a roller bandage to hold the ice pack in place unless there is a dislocation.

- Whenever you splint an arm or leg, leave the tips of the fingers or toes exposed so you can assess circulation by checking capillary refill.

Key Terms

Make sure you understand the following key terms:

acromioclavicular joint
palpable
tennis elbow
Colles's fracture
Smith's fracture
anatomical snuffbox
ischial tuberosity
patella

Critical Thinking Exercise

It is time for volleyball tryouts for your school's champi-
onship volleyball team. You are all working hard to impress
the coaches. A player from the opposing team spikes the
ball hard, drilling it at high speed toward the floor on your
side. Your teammate, Paula, dives to the floor in an
attempt to deflect the ball upward. Instead, her outstretched hand slams into the hardwood floor.

   You run quickly to Paula, who is complaining of pain in
her shoulder and is holding her elbow up into her side.
Her shoulder has an abnormal appearance.

1. How would you evaluate the potential injuries?

2. What immediate first aid action would you take?

3. How would you immobilize the injured area to prevent
    further injury?

Chapter 12 Self-Test

Student: _____   Date: _____

Course: _____   Section #: _____

Part 1   True/False

If you believe the statement is true, circle the T. If you believe the statement is false, circle the F.

T   F   **1.** You should provide slight traction or pressure for a dislocated shoulder.

T   F   **2.** The most common victims of dislocated elbow are those who support their weight on their hands, such as wrestlers or gymnasts.

T   F   **3.** The best way to assess fracture of the radial head is to have the victim rotate the forearm.

T   F   **4.** Ischial tuberosity fracture carries with it the classic "silver fork deformity."

T   F   **5.** Dislocation of the carpal bones causes deformity and swelling on the back of the wrist; to treat, immobilize with an air splint.

T   F   **6.** A twisted finger with the nailbed turned to one side is typically the result of metacarpal fracture.

T   F   **7.** You should assess for dislocated elbow by having the victim straighten the arm.

T   F   **8.** A victim may hear an audible "pop" during several different injuries, including dislocated patella and achilles tendon rupture.

T   F   **9.** The force that causes a sprained ankle can also fracture the bones of the lower leg.

Part 2   Multiple Choice

For each item, circle the correct answer or the phrase that best completes the statement.

1. A shoulder that appears almost flattened is an indication of
    a. fracture
    b. dislocation
    c. separation
    d. strain

2. A classic sign of a dislocated elbow is
    a. a shortened forearm
    b. pain while rotating the forearm
    c. compromised pulse at the wrist
    d. lack of swelling

3. The classic sign of Colles's fracture is
    a. compromised pulse at the wrist
    b. a golf-ball-sized lump on the back of the elbow
    c. the "silver fork deformity"
    d. inability to straighten the leg

4. Care for dislocated carpal bones by
    a. immobilizing with a ladder or vacuum splint
    b. immobilizing with an air splint
    c. reducing the dislocation
    d. none of the above

5. Swelling, pain, and a lump in the buttocks of a sprinter would probably indicate
    a. hamstring strain
    b. gluteus maximus strain
    c. contusion of the iliac crest
    d. ischial tuberosity fracture

6. To treat a dislocated patella
    a. splint in the position in which the leg was found
    b. use a pillow splint or vacuum splint
    c. apply ice packs or cold compresses
    d. all of the above

7. Splint a victim of a sprained knee ligament
    a. in the position in which the leg was found
    b. with the leg straightened
    c. with the knee flexed
    d. in the most comfortable position

8. To assess whether achilles tendon rupture is complete, squeeze the victim's calf muscle; if the rupture is complete,
    a. squeezing the muscle will cause severe pain
    b. you will hear a "pop"
    c. the foot will not flex
    d. there will be limited range of motion

Part 3 Matching

Match the injury with the appropriate treatment.

Injury

1. _____ Fractured clavicle
2. _____ Finger fracture with little deformity
3. _____ Radial head fracture
4. _____ Shoulder dislocation

First Aid Care

A. Immobilize in the position found
B. Use immobilization that provides slight traction on the injury site
C. Splint against the adjacent one
D. Use a combination of a splint and a sling

Part 4 What Would You Do If?

1. During an attempted tackle, a defensive lineman rams his helmet into the quarterback's hip. The quarterback limps from the field, but insists his leg is not broken.

2. A 20-year-old woman competing in a triathalon skids in the gravel rounding a curve and catapults over the handlebars of her bicycle, falling on her outstretched hand. There is only mild deformity and slight swelling over the lateral side of the elbow. What injury would you suspect? How would you assess it? If your hunch proved right, how would you care for the woman?

13

Head and Spine Injuries

Learning Objectives

When you have mastered the material in this chapter, you will be able to

1 Describe the appropriate first aid care for injury to the scalp

2 Describe the physiology of injury to the brain

3 List the four types of skull fracture

4 Describe appropriate assessment for victims of head injury

5 List the signs and symptoms of skull fracture

6 Distinguish between open and closed head injury

7 Discuss the signs and symptoms of both open and closed head injury

8 Describe and demonstrate the appropriate first aid care for head injury

9 Describe the common mechanisms of spinal injury

10 Describe the assessment of spinal injury victims

11 List the signs and symptoms of spinal injury

12 Describe and demonstrate the appropriate first aid care for spinal injury

13 Describe the technique for removing a helmet from a head- or spinal-injured victim

On the Scene

Fred Hansen and two of his colleagues from a local software company stopped by the community swimming pool to discuss some software needs with the city's recreation director. As they got out of the car, they saw a group of people gathered around an adolescent boy, who was lying still at the pool edge.

Fred and the other two men ran toward the group and asked what happened. "My friend was doing some dives off that board," said 13-year-old Mark Welling. "I think he hit his head on the bottom of the pool. Jake and I pulled him out."

Fourteen-year-old Lance Colledge was unconscious, but he was breathing and had a pulse. Fred immediately suspected a spine injury. The lifeguard on duty had already called EMS.

Fred grabbed a beach towel from a bystander; rolling it, he improvised a "collar" that would stabilize Lance's neck. As his colleague placed both hands on Lance's head and maintained it in a neutral position, Fred tucked the towel gently around Lance's neck, placing it firmly against both his chin and his collarbone.

By the time EMTs arrived, Fred had stabilized Lance's neck with the rolled towel and had covered him with a thick terrycloth robe to preserve his body heat and prevent shock.

Half a million americans suffer head injuries every year (see Figure 13-1); head injury is second only to stroke as a cause of major neurological trauma. While head injury constitutes only a small percentage of all injuries, it causes more than half of all fatalities from injuries.

Any trauma severe enough to cause injury to the head—including a simple fall—can also cause injury to the spine. Spinal injury can also result from any force that pushes the spine beyond its normal weight-bearing ability or its normal limits of motion. Spinal cord injuries are some of the most formidable and traumatic injuries you will face: spinal cord injury may affect other organ systems, and improper handling may paralyze the victim or may even lead to death.

This chapter outlines the specific assessment skills needed to evaluate victims of suspected head and spinal injuries and details the emergency care procedures that will enable you to prevent further injury for such victims.

13.1 Types of Head Injury

The brain is enclosed in the skull—a rigid, unyielding case. The skull is considered to be a closed container. If an injury to the brain were to occur that results in swelling of the brain tissue and bleeding within the skull, the closed skull would not allow the brain to expand with the swelling or bleeding. The pressure would increase inside the skull, and could compress the brain tissue. This leads to brain tissue dysfunction and if unrelieved, the pressure can cause death.

Head injuries can involve either injury to the scalp or injury to the brain itself.

Injury to the Scalp

Learning Objective 1 Describe the appropriate first aid care for injury to the scalp.

Motor vehicle crashes   50%

Assaults and violence   12%

Falls   21%

Sports and recreation   10%
Other causes   7%

FIGURE 13–1. Causes of head injuries

The scalp may be injured in the same way as any other soft tissue—it may be contused, lacerated, abraded, or avulsed.

Because of the rich supply of blood vessels to the scalp and the inelastic matrix of tissue that the vessels are in, injuries of the scalp tend to bleed very heavily. In addition, the underlying tougher tissue might be torn even when the skin stays intact; bleeding then occurs under the skin and may be confusing at first as you try to assess the victim. (The presence of blood under intact skin can mimic a depressed skull fracture; or it can fill the depressed skull fracture with blood, making it appear normal.)

To control bleeding of a scalp injury, apply gentle direct pressure with a dry sterile dressing, as with other soft-tissue injuries. Do not apply pressure directly over the area if you suspect a skull fracture, especially if a depression is present; doing so can drive bone fragments into the brain tissue. Instead, apply pressure over a broad area or around the edges of the wound.

If an object is impaled in the scalp, do not remove the impaled object; stabilize it with bulky dressings as described in Chapter 8.

Injury to the Brain

Learning Objective **2** Describe the physiology of injury to the brain.

Most brain injuries (see Figure 13-2) are caused by trauma, most often in a motor vehicle accident or fall. Nontraumatic brain injury may also be secondary—the brain can be injured as a result of inadequate blood flow and inadequate delivery of oxygen to the brain cells (poor perfusion). Establishing and maintaining good airway and adequate ventilation are extremely important in a head injury to prevent further brain injury. Because of the relatively large size of their heads and weakness of their necks, children are especially vulnerable to brain injury. One of the most common types of

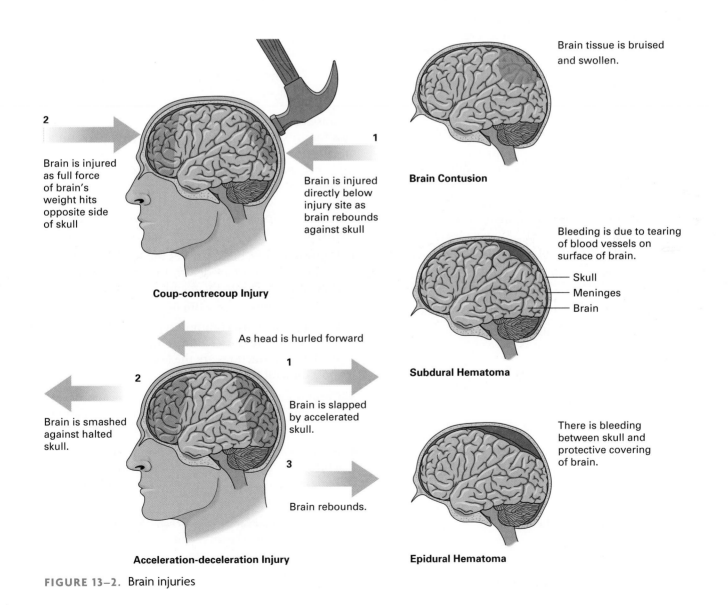

FIGURE 13-2. Brain injuries

injury is **coup-contrecoup**, a type of acceleration—deceleration injury—the head comes to a sudden stop, but the brain continues to move back and forth inside the skull, resulting in massive injury. There are actually two sites of injury: the point of impact, and the point on the opposite side where the brain hits the skull.

When the brain is injured, blood vessels in the brain increase in size (dilate) so that more blood can flow to the injured area. However, injured blood vessels in the brain may allow fluid from the blood to leak out of the vessel and into the affected area, which decreases perfusion in the brain. A decrease in brain perfusion causes carbon dioxide to build up in the brain tissue, which further dilates the blood vessels.

When blood vessel leakage occurs, swelling results. The swelling and the extra blood volume increase the pressure inside the skull, which may cause brain tissue to become compressed and cease functioning. Blood flow to the brain will decrease as pressure within the brain becomes greater. The brain stem can become compressed by swelling, affecting the heart, breathing, and blood pressure. If these systems fail, the brain will not be perfused or oxygenated and as a result will die.

Some brain injuries occur in the absence of trauma. A blood clot or rupture of a brain vessel with hemorrhaging (such as stroke) can cause brain injury through much the same process described above.

SIGNS AND SYMPTOMS OF BRAIN INJURY

Signs and symptoms might not occur immediately following brain injury; they usually become obvious as the brain swells inside the skull, which may take several hours. The hallmark sign is an altered mental status that does not improve, or a continuously deteriorating mental status. (see Figure 13-3).

Signs of increased pressure inside the skull include:

- Decreasing mental status or altered responsiveness; the victim is no longer alert, and may respond only to verbal stimuli or pain
- Combativeness and erratic behavior
- Nausea and/or vomiting
- Pupils that are not equal or reactive to light
- Double vision or other visual disturbances
- Headache, sometimes severe
- Loss of memory, confusion, or disorientation
- Weakness or loss of balance
- Seizures
- Evidence of trauma to the head
- Slow heart rate
- Irregular breathing pattern

FIRST AID CARE FOR BRAIN INJURY

Any victim with suspected brain injury needs *immediate* medical attention; as mentioned above, continued swelling of the brain can compress the brain stem, affecting breathing, heart function, and blood pressure. First Aiders really can't do anything to stop the swelling or to treat brain injury; the goal of first aid is to support the victim's vital functions until medical help arrives:

1. Suspect spine injury in any victim with suspected brain injury; stabilize the head and neck as described later in this chapter.

2. Establish and monitor the victim's ABCDs; ensure the airway is open, provide rescue breathing if the breathing is inadequate.

3. Anticipate vomiting; be prepared to keep the victim's head and neck stabilized as you roll the victim on his or her side to prevent aspiration.

4. Treat the victim for shock; keep the victim warm, but *do not elevate the legs.*

Injury to the Skull (Skull Fracture)

Learning Objective **3**　List the four types of skull fracture.

Because of the skull's shape (spherical) and its thickness (approximately ¼ inch), it is generally fractured only if the force to the head is extreme. Skull fracture itself presents little danger unless accompanied by brain injury, hematoma, cerebrospinal fluid leakage, or subsequent infection.

There are four basic types of skull fracture (see Figure 13-4 on page 224):

1. **Depressed**—An object strikes the skull, leaving an obvious depression or deformity; bone fragments are often driven into the membranes or the brain itself by the force of the impact.

2. **Linear**—The most common type of skull fracture, a linear fracture causes a thin-line crack in the skull. Linear fractures are the least serious and the most difficult to detect.

3. **Comminuted**—A comminuted fracture appears at the point of impact, with multiple cracks radiating from the center (it looks like a cracked eggshell).

4. **Basilar**—A basilar skull fracture occurs when there is a break in the base of the skull; it is often the result of a linear fracture that extends to the floor of the skull.

coup-contrecoup A mechanism of brain injury in which the head comes to a sudden stop but the brain continues to move back and forth inside the skull

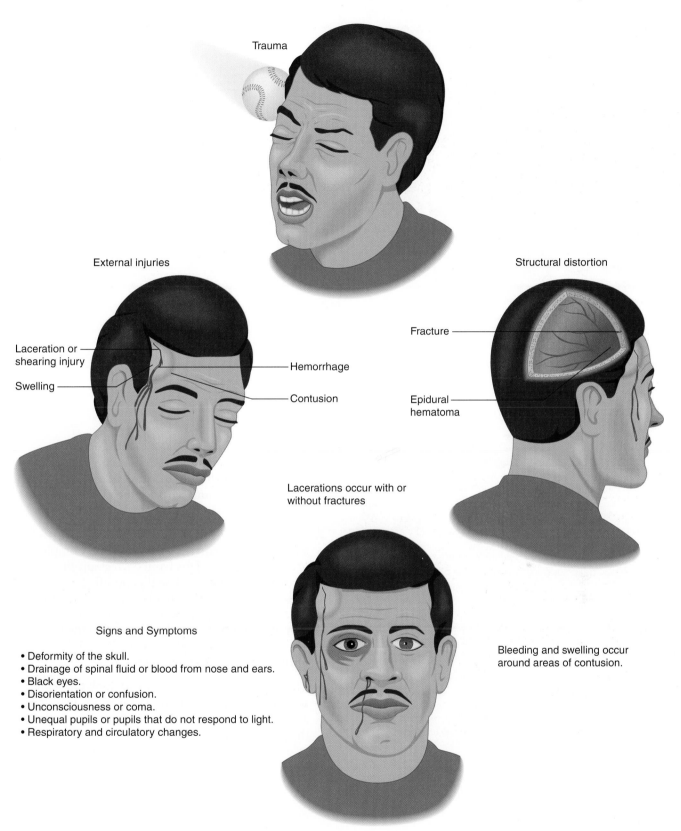

Trauma

External injuries

Laceration or shearing injury

Swelling

Hemorrhage

Contusion

Structural distortion

Fracture

Epidural hematoma

Lacerations occur with or without fractures

Signs and Symptoms

- Deformity of the skull.
- Drainage of spinal fluid or blood from nose and ears.
- Black eyes.
- Disorientation or confusion.
- Unconsciousness or coma.
- Unequal pupils or pupils that do not respond to light.
- Respiratory and circulatory changes.

Bleeding and swelling occur around areas of contusion.

FIGURE 13–3. Head injury and brain trauma

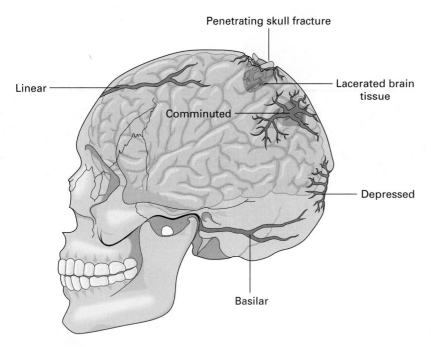

FIGURE 13–4. Types of skull fracture

13.2 Assessment, Signs, and Symptoms of Head Injury

Victim Assessment

Learning Objective **4** Describe appropriate assessment for victims of head injury.

To assess a victim of head injury:

1. Obtain a history that includes the mechanism of injury, whether the victim's level of consciousness has deteriorated, and whether the victim has been moved.

2. If possible, have someone stabilize the head, neck, and spine in a neutral in-line position. Complete a primary survey to detect and correct any life-threatening problems. Use the modified jaw-thrust maneuver to open the airway and provide artificial ventilation if needed; the most serious complication of head injury is lack of oxygen to the brain. *There must be absolutely no movement of the victim until the victim is immobilized.*

3. Check the head (see Figure 13-5); look for depressions, fractures, lacerations, deformities, bruising, and other obvious problems. Determine whether the pupils are equal and react to light, whether the face is symmetrical on both sides, and whether blood or fluid is dripping from the nose, ears, or mouth. *Never palpate a wound, probe a wound to determine its depth, separate the edges of a wound to explore it, or remove impaled objects.*

4. Maintain in-line stabilization, check the neck and spine for lacerations, bruises, swelling, protrusions, or other obvious deformities; ask the victim if there is pain, or muscle spasm.

5. Check the arms and legs for paralysis, weakness, or loss of sensation.

FIGURE 13–5. Carefully check the head for injuries. Instruct the victim not to move his or her head or neck.

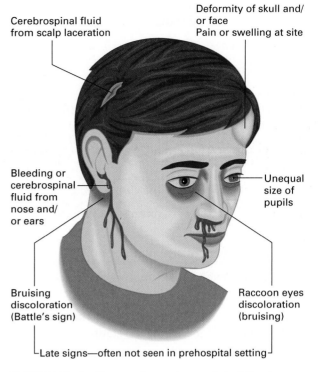

Cerebrospinal fluid from scalp laceration

Deformity of skull and/ or face
Pain or swelling at site

Bleeding or cerebrospinal fluid from nose and/ or ears

Unequal size of pupils

Bruising discoloration (Battle's sign)

Raccoon eyes discoloration (bruising)

Late signs—often not seen in prehospital setting

FIGURE 13–6. Signs and symptoms of skull fracture

Signs and Symptoms of Skull Fracture

> Learning Objective 5 List the signs and symptoms of skull fracture.

You should suspect a skull fracture with any significant force applied to the head; the mechanism of injury may make you suspicious of significant force applied to the head. Skull fracture can cause the following signs and symptoms (see Figure 13-6):

- Contusions, lacerations, or hematomas to the scalp

- Deformity of the skull

- Blood or cerebrospinal fluid (clear fluid) leaking from the ears, nose, or mouth.

- Bruising around the eyes in the absence of trauma to the eyes (**raccoon eyes**) is a very late sign

- Bruising behind the ears, or mastoid process (**Battle's sign**) is a very late sign

- Damage to the skull visible through lacerations in the scalp

- Pain, tenderness, or swelling at the site of injury

Closed and Open Head Injuries

> Learning Objective 6 Distinguish between open and closed head injury.

Injuries to the head can be open or closed. In closed head injuries, the scalp may be lacerated, but the skull is

not exposed and there is no opening to the brain. Brain damage, however, can nonetheless be extensive. In general, brain tissue is susceptible to the same kinds of injury as any soft tissue—contusion, laceration, and puncture wounds—even when the skull is not exposed.

An open head injury is accompanied by a break in the skull, such as that caused by fracture or an impaled object. It involves direct local damage to the involved tissue, but can also cause brain damage due to infection, laceration of the brain tissue, or puncture of the brain by objects that penetrate the skull.

Signs and Symptoms of Closed and Open Head Injuries

> Learning Objective 7 Discuss the signs and symptoms of both open and closed head injury.

The following are general signs and symptoms of closed head injury:

- Altered or decreasing mental status—the best indicator of a brain injury (A conscious victim

> **raccoon eyes** Bruising around the eyes in the absence of trauma to the eyes; a very late sign of skull fracture
>
> **Battle's sign** Bruising behind the ears (mastoid process); a very late sign of skull fracture

may be confused, disoriented, or suffering from a deteriorating mental status).

- Unresponsiveness

- Irregular breathing pattern

- Obvious signs of a mechanism of injury—contusions, lacerations, or hematomas to the scalp or deformity to the skull

- Blood or cerebrospinal fluid leaking from the ears or nose

- Bruising around the eyes (raccoon eyes)

- Bruising behind the ears, or mastoid process (Battle's sign)

- Loss of movement or sensation

- Nausea and/or vomiting; vomiting may be forceful or repeated

- Unequal pupil size (dilated) that does not react to light (fixed) with altered mental status

- Possible seizures

The following are general signs and symptoms of open head injury (see Figure 13-7):

- Obvious results of the mechanism of injury—contusions, lacerations, or hematomas to the scalp; deformity to the skull; or obvious penetrating injury

- A soft area or depression detected during palpation

- Brain tissue exposed through an open wound

- Bleeding from an open bone injury

PROGRESS CHECK

1. The most serious complication of head injury is _____ to the brain. *(contusion/laceration/lack of oxygen)*

2. During assessment, check for scalp and skull wounds by _____ . *(visually examining/probing/separating the edges of the wound)*

3. During assessment, check the arms and legs for paralysis and _____ . *(pulse/fractures/loss of sensation)*

4. In closed head injury, the _____ is not broken. *(scalp/skull/tough tissue)*

5. Raccoon eyes, a classic sign of skull fracture, involves bruising around the _____ . *(ears/eyes/mastoid process)*

6. Head injury is indicated by blood or _____ dripping from the ears, nose, or mouth. *(lymph fluid/cerebrospinal fluid/mucus)*

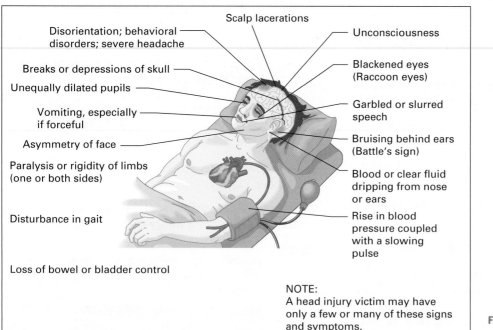

Disorientation; behavioral disorders; severe headache

Scalp lacerations

Unconsciousness

Breaks or depressions of skull

Unequally dilated pupils

Vomiting, especially if forceful

Asymmetry of face

Paralysis or rigidity of limbs (one or both sides)

Disturbance in gait

Loss of bowel or bladder control

Blackened eyes (Raccoon eyes)

Garbled or slurred speech

Bruising behind ears (Battle's sign)

Blood or clear fluid dripping from nose or ears

Rise in blood pressure coupled with a slowing pulse

NOTE:
A head injury victim may have only a few or many of these signs and symptoms.

FIGURE 13–7. Signs and symptoms of head injury

13.3 First Aid Care for Head Injury

Learning Objective **8** Describe and demonstrate the appropriate first aid care for head injury.

Before beginning any first aid care for head injury, assess the victim's mental status. Any victim who loses consciousness, even briefly, must be evaluated at a medical facility. A victim whose mental status deteriorates or does not improve needs immediate assessment and treatment by EMS.

Whenever you care for a victim of head injury (see Figures 13-8 and 13-9), always assume that a spinal injury also exists. Activate the EMS system, then:

1. The top priority is establishing and maintaining an open airway with adequate oxygenation. Use the modified jaw-thrust technique to open the airway, maintain a neutral in-line position of the head and neck, remove any foreign bodies from the mouth, and provide rescue breathing if breathing is inadequate.

   Closely monitor the airway, breathing, pulse, and mental status for deterioration; *you must seek additional medical care and prepare for immediate transport for any victim who displays any evidence of head injury or deteriorating mental status.* A victim of head injury may vomit, so be prepared to position the victim to keep the airway clear.

2. Control bleeding; face and scalp wounds may bleed heavily, but such bleeding is usually easy to control with direct pressure.

   - Do not apply pressure to an open or depressed skull injury.
   - Dress and bandage open head wounds as indicated in the discussion of treatment of soft-tissue injuries (see Chapter 7).

REMEMBER: Take spinal injury precautions in all cases of head trauma, as well as all cases of multiple trauma involving unconsciousness, particularly if resuscitative measures are required at the accident site.

FIGURE 13–9. Always take spinal injury precautions in victims with injury to the head.

- Do not attempt to stop the flow of blood or cerebrospinal fluid from the ears or nose (see Figure 13-10); instead, cover loosely with a sterile gauze dressing to absorb, but not stop, the flow.

FIGURE 13–8. Always suspect and assess for spinal injury in a victim with trauma to the head.

FIGURE 13–10. Blood and/or cerebrospinal fluid may come from the ears and/or nose of a victim of head injury. Cover lightly with dressing. Do not block the drainage.

3. Never try to remove a penetrating object; instead:
   - Immobilize it with soft, bulky dressings and dress the wound with sterile dressings.
   - If the object is too long to allow for victim transport, it will need to be stabilized and cut; wait for the arrival of emergency personnel.

4. If the victim sustained a medical or nontraumatic injury, place the victim on the left side; elevate the head slightly, keep the victim warm, but avoid overheating.

5. While waiting for emergency personnel to arrive:
   - Dress any facial and scalp wounds that have not been dressed.
   - Continue to monitor vital signs.
   - Stay alert to the possibility of vomiting or seizures; work quickly to prevent aspiration.
   - Continually monitor the airway and the victim's neurological status.

PROGRESS CHECK

1. The top priority in treating victims of head injury is establishing and maintaining _____ . *(an open airway/circulation/hemorrhage control)*

2. Use the modified _____ technique to open the airway. *(head-tilt/chin-lift/jaw-thrust)*

3. If there is blood or fluid dripping from the ear, _____ . *(control it with pressure/pack the ear with gauze/cover the ear loosely with gauze to absorb the flow)*

4. If you suspect a fracture beneath a bleeding scalp wound, _____ . *(do not apply pressure/apply pressure/use a compression bandage)*

5. _____ any object protruding from the head. *(Remove/Cut off/Stabilize and leave in place)*

13.4   Injuries to the Spine

The spine consists of a column of hollow vertebrae; the spinal cord, which controls many of the nervous functions of the body, passes through the channel formed by the hollow spaces. Injury to the spine can pinch or sever the spinal cord, resulting in permanent damage and disability.

Unless the spinal cord is injured, the victim may not show any signs of weakness, numbness, lack of sensation, or paralysis. A victim might actually suffer a spinal column (bony vertebrae) fracture without a spinal cord injury that can be easily converted to a spinal cord injury without the proper protection of the victim while on the scene. For example, a victim might have a fracture to his vertebrae in his neck from a fall off scaffolding at a work site. When you arrive at the victim's side to provide first aid, you lift his head to place a soft towel underneath it. By lifting his head, you may have moved the vertebrae out of line and caused the fractured vertebrae to compress or lacerate (cut) the spinal cord. The victim may now suffer permanent injury due to your improper movement of his head. Victims with suspected spine injuries must be kept still with their head, neck, and body in an in-line position and handled with extreme caution to protect the spine.

The four common causes of spinal cord injury are car accidents, shallow-water swimming/diving accidents, motorcycle accidents, and other injuries and falls. Many sports—including diving/swimming, skiing, sledding, and football—cause accidents that lead to spinal damage.

Some parts of the spine are far more susceptible to injury than others (see Figure 13-11 for spinal regions). Half of all spinal injuries occur in the neck, and half of those result in complete paralysis. Fewer injuries involve the thoracic vertebrae or the sacral and coccygeal vertebrae, which have little movement but are designed to bear weight (see Chapter 2).

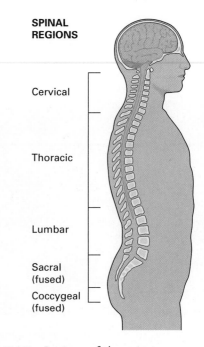

SPINAL REGIONS

Cervical

Thoracic

Lumbar

Sacral (fused)

Coccygeal (fused)

FIGURE 13–11. Regions of the spine

Mechanisms of Injury

> **Learning Objective 9** Describe the common mechanisms of spinal injury.

The basic mechanisms that cause spinal injury (see Figure 13-12 on page 230) include:

- Compression (the weight of the body is driven against the head, as in falls)
- Excessive flexion, extension, or rotation
- Lateral bending
- **Distraction** (a sudden "pulling apart" of the spine that stretches and tears the spinal cord, as in hangings)

In addition, bony spinal injuries occur when fragments of bone or pieces of disc injure the spinal cord. Spinal cord injuries in the absence of fractures are always a possibility in cases involving penetrating objects and in any instance of sudden, unexplained loss of movement or sensation.

You should suspect spinal injury in the following situations:

- Motor vehicle accidents
- Pedestrian-vehicle accidents
- Falls (even from a standing position to the ground)
  Blunt trauma
- Penetrating trauma to the head, neck, or torso
- Motorcycle accidents
- Hangings
- Diving accidents (especially in shallow water)
- Unwitnessed submersion incident
- Sports injury accidents that cause damage to helmets
  Violent injuries, assaults, and shootings
- Accident victims with an altered mental status

Complications of Spinal Injury

There are two major complications of spinal injury (see Figure 13-13 on page 231): inadequate breathing effort and paralysis.

INADEQUATE BREATHING EFFORT

Respiratory paralysis may occur with spine injury, and death may occur rapidly if respiratory assistance is delayed. A cervical spine injury may damage the nerve that controls the diaphragm. A victim who loses the contraction of the diaphragm will have shallow breathing with little movement of the chest or abdomen.

PARALYSIS

There is usually weakness, loss of sensation, or paralysis below the level of injury. In the conscious victim, paralysis of the arms or legs is considered the most reliable sign of spinal injury.

Victim Assessment

> **Learning Objective 10** Describe the assessment of spinal injury victims.

Caution: The extent of assessment should be based on the level of training the First Aider has had under the direction of a qualified and certified instructor.

To assess a responsive victim:

1. Note the mechanism of injury—especially the type of movement and amount of force that was involved in the injury. Even if a victim can move or walk around, spinal injury may exist—so always suspect spinal injury if the mechanism of injury suggests it.

2. Ask:
   - Does your neck or back hurt?
   - What happened?
   - Where does it hurt?
   - Can you move your hands and feet?
   - Can you feel me touching your fingers?
   - Can you feel me touching your toes?
   - Can you feel which toe I am pinching?
   - Can you feel which finger I am pinching?

3. Inspect the back for contusions, deformities, lacerations, punctures, penetrations, and swelling. If necessary, cut clothing away so you can see the area clearly (see Figures 13-14 through 13-22 on pages 231–232).

4. Palpate gently for areas of tenderness or deformity.

5. Assess equality of strength in the victim's extremities:
   - Have the victim grip and squeeze both your hands; note differences in strength.
   - Have the victim gently push his or her feet against your hands; note strength and equality.

> **distraction** The sudden pulling apart of the spine that stretches and tears the cord

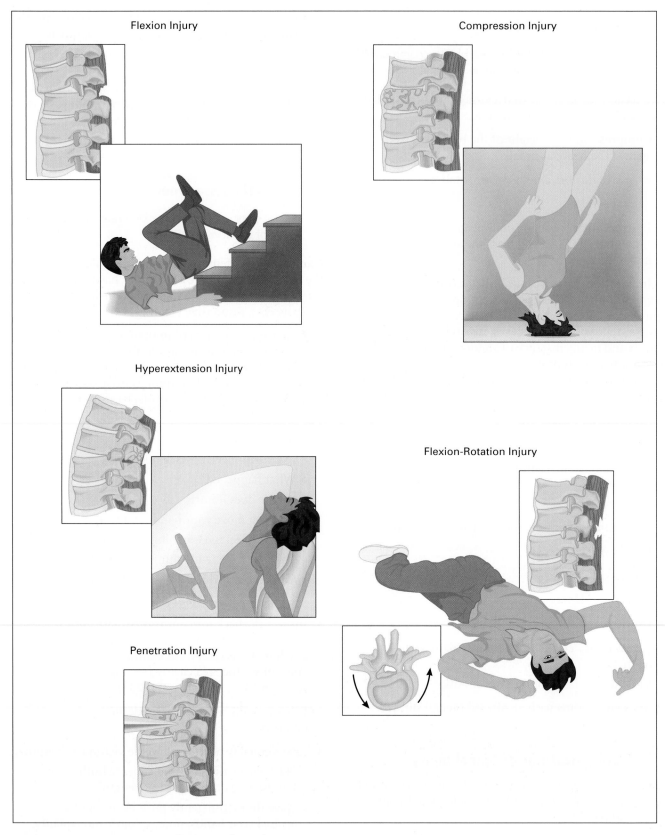

FIGURE 13–12. Common mechanisms of spinal injury

NOTE:

Persons with neck injuries may have paralyzed chest muscles and damage to nerves affecting size of blood vessels. Breathing can then be accomplished only by the diaphragm. Inadequate breathing and shock may occur.

Spine injuries are most common at the cervical level (A). The prime hazard is damage to the spinal cord (B), which may result from trauma per se or from well-meaning but injudicious management following the accident. RULE: In all cases of suspected spine injury, treat the victim as if there is a cervical fracture, unless proven otherwise.

REMEMBER: Take spinal injury precautions in all cases of head trauma, as well as all cases of multiple trauma involving unconsciousness, particularly if resuscitative measures are required at the accident site.

FIGURE 13–13. Considerations in cervical spine injury

FIGURE 13–14. Assess for cervical tenderness and deformity.

FIGURE 13–15. Assess for spinal column tenderness and deformity.

FIGURE 13–16. Use the toe touch and foot pinch to assess for light touch and pain sensation.

FIGURE 13–17. Use the foot wave to see if the feet and toes move.

FIGURE 13–18. Use the foot push to assess for equality of strength.

FIGURE 13–19. Use the finger touch and hand pinch to assess for light touch and pain sensation.

FIGURE 13–20. Use the hand wave to see if the hands and fingers move.

FIGURE 13–21. Use the hand squeeze to assess for equality of strength.

FIGURE 13–22. A victim with an altered mental status may respond only to painful stimuli. Note how the victim responds.

To assess an unresponsive victim:

1. Note the mechanism of injury. If the mechanism of injury suggests spinal injury and the victim is unconscious, assume spinal injury has occurred.

2. Inspect for contusions, deformities, lacerations, punctures, penetrations, or swelling; palpate for areas of deformity.

3. Ask others at the scene about the mechanism of injury and the victim's mental status before you arrived on the scene.

PROGRESS CHECK

1. The vertebrae most likely to be injured are the _____ . (thoracic/lumbar/cervical)

2. One mechanism of spinal injury is distraction, or _____ of the vertebrae. (compression/pulling apart/rotation)

3. The first step in assessment of spinal injury victims is to note the _____ . (mental status/loss of motor function/mechanism of injury)

4. If the victim is _____ and the mechanism of injury suggests it, suspect spinal injury. (paralyzed/unconscious/in pain)

13.5 Signs and Symptoms of Spinal Injury

Learning Objective 11 List the signs and symptoms of spinal injury.

Suspect spinal injury with any serious injury, even injuries to the arms and legs; spinal injury often accompanies head, neck, and back injuries.

Remember that a fracture of one spot on the spine may be associated with a fracture in other areas of the spine. Remember, too, that the ability to walk, move the arms and legs, feel sensation, or the lack of pain to the spinal column does not rule out the possibility of spinal column or spinal cord damage.

The general signs and symptoms of spinal injury include the following (see Figure 13-23):

- Tenderness in the area of the injury; lacerations, cuts, punctures, or bruises over or around the spine indicate forceful injury.

- Pain associated with movement; suspect spinal injury if the victim complains of pain when moving an apparently uninjured neck, shoulder, or leg. Pain from spinal injury may be localized, and the victim may be able to indicate exactly where it hurts. *Never ask the victim to move, never allow the victim to move, and never move the victim yourself to test for pain*; base your assessment on any movement that occurred before you arrived on the scene.

- Pain independent of movement or palpation along the spinal column or in the lower legs. Such pain is generally intermittent instead of constant, and it may occur anywhere along the spine between the top of the head and the tops of the legs. If the lower spinal column or cord is injured, the victim may feel pain in the legs.

- Obvious deformity of the spine upon palpation (not a usual sign). Never have the victim remove clothing so you can examine the back, because the movement may aggravate any existing injury. If necessary, cut clothing away.

- Soft-tissue injuries associated with trauma in the head and neck (causing cervical spine injury); shoulders, back, or abdomen (causing thoracic or lumbar injury); or the legs (causing lumbar or sacral injury).

- Numbness, weakness, or tingling in the arms or legs.

- Loss of sensation, weakness, or paralysis in the arms or legs. (Paralysis of the arms or legs is considered the most reliable sign of spinal injury.)

- Urinary or fecal incontinence.

- Impaired breathing, especially breathing that involves little or no chest movement and only slight abdominal movement.

STEPS FOR CHECKING SIGNS AND SYMPTOMS

PAIN. The victim may be aware of unprovoked pain in the area of injury.

TENDERNESS. Gently touching the suspected area may result in increased pain.

DEFORMITY. Deformity is rare although there may be an abnormal bend or bony prominence.

CUTS AND BRUISES. Victims with neck fractures may have cuts and bruises on the head, or face. Victims with injuries in other areas of the spine will have bruises on the shoulders, back, or abdomen.

PARALYSIS. If the victim is unable to move or feels no sensation in some part of his body, he may have a spinal fracture, with cord injury.

PAINFUL MOVEMENT. If the victim tries to move, the pain may increase—never try to move the injured area for the victim.

CONSCIOUS VICTIMS	UNCONSCIOUS VICTIMS
■ Ask: What happened? Where does it hurt? Can you move your hands and feet? Can you feel me touching your hands (feet)? Can you raise your legs and arms? ■ Look: for bruises, cuts, deformities. ■ Feel: for areas of tenderness, deformity, abnormal sensation. ■ The victim's strength can be determined by having the victim squeeze the rescuer's hand or by checking pressure against the foot.	■ Assess for breathing. ■ Look: for cuts, bruises, deformities. ■ Feel: for deformities, sensation. ■ Ask others: What happened? ■ Probe the soles of the feet, then the palms of the hands with a sharp object to check for response.

FIGURE 13–23. Signs of possible spinal cord injury

1. The ability to walk or move the arms and legs does not rule out _____ . *(priapism/ deformity/spinal injury)*

2. The most reliable sign of spinal injury in a conscious victim is _____ . *(priapism/ incontinence/paralysis of the extremities)*

3. Breathing that involves little or no chest movement indicates that the victim is breathing with only the _____ . *(abdomen/diaphragm/mouth)*

13.6 First Aid Care for Spinal Injury

Learning Objective **12** Describe and demonstrate the appropriate first aid care for spinal injury.

Caution: The first aid procedures discussed in this chapter should not be attempted unless you have adequate classroom and practical training under the direction of an authorized instructor.

The general rule for management of spinal injury is to support and immobilize the spine, the head, the torso, and the pelvis. Your goal is to end up with a victim who is properly immobilized on a backboard. It is better to overtreat than to risk further injury (see Figure 13-24).

Activate the EMS system, then:

1. Establish and maintain in-line stabilization.

   - Place the head in a neutral in-line position unless the victim complains of pain or the head is not easily moved into position.

   - If you encounter resistance, stabilize the neck in the position in which you found it.

   - Place the head in alignment with the spine.

   - Maintain a constant manual in-line stabilization (see Figure 13-25) until the victim is properly secured to a backboard with the head immobilized.

Always activate the EMS system first. Take every precaution against converting a spinal injury into cord damage. In vehicular accidents immobilize cervical spine (using spine board, cervical collar, rolled blanket, etc.) before removing victim. Advise the conscious victim not to move the head. A helmet should be removed unless here is difficulty in removing it. *Follow local protocol.* In such cases, immobilize victim on spine board with helmet in place.

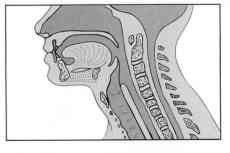

Is the victim experiencing respiratory difficulty? Remember that the airway has first priority. If resuscitative measures are indicated, support the head, immobilize the neck, and get help to move the victim to a flat surface. Check the mouth for obstruction (dentures, tongue, etc.), and ventilate, taking care to minimize motion of the neck. Control severe bleeding by direct pressure. If necessary, initiate CPR.

Keep in mind that respiratory paralysis may occur with cervical spine injury and that death may occur rapidly if respiratory assistance is delayed. Unless it is necessary to change a victim's position to maintain an open airway or for some other compelling reason, it is best to splint the neck or back in the original position of deformity.

Be alert for shock and vomiting. If necessary, administer artificial ventilation.

Immobilize victim before moving. As soon as possible, transfer to a firm stretcher or spine board and restrict head movement with tape, sandbags, collar, rolled towels, and/or blankets.

Provide emotional support.

Always support the head in neutral alignment with body. Avoid flexion, extension, lateral movement, rotation, and traction.

FIGURE 13–24. First aid care for suspected spinal injury

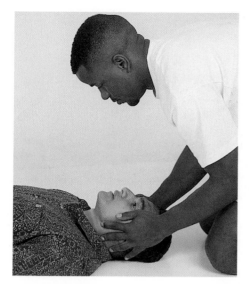

FIGURE 13–25. Maintaining neutral in-line stabilization of the head and neck

Prevent movement of the victim's head by one of the following methods:

- Having a person hold the head and neck in a neutral in-line position.
- Kneel with the victim's head held firmly between your knees.

2. Establish and maintain an open airway and adequate ventilation. Use the modified jaw-thrust technique to open the airway and provide rescue breathing if breathing is inadequate.

3. Perform the initial assessment; check pulse and circulation; perform CPR if necessary, but do not move the victim. Control hemorrhage, but never try to stop the flow of blood or fluid from the ears, nose, or mouth. Never apply pressure to a bleeding head wound if you suspect skull fracture.

Helmet Removal

Learning Objective **13** Describe the technique for removing a helmet from a head- or spinal-injured victim.

Caution: Never attempt to remove a helmet unless you have been trained in these advanced techniques by a certified instructor.

Thorough assessment of any victim is difficult, and that especially applies to a victim who is wearing a helmet. You need to assess the fit of the helmet and movement of the victim's head within the helmet, and determine your ability to gain access to airway and breathing.

You should leave the helmet in place if:

- The helmet fits well, and there is little or no movement of the victim's head inside the helmet.
- There are no impending airway or breathing problems.
- Removal of the helmet would cause further injury to the victim.
- You can properly immobilize the spine with the helmet in place.
- The helmet doesn't interfere with your ability to assess and reassess airway and breathing.

You should remove the helmet if:

- The helmet interferes with your ability to assess or reassess airway and breathing.
- The helmet interferes with your ability to manage the airway or breathing adequately.
- The helmet does not fit well and allows excessive movement of the head inside the helmet.
- The helmet interferes with proper spinal immobilization.
- The victim is in cardiac arrest.

There are two general types of helmets: sports helmets (such as those worn for football) and motorcycle helmets. Generally, sports helmets have an opening in the front and allow much easier access to the airway. Motorcycle helmets, on the other hand, generally cover the full face and have a shield that prevents access to the airway. Football helmets should be left in place; however, the face shield should be removed if the victim requires immediate access to the airway or breathing. Football shoulder pads must also remain in place. The victim will be immobilized to the backboard without removing helmet and shoulder pads. The face shield must be removed if the victim is to be transported.

The technique for removal of a helmet depends on the type of helmet the victim is wearing. The following are general rules for removal of a helmet (see Figures 13-26 through 13-29 on page 236)

1. Take the victim's eyeglasses off before you attempt to remove the helmet.

2. One First Aider should stabilize the helmet by placing hands on each side of the helmet, fingers on the mandible (lower jaw) to prevent movement.

3. A second First Aider should loosen the chin strap.

4. The second First Aider should place one hand on the mandible at the angle of the jaw, and the other hand at the back of the head.

FIGURE 13–26. The first First Aider takes a position above or behind the victim and places his or her hands on each side of the neck at the base of the skull, applying steady stabilization with the victim's neck in a neutral position. The First Aider may use the index fingers and the thumbs to perform a jaw-thrust while doing this.

FIGURE 13–27. The second First Aider takes a position over or to the side of the victim and removes or cuts the chin strap.

FIGURE 13–28. The first First Aider now removes the helmet by pulling out laterally on each side to clear the ears and then up to remove. Full face helmets will have to be tilted back to clear the nose (tilt the helmet, not the head). If the victim has glasses on, the first First Aider should remove them through the visual opening before removing the full face helmet. The second First Aider maintains steady stabilization during this procedure.

FIGURE 13–29. The second First Aider now applies a suitable cervical spine immobilization collar, and the victim is secured to a long board.

5. The First Aider holding the helmet should pull the sides of the helmet apart (to provide clearance for the ears), gently slip the helmet halfway off the victim's head, then stop.

6. The First Aider who is maintaining stabilization of the neck should reposition, sliding the hand under the victim's head to secure the head from falling back after the helmet is completely removed.

7. The first First Aider should remove the helmet completely.

8. The victim should then be immobilized as described on pages 234–235.

The victim should then be immobilized as described on pages 234–235.

PROGRESS CHECK

1. The general rule for management of spinal injury is to _____ the spine, head, torso, and pelvis. *(reduce/straighten/immobilize)*

2. The first priority in caring for spinal injury is to ensure adequate _____ . *(airway and ventilation/circulation/immobilization)*

Summary

- In open head injury, the skull is fractured, causing exposure of the brain; in closed head injury, the scalp may be lacerated but the skull is intact.

- Skull fracture itself does not cause disability and death; the underlying damage is what leads to serious consequences.

- There are four types of skull fracture—depressed, linear, comminuted, and basilar.

- You should suspect skull fracture with any significant trauma to the head.

- Never attempt to stop the flow of blood or fluid from the nose, ears, or mouth; cover loosely with a piece of gauze that will absorb, but not block, the flow.

- The top priority in treating head injuries is to establish and maintain an open airway with adequate breathing and oxygenation; the most common cause of death following head injury is oxygen deficiency in the brain.

- Head and scalp wounds may bleed heavily; don't apply direct pressure on a wound if you suspect underlying damage to the skull.

- The cervical vertebrae are most prone to injury; the lumbar are least.

- The basic mechanisms of spinal injury are compression, distraction, rotation, flexion, and extension.

- Paralysis in a responsive victim is the most reliable sign of spinal injury.

- The general rule for management of spinal injury is to support and immobilize the spine, head, torso, and pelvis.

- The first priority in treating spinal injury is to stabilize the spine and ensure an adequate airway and ventilation.

Key Terms

Make sure you understand the following key terms:

coup-contrecoup
raccoon eyes
Battle's sign
distraction

Critical Thinking Exercise

You are out cutting the lawn when you notice your neighbor fall from a ladder from the top of his two-story home. You rush over to help him. He is lying on his back, and his eyes are not open. He is not responding to you when you call his name. There is blood coming from his right ear. His breathing is irregular and shallow.

1. What injuries do you suspect he could have suffered?

2. What immediate first aid would you provide to the victim?

3. How would you protect the spine from further injury?

Chapter 13 Self-Test

Student: _____ Date: _____

Course: _____ Section #: _____

Part 1   True/False

If you believe the statement is true, circle the T. If you believe the statement is false, circle the F.

T   F   **1.** In a head-injured victim, use the head-tilt/chin-lift maneuver to open the airway.

T   F   **2.** Forceful vomiting may be a sign of head injury.

T   F   **3.** A basilar skull fracture is the most common and least serious.

T   F   **4.** Face and scalp wounds may bleed heavily but are usually easy to control.

T   F   **5.** It is not possible for a spine-injured victim to walk around.

T   F   **6.** Spinal-injury precautions should be taken in all cases of head trauma.

T   F   **7.** The airway is the first priority in a spine-injured victim.

T   F   **8.** Always pad behind the neck of the victim on a rigid support.

T   F   **9.** Any trauma severe enough to cause injury to the brain can also cause injury to the spine.

T   F   **10.** With proper precautions, one First Aider can safely remove a victim's helmet.

Part 2   Multiple Choice

For each item, circle the correct answer or the phrase that best completes the statement.

1. If a victim has blood or cerebrospinal fluid draining from the ears but shows no indication of spinal injury, the first step in first aid care is to

   a. stabilize the neck
   b. stop the flow of blood and cerebrospinal fluid
   c. complete the primary survey
   d. establish and maintain an open airway

2. Which of the following methods of maintaining an open airway should be used on an unresponsive victim with a head injury?

   a. chin-lift only
   b. head-tilt/chin-lift
   c. modified jaw-thrust
   d. head-tilt/neck-lift

3. When a foreign object is impaled in the skull

   a. do not remove the object, but carefully stabilize it
   b. remove the object and apply a loose sterile dressing
   c. do not remove the object unless it will hinder transport
   d. remove the object and pack the wound with sterile pads

4. With a comminuted skull fracture

   a. the fracture is not in the area of impact or injury
   b. the skull is depressed
   c. scalp laceration and brain laceration are also present
   d. multiple cracks radiate from the center of impact

5. What is the most common characteristic of Battle's sign?

   a. unequal dilation of the pupils
   b. discoloration of the soft tissue under the eyes
   c. a bruise-like mark behind either ear
   d. one eye that appears sunken

6. Which of the following occurs in coup-contrecoup injury to the brain?

   a. the brain is slapped against the skull as the head is hurled forward
   b. the brain rebounds against the opposite side of the skull
   c. the skull stops suddenly and the brain is smashed against it
   d. all of the above

7. Which of the following is *not* a sign of spinal injury?

   a. numbness and tingling in the arms and/or legs
   b. loss of response to pain
   c. loss of bowel and bladder control
   d. position of the legs

8. Check for spinal-cord damage in a responsive victim by

   a. asking the victim to wiggle fingers and toes
   b. asking the victim to speak
   c. asking the victim to read
   d. checking reflexes at the knees or elbows

1. A 5-year-old child falls off a high fence, hitting his head on a concrete driveway. He has an open wound on the forehead, he is unconscious, and he has blood-tinged fluid draining from his left ear.

2. You are at a park where a teenaged boy has been hit in the head with a baseball. He is in a prone position and has a large swelling on the side of his head. Bystanders say that he was unconscious, but he is conscious now. He seems confused, restless, and irritable and is vomiting.

3. You are at the scene of an automobile accident and find a woman who was thrown out of one of the vehicles. She is in a sitting position, has a large forehead laceration, and is complaining of neck pain.

Part 4   Skills Review

The following photographs show steps in the removal of a helmet. Number the photographs from 1 to 4 to show the correct order of the sequence.

_____   _____   _____   _____

14

Poisoning Emergencies

Learning Objectives

When you have mastered the material in this chapter, you will be able to

1 Identify the ways in which poisons can enter the body

2 List the signs and symptoms of ingestion (swallowing) of poison

3 Describe and demonstrate first aid care for victims of ingested poisons

4 Discuss the guidelines for use of activated charcoal

5 List the signs and symptoms of inhalation (breathing) of poison

6 List the signs and symptoms of carbon monoxide poisoning

7 Describe and demonstrate first aid care for victims of inhaled poisons

8 List the signs and symptoms of injection of poison

9 Describe and demonstrate first aid care for victims of injected poisons

10 List the signs and symptoms of absorption of poison

11 Describe and demonstrate first aid care for victims of absorbed poisons

On the Scene

Cliff Harding was raking leaves in his front yard when he heard 2-year-old Joshua Bandley screaming in the garage next door. Running to the garage, Cliff found the toddler wiping frantically at his mouth. Next to him on the garage floor was a soda pop bottle. Sniffing at the mouth of the bottle, Cliff knew some kind of insecticide had been stored inside.

As Cliff assessed the situation, Joshua began vomiting. Cliff realized the toddler's breathing rate was slowing and that he was showing signs of shock. When Joshua's mother ran into the garage in response to her child's screams, Cliff sent her to call for emergency personnel.

Cliff positioned Joshua on his side, covered him with a jacket, and—still wearing garden gloves—wiped the remaining vomitus from Joshua's mouth to keep his airway clear. Cliff monitored Joshua's breathing and kept him on his side with his face pointed downward until emergency personnel arrived a few minutes later.

Each year in the United States, between one and two million poisonings occur, 90 percent of them in the home. Only a small percentage are fatal; still, thousands of people die from suicidal or accidental poisonings. Poisoning is the third most common cause of accidental death in the United States, and is a leading cause of deaths among children.

In fact, most unintentional poisoning occurs in children younger than 5 years old. Although the death rate among children has decreased slightly over the past three decades, it has increased among adults, mostly because of drug use and suicide. In addition to the fatalities, approximately one million cases of nonfatal poisoning occur because of exposure to substances such as industrial chemicals, cleaning agents, plant and insect sprays, and medications—in fact, two-thirds of all poisonings in all age groups involve drugs.

A poison is any substance—liquid, solid, or gas—that impairs health or causes death by its chemical action when it enters the body in relatively small amounts or comes into contact with the surface of the skin. Some substances that are otherwise harmless become deadly if used incorrectly. For example, half of all fatal drug overdoses occur when people abuse or misuse prescription drugs.

Poisons may enter the body in four ways (see Figure 14-1):

1. Swallowing (**ingesting**) substances such as medications, household cleaners, or chemicals

2. Inhaling noxious dusts, gases, fumes, or mists

3. Penetrating the skin, such as by injection with hypodermic needles or by animal, snake, or insect bites

4. Absorbing through the skin (as with poisonous liquids) or touching the skin (as with poisonous plants)

This chapter discusses the challenges involved in caring for victims who have swallowed, inhaled, injected, or absorbed poisons; outlines first aid care; and provides the latest guidelines on the use of activated charcoal. First aid treatment for poisoning is extremely important, as there are very few antidotes, and antidotes are not available for most poisons.

14.1 Ingested Poisons

The most common items that can cause poisoning when swallowed are aspirin, acetaminophen, alcohol, detergents/soaps, household cleaning products, and

Learning Objective 1 Identify the ways in which poisons can enter the body.

ingesting Taking a substance into the body through the mouth

Poisons May Enter the Body Through

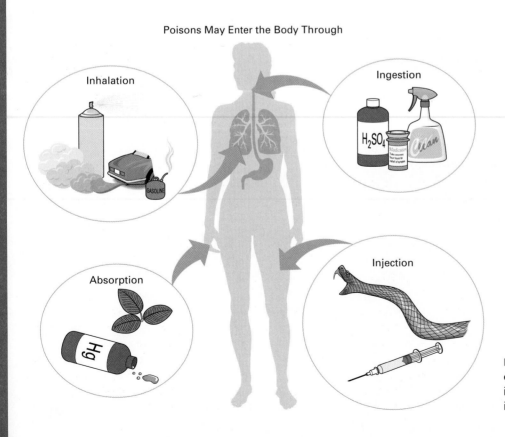

FIGURE 14–1. Poisons may enter the body by ingestion, inhalation, absorption, or injection.

FIGURE 14—2. Poisoning is the number-one cause of accidental death among children.

petroleum distillates. Children are frequently poisoned (see Figure 14-2) by swallowing household products or by eating houseplants or outdoor plants; half of all plant poisonings are caused by mushrooms. Most of the time, the amount of toxin is too low or the amount of poison swallowed is too little to result in severe poisoning. Even with that in mind, however, the potential for fatal or severe poisoning always exists, so first aid care is always appropriate.

Poisonous plants are not necessarily exotic—they include common household and backyard plants, such as morning glory, rhubarb leaves, buttercup, daisy, daffodil, lily of the valley, narcissus, tulip, azalea, iris, hyacinth, laurel, philodendron, dieffenbachia, Jerusalem cherry, snowdrop, oleander, rhododendron, wisteria, and certain parts of the tomato, potato, asparagus, and petunia plants. The berries of holly, mistletoe, and English ivy are poisonous, as is the sap of the poinsettia. The most poisonous wild plant is water hemlock; others include nightshade and mountain laurel. Parts of some common foods are even poisonous. The pits of cherries, peaches, apricots, and other fruit have enough cyanide to cause death. So do the seeds of apples and some other fruits.

Many things that are safe in small amounts can be poisonous if swallowed in large amounts. Medicines, whether over-the-counter or prescription, can be poisonous if they are not used according to label directions.

Ingested poisons usually remain in the stomach only a short time; most absorption takes place after the poison has passed into the small intestine. The goal of first aid care for swallowed poisons, then, is to rid the body of poison before it enters the intestinal tract.

Poison Control Centers

Poison control centers are specialized health-care centers that provide information and advice about care for people who have been poisoned. They answer more than two million calls a year; they have been set up across the United States and Canada and are sometimes housed in hospital emergency rooms. Officials at the center can help you set priorities and formulate an effective first aid plan and can provide information about any available antidote that may be appropriate.

You can get the number of your local Poison Control Center from the phone book, a doctor, a hospital, or EMS personnel. Calls to Poison Control Centers are toll-free, and most centers are staffed 24 hours a day by experienced professionals. Each center is also connected to a network of nationwide consultants who can answer questions about almost any toxin. In addition, information on the Poison Control Center's computer is updated every 90 days to provide the latest information on treatment options and antidotes. Finally, centers provide follow-up telephone calls, monitoring the victim's progress and making treatment suggestions until the victim is either hospitalized or free of symptoms.

If the poisoning victim is conscious, call Poison Control before you do anything else. Be prepared to tell poison center officials the victim's approximate age and weight. Summarize the victim's condition, including level of consciousness, level of activity, skin color, vomiting, and so on. Give as many specifics about the poison as you can.

If the victim is unconscious, activate the EMS before calling Poison Control.

The Importance of Taking a History

Getting a history from a poisoning victim can be difficult, and the history you do get might not be accurate—the victim might be misinformed, might be subject to a drug-induced confusion, or might be deliberately trying to deceive you. In addition, some poisons act so slowly that signs and symptoms might not be obvious at first. To give correct first aid care to a poisoning victim, however, you need a relevant history. Finding out that the poisoning has occurred is the most important part of first aid care for poisoning.

If the victim is a child, other children in the house may have also eaten the poison, so assess all children carefully. Interview family members and witnesses. Quickly look for clues at the scene—overturned or empty medicine bottles, scattered pills or capsules, recently emptied containers, spilled chemicals, spilled cleaning solvents, an overturned plant or pieces of plant, the remains of food or drink, or vomitus.

Ask the victim or bystanders the following questions:

- What was swallowed?

- When was it swallowed?

- How much was swallowed?

- Has anyone tried to induce vomiting? Has anything been given as an antidote?

- Does the victim have a history that suggests a possible suicide attempt?

- Does the victim have an underlying medical illness, allergy, chronic drug use, or addiction?

Signs and Symptoms

> Learning Objective 2 List the signs and symptoms of ingestion (swallowing) of poison.

People who have swallowed poisons usually look ill; in addition, you may find a container of a potentially poisonous substance near the victim. The signs and symptoms of poisoning by ingestion vary, depending on what was ingested (see Figure 14-3); the following are the most common:

- Nausea, vomiting, and diarrhea

- Excessive salivation

- Varying levels of unconsciousness, from drowsiness to unconsciousness

- Abdominal pain, tenderness, bloating, and/or cramps

- Burns or stains around the mouth, pain in the mouth or throat, and/or pain during swallowing (corrosive poisons may corrode, burn, or destroy the tissues of the mouth, throat, and stomach)

- Unusual breath or body odors; characteristic chemical odors (such as turpentine) on the breath

If you have even slight suspicion that a person has been poisoned, give first aid care.

POSSIBLE INDICATORS OF CHILDHOOD POISONING

PAY PARTICULAR ATTENTION TO

The child who has swallowed a poison before

The level of consciousness, including any behavioral changes (clumsiness? drowsiness? coma? convulsions? mental disturbances? delirium?)

Skin and mucosa findings (color, temperature of skin, lips, mucous membranes)

Temperature, blood pressure, pulse rate, respiratory alterations

Paralysis?

Constriction   Dilation

The size and reaction of pupils (constriction? dilation?)

Mouth signs (burns? discoloration? dryness? excessive salivation? stains? characteristic breath odors? pain on swallowing?)

Nausea, vomiting (appearance? odor? blood present?)

Diarrhea? odor? appearance? blood present?

FIGURE 14–3. Annually, thousands of U.S. children require some treatment for poisoning.

First Aid Care

Learning Objective **3** Describe and demonstrate first aid care for victims of ingested poisons.

Immediately call Poison Control, activate the EMS system, then follow these steps:

1. Maintain the airway and monitor the victim's airway, breathing, circulation, and disabilities (ABCDs). Protect yourself from injury by wearing gloves to remove any remaining pills, tablets, capsules, or other fragments from the victim's mouth. Secretions may be profuse following the ingestion of certain poisons, so keep the victim's face pointed downward to facilitate drainage.

2. If the poison was a corrosive (acid) or caustic (alkali), immediately give the victim one or two 8-ounce glasses of *cold* water or milk to dilute the poison as instructed by Poison Control. Cold water or milk absorbs heat better than room-temperature or warm liquids. *Do not give water or milk in any other case unless you are told to do so by the Poison Control Center.* Water or milk may cause a dry poison (such as a tablet) to dissolve, and fills up the stomach, forcing stomach contents more quickly into the small intestine, where most of the absorption of poison into the bloodstream takes place.

3. Place the victim on his or her left side so that gravity will delay the poison from entering the small intestine, where most substances are absorbed into the bloodstream. Positioning the victim on his or her left side can delay movement of the poison into the small intestine by as long as 2 hours.

4. Call Poison Control; an estimated three-fourths of all ingested poison emergencies can be successfully handled with instructions given over the phone. Don't simply follow a container's label, which may be outdated or incorrect. In most areas, you will be instructed to administer activated charcoal to absorb the poison; details on activated charcoal are found later in this chapter.

5. *With the exception of an acid or alkali poisoning, never give a poisoning victim anything to eat or drink unless you are told to do so by Poison Control or by a medical professional.*

6. *Never induce vomiting.*

7. Send suspected poisons, containers, plant parts, or other specimens with the victim to the receiving facility. If the victim has vomited, send a sample of the vomitus in a clean, closed container to the receiving facility.

All poisoned victims need to see a physician, even if it appears that all signs and symptoms have been controlled and the emergency is over.

Food Poisoning

A specific kind of poisoning is *food poisoning*, ingestion of food that contains bacteria or the toxins that bacteria produce or that has been contaminated by chemicals (including the lead in water pipes that deliver the water used for cooking). Most commonly, bacterial contamination occurs when food is allowed to sit at room temperature too long; most often at fault are foods containing raw egg, meat, and dairy products. The incidence of food poisoning is increasing dramatically; each year, some 33 million Americans develop gastrointestinal disease as a result of food poisoning.

There are several main types of food poisoning, as detailed in this section.

Botulism. The most fatal type of food poisoning, botulism is a rare but serious illness caused by a nerve toxin that is produced by the bacterium *Clostridium botulinum* (Because the bacteria is found in the soil, a separate type of botulism also results when wounds are contaminated by soil that contains the bacteria.) An average of 110 cases of botulism are reported in the United States each year; of these, approximately one-fourth are caused by eating contaminated food.

Most commonly, botulism results from improperly processed canned foods (usually home-canned foods). The most likely home-canned foods affected are those with low acid content, such as asparagus, green beans, beets, and corn. However, there have also been outbreaks of botulism from more unusual foods, such as chopped garlic in oil, chili peppers, tomatoes, improperly handled baked potatoes wrapped in aluminum foil, and home-canned or fermented fish.

The classic symptoms of botulism include:

- Double or blurred vision
- Drooping eyelids
- Slurred speech
- Difficulty swallowing
- Dry mouth
- Muscle weakness

The classic symptoms are all symptoms of the muscle paralysis caused by the bacterial toxin. If untreated, the infection may progress to cause paralysis of the muscles in the arms, legs, and trunk and those that control breathing. Symptoms of botulism generally begin 18 to 36 hours after eating a contaminated food, but they can occur as early as 6 hours or as late as 10 days after eating contaminated food.

Salmonella (Salmonellosis). Salmonellosis—more commonly referred to as salmonella—is caused by infection with the bacteria *Salmonella*. The *Salmonella* germ is actually a group of bacteria that live in the intestinal tracts of humans and other animals, including birds. *Salmonella* may also be found in the feces of some pets, especially those with diarrhea, and people can become infected if they do not wash their hands after contact with these feces. (Reptiles are particularly likely to harbor *Salmonella*, and people should always wash their hands immediately after handling a reptile, even if the reptile is healthy.) Most often, food becomes contaminated by the unwashed hands of an infected food handler, who forgot to wash his or her hands with soap after using the bathroom.

Foods contaminated with *Salmonella* usually look and smell normal. The most frequently contaminated foods are of animal origin, such as beef, poultry, milk, or eggs—but all foods, including vegetables, may become contaminated. Thorough cooking kills *Salmonella*.

The most common symptoms of salmonellosis include:

- Diarrhea, usually with abdominal cramping

- Fever

Symptoms usually develop 12 to 72 hours after eating the contaminated food. The illness usually lasts 4 to 7 days, and most people recover without treatment. However, if the diarrhea becomes severe, the victim may need to be hospitalized. In some, the *Salmonella* infection may spread from the intestines to the bloodstream, and then to other body sites; in these cases, prompt antibiotic treatment is needed.

Staph Food Poisoning. Staph food poisoning results from eating foods contaminated by *Staphylococcus aureus* bacteria. Most commonly, staph gets into food when the people handling it touch pimples, boils, rashes, infected eyes, infected fingers, or nasal secretions, and then don't wash their hands before touching the food. If staph bacteria get into foods that are not immediately cooked or refrigerated, the bacteria multiply and produce a toxin that will not be destroyed by cooking. (Body temperature is the ideal temperature in which staph bacteria grow.)

The most commonly affected foods include sandwiches; sliced ham, poultry, or other meats; potato salads and egg salads; salad dressings; and cream-filled pastries and custards.

Staph food poisoning causes rapid and dramatic symptoms, including:

- Severe nausea

- Vomiting

- Abdominal cramps

- Diarrhea

- Lack of fever (the temperature may actually be slightly lower than normal)

Staph food poisoning symptoms usually begin within 4 to 8 hours after eating contaminated food—and sometimes within 30 minutes. Its rapid onset makes it easy to distinguish it from the other forms of food poisoning, which take longer to develop.

First Aid Care

To care for a victim of suspected food poisoning, do not give the victim anything by mouth. Seek medical help as soon as possible, since only a physician can properly diagnose food poisoning and since some victims may need advanced treatment.

Syrup of Ipecac

Beginning in 1965 and until recently, the Poison Control Center and physicians advised First Aiders to induce vomiting if a victim swallowed poison—and the recommended way to induce vomiting was with syrup of ipecac. However, in November 2003, the American Academy of Pediatrics (AAP) advised that syrup of ipecac no longer be used to induce vomiting, and advised that people discard any syrup of ipecac they had on hand.

According to the Academy, syrup of ipecac does not improve the outcome for victims of poisoning. In addition, the Academy now advises against inducing vomiting in people who have swallowed poison. Hospitals and emergency clinics throughout the country now use activated charcoal to absorb ingested poisons instead of trying to induce vomiting. (Activated charcoal is discussed in the next section.) The United States Food and Drug Administration has advised that syrup of ipecac no longer have over-the-counter status.

PROGRESS CHECK

1. One of the most common agents involved in poisoning by ingestion is _____ . *(Tabasco sauce/motor oil/aspirin)*

2. While the signs and symptoms of ingestion poisoning vary, it often causes _____ . *(nausea/cyanosis/paralysis)*

3. The top priority in managing ingestion poisoning is maintaining the _____ . *(airway/circulation/level of consciousness)*

4. Syrup of ipecac _____ . *(should only be used in children/should be used immediately regardless of the poison/should not be used)*

14.2 Activated Charcoal

The medication of choice in the first aid care of swallowed poisons is **activated charcoal**, the single most effective treatment for ingested poison. Poison Control Centers, hospitals, and physicians recommend the aggressive use of activated charcoal in such cases. Simply, activated charcoal acts like a sponge to help keep the poison in the digestive system until it is eliminated from the body, preventing absorption in the bloodstream.

Activated charcoal is a special distilled charcoal made of organic vegetable matter (most often wood pulp) that is burned at high temperatures and exposed to strong acids and intense steam. Activated charcoal can absorb many times its weight in contaminants because of its porous surface. (See Figure 14-4.) It is the single most effective first aid treatment for swallowed poison. Activated charcoal is an odorless, tasteless powder or liquid that works best when used promptly, but it can still be effective after several hours—as long as 4 hours after ingestion for some poisons.

Activated charcoal binds to poisons in the stomach, prevents their absorption into the body, and enhances their elimination from the body. Some commercially available activated charcoal products also contain a laxative agent that helps speed the charcoal through the intestinal tract, further limiting any absorption into the body. Activated charcoal does not bind to alcohol, acids, alkalies, potassium, DDT, ferrous sulfate, kerosene, gasoline, caustics, or metals, such as iron.

Some of the more well-known trade names of activated charcoal are SuperChar, InstaChar, Actidose, and LiquiChar. It is generally available at pharmacies, though it may have to be ordered. You can *not* use regular charcoal in place of activated charcoal to treat poisoning.

FIGURE 14–4. Activated charcoal should be used only for victims who have swallowed a poison.

Activated charcoal should be used for victims who have ingested poisons by mouth. Poison Control may instruct you to give several repeat doses over a period of 4 to 6 hours, which may speed the elimination of certain poisons more than a single dose. It has been shown that repeated doses every 2 to 6 hours are more effective than a single dose.

Do *not* give activated charcoal to a victim who:

- Is not fully conscious (has an altered mental status)
- Has swallowed acids or alkalies
- Is unable to swallow

Dosage

> Learning Objective 4 Discuss the guidelines for the use of activated charcoal.

For first aid, use activated charcoal that has been pre-mixed with water instead of charcoal in a powder form; the most common brands contain 12.5 grams of activated charcoal mixed with water in a plastic bottle. (Powdered activated charcoal must be mixed with water and is more difficult to use.)

Unless directed otherwise by Poison Control, give both adults and children 1 gram of activated charcoal per kilogram of body weight. The usual adult dose is 25 to 50 grams. The usual dose for infants and children is 12.5 to 25 grams.

Administration

Directions that follow are general. Consult Poison Control or a medical professional for direction before administering activated charcoal to any victim. To administer activated charcoal (see Figure 14-5):

1. Shake the container of activated charcoal thoroughly; if it is too thick to shake well, remove the cap and stir it until well mixed. The activated charcoal settles to the bottom of the bottle, and needs to be evenly distributed.

2. Activated charcoal looks like mud; you may have an easier time persuading the victim to drink it if you use a straw and a covered, opaque container so the victim can't see it. Don't mix the activated charcoal with anything else in an effort to make it more acceptable to the victim; you could make it less absorbent.

> **activated charcoal** A special steam-distilled charcoal that can absorb many times its weight in contaminants because of its porous surface

FIGURE 14–5. Administering activated charcoal to a victim who has swallowed a poison.

3. If the victim takes a long time to drink the activated charcoal, it will settle. Make sure you shake or stir it again before letting the victim finish the dose.

4. Record the time the victim took the activated charcoal and the specifics about the dose.

5. If the victim vomits, repeat the dose once.

Once you have given a victim activated charcoal, don't let the victim have milk, ice cream, or sherbet; all decrease the effectiveness of the activated charcoal.

PROGRESS CHECK

1. Activated charcoal absorbs poison because of its _____ . *(chemical composition/additives/porous surface)*

2. Activated charcoal works by _____ poisons. *(absorbing/binding/neutralizing)*

3. You should not use activated charcoal for a victim who ingested _____ . *(morning glory/detergent/gasoline)*

4. Don't give activated charcoal to someone who is not fully _____ . *(alert/compromised/able to consent)*

5. Use the _____ form of activated charcoal whenever possible. *(powdered/premixed/premeasured)*

14.3 Inhaled Poisons

Almost 8,000 people die each year in the United States from inhaling poisonous vapors and fumes, some of which are present without any sign. Most toxic inhalation (taking toxins into the body through the lungs) occurs as a result of fire; other common inhaled poisons include chemicals at industrial sites, fumes from drugs (such as crack cocaine), fumes from liquid chemicals, chlorine, ammonia, gases used for medical purposes, solvents used in dry cleaning, sewer gas, carbon dioxide caused by decomposition, and carbon monoxide generated by the incomplete combustion of natural gas.

Immediate first aid is critical, because the body absorbs inhaled poisons rapidly. The longer the exposure without first aid care, the poorer the prognosis. It is also especially important to protect yourself from inhaling the same poison as the victim while you are giving first aid.

Carbon Monoxide Poisoning

Of special concern is **carbon monoxide** poisoning. Carbon monoxide causes half of all poisoning deaths in the United States each year, is the leading cause of poisoning deaths, and is the leading cause of death among people who inhale the smoke from fires. Approximately 1,500 die each year in the United States from carbon monoxide poisoning, and an additional 10,000 require hospitalization.

Carbon monoxide—formed by the incomplete combustion of gasoline, coal, kerosene, plastic, wood, and natural gas—is common in the environment and is completely nonirritating, tasteless, colorless, and odorless. It causes a life-threatening lack of oxygen in two ways. First, it reduces the amount of oxygen carried to cells in the body by the red blood cells; instead of binding to oxygen in the bloodstream, they are 200 times more likely to bind to any carbon monoxide in the bloodstream. Second, it inhibits the ability of body cells to utilize what little oxygen is delivered. The brain and heart sustain the greatest damage.

The primary sources of carbon monoxide are home-heating devices (including furnaces and wood-burning fireplaces) and automobile exhaust fumes (which often enter the car through rust holes in the exhaust system). Because of exhaust fumes, it is extremely dangerous to ride in the back of an enclosed pickup truck. Other common sources of carbon monoxide are tobacco smoke, barbecue grills and charcoal briquettes, kitchen stoves, gas lamps, recreational fires (including sterno and hibachi), propane-powered industrial equipment, and faulty water heaters, kerosene heaters, and space heaters.

---

inhalation The act of breathing in (inspiration), or the drawing of air or other gases into the lungs

carbon monoxide An odorless, tasteless, colorless toxic gas that results from incomplete combustion

It takes only a few minutes to die from carbon monoxide poisoning. Death is so certain, in fact, that more than half of all suicides in the United States each year are committed with automobile exhaust, which is 7 percent carbon monoxide.

Signs and Symptoms

> **Learning Objective 5** List the signs and symptoms of inhalation (breathing) of poison.

The signs and symptoms of carbon monoxide poisoning generally worsen or improve at certain times of the day or in certain places. Additionally, people around the victim are usually ill with the same signs and symptoms in the same circumstances—and pets may also appear to be ill. General signs and symptoms of inhalation poisoning characteristically come and go and include the following:

- Difficulty breathing or shortness of breath

- Chest pain or tightness; a burning sensation in the chest or throat

- Nausea and vomiting

- Visual changes (blurred or double vision)

- Muscle weakness

- Cough, harsh vibrating sound when breathing, wheezing, or other abnormal breathing sounds

- Hoarseness

- Dizziness

- Headache, often severe

- Ringing in the ears (tinnitus)

- Seizures

- Altered mental status or confusion

- Signs of respiratory tract burns, such as singed nasal hairs, soot in the saliva, or soot in the throat

> **Learning Objective 6** List the signs and symptoms of carbon monoxide poisoning.

The signs and symptoms of carbon monoxide poisoning (see Figure 14-6) change with length of exposure and intensity of poisoning. They also change in certain situations (diminishing when you go outside, for example), during certain times of the day (worse when the furnace is running, or when meals are being prepared on a gas stove), and so on. A characteristic sign is that pets in the household also become ill. Carbon monoxide poisoning can initially produce flu-like symptoms, but there are several important differences: carbon monoxide poisoning does not cause a fever, generalized body

Cherry red skin color also may appear, but it is not a reliable indicator. It usually occurs at high levels of exposure at late stages only.

FIGURE 14–6. Signs and symptoms of carbon monoxide poisoning

aches, or swollen lymph glands. One of the things that makes carbon monoxide poisoning—especially from chronic exposure—so dangerous is that it may easily be mistaken for something else.

Low levels of carbon monoxide cause throbbing headache, ringing in the ears, muscle weakness, shortness of breath, nausea, irritability, confusion, loss of judgment, and difficulty concentrating.

Moderate levels of carbon monoxide cause severe headache, severe nausea and vomiting, dizziness, yawning, visual disturbances, and difficulty thinking.

High levels of carbon monoxide cause lethargy and stupor, fainting on exertion, chest pain, heart arrhythmias, temporary loss of vision, convulsions, and coma.

Skin color is normal at first, but becomes pale and then bluish as poisoning progresses. The mucous membranes and skin generally do not become bright cherry-red in color until the victim is dead.

You should consider carbon monoxide poisoning whenever you encounter unexplained flu symptoms (such as headache, nausea, vomiting, and confusion)—especially if the symptoms are shared by other people and pets in the same environment.

First Aid Care

> **Learning Objective 7** Describe and demonstrate first aid care for victims of inhaled poisons.

All victims of inhaled poisons need to be given oxygen as soon as possible, so activate the EMS system *immediately*, then:

1. *Immediately* move the victim into fresh air. Protect yourself—a trained First Aider should remove the victim from the poisonous environment. Never enter an area that might be contaminated. If you suspect that someone has suffered carbon monoxide poisoning, evacuate everyone from the enclosed space—even people who apparently have no symptoms. Ideally, victims should be moved at least 150 feet from the suspected source of the carbon monoxide into open air.

2. Monitor the victim's airway, breathing, circulation, and disability (ABCDs) as explained in Chapter 3. If there are no contraindicating injuries and the victim is conscious, have the victim lie down with head elevated; loosen all tight-fitting clothing, especially around the neck and over the chest. If the victim is unresponsive, place the victim on his or her left side.

3. If the victim is not breathing, start artificial ventilation immediately; do not interrupt it for any reason. Continue until the victim is breathing spontaneously or you are relieved by emergency personnel.

All victims of carbon monoxide poisoning must receive medical care; 45 percent develop delayed neurological complications after initial recovery. A carbon monoxide victim needs medical treatment immediately, even if the victim seems to have recovered. (Remember that awakening or seeming alertness can be false signs of recovery.) Additionally, emergency medical personnel can administer 100 percent oxygen, which speeds recovery. In a conscious victim of carbon monoxide poisoning, it takes 4 to 5 hours on room air to reverse the effects of the poisoning—but it takes only half an hour of 100 percent oxygen to accomplish the same thing.

PROGRESS CHECK

1. Most cases of toxic inhalation occur as a result of _____ . *(automobile exhaust/carbon monoxide/fire)*

2. The most common gas that causes poisoning is _____ . *(sulphur dioxide/nitrous oxide/carbon monoxide)*

3. Carbon monoxide is difficult to detect because it is completely colorless and _____ . *(pervasive/odorless/combustible)*

4. Carbon monoxide poisoning causes symptoms similar to _____ symptoms. *(flu/emphysema/respiratory arrest)*

5. _____ victims of carbon monoxide poisoning need medical care, even if they seem to have recovered. *(No/About half/All)*

14.4 Injected Poisons

Injected poisons are those that enter the body through a break in the skin—sometimes by intentional injection, other times by the bites or stings of animals and insects.

Substances, such as illicit drugs, may be injected under the skin, into the muscle, or directly into the bloodstream. More detailed information on specific drug-related emergencies is found in Chapter 15.

The most common sources of injected poisons are animal and insect bites and stings. Most common are stings from bees, wasps, hornets, yellow jackets, and ants; others include the bites of spiders, ticks, snakes, and the stings of marine animals (such as jellyfish, coral, anemones, and stingrays). (See Chapter 23.)

Injected poisons generally cause an immediate reaction at the injection site followed by a delayed widespread reaction throughout the body. Of special note is the threat of anaphylactic shock following the allergic reaction to an insect bite or sting (see Chapter 6).

Signs and Symptoms

Learning Objective 8 List the signs and symptoms of injection of poison.

General signs and symptoms of toxic injection include:

- Weakness
- Dizziness
- Chills and fever
- Nausea and/or vomiting

Specific signs and symptoms and first aid care of anaphylactic shock are listed in Chapter 6.

First Aid Care

Learning Objective 9 Describe and demonstrate first aid care for victims of injected poisons.

Activate the EMS system, then follow these steps:

1. Maintain the victim's airway.

2. Be alert for vomiting; keep the victim sitting if possible to prevent the victim from inhaling vomit.

3. In the case of an animal or insect bite or sting, protect yourself from injury and protect the victim from repeated injection. Bees can sting only once, then lose their stinger, but wasps, hornets, and yellow jackets can sting repeatedly. (See Chapter 23.)

4. If the victim was bitten or stung, identify the insect, reptile, or animal that caused the injury, if possible; if you killed it, send it to the receiving facility with the victim.

PROGRESS CHECK

1. The most common source of injected poison is _____ . (illicit drugs/marine animals/insect stings)

2. Injected poisons cause a reaction at the injection site followed by a delayed _____ reaction. (systemic/respiratory/circulatory)

3. The greatest danger from insect stings is _____ . (systemic poisoning/lack of antitoxins/anaphylactic shock)

4. The highest priority in caring for a victim of injected poison is _____ . (removing the stinger/maintaining the airway/placement of a constricting band)

14.5 Absorbed Poisons

Absorption of poisons—usually dry or wet chemicals or poisons from plants that enter through the skin—generally causes burns, lesions, and inflammation. Chemicals that are splashed into the eyes cause extreme burning pain, excessive tearing, and the inability to open the eye.

Skin reactions range from mild irritation to severe chemical burns. Absorbed poisons often cause both local and systemwide reactions, which can be severe—exposure of as little as 2.5 percent of the body surface to 100 percent hydrofluoric acid, for example, can cause death.

A fairly common type of absorbed poisoning comes from skin contact with a poisonous plant (see Figures 14-7 through 14-10 on page 252)—usually poison ivy, poison sumac, or poison oak. (More than 60 plants can cause allergic reaction that mimics poisoning.) You don't need direct contact with poison ivy in order to have a reaction from it: the poisonous element, **urushiol,** can be carried on animal fur, tools, and clothing. If poison ivy is burned, molecules of urushiol are emitted in the smoke and can be breathed in or absorbed through the skin. Urushiol, which is actually a resin found in the plant, is a colorless or sometimes slightly light yellow oil that runs just under the surface of the plant; it is easily released and immediately oozes to the surface of the plant if a person or animal brushes up against the plant. It generally can't be seen on the skin, and can stay active for months—sometimes years. An estimated half of all people in the United States are sensitive to poison ivy, and of those, one-fourth have such severe reactions that they require medical treatment. Poison ivy is common throughout most of the United States. Poison sumac grows mostly in the swampy areas of the eastern United States, while poison oak grows mostly along the coastlines and in the south central region of the country.

The stems and leaves of the stinging nettle are covered with fine, hollow stinging "hairs." Unlike poison ivy, which generally causes an allergic response, the effect of stinging nettle is due to its irritating sap, which is injected into the skin by the hairs. An allergic reaction to stinging nettle is rare. The primary symptom of contact with stinging nettle is immediate, intense, burning or stinging pain; depending on how sensitive the victim is, the stinging nettle may also cause redness and itching that can last for several hours.

Other plants that can cause mild to severe skin irritation (dermatitis) include crown of thorns, buttercup, mayapple, marsh marigold, candelabra cactus, brown-eyed Susan, shasta daisy, and chrysanthemum. Approximately one-fourth of those who contact poisonous plants require medical care.

Signs and Symptoms

Learning Objective **10** List the signs and symptoms of absorption of poison.

Signs and symptoms of absorbed poison include:

- Exposure to a poisonous substance
- Traces of liquid or powder on the skin
- Burns
- Itching and/or irritation
- Redness

absorption Taking a substance into the body through the skin

urushiol The toxic element of poison ivy, which can be carried on animal fur, tools, clothing, and, when the plant is burned, in the air

FIGURE 14–7. Poison ivy

FIGURE 14–8. Poison sumac

FIGURE 14–9. Poison oak

FIGURE 14–10. Blisters from contact with a poisonous plant

Signs and symptoms of contact with a poisonous plant include:

- Fluid-filled, oozing blisters
- Itching and burning
- Swelling
- Possible pain
- A rash lasting from 1 to 3 weeks
- Secondary infections from an irritated rash

First Aid Care

> Learning Objective 11 Describe and demonstrate first aid care for victims of absorbed poisons.

The more skin that is affected by poison, the greater the need for medical attention. Make sure the victim sees a doctor if the face or large areas of skin are affected. If a victim has absorbed poison through the skin:

1. Protecting your hands with gloves, move the victim from the source of the poison and remove the victim's contaminated clothing and jewelry. If swelling occurs, remove any noncontaminated clothing or jewelry that constricts.

2. Brush any dry chemicals or solid poisons from the skin, taking extreme care not to scrape the skin.

3. Irrigate the affected area with clean water for at least 20 minutes or until medical help arrives. (A shower or garden hose is ideal.) Carefully check "hidden" areas, such as the nailbeds, skin creases, areas between the fingers and toes, and any hair. If the victim was poisoned by dry chemicals, wash them from the skin only if you have access to a continuous stream of running water.

4. If the victim has been in contact with a poisonous plant, decontaminate the skin immediately by washing it with soap and water or by rinsing it with liberal amounts of rubbing alcohol. (If you use too little alcohol, you may actually cause the oil to spread, increasing the area of injury.) For a mild reaction, have the victim soak in a lukewarm bath sprinkled with two cups of colloidal oatmeal

(available in commercial preparations to relieve itching), apply calamine lotion, take diphenhydramine HCl (Benadryl), or apply a paste of water and baking soda (three parts of baking soda to one part of water). For a moderate reaction, have the victim take a hot shower, with water hot enough to redden but not burn the skin—the release of histamines will cause intense itching for a few minutes followed by relief for as long as 8 hours. For more severe reactions, seek medical help; the victim may need prescription ointment or oral medication.

5. To relieve the reaction from stinging nettle, wash the area well with soap and water, rinse thoroughly, and apply wet, cold compresses to relieve pain and itching. You can also use a colloidal oatmeal paste, 1 percent over-the-counter cortisone cream, calamine lotion, or over-the-counter antihistamine medication.

6. If any reaction is severe, activate the EMS system or transport the victim to a medical facility.

If there are any chemicals on the skin or in the eye, activate the EMS system immediately. If poison has been splashed into the eye, follow the guidelines listed in Chapter 8 for treatment of chemical burns to the eye.

Table 14-1 summarizes the signs, symptoms, and first aid care for common poisons.

PROGRESS CHECK

1. Absorbed poisons enter the body through the _____ . *(alveoli/skin/small intestine)*

2. The poisonous element in poison _____ can be breathed in from smoke or carried on an animal's fur. *(oak/ivy/sumac)*

3. If there is a liquid poison on the victim's skin, _____ for at least 20 minutes. *(keep the victim quiet/irrigate with running water/monitor the victim's status)*

TABLE 14–1	Poisons: Signs and Symptoms, and First Aid Care	
Poison	**Signs and Symptoms**	**First Aid Care**
Ingested poisons (medications, alcohol, detergents, household cleaning products, petroleum distillates, poisonous plants)	• Nausea, vomiting • Diarrhea • Excessive salivation • Altered consciousness • Abdominal pain, cramps • Burns or stains around the mouth • Pain in mouth/throat • Unusual breath/body odors	• Call Poison Control and follow instructions • Maintain airway • If poison was acid or alkali, give cold milk or water; otherwise, give nothing by mouth • Place victim on left side • *Never induce vomiting* • Give activated charcoal
Botulism food poisoning	Within 18–36 hours: • Double or blurred vision • Drooping eyelids • Slurred speech • Difficulty swallowing • Dry mouth • Muscle weakness	• Consult medical help
Salmonella food poisoning	Within 12–72 hours: • Diarrhea • Abdominal cramps • Fever	• Consult medical help
Staph food poisoning	Rapid onset: • Severe nausea • Vomiting • Abdominal cramps • Diarrhea • Lack of fever	• Consult medical help

(Continued)

TABLE 14-1	Poisons: Signs and Symptoms, and First Aid Care (Continued)	
Poison	**Signs and Symptoms**	**First Aid Care**
Carbon monoxide poisoning	• Difficulty breathing, shortness of breath • Chest pain/tightness • Nausea/vomiting • Blurred/double vision • Muscle weakness • Cough/hoarseness • Dizziness • Headache, often severe • Ringing in ears • Seizures • Altered mental status	• *Immediately* move victim into fresh air • Monitor airway, breathing, and circulation • Seek medical help immediately
Insect stings/bites	• Weakness • Dizziness • Fever, chills • Nausea/vomiting	• Maintain airway and circulation • Protect from further injury • Seek medical help
Poison ivy/oak/sumac	• Blistering • Redness • Itching or burning	• Wash with soap and water or irrigate with rubbing alcohol • Bathe in lukewarm tub with colloidal oatmeal • Use baking soda/water paste (3:1) • Shower in hot water (redden skin) every 8 hours
Stinging nettle	• Immediate, intense burning or stinging pain • Redness and/or itching	• Wash with soap and water • Apply cold, wet compresses • Use colloidal oatmeal paste, calamine, or over-the-counter antihistamines

Summary

- Poisons can enter the body through ingestion, inhalation, injection, or absorption.

- Ingested poisons usually only remain in the stomach a short time; most absorption takes place after the poison passes into the small intestine. Therefore, care is aimed at getting the substance out of the body as quickly as possible.

- Activated charcoal is the treatment of choice for victims of swallowed poison; it works by absorbing many times its weight in contaminants.

- You should not administer activated charcoal to a victim who has swallowed alcohol, kerosene, gasoline, acids, or alkalies or a victim who is not fully alert.

- If possible, use the premixed form of activated charcoal.

- Poison Control centers are professionally staffed, 24-hour-a-day referral centers that can provide information on care and antidotes.

- Most toxic inhalation occurs as a result of fire; the most common gas that causes poisoning is carbon monoxide.

- Because carbon monoxide is completely colorless, odorless, and tasteless, it cannot be detected without specialized equipment.

- Symptoms of carbon monoxide poisoning are similar to those caused by the flu, except there is no fever, body ache, and swollen glands; suspect carbon monoxide poisoning in cases where there are unexplained flu symptoms.

- The greatest danger from injected poison is anaphylactic shock.

- You do not actually have to contact poison ivy to have a reaction; urushiol, the poisonous element, can be carried on animal fur, tools, clothing—and, if the poison ivy is burned, in smoke.

Key Terms

Make sure you understand the following key terms:

ingesting
activated charcoal
inhalation
carbon monoxide
absorption
urushiol

Critical Thinking Exercise

You are raking leaves in your backyard on a crisp, clear autumn morning. Suddenly a toddler's scream pierces the still autumn air. You quickly locate the source of the screaming as coming from the neighbor's garage. You immediately dash toward the garage and upon entering, see a toddler sitting on the floor, wiping at his mouth between screams. Next to the little boy on the garage floor lies a soda pop bottle. With a hand on the little boy, you pick up the bottle and smell the contents. It is the aroma of some kind of insecticide.

1. What is your first immediate action to aid the little boy?

2. What follow-up first aid would you administer?

3. Are there any follow-up procedures you would recommend?

14 Chapter 14 Self-Test

Student: _____ Date: _____

Course: _____ Section #: _____

Part 1   True/False

If you believe the statement is true, circle the T. If you believe the statement is false, circle the F.

T F **1.** Ingestion of poisonous plants is a common poisoning emergency in children.

T F **2.** A victim of inhaled poison should be given activated charcoal.

T F **3.** Cherry-red lips are a common early sign of carbon monoxide poisoning.

T F **4.** A throbbing headache is a symptom of low-level carbon monoxide poisoning.

T F **5.** Activated charcoal should be used only if the victim vomits.

T F **6.** A victim of poisoning should be kept in a sitting position.

T F **7.** Initial symptoms of carbon monoxide poisoning include headache, weakness, agitation, confusion, and dizziness.

T F **8.** For first aid, you should use powdered activated charcoal so you can determine the strength of dosage.

T F **9.** Activated charcoal will not bind to alcohol, kerosene, or gasoline.

T F **10.** Activated charcoal should be used in cases of ingested poisoning because of its ability to neutralize poisons.

Part 2   Multiple Choice

For each item, circle the correct answer or the phrase that best completes the statement.

1. Poisoning is the _____ common cause of accidental death in the United States.

a. most
b. third most
c. fifth most
d. second most

2. Which of the following is *not* a way that poisons may enter the body?

a. absorption
b. emesis
c. inhalation
d. injection

3. The common signs and symptoms of poisoning by ingestion are

a. nausea, vomiting, diarrhea
b. severe abdominal pain or cramps
c. excessive salivation
d. all of the above

4. It is critical that care be given immediately to the person who has inhaled poison because

a. inhaled poisons are more toxic than ingested poisons
b. the body absorbs inhaled poisons rapidly
c. inhaled poisons remain in the system longer than ingested poisons
d. the victim may experience convulsions, which makes treatment difficult

5. Which of the following is a characteristic symptom of carbon monoxide poisoning?

a. headache
b. cool, pale skin
c. complaints of a strange taste in the mouth
d. stains around the mouth

6. What is the initial first aid care procedure for inhalation poisonings?

a. remove the victim to fresh air
b. begin mouth-to-mouth resuscitation
c. treat the victim for shock
d. seek medical care immediately

7. The First Aider's primary responsibility in the first aid care of poisoning is to
   a. maintain the airway and prevent aspiration of vomitus
   b. determine what substance caused the poisoning
   c. assess the level of consciousness
   d. assess respirations

8. After a poisoning victim vomits, give the victim
   a. activated charcoal
   b. lemon juice in a glass of water
   c. raw egg to coat the stomach
   d. syrup of ipecac and water

Part 3 Matching

For each poisoning situation, indicate whether activated charcoal should be used.

Poisoning Situation

1. _____ A stuporous or comatose victim
2. _____ A victim who swallowed silver nitrate
3. _____ A victim who swallowed strychnine
4. _____ A victim who swallowed acid
5. _____ A victim who swallowed kerosene
6. _____ A victim who swallowed insecticide
7. _____ A victim who swallowed gasoline

First Aid Care

A. Give activated charcoal.
B. Do not give activated charcoal.

Part 4 What Would You Do If?

A teenaged boy is found in his garage with the car running and the doors closed. When you arrive, he has been removed from the garage. He is unconscious, has a rapid heart and breathing rate, and has bluish-colored skin.

15

Drug and Alcohol Emergencies

Learning Objectives

When you have mastered the material in this chapter, you will be able to

1 Determine if an emergency is drug or alcohol related

2 Determine if a drug- or alcohol-related emergency is life threatening

3 List the signs and symptoms of acute alcohol intoxication

4 List the signs and symptoms of withdrawal syndrome

5 Identify assessment techniques to use in drug and alcohol emergencies

6 Describe and demonstrate the general guidelines for managing a drug- or alcohol-related emergency

7 Describe and demonstrate the guidelines for managing a violent victim of drug overdose

8 Describe and demonstrate the guidelines for managing an overdose

9 Describe and demonstrate the talk-down technique

10 Describe four classifications of illegal drugs

11 Describe the care for victims who have taken a drug

On the Scene

Early in the morning of January 27, 2006, Connor Wilson answered his apartment door to find his distraught neighbor. "My roommate passed out!" she cried. "I think she took something!"

When he arrived at the apartment, Connor found 23 year-old Anne Rhodes unconscious in the hallway next to the bathroom. Placing his hand on her wrist to determine a pulse, he found that she was feverish; her pulse was irregular, and her breathing was shallow but adequate.

Instructing the roommate to call 9-1-1, Connor used a head-tilt/chin-lift maneuver to open Anne's airway and check for foreign objects; there were none. He then gently turned Anne on her side and positioned her face downward in case she vomited. Monitoring Anne's breathing constantly in case she needed rescue breathing, Connor had her roommate rinse several washcloths in cool water and sponge Anne off in an effort to bring her temperature down.

By the time ambulance personnel arrived, Connor had started rescue breathing. EMTs took over, stabilizing Anne and transporting her to a nearby hospital for treatment of an accidental drug overdose.

rugs and alcohol are misused and abused by a variety of people. Alcoholism—which is treatable but not curable, and fatal if not treated—strikes all classes and almost every age group. Alcohol is the most abused drug in the United States: two-thirds of all adults are "social drinkers," and there are more than 100 million drinkers, 20 percent of whom are alcoholics.

Each year, alcohol is directly involved in thousands of automobile accidents that result in death and injury. It is a factor in 40 percent of all motor vehicle accidents and in 78 percent of all fatal injuries of drivers over the age of 25. It is a factor in half of all arrests for criminal activity. Because of its deleterious effects on the liver, pancreas, central nervous system, and other body organs, alcohol dramatically reduces the average life span of an alcoholic.

Drug abusers are more prone to certain injuries, illnesses, and infectious diseases. Most prominent among these are AIDS, hepatitis, endocarditis, phlebitis, paranoia, depression, and injuries from falls. In addition, drug abusers are often the victims of homicide, and they may be the victims of accidental overdose or intentional suicide.

This chapter helps you determine when an emergency is drug or alcohol related and details the steps you should take to deal with both drug and alcohol emergencies.

15.1 The Nature of Drug and Alcohol Emergencies

Many emergencies involve drug overdose—poisoning by a drug. Most drug overdoses involve habitual drug users, but drug overdose can also be accidental (the result of miscalculation, confusion, or using more than one drug) or intentional (usually a suicide attempt). Drug and alcohol abuse can have both immediate and long-term effects (see Figures 15-1 through 15-9).

It is usually not possible to determine in the field which drug a victim has taken. Many users take a combination of drugs (sometimes without knowing it), and many drugs purchased on the street are adulterated with white, powdery substances such as starch, talc, sugar, or sawdust. (Some estimate that cocaine sold on the street is often diluted up to 75 percent with sucrose, talc, or starch.)

Even if the victim can tell you what he or she took, that self-assessment might not be accurate—the victim may have been misled by the person who sold the drug. For example, only a small percentage of all the drugs that contain PCP are actually sold on the street as PCP.

FIGURE 15–1. Heart damage caused by fungus introduced during drug injection

FIGURE 15–2. Bullet wound to brain, alcohol related

FIGURE 15–3. Chronic gastric ulcer from alcohol use

FIGURE 15–4. Alcoholic cirrhosis of liver

FIGURE 15–5. Enlarged, weak heart, alcohol induced

FIGURE 15–6. Ruptured vein in esophagus, causing severe internal bleeding, alcohol induced

FIGURE 15–7. Dilated esophageal veins from chronic alcohol use

FIGURE 15–8. Internal bleeding from an ulcer caused by chronic alcohol use

FIGURE 15–9. Brain damage (cerebellum) from chronic alcohol use

Determining Whether an Emergency Is Drug or Alcohol Related

> Learning Objective 1 Determine if an emergency is drug or alcohol related.

Because drugs and alcohol produce signs that mimic a number of system disorders or diseases, it can be difficult to assess a drug or alcohol emergency properly, especially if the victim is unconscious.

If you suspect an unconscious victim might be experiencing a drug or alcohol emergency, do the following:

- Inspect the area immediately around the victim for evidence of drug or alcohol use—empty or partially filled pill bottles, syringes, empty liquor bottles, and so on. The victim may have drugs on his person. Check for these only if the patient's condition allows, and you are permitted to do so.

- Check the victim's mouth for signs of partially dissolved pills or tablets; if you find any, remove them.

- Smell the victim's breath for traces of alcohol. (Do not confuse a musky, fruity, or acetone odor for alcohol—all three can indicate diabetic coma.)

- Ask the victim's friends or family members or any witnesses what they know about the incident.

If the victim is conscious, watch for an unsteady, staggering gait or a pronounced lack of coordination. Remember that many serious diseases (such as diabetes and epilepsy) resemble drug overdose or abuse. Don't assume that ingested drugs are the only reason a person is stuporous or has slurred speech. *Never jump to conclusions.*

Determining if a Drug or Alcohol Related Emergency Is Life Threatening

> Learning Objective 2 Determine if a drug- or alcohol-related emergency is life threatening.

The following six signs and symptoms indicate a life-threatening emergency (see Figure 15-10 on page 262):

1. Unconsciousness—the victim cannot be awakened or, if awakened, lapses back into unconsciousness almost immediately.

2. Breathing difficulties—the victim's breathing may have stopped, may be weak and shallow, or may be weak and strong in cycles. The victim's exhalations may be raspy, rattling, or noisy. The victim's skin may be cyanotic, indicating lack of oxygen.

3. Fever—any temperature above 100°F (38°C) may indicate a dangerous situation when drugs and/or alcohol are involved.

4. Abnormal or irregular pulse—any pulse less than 60 or more than 100 beats per minute may indicate danger, as does a pulse that is irregular (not rhythmical).

5. Vomiting while not fully conscious

6. Convulsions—an impending convulsion may be indicated by twitching of the face, trunk, arms, or legs; muscle rigidity; or muscle spasm.

PROGRESS CHECK

1. Alcohol on the breath does not smell musky, fruity, or acetone; those odors are caused by _____ . *(insulin shock/hypoglycemia/ diabetic coma)*

2. A life-threatening emergency is indicated by a pulse lower than _____ beats per minute. *(50/60/70)*

3. A fever higher than _____ F indicates a life-threatening emergency if drugs are involved. *(99/100/101)*

DRUG AND ALCOHOL EMERGENCY INDICATORS

1. Unconsciousness

2. Respiratory difficulties

3. Raised temperature

4. High or low pulse rate or irregular pulse rate

5. Vomiting while semiconscious

6. Convulsions or seizures

FIGURE 15–10. First aid care and medical assistance are needed immediately if any of the six danger signs are present—no matter what the cause.

15.2 Alcohol Emergencies

Alcohol is a central nervous system depressant that in moderate doses causes stupor, and in large doses can cause coma or death.

Alcohol is completely absorbed from the stomach and intestinal tract within 2 hours of the time it is ingested—and sometimes as quickly as within 30 minutes. Once absorbed from the stomach, it is distributed to all body tissues relatively quickly. It is concentrated, however, in the blood and brain, with brain concentrations rapidly approaching those found in the blood.

The alcoholic syndrome usually consists of problem drinking—during which alcohol is used frequently to relieve tensions or other emotional difficulties—and true addiction, in which abstinence from drinking causes major withdrawal symptoms. Frequently, alcoholics are dependent on other drugs as well, especially those in the sedative, narcotic, and tranquilizer categories.

Alcoholics might begin drinking early in the day, be more prone to drink alone or secretly, and might periodically go on prolonged binges characterized by loss of memory (*blackout periods*). Abstinence from alcohol is likely to produce withdrawal symptoms, such as tremulousness, anxiety, or delirium tremens (DTs).

As the alcoholic becomes more dependent on alcohol, performance at work and relationships with friends and family are likely to deteriorate. Absences from work, emotional disturbances, and automobile accidents become more frequent.

Acute Intoxication

Learning Objective **3** List the signs and symptoms of acute alcohol intoxication.

The degree of acute intoxication depends on the amount of alcohol consumed. Signs and symptoms (see Figure 15-11) include:

ALCOHOL EMERGENCIES

CAUTION: Do not immediately decide that a patient with apparent alcohol on the breath is drunk. The signs may indicate an illness or injury such as epilepsy, diabetes, or head injury.

SIGNS OF INTOXICATION
- Odor of alcohol on the breath
- Swaying and unsteadiness
- Slurred speech
- Nausea and vomiting
- Flushed face
- Drowsiness
- Violent, destructive, or erratic behavior
- Self-injury, usually without realizing it

EFFECTS
- Alcohol is a depressant. It affects judgment, vision, reaction time, and coordination.
- When taken with other depressants, the result can be greater than the combined effects of the two drugs.
- In very large quantities, alcohol can paralyze the respiratory center of the brain and cause death.

MANAGEMENT
- Give the same attention as you would to any patient with an illness or injury.
- Monitor the patient's vital signs constantly. Provide life support when necessary.
- Position the patient to avoid aspiration of vomit.
- Protect the patient from hurting him- or herself.

FIGURE 15–11. The signs, effects, and management of alcohol emergencies

- Drowsiness
- Disordered speech and gait
- Violence
- Destructive or erratic behavior

Note: Acute intoxication often mimics insulin shock. Always suspect diabetes; when in doubt, give sugar.

Also be alert to the possibility that the victim might have taken a combination of alcohol and sedative drugs. Check the victim and surroundings for evidence of medications, which may significantly complicate the picture.

Binge Drinking

Another problem with alcohol is *binge drinking.* Common on college campuses, binge drinking is defined simply as drinking with the intent of becoming intoxicated. The consumption of large quantities of an alcoholic beverage (or mixing alcoholic beverages) with resulting stupor, unresponsiveness, and vomiting has frequently caused deaths on and around college campuses.

Withdrawal Syndrome

Learning Objective 4   List the signs and symptoms of withdrawal syndrome.

Withdrawal syndrome occurs after a cutback in the amount of alcohol a person is used to; it does not require that the alcoholic stop drinking completely. Withdrawal syndrome can also occur when blood alcohol levels begin to fall after severe intoxication. Withdrawal syndrome is dose dependent: the more the alcoholic was drinking, the more severe the syndrome will be.

There are four general stages of alcohol withdrawal (see Figure 15-12 on page 264):

1. Stage 1, which occurs within about 8 hours of a cutback in alcohol, is characterized by nausea, insomnia, sweating, and tremors.

2. Stage 2, which occurs within 8 to 72 hours, is characterized by a worsening of Stage 1 symptoms, plus vomiting and illusions or hallucinations.

3. Stage 3, which usually occurs within 48 hours, is characterized by major seizures.

4. Stage 4 is characterized by delirium tremens.

withdrawal syndrome A four-stage syndrome that occurs after a cutback in the amount of alcohol a person is used to or when blood alcohol levels start to fall after severe intoxication

Delirium tremens constitutes the most extreme form of alcohol withdrawal syndrome. Less severe forms include alcoholic tremulousness, alcoholic hallucinosis, and withdrawal seizures, which generally (but not always) precede delirium tremens.

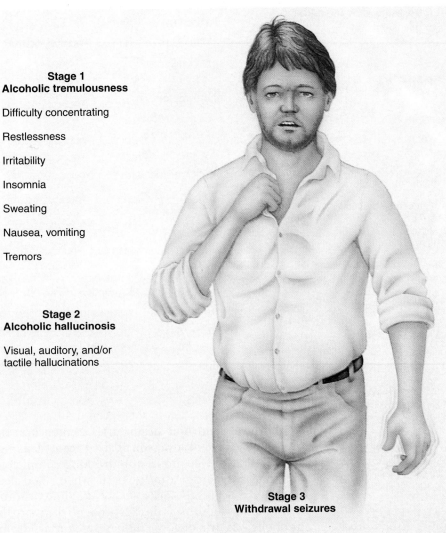

**Stage 1
Alcoholic tremulousness**

Difficulty concentrating

Restlessness

Irritability

Insomnia

Sweating

Nausea, vomiting

Tremors

**Stage 2
Alcoholic hallucinosis**

Visual, auditory, and/or tactile hallucinations

**Stage 4
Delirium tremens**

Confusion

Inattentiveness

Disorientation

Fever

Nausea, vomiting

Incoherence

Hyperirritability

Relentless insomnia

**Stage 3
Withdrawal seizures**

Seizures are characterized by muscle rigidity and relaxation that usually alternate rhythmically in rapid succession; victims typically experience two to six seizures in a row.

FIGURE 15–12. Stages of withdrawal

Withdrawal syndrome, which can mimic a number of psychiatric disorders, is characterized by the following signs and symptoms:

- Insomnia
- Muscular weakness
- Fever
- Seizures
- Disorientation, confusion, and thought-process disorders
- Hallucinations
- Anorexia
- Nausea and vomiting
- Sweating
- Rapid heartbeat

Delirium Tremens

Delirium tremens (DTs)—a severe, life-threatening condition with a mortality rate of approximately 15 percent—can occur between 1 and 14 days after the victim's last drink, most commonly within 2 to 5 days. A single episode of DTs lasts between 1 and 3 days; multiple episodes can last as long as a month. DTs should be suspected in any victim with delirium of unknown cause.

DTs are characterized by these signs and symptoms:

- Severe confusion
- Loss of memory
- Tremors
- Restlessness
- Extremely high fever
- Dilated pupils
- Profuse sweating
- Insomnia
- Nausea
- Diarrhea
- Hallucinations, mostly of a frightening nature (such as delusions of snakes, spiders, or rats)

Seizures are very common in alcoholic withdrawal, but not in DTs. However, approximately one-third of all those who have seizures in early withdrawal will progress to DTs if left untreated or if treated inadequately.

15.3   Assessment and Management

Observation and Assessment

> **Learning Objective 5** Identify assessment techniques to use in drug and alcohol emergencies.

The most important information to be gathered during assessment of the drug/alcohol victim is severity of intoxication and level of consciousness.

SEVERITY OF INTOXICATION

Determine the severity of intoxication by observing:

- Whether the victim is awake and will answer questions
- Whether the victim withdraws from painful stimuli
- Whether respirations are adequate
- Whether the circulatory system is functioning properly (as indicated by pulse and skin color)

delirium tremens A life-threatening condition causing delirium that usually occurs within 5 days of an alcoholic's last drink

LEVEL OF CONSCIOUSNESS

Typically, victims fall into one of three categories:

- Awake, claiming to have ingested a medicine—the victim answers questions and is alert and aware.

- Responsive verbally or to pain—the victim will respond appropriately to verbal or noxious stimuli but will stop responding when the stimuli are removed.

- Unresponsive—the victim cannot be aroused to consciousness by verbal or noxious stimuli.

OBTAINING A HISTORY

Obtain a history by asking the following questions:

- What was taken? If you can, find the drug container and its contents so it can be transported with the victim.

- When was it taken?

- How much was taken?

- Was anything else taken (other drugs or alcohol)?

- What has been done to try to correct the situation? Has vomiting been induced? (Street resuscitation procedures are frequently as dangerous as the overdose itself, so it is important to find out exactly what has been done for the victim.)

Signs That Immediate Medical Attention Is Needed

The following signs and symptoms indicate that medical attention is needed immediately:

- Nervous system depression (sleepiness, coma, lethargy, and decreased response to pain)

- Tremors (especially if the victim is suffering withdrawal)

- Withdrawal accompanied by pain

- Digestive problems that include vomiting, bleeding, and dehydration

- Slow or absent breathing

- Grand mal seizures

- Delirium tremens

- Disturbances of vision, mental confusion, and muscular incoordination

- Disinterested behavior and loss of memory

General Guidelines for Managing a Drug/Alcohol Crisis

> **Learning Objective 6** Describe and demonstrate the general guidelines for managing a drug or alcohol related emergency.

Crisis intervention is, by definition, short term. It involves alleviating the pain and confusion of victims in a specific event or circumstance. The goal of crisis intervention is to establish and maintain rapport, create trust, and build a short-term working relationship that will lower anxiety, produce a clearer understanding of the problem at hand, and identify the resources necessary to cope with it (see Figure 15-13).

Follow these guidelines:

1. Assure your own personal safety.

2. Provide a reality base.
   - Identify yourself and your position.
   - Use the victim's name.
   - Anticipate the concerns of the victim, family, and friends.
   - Based on the victim's response, introduce as much familiarity as possible—persons, objects, newspapers, or TV programs.
   - Be calm and self-assured.

3. Provide appropriate nonverbal support.
   - Maintain eye contact.
   - Maintain a relaxed body posture.
   - Be quiet, calm, and gentle.
   - Touch the victim if it seems appropriate.

4. Encourage communication.
   - Communicate directly with the victim, not through others.

FIGURE 15–13. Reassure the victim. Explain who you are and that you are trying to help.

- Ask clear, simple questions.
- Ask questions slowly, one at a time.
- Try not to ask questions that require a simple yes or no.
- Tolerate repetition; do not become impatient.

5. Foster confidence.

- Be nonjudgmental; don't accuse the victim.
- Help the victim gain confidence in you.
- Listen carefully.
- Respond to feelings; let the victim know that you understand his or her feelings.
- Identify and reinforce progress.

Managing a Violent Drug/Alcohol Victim

> **Learning Objective 7** Describe and demonstrate the guidelines for managing a violent victim of drug overdose.

The following indicate that a victim is about to lose control and become violent (see Figure 15-14):

- Extreme agitation, including shouting or screaming, excessive energy (fidgeting, pacing), threats or violent movements (punching walls or swinging)
- Sweating
- Excessive talking (rapid, loud, or uncontrolled speech)

Be alert to signals of danger or violence and take evasive action. Leave the scene and call for police and EMS. Do not enter a scene with a victim who appears violent or potentially violent. Only attempt to restrain a violent victim if you are trained and authorized to do so.

FIGURE 15–14. Agitation, perspiration, and excessive talking might indicate that a victim is about to lose control.

To prevent a victim from becoming violent, take these steps:

1. Do not invade the person's personal space (moving closer than 3 feet to the victim). Getting too close may seem threatening.

2. Use a calming voice and compassionate tone.

3. Do not place objects between the victim and the door or appear as if you are blocking his or her escape.

4. Move dangerous objects out of sight and reach of the victim.

If a victim is violent:

1. Leave the scene and notify law enforcement authorities.

2. Do not attempt restraint unless you are trained and authorized to do so and you have sufficient people to do so effectively.

3. Leave the scene at any time weapons of any type are used or threatened.

For information on how to restrain a violent victim, see Chapter 28.

First Aid Care

The immediate objective in first aid care of the drug or alcohol victim is to assess cardiopulmonary functioning and to stabilize basic life support functions. The primary concern in acute intoxication is maintaining an airway.

A drug or alcohol victim in a coma or with cardiac complications should be given the same first aid care as any other comatose victim.

Hyperventilation, common in drug-abuse victims, can indicate severe pain, drug withdrawal, or aspirin poisoning. In a drug emergency, treat hyperventilation as a medical disorder, not as anxiety hyperventilation. (See Chapter 17.) Do not have the victim breathe into a paper bag.

First Aid Care for Overdose

> **Learning Objective 8** Describe and demonstrate the guidelines for managing an overdose.

The general goals in handling a victim of overdose are to protect both victim and First Aiders, to calm the victim, and to prevent physical injury, aspiration, and hypothermia. Activate the EMS system; then follow these steps:

1. Be prepared for cardiac arrest. Constantly monitor vital signs; your primary priority is to maintain an open airway.

2. Do not panic; treat the victim calmly. Move a victim who is inhaling a harmful substance or who is in immediate danger from surroundings. Do not place yourself in danger.

3. If the person is conscious, try to get the victim to sit or lie down. Do not use restraints unless the victim poses a risk to safety.

4. Establish and maintain a clear airway. Remove anything from the mouth or throat that might pose a breathing hazard, including false teeth, blood, mucus, or vomitus. Administer artificial ventilation if needed.

5. Turn the victim's head to the side or toward the ground in case of vomiting. Report any blood in the vomitus; bright red blood in the vomitus can be a sign of ruptured blood vessels in the stomach or esophagus.

6. Monitor the victim's vital signs frequently; overdose victims can be conscious one minute and lapse into a coma the next. In case of respiratory or cardiac complications, treat life-threatening situations immediately.

7. Try to maintain proper body temperature. If the temperature goes over 104°F, sponge the victim with tepid water.

8. Take measures to correct or prevent shock, which can result from vomiting, profuse sweating, or inadequate fluid intake. Be alert for allergic reactions.

9. Reduce stimuli as much as possible; lower the lights if you can, and let the victim rest in a calm, quiet atmosphere. If the victim is agitated, move the victim to a quiet place for observation.

10. Carefully explain each step of care so that you can help reduce paranoia.

If there is time before the victim is transported, search the area around the victim for tablets, capsules, pill bottles or boxes (especially empty ones), syringes, other drug paraphernalia, ampules, prescriptions, hospital attendance cards, or physician's notes that might help you identify what drug the victim has taken. Any such evidence should be transported with the victim.

The Talk-Down Technique

Learning Objective 9 Describe and demonstrate the talk-down technique.

The dangers associated with the use of hallucinogens and marijuana are primarily psychological in nature. These may be evident as intense anxiety or panic states (bad trips), depressive or paranoid reactions, mood changes, disorientation, and an inability to distinguish between reality and fantasy. Some prolonged psychotic reactions to psychedelic drugs have been reported, particularly in persons who are already psychologically disturbed.

The talk-down technique is the preferred method for handling bad trips. This technique involves nonmoralizing, comforting, personal support from an experienced individual. It is aided by limiting external stimulation, such as intense light or loud sounds, and having the person lie down and relax. The goal of talking down is to reduce the victim's anxiety, panic, depression, or confusion.

Never use the talk-down technique for victims who have used PCP, because it may further aggravate them. To use the technique in other situations, follow these steps (see Figure 15-15):

1. Make the victim feel welcome. Remain relaxed and sympathetic. Because a victim can become suddenly hostile, have a companion with you. Be calm, but be authoritative.

2. Reassure the victim that his or her strange mental condition is caused by the drug and will not last forever. Help the victim realize he or she is not mentally ill.

3. Identify yourself clearly. Tell the victim who you are and what you are doing to help. Be careful not to invade the victim's "personal space" until you have established rapport; try to stay approximately 8 to 10 feet away until you sense that the victim has some trust in you. Never touch the victim until he or she gives you permission or unless the victim suddenly poses a threat to safety (his or her own or someone else's).

4. Help the victim verbalize what is happening. Review for the victim what is going on; ask questions. Outline the probable schedule of events, if appropriate.

5. Reiterate simple and concrete statements; repeat and confirm what the victim says. Orient the victim to time and place: be absolutely clear in letting the victim know where he or she is, what is happening, and who is present. Help the victim identify surrounding objects that should be familiar—a process that helps with self-identification. Listen for clues that will let you know whether the victim is anxious; if so, discuss those anxieties. Help the victim work through them and to conquer guilt feelings.

6. Forewarn the victim about what will happen as the drug begins to wear off. There may be confusion one minute, mental clarity the next. Again, help the victim understand that these changes are due to the drug, not to mental illness.

FIGURE 15–15. Use the talk-down technique to help calm an anxious victim.

Once the victim is calm, transport the person to a medical facility.

PROGRESS CHECK

1. The most important information to gather during assessment of a drug/alcohol victim is severity of intoxication and _____ . *(history/chief complaint/level of consciousness)*

2. _____ is a sign that medical attention is needed immediately. *(Grand mal seizure/Vomiting/Rapid heartbeat)*

3. One way to provide a reality base is to _____ . *(maintain eye contact/listen carefully/use the victim's name)*

4. You can provide nonverbal support by _____ . *(touching the victim/letting the victim watch TV/listening carefully)*

5. You can encourage communication by _____ . *(responding to feelings/maintaining a relaxed body posture/asking questions slowly)*

6. The primary goals of care are to monitor vital signs and _____ . *(prevent shock/provide basic life support/prevent aspiration)*

7. The top priority in caring for victims of drug/alcohol emergencies is to _____ . *(maintain the airway/maintain circulation/maintain consciousness)*

8. The talk-down technique should not be used if the victim took _____ . *(cocaine/PCP/alcohol)*

15.4 Drugs of Concern

Learning Objective 10 Describe four classifications of illegal drugs.

There are numerous illegal drugs available. Additionally, many legal prescription drugs (e.g., painkillers) can be used improperly and become addictive. This section will provide an overview of some of the drugs available on the street today.

Hallucinogens

Lysergic acid diethylamide (LSD) is a liquid that is placed on paper. These small strips of paper (known as *blotter acid*) are placed in the mouth where saliva liberates the acid from the paper and moves it to absorption in the bloodstream. LSD causes hallucinations ranging from mild visual or auditory hallucinations to dramatic hallucinations accompanied by fear or paranoia. These unpleasant hallucinogenic reactions are referred to as *bad trips*.

Phencyclidine (**PCP**) is a hallucinogen known for more severe hallucinations, violent outbursts, lack of response to pain and extreme agitation.

Ketamine is another substance which can cause hallucinations. Called *Special K* on the street, the drug is legally used as a large-animal tranquilizer. There is some human use as an anesthetic and pain-killer, but these uses are limited due to hallucinations caused by the drug.

Stimulants

Cocaine is one of the more common illegal stimulants on the street today. It can be smoked (crack cocaine), snorted, or injected (cocaine powder). Cocaine causes an immediate euphoria and is highly addictive. Cocaine can cause a rapid and dangerous rise in pulse and blood pressure and can lead to seizures, stroke, or death.

Methamphetamine is also a stimulant in the amphetamine class of drugs. Unlike cocaine, which is derived from the coca plant, methamphetamine is a chemical mixture created illegally in clandestine drug labs. Methamphetamine can be smoked or injected and causes reactions similar to cocaine.

Ritalin, a drug used for attention deficit hyperactivity disorder (ADHD), is a stimulant that can be taken orally in pill form or ground up and snorted.

PCP Phencyclidine, a hallucinogenic drug that acts as an anesthetic

Depressants/Narcotics

Heroin is a narcotic and central nervous system depressant. It is most commonly injected into a vein. Very pure forms may be snorted. Once it enters the body, it causes a "rush," followed by a period of drowsiness and sometimes sleep. As a depressant, heroin can cause severe respiratory depression and can stop breathing completely. Coma and death follow.

Oxycontin is a legal narcotic pain reliever used for chronic pain. It is designed to provide long-acting pain relief. The drug is abused by crushing it and snorting the powder. This allows the abuser to get the full dose of the drug right away, bypassing the long-acting effect.

There are other depressant drugs that are not narcotics. Drugs such as antianxiety agents (Xanax), Valium (Diazepam), and sleeping pills can cause respiratory depression, coma, and death.

Other Drugs of Abuse

Substances such as rohypnol, ecstasy and GHB are sometimes referred to as *club drugs* because they were first observed in clubs and at rave parties. Use of these drugs is not limited to clubs or parties and is increasingly common.

Rohypnol (roofies) gained most notoriety as a *date rape drug* because it causes both sedation and amnesia. People who are given this drug will not remember most events that occur while under its effect. It comes in a tablet form that will dissolve easily in carbonated beverages. It is from a group a drugs similar to Valium. Rohypnol is no longer produced in the United States.

Ecstasy (XTC, X, MDMA) is chemically called methylenedioxymethamphetamine, which is a stimulant with some hallucinogenic properties. Usually found in tablet form, it lasts for about 3 to 6 hours and is often taken in combination with other substances.

GHB (Georgia home boy, grevious bodily harm, goop) is gammahydroxybutyrate. It is a depressant with some hallucinogenic properties. It is often found in liquid form and is added to beverages. The drug achieves onset in 10 to 20 minutes and can last 4 hours, depending on the dose.

Care for Drug Use and Overdose

Learning Objective 11 Describe the care for victims who have taken a drug.

Regardless of the substance ingested, there are certain principles of care that apply to all cases of drug abuse and overdose:

1. Assure your personal safety. Drug use can cause erratic and dangerous behavior. Call for law enforcement assistance.

2. Activate the EMS system.

3. Monitor the victim's airway, breathing, and circulation. Drugs can cause unresponsiveness (coma), respiratory depression, and respiratory arrest. Vomiting and seizures may occur. Protect the airway and provide ventilation and CPR as needed.

4. Provide supportive care such as the talk-down techniques discussed earlier in the chapter and prevent further injury.

5. Monitor vital signs until EMTs arrive.

PROGRESS CHECK

1. LSD is a/an _____ . (hallucinogen/amphetamine/narcotic)

2. A drug used as a date rape drug is _____ . (PCP/cocaine/Rohypnol)

3. Ecstasy is a drug with _____ properties. (depressant/stimulant/narcotic)

Summary

- Because many serious diseases resemble drug and alcohol overdose, it is important to assess the situation carefully to determine whether an emergency is drug or alcohol related.
- A musky, fruity, or acetone odor on the breath is a sign of diabetic coma, not alcohol intoxication.
- Six signs and symptoms indicate that a drug/alcohol emergency is life-threatening: unconsciousness, breathing difficulties, fever, abnormal or irregular pulse, vomiting while not fully conscious, and seizures.
- Acute alcohol intoxication has many of the same signs and symptoms of insulin shock; when in doubt, give sugar.
- Withdrawal syndrome occurs after a cutback in the amount of alcohol a person is used to, or when blood alcohol levels start to fall after severe intoxication; it can progress to delirium tremens.

- Delirium tremens, characterized by severe confusion and often frightening hallucinations, is a life-threatening condition.

- The general guidelines for managing a drug/alcohol crisis are to provide a reality base, provide appropriate nonverbal support, encourage communication, and foster confidence.

- To manage a violent victim of drug overdose, watch for the signs that a person is about to lose control—high degrees of agitation, sweating, and excessive talking while struggling with violent impulses.

- Handle a victim of drug or alcohol overdose much as you would a victim with any other medical problem; top priorities are breathing and circulation.

- The talk-down technique involves nonmoralizing, comforting, personal support from an experienced individual and is recommended for handling bad trips caused by any drug other than PCP.

Key Terms

Make sure you understand the following key terms:

withdrawal syndrome
delirium tremens
PCP

Critical Thinking Exercise

You are at a party and you hear a crash. Two people are helping up a friend who fell and knocked over a small end table. He doesn't appear hurt but you notice he is staggering and mumbling incoherently. You overhear someone say "He's not bad when he's drunk, but he should stay off the ecstasy. He gets really stupid. Let's see if we can put him to bed to sleep it off."

1. Should this person be put to bed to "sleep it off"? What risks would this pose to the patient?

2. List some medical conditions that this patient could experience as a result of his condition.

3. If you offered to help the patient and he became a bit belligerent, explain how you would calm him down.

15 Chapter 15 Self-Test

Student: _____   Date: _____

Course: _____   Section #: _____

Part 1   True/False

If you believe the statement is true, circle the T. If you believe the statement is false, circle the F.

T   F   **1.**   First aid care for a drug overdose depends entirely on what kind of drug was used.

T   F   **2.**   Seizures are rare in alcoholic withdrawal.

T   F   **3.**   The most severe reactions from PCP use include paranoia and memory loss.

T   F   **4.**   Hyperventilating drug-emergency victims should be encouraged to breathe into a paper bag.

T   F   **5.**   DTs that occur more than 1 day after the last drink are rarely life threatening.

Part 2   Multiple Choice

For each item, circle the correct answer or the phrase that best completes the statement.

1. A common emergency among drug-abuse victims is
   a. hyperventilation
   b. cardiac arrhythmias
   c. convulsions
   d. tremors

2. Hyperventilation in a drug emergency should be treated by
   a. removing the victim from the crisis situation as soon as possible
   b. quieting the victim and leaving the victim alone to calm down
   c. encouraging the victim to place the head lower than the knees
   d. having the victim breathe into a paper bag

3. A pulse rate _____ may indicate danger in a drug/alcohol emergency in an adult.
   a. below 60 or above 100
   b. below 60 or above 130
   c. below 60 or above 120
   d. below 80 or above 100

4. Which of the following may indicate that a drug/alcohol emergency is life threatening?
   a. pancreatitis
   b. impaired coordination
   c. vomiting while not fully conscious
   d. disturbance of vision

5. Which of the following is not a guideline for dealing with an overdose victim?
   a. maintain a clear airway
   b. throw a little cold water on a semiconscious victim
   c. try to get the victim to sit or lie down
   d. be firm but friendly

6. What is the preferred method for handling a victim experiencing a bad trip?
   a. throw cold water on the victim
   b. use the talk-down technique
   c. get the victim to walk around
   d. put the victim in an isolated room

7. The signs of acute intoxication may be mimicked by a victim of
   a. diabetic coma (hyperglycemia)
   b. insulin shock (hypoglycemia)
   c. epilepsy
   d. violence

8. Which of the following indicates that medical attention is needed immediately for an alcohol-abuse victim?
   a. grand mal seizure
   b. high blood pressure
   c. vomiting
   d. increased breathing rate

9. Delirium tremens occur as a result of
   a. alcohol overdose
   b. alcohol taken with tranquilizers
   c. high alcohol concentrations ingested very quickly
   d. alcohol withdrawal

10. Which of the following is not a symptom of delirium tremens?
   a. confusion
   b. hallucinations
   c. shaking hands
   d. deep, comatose sleep

Part 3 What Would You Do If?

You find an older man unconscious in an alley. He smells of alcohol and exhibits respiratory depression and signs of shock.

16

Cardiovascular and Stroke Emergencies

Learning Objectives

When you have mastered the material in this chapter, you will be able to:

1 Identify the two types of coronary artery disease

2 Describe the physiological process involved in angina pectoris

3 List the signs and symptoms of angina pectoris

4 Describe the physiological process involved in congestive heart failure

5 List the signs and symptoms of congestive heart failure

6 Describe the physiological process involved in myocardial infarction

7 List the signs and symptoms of myocardial infarction

8 Describe and demonstrate the first aid care of a victim who does not have a pulse

9 Describe and demonstrate the first aid care of a victim who is responsive

10 Explain the guidelines for use of nitroglycerin

11 Describe and demonstrate how to help a victim use physician-prescribed nitroglycerin

12 Describe the physiological processes in the brain that cause stroke

13 List the signs and symptoms of stroke

14 Describe and demonstrate the first aid care of a stroke victim

Seventy-year-old Harold Hawker was raking leaves under a stand of maples when he suddenly felt nauseous and light-headed. As he walked toward a garden bench at the edge of his yard, he began to feel a squeezing, burning, heavy sensation in the center of his chest. As he slumped onto the bench, he called out to his neighbor, Phyllis Gibb, who was raking leaves in her own yard.

When Phyllis reached Harold, the pain in his chest had become intense. He was still complaining of nausea, and his skin was cool and moist. He was struggling with shortness of breath, and he told Phyllis he felt extremely weak. She noticed that his brow was covered with profuse perspiration, despite the cool weather.

Phyllis told Harold to keep still, ran back to her own yard, and asked her teenage son to call for paramedics. She returned to Harold and verified that he was still breathing and had a pulse. Reassuring him, she helped him to a sitting position, which enabled him to breathe a little more easily. Phyllis unbuttoned Harold's top two shirt buttons, then draped her own sweater across his shoulders to help him keep warm. Phyllis continued to reassure and calm Harold while they both waited for emergency personnel to arrive. EMTs treated Harold and transported him to a nearby hospital where it was confirmed he had a minor heart attack. Phyllis waited for Harold's wife to return from the grocery store.

Heart attacks and associated heart disease are the number-one killer in the United States. About 350,000 Americans die each year of cardiovascular disease, and nearly 29 million more Americans suffer from some form of the disease. The most common problem is coronary artery disease, which usually causes angina pectoris and, left untreated, may eventually lead to acute myocardial infarction (heart attack).

Because of the critical nature of heart disease emergencies, you should treat every adult with chest pain as a heart attack victim until proven otherwise.

This chapter lists the signs and symptoms associated with cardiovascular emergencies and outlines life-sustaining care you can provide until emergency personnel arrive at the scene.

16.1 Coronary Artery Disease

> Learning Objective 1 Identify the two types of coronary artery disease.

As the name implies, **coronary artery disease** affects the arteries that supply the heart with blood by injuring the inner lining of the arterial walls. The two types of coronary artery disease are **atherosclerosis** and **arteriosclerosis**. In coronary artery disease, the opening of the coronary artery is narrowed, restricting the amount of blood that can reach and nourish the heart muscle (see Figures 16-1, 16-3, 16-4, and 16-5). Roughened interior surfaces on the artery cause buildup of additional debris, further narrowing the artery. Eventually, the victim may experience chest pain or a heart attack, because the coronary artery eventually becomes blocked (Figure 16-6). Figure 16-2 outlines cardiac risk factors.

Atherosclerosis

Atherosclerosis results when fatty substances—called **plaque**—and other debris are deposited on the inner lining of the arterial wall. As a result, the opening of the artery is narrowed, reducing the flow of blood through the affected artery.

Arteriosclerosis

Arteriosclerosis occurs when calcium is deposited in the walls of the arteries, resulting in loss of arterial elasticity and an increase in blood pressure. The plaque deposits of atherosclerosis can also cause arteriosclerosis, or "hardening of the arteries." Arteriosclerosis generally affects other arteries in addition to the coronary arteries, and may lead to hypertension, kidney disease, or stroke.

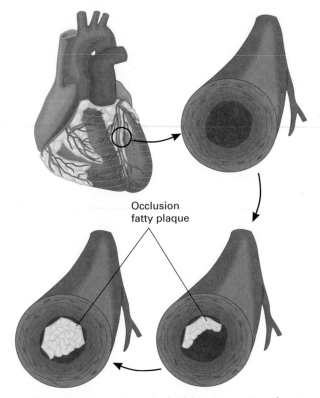

Occlusion
fatty plaque

FIGURE 16–1. Fatty deposits build up in arteries, depriving the heart muscle of blood and oxygen.

PROGRESS CHECK

1. _____ results when fatty substances are deposited on the inner lining of the arterial walls. *(Arteriosclerosis/Atherosclerosis/Angina pectoris)*

2. _____ occurs when arteries lose their elasticity. *(Arteriosclerosis/Atherosclerosis/Angina pectoris)*

3. Coronary artery disease affects the arteries that supply the _____ . *(heart/lungs/brain)*

4. Heart attack occurs when the coronary artery becomes _____ . *(constricted/dilated/blocked)*

coronary artery disease A condition in which a coronary artery has been damaged

atherosclerosis A condition in which fatty substances and other debris are deposited on the arterial walls

arteriosclerosis A disease condition in which the arteries lose their elasticity

plaque Fatty deposits on the arterial walls

CARDIAC RISK FACTORS

Physical inactivity
Sedentary lifestyle

Obesity

Cigarette smoking

High serum cholesterol
and triglycerides

Diabetes

Prolonged tension,
frustration, or hostility

Age (incidence increases
over 30 years of age)

High blood pressure

Male gender

Oral contraceptive
use in women over 40

Family history of premature coronary heart disease (usually under age 60)

FIGURE 16–2. Each additional risk factor increases the likelihood of premature myocardial infarction. The risk for a victim who has high cholesterol levels and high blood pressure and who is a heavy smoker is 10 times that of someone without those risk factors.

FIGURE 16–3. Inside surface of a normal artery

FIGURE 16–4. Artery damaged by coronary artery disease

FIGURE 16–5. Severe atherosclerosis (inside surface of artery)

FIGURE 16–6. Myocardial infarction

16.2 Angina Pectoris, Congestive Heart Failure, and Myocardial Infarction

Angina Pectoris

> Learning Objective **2** Describe the physiological process involved in angina pectoris.

Angina pectoris literally means "pain in the chest" and is actually a set of signs and symptoms that can occur in a victim with serious coronary artery disease.

Angina occurs when the heart's demand for oxygen is temporarily greater than what it is receiving. Because of the disease, the coronary arteries are narrowed, and only a limited supply of oxygen-rich blood can be delivered to the heart.

Like any muscle, the heart relies on a constant supply of oxygen to function. When the demand for oxygenated blood is greater than the diseased or constricted arteries can provide, the victim experiences angina pectoris—a brief feeling of pain or discomfort that signals the heart's need for oxygen.

Most often angina pectoris occurs because the victim has increased the heart's workload and thus its demand for oxygen, usually by physical activity or emotional excitement, and often in cold weather. When the heart's workload is increased, it needs greater amounts of blood, which the diseased arteries are unable to deliver.

Angina is reversible and produces no permanent damage to the heart. Pain is generally relieved by rest, usually within a few minutes after the victim stops the activity, calms down, moves indoors, or takes nitroglycerin as prescribed by a physician.

SIGNS AND SYMPTOMS

> Learning Objective **3** List the signs and symptoms of angina pectoris.

The most common symptom of angina is chest pain; it may range from a mild ache to a severe crushing pain. It appears suddenly, but is usually associated with physical exertion. The pain is located under the sternum, but may also radiate to the jaw, neck, left shoulder, left arm, and left hand.

Other common signs and symptoms include:

- Dyspnea (shortness of breath)
- Profuse perspiration
- Light-headedness
- Palpitations
- Nausea and/or vomiting
- Pale, cool, moist skin

Remember: It is impossible for a First Aider to tell the difference between the pain of angina pectoris and that of heart attack. All victims with chest pain should be treated for heart attack and should be transported to a medical facility for evaluation.

Congestive Heart Failure

> Learning Objective **4** Describe the physiological process involved in congestive heart failure.

Congestive heart failure results when the left ventricle can no longer pump blood effectively to the body. While there are a number of causes, the most common include heart attack, high blood pressure, chronic obstructive pulmonary disease, coronary artery disease, and heart valve damage.

As congestive heart failure progresses, fluid builds up behind the failing left side of the heart. This increases pressure in the pulmonary capillaries, causing plasma to seep out of the capillaries and into the surrounding lung tissue, a condition called **pulmonary edema**. If pulmonary edema is not corrected, severe respiratory distress follows. Congestive heart failure gradually reduces the lungs' oxygen capacity, and death occurs.

Congestive heart failure is a true medical emergency—a stable victim can suddenly and rapidly deteriorate without warning.

SIGNS AND SYMPTOMS

> Learning Objective **5** List the signs and symptoms of congestive heart failure.

Pain may or may not occur with congestive heart failure, usually depending on whether heart attack has also occurred. The most dramatic sign of congestive heart failure is pulmonary edema, resulting in severe shortness of breath. Other signs and symptoms include the following (see Figure 16-7):

- Wheezing
- Profuse sweating

> **angina pectoris** Chest pain caused when the heart's need for oxygen is not met
> **pulmonary edema** A condition in which plasma (fluid) seeps out of the capillaries into the lungs as a result of pressure from a failing heart

SIGNS AND SYMPTOMS OF
CONGESTIVE HEART FAILURE

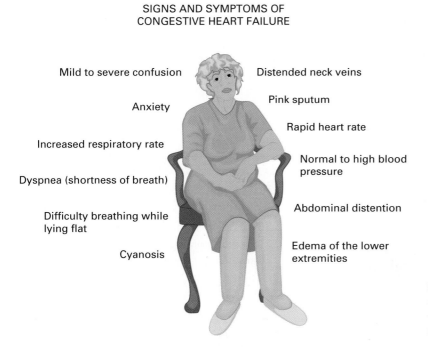

Mild to severe confusion

Anxiety

Increased respiratory rate

Dyspnea (shortness of breath)

Difficulty breathing while lying flat

Cyanosis

Distended neck veins

Pink sputum

Rapid heart rate

Normal to high blood pressure

Abdominal distention

Edema of the lower extremities

FIGURE 16–7. Although these signs and symptoms are most common, the victim of congestive heart failure may have any combination of symptoms or only one or two.

- Rapid heart rate

- Increased respiratory rate with fast, labored breathing

- Paleness or cyanosis

- Difficulty breathing while lying flat

- Swelling of the feet and lower legs

- Anxiety

- Mild to severe confusion

- A desire to sit upright

- Abdominal distension

- Distended neck veins

- Apprehension or agitation, coupled with the feeling of being smothered

Remember: Although these signs and symptoms are the most common, the victim might have any combination of them, and some victims have only one or two.

Myocardial Infarction

Learning Objective **6** Describe the physiological process involved in myocardial infarction.

Most often called a *heart attack*, **myocardial infarction** means the death of the **myocardium**, or heart muscle. When blood supply to part of the heart is significantly

reduced or is stopped completely, the affected part dies.

Myocardial infarction is most often associated with coronary artery disease—most frequently, with a thrombus or clot in a coronary artery already diseased by atherosclerosis. It can also result from a spasm in the coronary artery or when the heart's need for oxygen exceeds its supply for an extended period of time.

SIGNS AND SYMPTOMS

Learning Objective **7** List the signs and symptoms of myocardial infarction.

The signs and symptoms of myocardial infarction vary, depending on the amount of heart damage and how the autonomic nervous system responds to the damage.

It can be very difficult to determine whether someone has suffered a heart attack without sophisticated diagnostic equipment. The major symptom of myocardial infarction is chest pain (see Figure 16-8, page 280) that may range from mild discomfort to severe crushing pain; it can also be an uncomfortable squeezing, pressure, or sensation of fullness. *Note that 25 percent of all myocardial infarction victims have no chest pain at all.*

myocardial infarction Heart attack, caused when the blood supply to the heart is restricted or cut off
myocardium The heart muscle

FIGURE 16-8. The major symptom of myocardial infarction is chest pain.

A heart attack without pain is called a **silent myocardial infarction**. These silent myocardial infarctions are most often seen in women, diabetics, and the elderly. The most common symptoms of myocardial infarction in these patients are fatigue and difficulty breathing.

When present, the pain lasts for longer than a few minutes. The classic location of the pain is the center of the chest; it often radiates to the neck, jaw, left shoulder, and left arm (see Figure 16-9). *Any adult with chest pain should be suspected of suffering myocardial infarction unless proven otherwise.*

The most common signs and symptoms of myocardial infarction include the following, but not all these occur with every heart attack:

- Shortness of breath
- Profuse sweating
- Cool, pale, moist skin
- Cyanosis
- Nausea and/or vomiting
- Weakness
- Light-headedness
- Anxiety
- Feeling of impending doom
- Pulse exceeding 100 beats per minute
- A pulse of less than 60 beats per minute
- Fainting

Many cases of chest pain are actually unrelated to the heart. Chest pain can be caused by a respiratory infection (such as bronchitis or pneumonia), pleuritis (which causes the lining of the lung to separate), overexertion, injuries to the ribs, strained muscles in the chest or back, or indigestion.

> **PROGRESS CHECK**
>
> 1. Angina pectoris occurs when the heart's demand for _____ exceeds its supply. *(blood/oxygen/rest)*
>
> 2. The most common symptom of angina pectoris is _____ . *(light-headedness/ profuse perspiration/chest pain)*
>
> 3. Congestive heart failure occurs when the heart's ability to _____ does not meet the demands of the body. *(pump blood/ oxygenate blood/circulate blood to the lungs)*
>
> 4. The most common cause of congestive heart failure is _____ . *(diabetes/stroke/ heart attack)*
>
> 5. The most dramatic sign of congestive heart failure is _____ . *(pulmonary edema/ swollen ankles/distended neck veins)*
>
> 6. Myocardial infarction literally means death of the _____ . *(pericardium/myocardium/ epicardium)*
>
> 7. The major symptom of myocardial infarction is _____ . *(dyspnea/nausea/chest pain)*
>
> 8. Approximately _____ percent of all myocardial infarction victims do not experience chest pain. *(10/25/50)*

16.3 First Aid Care

Time is critical in the treatment of cardiac emergencies. Activate the EMS system as soon as possible. Many heart attacks can be treated with excellent results if the patient reaches the hospital soon enough.

Treatment varies depending on whether the victim has absent circulation or the victim is responsive with a

silent myocardial infarction A heart attack that does not cause chest pain

Location of Pain and Discomfort in Heart Attack

Just under sternum, midchest, or the entire upper chest

Midchest, neck, and jaw

Midchest and on left more frequently, the shoulder and inside arms

Upper abdomen, often mistaken for indigestion

Larger area of the chest, plus neck, jaw, and inside arms

Jaw from ear to ear, in both sides of upper neck, and in lower center neck

Shoulder (usually left) and inside arm to the waist, plus opposite arm, inside to elbow

Between the shoulder blades

FIGURE 16–9. Pain or discomfort can occur in any one location or any combination of locations.

known history of cardiac problems. Not all patients who have heart attacks go into cardiac arrest and require CPR and defibrillation.

First Aid Care—Pulse Is Absent

Learning Objective **8** Describe and demonstrate the first aid care of a victim who does not have a pulse.

For details on CPR, see Chapter 5.

First Aid Care—Responsive Victim

Learning Objective **9** Describe and demonstrate the first aid care of a victim who is responsive.

To treat a responsive victim, activate the EMS system; then:

1. Perform an initial assessment. Note the type, location, and intensity of any pain and the presence of other signs and symptoms characteristic of cardiac compromise.

2. If the victim complains of chest pain or discomfort, monitor vital signs continuously; provide rescue breathing if it becomes appropriate (see Figure 16-10, page 282).

3. If the victim has physician-prescribed **nitroglycerin**, help the victim take one dose of the medication *if you are allowed to do so in your area and if the victim has not already taken it.*

   ■ Repeat the dose in 5 minutes if pain is not relieved.

   ■ Give as many as three doses, each 5 minutes apart. Reassess vital signs and chest pain after each dose.

nitroglycerin Medication prescribed to ease the pain of angina pectoris

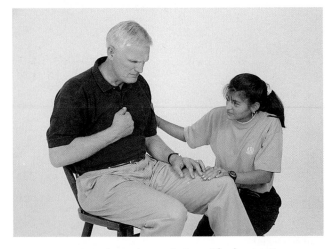

FIGURE 16–10. Assessing a victim with chest pain

4. Don't let the victim move on his or her own; reassure and comfort the victim, and place the victim in the position of greatest comfort (usually semisitting, with legs up and bent at the knees).

5. Loosen restrictive clothing at the neck and midriff, and keep the victim warm, but do not overheat.

6. Monitor vital signs continuously, and be prepared to start CPR if needed.

Cautions about Nitroglycerin

Learning Objective 10 Explain the guidelines for the use of nitroglycerin.

The most commonly prescribed medication for those with a history of cardiac compromise is nitroglycerin, known by the trade names of Nitro-bid, Nitrong, and Nitro-stat.

If allowed to do so in your area, you can help the victim take the nitroglycerin if all of the following criteria exist:

- The victim has chest pain.
- The nitroglycerin was prescribed for the victim by a physician.
- You have specific authorization to assist the victim in taking the nitroglycerin.

You should not allow the victim to take nitroglycerin if any of the following exist:

- The victim has low blood pressure (systolic pressure below 100 mmHg).
- The patient has a very slow pulse (< 50) or very rapid pulse (> 100).

- You suspect or know that the victim has a head injury.
- The victim is an infant or child.
- The victim already took the maximum prescribed dose before you arrived on the scene.

Learning Objective 11 Describe and demonstrate how to help a victim use physician-prescribed nitroglycerin.

Nitroglycerin is available in two different forms, tablets and spray, both of which are administered under the tongue. If you are authorized to help the victim:

1. Take the victim's blood pressure; the systolic pressure must be more than 100 mmHg if you are to use nitroglycerin.

2. Verify that you have the right victim, the right medication (nitroglycerin), the right form of medication (tablets or spray), and that the victim is alert and responsive.

3. Check the expiration date on the victim's prescription to verify that the medication is still potent. Potent nitroglycerin will have a bitter taste and may cause a headache.

4. Ask the victim to lift his or her tongue; wearing latex gloves, place the tablet or spray under the tongue, or have the victim place the tablet or spray under the tongue.

5. Have the victim keep his or her mouth closed (without swallowing) until the tablet has dissolved and been absorbed by the tissues under the tongue.

6. Within 2 minutes, check the victim's blood pressure; perform a reassessment.

PROGRESS CHECK

1. If the victim does not have a pulse, immediately begin _____ . (monitoring vital signs/CPR/rescue breathing)

2. If the victim is responsive, keep the victim in a _____ position. (comfortable/supine/prone)

3. Do not let the victim _____ . (eat/drink/move around)

4. If the victim has physician-prescribed _____ , help the victim use it. (pain medication/high blood pressure medication/nitroglycerin)

16.4 Stroke

Stroke (cerebrovascular accident, or CVA) is defined as any disease process that impairs circulation to the brain. Without adequate blood circulation, brain cells are deprived of oxygen and die within minutes; dead brain cells are never replaced and do not regenerate. The third most common cause of death in this country, stroke affects more than half a million Americans each year. More than half of those die, and many others suffer permanent physiological damage.

The characteristics of stroke depend on the extent of the stroke, the site of the stroke, and the amount of brain damage that results. The outcome depends on the age of the victim, the location and function of brain cells that were damaged, the extent of the damage, and how rapidly other areas of brain tissue are able to take over the work of the damaged cells.

Causes of Stroke

> Learning Objective **12** Describe the physiological processes in the brain that cause stroke.

Stroke, also known as cerebrovascular accident (CVA), occurs when blood flow to the brain is interrupted long enough to cause damage, resulting in the sudden onset of brain dysfunction. There are four general causes of stroke (Figure 16-11):

- Thrombus
- Embolus
- Hemorrhage
- Compression

> **stroke** Any disease process that impairs circulation to the brain

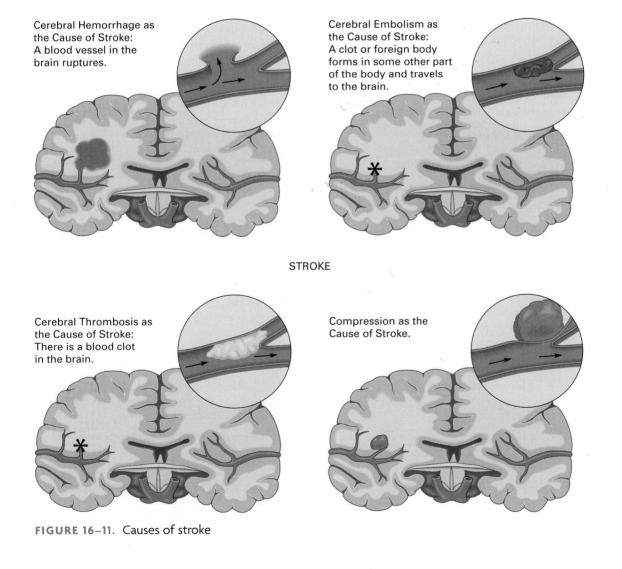

Cerebral Hemorrhage as the Cause of Stroke: A blood vessel in the brain ruptures.

Cerebral Embolism as the Cause of Stroke: A clot or foreign body forms in some other part of the body and travels to the brain.

STROKE

Cerebral Thrombosis as the Cause of Stroke: There is a blood clot in the brain.

Compression as the Cause of Stroke.

FIGURE 16–11. Causes of stroke

THROMBUS

Approximately 80 percent of all strokes occur when a cerebral artery is blocked by a clot (**thrombus**) that lodges inside the brain. A thrombotic stroke is also called an **ischemic stroke**. Most occur in those over the age of 50, and the incidence increases with age. Clots generally do not form in healthy arteries, but rather around the hardened, thickened walls of arteries damaged by atherosclerosis.

Many thrombotic strokes are preceded by one or more **transient ischemic attacks** (TIAs), brief spells similar to strokes that occur when the blockage is partial or lasts only a few minutes. TIAs may occur in a series over a period of days, usually getting worse with time; brain cells are injured, but they do not die.

The symptoms of a TIA last for less than 24 hours and usually for less than 1 hour; TIAs do not cause nausea or vomiting, and headache is not often present. The most common signs and symptoms of TIAs are the same as those of stroke, and include:

- Blindness in one eye
- Dizziness
- Light-headedness
- Fainting
- Difficulty performing familiar acts
- Temporary paralysis of the face
- Temporary paralysis of one side of the body
- Difficulty pronouncing or understanding words
- Inability to recognize familiar objects

EMBOLUS

A stroke may also result when a clot develops elsewhere in the body, travels through the bloodstream, and becomes lodged in one of the cerebral arteries—a condition called **cerebral embolism**. Of all strokes, these have the most rapid onset; they often occur in young or middle-aged adults and are most common among people with existing heart disease.

HEMORRHAGE

In about 20 percent of all strokes, a diseased blood vessel in the brain bursts, flooding the surrounding brain tissue with blood (Figure 16–12). Bleeding can either be into the brain tissue itself or into the spinal fluid that surrounds the brain. Hemorrhage is the most dramatic form of stroke, and 80 percent of its victims die. Onset is abrupt.

FIGURE 16–12. Brain of a victim of cerebrovascular accident (stroke) from cerebral hemorrhage

COMPRESSION

A small percentage of strokes occur when extreme pressure is applied to a cerebral artery, cutting off blood supply to adjacent brain tissue and nerves. Pressure can be caused by a brain tumor, displaced brain tissue following hemorrhage somewhere else in the brain, or a clot that forms outside the artery from blood leakage.

Signs and Symptoms

Learning Objective **13** List the signs and symptoms of stroke.

The signs and symptoms of stroke depend on the cause, location, and severity of the stroke. A stroke caused by thrombus results in lessening of bodily functions without accompanying pain or seizures; onset is gradual and progresses in a step-like way. A stroke caused by cerebral hemorrhage produces sudden headache followed by a sudden change in mental status and coma.

thrombus A clot that forms in a cerebral artery

ischemic stroke A stroke caused by a clot inside the brain

transient ischemic attack Brief attacks similar to strokes that occur when arterial blockage is partial or brief

cerebral embolism A clot that forms elsewhere in the body, travels through the bloodstream, and lodges in a cerebral artery

GENERAL SIGNS AND SYMPTOMS OF STROKE

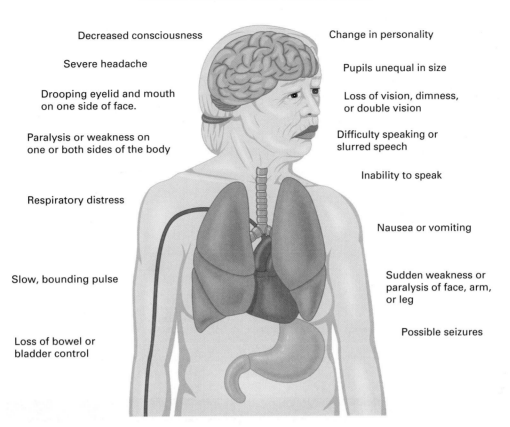

Decreased consciousness

Severe headache

Drooping eyelid and mouth on one side of face.

Paralysis or weakness on one or both sides of the body

Respiratory distress

Slow, bounding pulse

Loss of bowel or bladder control

Change in personality

Pupils unequal in size

Loss of vision, dimness, or double vision

Difficulty speaking or slurred speech

Inability to speak

Nausea or vomiting

Sudden weakness or paralysis of face, arm, or leg

Possible seizures

FIGURE 16–13. One or more signs or symptoms may be sufficient reason to begin first aid care.

The general signs and symptoms of stroke occur suddenly and may include the following (Figure 16-13):

- Altered level of consciousness—dizziness, confusion, unsteadiness, change in personality, change in the level of mental ability, seizures, decreased consciousness, or coma

- Motor function problems—weakness of the arms, legs, or face; numbness or paralysis of the face, arms, or legs, often on only one side; one-sided weakness or numbness that gradually spreads; mouth drawn to one side or drooping; paralysis of facial muscles

- Sensory function problems—loss of vision, temporary dimness of vision, or double vision

- Altered communication abilities—inability to speak, trouble speaking or understanding speech, or stuttering

- Headache that is sudden, severe, or accompanied by a stiff neck

- Flushed or pale face

- Respiratory distress

- Constricted pupils, or pupils unequal in size or reaction

- Loss of bowel or bladder control

- Nausea and/or vomiting

It is important to note the victim's state of consciousness. Only massive strokes or those involving the brain stem render the victim completely unconscious. The most critical stroke victim is the one who loses consciousness completely and becomes limp on one side; these signs indicate major brain injury.

First Aid Care for Stroke

Learning Objective **14** Describe and demonstrate the first aid care of a stroke victim.

Remember: It is not important to determine at the scene the kind of stroke that occurred. First aid care is the same, regardless of what caused the stroke, and is limited to support of the victim.

To treat a victim of stroke, activate the EMS system; then follow these steps:

1. Handle the victim calmly and carefully; be particularly gentle with paralyzed parts. Say nothing to increase the victim's anxiety (remember that a victim who can't communicate can still hear you); anxiety can considerably worsen a stroke.

2. If the victim is conscious, position him or her on the back with the head and shoulders slightly raised; keep the head in a neutral, forward-facing position. If the victim is unconscious, place him or her on the left side.

3. Assess airway and respiration.

4. If the victim develops difficulty breathing or becomes unconscious, turn him or her on the side with the paralyzed side down and well cushioned. If the victim vomits, clear the airway and allow drainage.

5. Keep the victim warm, but don't overheat.

6. Keep the victim quiet and shielded from onlookers.

7. Never give the victim anything to eat or drink.

PROGRESS CHECK

1. Stroke occurs when _____ to the brain is impaired. *(blood pressure/blood circulation/nerve impulse)*

2. Most strokes are caused by _____. *(embolus/thrombus/hemorrhage)*

3. The most serious strokes are characterized by _____. *(paralysis/loss of vision/total loss of consciousness)*

4. Position a stroke victim _____. *(on the side/flat on the back/on the back with head and shoulders elevated)*

Summary

- Coronary artery disease affects the artery that supplies the heart with blood; when the blood supply is compromised, angina pectoris or myocardial infarction can result.

- Angina pectoris occurs when the heart's need for oxygen exceeds its supply; it is reversible and is usually relieved by rest.

- Congestive heart failure is a true medical emergency. The left ventricle begins to fail. The body receives less oxygen and blood backs up in the lungs, causing pulmonary edema.

- Myocardial infarction, or heart attack, causes death of the myocardium (the heart muscle); it occurs when the blood supply to the heart is severely restricted or cut off completely.

- All victims of chest pain should be suspected of having suffered myocardial infarction.

- The most classic symptom of both angina pectoris and myocardial infarction is chest pain; the most dramatic symptom of congestive heart failure is pulmonary edema.

- Not all patients experience chest pain. In some patients, difficulty breathing and fatigue are signs of a heart attack.

- To care for a cardiac victim without a pulse, initiate defibrillation and CPR as described in Chapter 5.

- To care for a responsive cardiac victim, keep the victim still, monitor vital signs continuously, place the victim in a position of comfort, and keep the victim warm.

- Stroke occurs when blood circulation to the brain is impaired; it can be caused by a clot that forms in a cerebral artery, a clot that forms elsewhere and gets lodged in a cerebral artery, a cerebral vessel that bursts and bleeds into brain tissue, or severe compression of a cerebral artery.

- The signs and symptoms of stroke depend on the cause, location, and severity of the stroke. Most strokes do not cause headache. Subtle changes, such as drooping of facial muscles or confusion, are more common.

Key Terms

Make sure you understand the following key terms:

coronary artery disease	myocardial infarction
atherosclerosis	myocardium
arteriosclerosis	silent myocardial infarction
plaque	nitroglycerin
angina pectoris	stroke
pulmonary edema	thrombus

ischemic stroke   cerebral embolism
transient ischemic attack

Critical Thinking Exercise

You are visiting your grandmother at her assisted living facility when her neighbor, Mrs. Murdoch, comes to the door. "Ingrid, I don't feel very well."

Your grandmother invites her in and finds that Mrs. Murdock is 83, a bit nauseous, feels weak, and, although she doesn't seem to realize it, is a bit short of breath. You notice her skin is somewhat ashen and moist.

1. Could this be a heart problem? Why or why not?

2. Your grandmother tells Mrs. Murdock to lie down. When Mrs. Murdock does this she become anxious and says she feels worse. What should you do?

3. What care should you give Mrs. Murdock while you wait for EMS?

16 Chapter 16 Self-Test

Student: _____ Date: _____

Course: _____ Section #: _____

Part 1 True/False

If you believe the statement is true, circle the T. If you believe the statement is false, circle the F.

(T) F **1.** Atherosclerosis results when fatty substances and other debris are deposited on the inner lining of the arterial wall.

T (F) **2.** Angina does not always cause pain.

T F **3.** Angina pain is usually relieved by rest.

T F **4.** Angina pain is usually on the left side.

T F **5.** It is quite easy to differentiate between the pain of angina pectoris and myocardial infarction.

T F **6.** About 25 percent of all myocardial infarction victims have no chest pain.

(T) F **7.** The pain of myocardial infarction lasts longer than 30 minutes and is usually under the sternum, radiating to the neck, jaw, left shoulder, and left arm.

T F **8.** Congestive heart failure with respiratory difficulty is life threatening and requires immediate care.

T F **9.** The major symptom of myocardial infarction is cyanosis.

T F **10.** Victims of heart disease emergencies should be put in a prone position.

Part 2 Multiple Choice

For each item, circle the correct answer or the phrase that best completes the statement.

1. The signs and symptoms of myocardial infarction include all of the following except

a. pale skin color
b. shortness of breath
c. a pulse rate of 70–80 beats per minute
d. feeling of impending doom

2. Most acute heart attacks are caused by blockage of the _____ artery.

a. cephalic
b. coronary
c. coronal
d. carotid

3. The buildup of fatty deposits in the arteries is called

a. atherosclerosis
b. angina pectoris
c. coronary thrombosis
d. cholesterol

4. Angina pectoris

a. is often accompanied by weakness and nausea
b. is a term that describes any kind of chest pain

c. usually lasts longer than 30 minutes
d. is pain in the heart caused by insufficient oxygen

5. Which of the following heart conditions would probably develop over a period of several months?

a. acute myocardial infarction
b. heart attack
c. cardiogenic shock
d. congestive heart failure

6. Which of the following is not a first aid care measure for a cardiac victim?

a. loosen restrictive clothing
b. place the victim in a sitting position
c. have the victim cease all movement
d. do not help the victim administer medication until a physician has evaluated the victim

7. Dyspnea means

a. shortness of breath while lying down
b. profuse sweating
c. lack of oxygen
d. shortness of breath

8. A victim with swelling in the lower legs and frothy, pink sputum would be manifesting symptoms of

    a. angina pectoris
    b. cardiac arrest
    c. congestive heart failure
    d. none of the above

9. Which of the following is not a cause of stroke?

    a. a blood clot in a cerebral artery
    b. a blood clot that forms elsewhere, then gets lodged in a cerebral artery

    c. a blood clot in the heart
    d. bleeding into brain tissue

10. A victim of stroke should be positioned

    a. flat on the back
    b. on the back with the feet raised
    c. on the back with the head and shoulders elevated
    d. on the side

Part 3   What Would You Do If?

You are called to the home of a middle-aged woman who is experiencing severe dyspnea and a rapid heart rate. She has lower-extremity edema and distended neck veins, and seems confused.

17

Respiratory Emergencies

On the Scene

Bess Adams was hosting a birthday party for her 9-year-old son. A friend of the family had come in cowboy garb and had brought a horse so the children could take turns riding around the block.

About 15 minutes after Cody Reese finished his ride, Bess noticed that he was struggling to breathe. He was making a whistling, high-pitched wheezing sound as he tried to exhale and using the muscles of his neck and shoulders to assist his breathing. Even with all his effort to breathe, he was moving very little air in and out.

Recognizing the signs of asthma, Bess called Cody's mother, who confirmed that Cody had both asthma and an allergy to horse hair. Cody's mother knew from the description of his symptoms that his attack was severe; she told Bess to call for help while she drove over with Cody's inhaler. Bess called 9-1-1, then asked her teenage daughter to take the other children to the backyard and supervise the other party activities. Bess led Cody to the couch and tried to calm him where it was quiet. Because his airway was clear, though constricted, and he was still able to move some air, Bess helped him into the most comfortable position on the couch—sitting upright and leaning forward. Bess monitored his breathing carefully until emergency personnel arrived.

Vital to survival is the body's ability to deliver sufficient amounts of freshly oxygenated blood to all cells. Without enough oxygen, some cells—such as those in the heart and brain—can die within minutes.

A variety of diseases and injuries can interfere with the body's ability to get enough oxygen. Rapid medical attention in these cases is essential to saving life and preventing cell death from oxygen starvation.

This chapter explains some of the major diseases that cause respiratory emergencies and outlines appropriate first aid care for each.

17.1 Dyspnea

> Learning Objective **1** Understand the physiology of dyspnea.

Dyspnea, one of the most common medical complaints, is defined as a sensation of shortness of breath—a feeling of air hunger accompanied by labored breathing. Patients won't use the word "dyspnea." The patients you encounter may report being "short of breath," "unable to breathe," or "unable to catch my breath." The common problem of all these patients is that the body perceives the need for more oxygen than it is receiving.

Dyspnea is not a disease in itself but is a symptom of a number of diseases. Breathing will generally be rapid and shallow, but victims may feel short of breath whether they are breathing rapidly or slowly. Remember, shortness of breath is normal following exercise, fatigue, coughing, or the production of excess sputum. In these cases, the condition is not considered true dyspnea.

First Aid Care

> Learning Objective **2** Describe the first aid care of dyspnea.

Activate the EMS system immediately; then:

1. Maintain an open airway. Dyspnea may be caused by aspiration of a foreign body, so consider aspiration and clear the airway if necessary.

2. Ventilate or provide assisted ventilations if necessary.

3. If the victim is breathing adequately, place in a position of comfort.

PROGRESS CHECK

1. Dyspnea is defined as _____ . (*labored breathing/air hunger/shortness of breath*)

2. Victims of dyspnea may be breathing rapidly or slowly, but always feel _____ . (*dizzy/short of breath/faint*)

3. Dyspnea is not a _____, but is a symptom of a number of diseases. (*disease itself/medical emergency/respiratory syndrome*)

4. Because dyspnea can be caused by _____, always check the airway. (*aspiration/internal bleeding/bronchitis*)

17.2 Chronic Obstructive Pulmonary Disease

More than 90 percent of those with **chronic obstructive pulmonary disease** (COPD) have emphysema, chronic bronchitis, or both. The most important known factor in COPD is cigarette smoking; most COPD victims are also prone to allergies and a variety of infections.

Emphysema and chronic bronchitis (Figure 17-1) represent two extremes of a whole spectrum of problems. Many victims fall somewhere in between the two extremes, manifesting signs and symptoms of both disorders.

Emphysema

> Learning Objective **3** Understand the physiology of emphysema.

Emphysema is characterized by distension of the air sacs (groups of alveoli) beyond the bronchioles, with destructive changes in their walls. Basically, the alveoli lose their elasticity, become distended with trapped air, and stop functioning. When air is trapped in the alveoli, the walls eventually break down and the total

> **dyspnea** Shortness of breath or difficulty in breathing
> **chronic obstructive pulmonary disease** A range of diseases including emphysema, chronic bronchitis, and asthma
> **emphysema** A respiratory disease characterized by overinflated alveoli

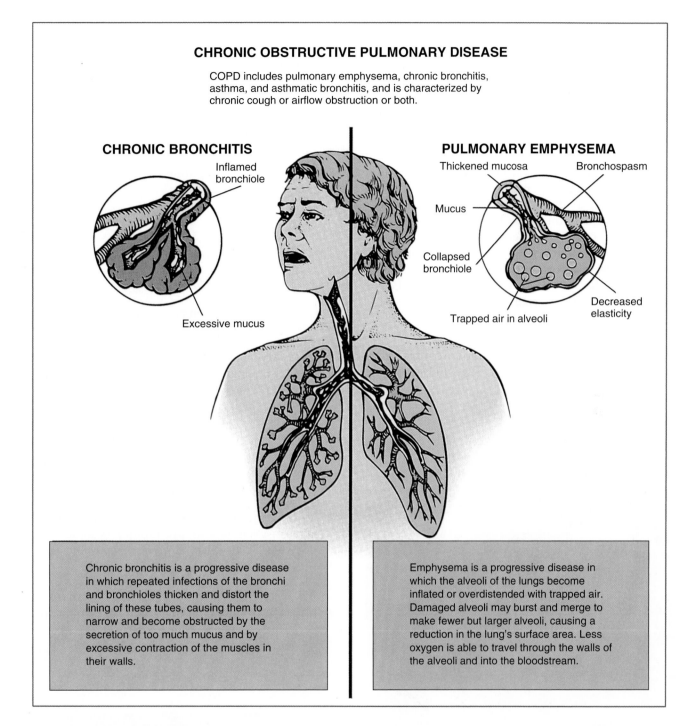

CHRONIC OBSTRUCTIVE PULMONARY DISEASE

COPD includes pulmonary emphysema, chronic bronchitis, asthma, and asthmatic bronchitis, and is characterized by chronic cough or airflow obstruction or both.

CHRONIC BRONCHITIS

Inflamed bronchiole

Excessive mucus

PULMONARY EMPHYSEMA

Thickened mucosa

Bronchospasm

Mucus

Collapsed bronchiole

Trapped air in alveoli

Decreased elasticity

Chronic bronchitis is a progressive disease in which repeated infections of the bronchi and bronchioles thicken and distort the lining of these tubes, causing them to narrow and become obstructed by the secretion of too much mucus and by excessive contraction of the muscles in their walls.

Emphysema is a progressive disease in which the alveoli of the lungs become inflated or overdistended with trapped air. Damaged alveoli may burst and merge to make fewer but larger alveoli, causing a reduction in the lung's surface area. Less oxygen is able to travel through the walls of the alveoli and into the bloodstream.

FIGURE 17–1. Forms of COPD

number of alveoli decreases, making it more difficult for the victim to breathe.

SIGNS AND SYMPTOMS

Because victims of emphysema are usually not cyanotic, they are referred to as **pink puffers**. Signs and symptoms may include:

- Evidence of weight loss

- History of increasing dyspnea on exertion
- Progressive limitation of activity
- Production of only small amounts of mucus with coughing
- Prolonged and difficult exhalation

pink puffer A victim of emphysema

- Lungs remain expanded even after exhalation
- Barrel-shaped chest (see Figure 17-2)

Chronic Bronchitis

Chronic bronchitis is characterized by inflammation, edema, and excessive mucus production in the bronchial tree. By definition, chronic bronchitis features a productive cough that has persisted for at least 3 months out of the year over the past 2 years.

The typical victim with chronic bronchitis has invariably been a heavy cigarette smoker with many respiratory infections. There is a tendency toward associated heart disease and right-heart failure.

SIGNS AND SYMPTOMS

Because victims of chronic bronchitis are often cyanotic, they are called **blue bloaters**. Signs and symptoms include:

FIGURE 17-2. Victims of emphysema and chronic bronchitis often lean forward in an attempt to breathe.

- Coughing that produces thick mucus
- Use of neck and chest muscles to assist breathing
- Cyanosis
- Swelling of the hands, feet, and ankles
- Distended neck veins
- High-pitched wheezing during both inhalation and exhalation
- Low-pitched snoring sounds during both inhalation and exhalation

First Aid Care for COPD

The number-one goal of first aid care for COPD is to enhance oxygenation; without it, the victim may die. The major threat to life in COPD is a lack of oxygen. To care for COPD, activate the EMS system; then:

1. Establish an airway.

2. Help the victim into the most comfortable position—usually sitting or semisitting.

3. If the victim is unconscious, administer artificial ventilation if necessary.

4. Monitor the victim's respiratory rate and depth, and assist ventilations if respiration becomes depressed. *Watch the victim closely for changes in rate and depth.*

5. Maintain the victim's body temperature.

6. Loosen restrictive clothing, comfort and reassure the victim, and encourage the victim to cough up secretions.

blue bloater A victim of chronic bronchitis

3. Because the walls of the alveoli have broken down in victims of emphysema, air is _____ in the lungs. *(trapped/concentrated/leaking)*

4. The number-one goal of care for COPD is to _____. *(prevent aspiration/enhance oxygenation/assist ventilation)*

17.3 Asthma

Asthma, which affects more than 10 million people in the United States, is characterized by an increased sensitivity of the trachea, bronchi, and bronchioles to various stimuli, with widespread reversible narrowing of the airways.

It is a chronic inflammatory disease, and occurs in two general degrees:

1. Acute asthma, consisting of periodic attacks and symptom-free periods between attacks

2. Status asthmaticus, consisting of a prolonged and life-threatening attack

There are also generally two different kinds of asthma. Extrinsic asthma, or *allergic* asthma, is usually a reaction to dust, pollen, or other irritants. It is often seasonal, occurs most often in children, and often clears up after adolescence. Intrinsic, or *nonallergenic*, asthma is most common in adults and occurs most often in response to emotion, industrial or other fumes, strong odors, strong perfumes, viral infections, aspirin and other medications, cold air, air pollution, or some other irritant.

The acute asthma attack varies in duration, intensity, and frequency and reflects airway obstruction due to one of the following:

- **Bronchospasm** (generalized spasm of the bronchi)
- Swelling of the mucous membranes in the bronchial walls
- Plugging of the bronchi by thick mucus secretions

SIGNS AND SYMPTOMS

Learning Objective 6 List the signs and symptoms of asthma.

The signs and symptoms of asthma can range from mild to severe, and can be life-threatening. A typical acute attack may feature the following signs and symptoms:

- Victim sitting upright, often leaning forward with nostrils flared, fighting to breathe
- Spasmodic, unproductive cough
- Whistling, high-pitched wheezing, usually during exhalation
- Very little movement of air during breathing, even when the victim is at rest
- Hyperinflated chest with air trapped in the lungs because of increased obstruction during exhalation
- Rapid, shallow respirations
- Rapid pulse (often more than 120 beats per minute)
- Fatigue
- Use of accessory muscles in the neck and shoulders to aid breathing

First Aid Care

Learning Objective 7 Describe and demonstrate the first aid care for a victim with asthma.

The three goals of first aid care for an acute asthma attack are to improve oxygenation, relieve bronchospasm, and improve the victim's ventilation. Activate the EMS system; then:

1. Establish an airway and assist ventilations if necessary.

2. Stay calm and keep the victim as calm as possible; stress and emotional intensity worsen the asthma attack. Keep the victim in a position of comfort, usually sitting up.

3. *If you are allowed to do so in your area,* help the victim use any asthma medication he or she may have (often an inhaler).

Status Asthmaticus

Status asthmaticus is a severe, prolonged asthma attack that does not respond to aggressive treatment and that represents a *dire medical emergency*.

SIGNS AND SYMPTOMS

Wheezing is not a reliable sign of status asthmaticus: *There may be no wheezing at all.* In fact, breath sounds may be almost absent. Other signs and symptoms may include the following (see Figure 17-3, page 296):

- Severe inflation of the chest due to continued trapping of air in the lungs

bronchospasm Generalized spasm of the bronchi
status asthmaticus A severe, prolonged asthma attack that represents a dire medical emergency

STATUS ASTHMATICUS
Status asthmaticus is a severe prolonged asthma attack.

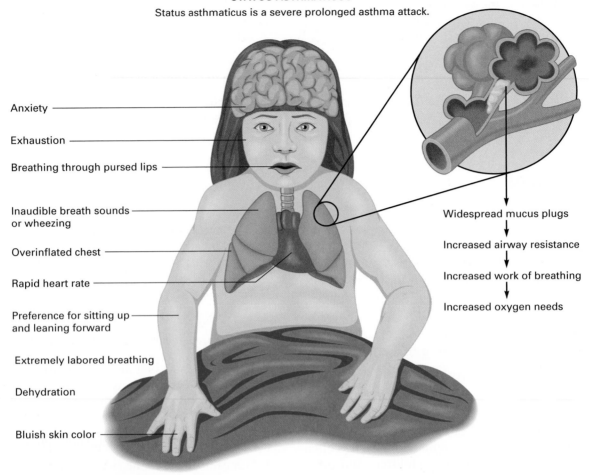

Anxiety

Exhaustion

Breathing through pursed lips

Inaudible breath sounds
or wheezing

Overinflated chest

Rapid heart rate

Preference for sitting up
and leaning forward

Extremely labored breathing

Dehydration

Bluish skin color

Walking and talking only with greatest effort

Widespread mucus plugs

Increased airway resistance

Increased work of breathing

Increased oxygen needs

FIGURE 17–3. Status asthmaticus is a dire medical emergency.

- Bluish discoloration of the skin

- Walking and talking only with the greatest effort

- Extremely labored breathing, with the victim fighting to move air and using accessory muscles to breathe

- Inaudible breath sounds

- Exhaustion

Don't be fooled by a victim who seems to be suffering from status asthmaticus but who then seems to begin to recover; *the victim could still be in grave danger.*

FIRST AID CARE

To care for the victim of status asthmaticus, follow the same general guidelines as for acute asthma, *but increase your urgency in establishing care and activating the EMS system.*

One note of caution: All that wheezes is not asthma. Many other diseases and injuries—such as heart failure, pneumonia, smoke inhalation, partial airway obstruction, cystic fibrosis, upper-airway inflammation, and anaphylactic shock—cause wheezing.

PROGRESS CHECK

1. The main physiological event in asthma is _____ of the airway. *(obstruction/narrowing/complete blockage)*

2. A prolonged, life-threatening asthma attack is called _____ . *(acute asthma/bronchial asthma/status asthmaticus)*

3. There are two different kinds of asthma—one most often caused by infection or emotion and the other most often caused by _____ . *(allergy/aspirin/cold air)*

4. In a typical attack, the victim's cough is _____ . *(productive/unproductive/intermittent)*

5. The three goals of first aid care for asthma are to improve oxygenation, relieve bronchospasm, and improve _____ . *(circulation/metabolism/ventilation)*

6. Status asthmaticus is usually characterized by _____ . *(severe wheezing/low-pitched snoring/absent breath sounds)*

17.4 Pneumonia

Pneumonia is a medical term used to describe a group of illnesses characterized by lung inflammation and fluid- or pus-filled alveoli, leading to inadequately oxygenated blood. Pneumonia is most frequently caused by a bacterial or viral infection, but can also be caused by inhaled irritants or aspirated materials.

Signs and Symptoms

Learning Objective **8** List the signs and symptoms of pneumonia.

Victims of pneumonia generally appear very ill; most complain of fever and chills that "shake the bed"; fever usually exceeds 101°F. Signs and symptoms depend on the lobe of the lung that is affected, and may include:

- Chest pain, usually worse when breathing
- Dyspnea
- Rapid respiration
- Respiratory distress
- Noisy breathing
- Productive cough, usually with yellow sputum or mucus that is sometimes streaked with blood
- Hot, dry skin

First Aid Care

Learning Objective **9** Describe and demonstrate the first aid care for a victim with pneumonia.

1. Place the victim in a position of comfort that enables the victim to breathe with the least distress; most prefer an upright or semisitting position.

2. Maintain an open airway.

3. Transport the victim to a physician.

17.5 Hyperventilation

Hyperventilation is a condition characterized by "overbreathing," or breathing too rapidly and too deeply. It is normal under a variety of conditions (such as following exercise), as long as breathing quickly returns to a normal rate.

Hyperventilation syndrome, on the other hand, is an abnormal state in which rapid breathing persists. The causes of hyperventilation syndrome are varied, but usually involve anxiety or emotional stress.

If caused by anxiety or stress, hyperventilation syndrome is relatively benign. If caused by an underlying medical condition—such as diabetic coma, asthma, aspirin overdose, or increased pressure in the skull—the outcome can be catastrophic.

Signs and Symptoms

Learning Objective **10** List the signs and symptoms of hyperventilation.

Hyperventilation involves breathing at a rate faster than 40 breaths per minute. Overbreathing lowers the carbon dioxide in the blood to an abnormal level, causing the following signs and symptoms:

- Marked anxiety, leading to panic
- Air hunger
- Giddiness or unusual behavior

hyperventilation A condition characterized by overbreathing or breathing too rapidly

hyperventilation syndrome An abnormal state in which rapid breathing persists

- Fatigue
- Abdominal discomfort or bloating
- Drawing up of the hands at the wrists and knuckles with flexed fingers (**carpopedal spasm**)
- Dyspnea
- Dizziness or light-headedness
- Blurring of vision
- Dryness or bitter taste in the mouth
- Numbness and/or tingling of the hands and feet or the area around the mouth
- Tightness or a "lump" in the throat
- Pounding of the heart with stabbing pains in the chest
- Great weakness
- A feeling of impending doom
- Fainting
- Deep, sighing, rapid respirations with a rapid pulse

First Aid Care

> Learning Objective **11** Describe and demonstrate the first aid care for a victim with hyperventilation.

Before starting any first aid care, rule out any medical causes for rapid breathing, such as diabetic coma, trauma, or asthma. If they exist, care for them appropriately. If you are certain the hyperventilation has no medical causes:

1. Remain calm and reassuring; listen carefully, show understanding and consideration, and try to calm the victim down.

2. Try to talk the victim into slowing the breathing rate. Have the victim breathe with his or her abdominal muscles as much as possible; instruct the victim to breathe in through the nose, hold the breath for a few seconds, then breathe out as slowly as possible through pursed lips.

3. Explain to the victim what happened, and reassure the victim that it is not serious.

4. Transport the victim to an emergency room or activate the EMS system.

Do not have the victim breathe into a paper bag; doing so does not balance blood gases, and can seriously stress the heart and lungs.

PROGRESS CHECK

1. Hyperventilation syndrome is an abnormal state in which rapid breathing _____. *(occurs periodically/comes in cycles/persists)*

2. Hyperventilation is fairly benign unless caused by _____. *(anxiety/severe fright/an underlying medical condition)*

3. Hyperventilation is characterized by _____ during breathing. *(deep sighs/wheezing/rales)*

4. To care for hyperventilation not caused by a medical condition, _____. *(have the victim breathe into a paper bag/ calm the victim/give artificial ventilation)*

carpopedal spasm Drawing up of the hands at the wrists and knuckles with flexed fingers

Summary

- Dyspnea, one of the most common medical complaints, is characterized by shortness of breath; make sure you rule out airway obstruction.
- Chronic obstructive pulmonary disease encompasses emphysema, chronic bronchitis, and asthma.
- In emphysema, damaged alveoli break down and fill with trapped air; in chronic bronchitis, repeated infections thicken and distort the lining of the bronchioles.

- In asthma, there is a generalized spasm of the bronchi, swelling of the mucous membranes in the bronchial walls, and plugging of the bronchi by thick mucus secretions.
- The three goals of first aid care for asthma are to improve oxygenation, relieve bronchospasm, and improve the victim's ventilation.
- Status asthmaticus, a prolonged, severe asthma attack, represents a dire medical emergency.

- Pneumonia is a group of illnesses that cause lung inflammation; the most characteristic sign is high fever and chills.

- Hyperventilation is fairly benign unless it is caused by an underlying medical condition.

- Never treat hyperventilation by having a victim breathe into a paper bag.

Key Terms

Make sure you understand the following key terms:

dyspnea
chronic obstructive pulmonary disease
emphysema
pink puffers
blue bloaters
bronchospasm
status asthmaticus
hyperventilation
hyperventilation syndrome
carpopedal spasm

Critical Thinking Exercise

You are at the basketball court with some friends when you notice a man on the opposite court having difficulty breathing. He is about 24 years old and leaning forward with his hands on his knees. As you approach, you hear wheezing. He is sweaty, pale, and very anxious. He tells you he has some condition where he has attacks but is having trouble remembering the name. He thinks he has an inhaler in his car.

1. What condition do you think this patient has? Why?

2. What would comprise your care for this condition?

3. If someone retrieved the inhaler from his car, would you give it to him to use?

Chapter 17 Self-Test

Student: _____ Date: _____

Course: _____ Section #: _____

Part 1   True/False

If you believe the statement is true, circle the T. If you believe the statement is false, circle the F.

(T) F   **1.** Dyspnea is not a disease itself, but a symptom of a number of other diseases.

(T) F   **2.** Dyspnea is a feeling of air hunger accompanied by labored breathing.

T (F)   **3.** Victims with emphysema are usually cyanotic.

(T) F   **4.** The victim with emphysema usually appears thin and wasted with a barrel-shaped chest.

(T) F   **5.** The chronic bronchitis victim uses the neck and chest muscles to assist in breathing.

(T) F   **6.** The number-one goal of first aid care for COPD is to enhance oxygenation.

T (F)   **7.** One of the three main goals of first aid care for asthma is to treat for shock.

T (F)   **8.** Have a hyperventilation victim breathe into a paper bag.

(T)(F)   **9.** The major threat to life for a COPD victim is a lack of oxygen.

Part 2   Multiple Choice

For each item, circle the correct answer or the phrase that best completes the statement.

1. Dyspnea means
   a. painful, rapid breathing
   b. excess sputum production
   c. shortness of breath
   d. fatigue

2. Which of the following is not a category of COPD?
   a. emphysema
   b. asthma
   c. chronic bronchitis
   d. atherosclerosis

3. Initial care for a person who is hyperventilating includes
   a. establishing an airway
   b. encouraging the victim to take rapid, shallow breaths
   c. loosening tight clothing
   d. calming and reassuring the victim

4. In status asthmaticus
   a. the victim is not in much danger
   b. the chest is sunken

   c. wheezing is very audible
   d. the victim uses accessory muscles of respiration

5. Which of the following is *not* a symptom of hyperventilation?
   a. slow heart rate
   b. fainting
   c. tingling in the hands and feet
   d. a feeling of weakness

6. First aid care for COPD victims is aimed primarily at
   a. causing expectoration of sputum
   b. enhancing oxygenation
   c. humidifying the air
   d. transporting the victim as soon as possible

7. Pink puffers and blue bloaters are
   a. newborns with breathing difficulties
   b. victims of heart disease
   c. victims with COPD
   d. all of the above

Part 3   Matching

Match the descriptions in the left column with the conditions in the right column.

Description

1. _____ C _____ Pink puffers
2. _____ F _____ Represents a dire medical emergency
3. _____ A _____ Sensation of shortness of breath
4. _____ G _____ Most frequently caused by a bacterial or viral infection
5. _____ H _____ Rapid, deep, abnormal breathing
6. _____ B _____ Characterized by chronic cough, airflow obstruction, or both
7. _____ E _____ Usually brought on by allergic reaction, respiratory infection, or emotional stress
8. _____ D _____ Blue bloater

Condition

A. Dyspnea
B. COPD
C. Emphysema
D. Chronic bronchitis
E. Asthma
F. Status asthmaticus
G. Pneumonia
H. Hyperventilation

Part 4   What Would You Do If?

1. You are at the home of a middle-aged man and find him sitting on the edge of his bed, gasping for air. He has distended neck veins and audible wheezes, and is cyanotic.

2. You are at a college dormitory where you find a woman having an asthma attack. She is fighting to breathe and has audible wheezes. The attack has been severe and prolonged, and the victim is exhausted.

18

Diabetic Emergencies

On the Scene

Twenty-nine-old Steve Cox returned to his desk at the university advisement center after playing an especially fast-paced game of basketball during his lunch hour. About half an hour later, when co-worker Julia Gallagher entered his office to discuss a meeting scheduled for that afternoon, Steve snarled angrily at her and ordered her from his office.

Knowing he was an insulin-dependent diabetic, Julia took as close a look at Steve as she could from across his desk. Though his office was almost cool, he was perspiring heavily; his breathing was rapid, his hands were trembling, and his pupils were dilated.

"Steve, have you eaten today?" she asked. "Breakfast," he replied coolly. "What about lunch?" she asked again. "Nope. Played basketball." The brusque replies were unusual for Steve, who was normally a warm, talkative person. "Have you taken your insulin today?" she coaxed. "Yup."

Suspecting Steve's blood sugar level was becoming too low, Julia stepped into the doorway and sent a co-worker to the vending machine for a drink with sugar. She asked another co-worker to call the university's emergency services personnel.

With some coaxing, she persuaded Steve to drink the fruit punch while she monitored his vital signs. By the time emergency personnel arrived a few minutes later, his symptoms were easing and his mental status was returning to normal.

onservatively estimated, three are more than 14 million diabetics in the United States. In approximately half of these cases, diabetes mellitus has not been diagnosed or recognized, so the victims are completely unaware of the disease. Unfortunately, the first indication of the disease may be a life-threatening medical emergency, such as severely elevated blood sugar level (hyperglycemia) or severely low blood sugar level (hypoglycemia).

This chapter gives basic background information about diabetes, differentiates between hyperglycemia and hypoglycemia, and details how to care for each.

18.1 Diabetes

> **Learning Objective 1** Understand the basic pathophysiology of diabetes mellitus.

Insulin is a hormone needed to facilitate the movement of **glucose** (sugar) out of the bloodstream, across cell membranes, and into the cells. Without glucose, cells are not able to meet their energy needs.

In people with diabetes mellitus, sugar accumulates in the bloodstream because insulin does not move it into the body cells (see Figure 18-1). It is a paradoxical situation: The diabetic has extremely elevated levels of sugar in the blood, but a severely depleted supply of sugar in the cells, where it is critically needed. All organ systems are affected except the brain, initially, since it does not require insulin to move glucose into the brain cells.

When glucose does not get delivered to the cells, the cells resort to using fat and proteins as fuel, eventually robbing the muscles and vital organs of their mass. The sugar continues to build up in the blood. The kidneys start spilling sugar into the urine, which draws large amounts of water into the urine.

Diabetes mellitus can cause long-term complications in a number of body systems. Common complications include circulatory problems, blindness (due to degeneration of the small blood vessels in the retina), and nervous system problems, including lack of sensation in the hands and feet, delayed emptying of the stomach, and sexual dysfunction and impotence. Two major complications include stroke and heart attack that result from the diseased vessels.

There are two basic types of diabetes:

- **Type I diabetes,** or insulin-dependent diabetes (IDDM), in which the victim has little or no ability to produce insulin. Type I usually begins in childhood (previously referred to as "juvenile-onset"), and victims require daily insulin injections.

- **Type II diabetes,** or non-insulin dependent diabetes mellitus (NIDDM), previously called "adult-onset diabetes," in which the victim produces insulin but either not enough insulin or the cells do not respond to it. Type II diabetes is generally controlled by diet, exercise, and/or oral medication.

Another type of diabetes, which is usually not permanent, is **gestational diabetes.** Gestational diabetes develops during pregnancy and occurs when the hormones in the placenta cause the body to resist the action of insulin. It is almost always treated with diet, though some women require medication to control gestational diabetes. Women with gestational diabetes tend to deliver very large babies. Gestational diabetes usually ends when the baby is born, and may or may not occur in subsequent pregnancies.

Diabetics face a grave physical situation when their blood glucose level is too high or too low: Either condition can cause alterations in consciousness, and both can be life threatening if not treated promptly.

PROGRESS CHECK

1. Insulin is needed to move _____ out of the bloodstream. *(oxygen/glucose/carbon dioxide)*

2. Cells need glucose to meet their _____ needs. *(energy/metabolic/elimination)*

3. In diabetes mellitus, sugars accumulate in the _____ . *(kidneys/liver/bloodstream)*

4. _____ diabetes mellitus usually starts later in life and occurs because the cells do not respond to the insulin. *(Type I/Type II)*

5. _____ diabetes mellitus results when the body produces little or no insulin. *(Type I/Type II)*

insulin A hormone needed to facilitate movement of glucose out of the bloodstream, across the cell membranes, and into the cells

glucose Sugar

Type I diabetes Diabetes that results when the body produces little or no insulin

Type II diabetes Diabetes that results when the body does not produce enough insulin or the cells do not respond as well to the insulin

gestational diabetes Temporary diabetes that develops in a pregnant woman

NORMAL VS. DIABETIC USE OF SUGAR

FIGURE 18–1. Diabetes has long been recognized as a serious metabolic disorder.

18.2 Understanding the Differences between Hyperglycemic and Hypoglycemic Emergencies

> Learning Objective **2** Differentiate between hyperglycemia (high blood sugar level) and hypoglycemia (low blood sugar level).

Hyperglycemia, once known as diabetic coma, and **hypoglycemia,** once known as insulin shock, are grave medical emergencies that can be life threatening if not treated promptly. However, there are significant differences in the causes, onset, and signs and symptoms of each condition.

> Learning Objective **3** List the signs and symptoms of hyperglycemia (high blood sugar level).

> Learning Objective **4** List the signs and symptoms of hypoglycemia (low blood sugar level).

Figures 18-2 through 18-4 on pages 306–308 illustrate the signs and symptoms of hypoglycemia and hyperglycemia.

> **PROGRESS CHECK**
>
> 1. _____ is caused by too little insulin and too much blood sugar. *(Hypoglycemia/Hyperglycemia)*
> 2. _____ is caused by too much insulin and too little blood sugar. *(Hypoglycemia/Hyperglycemia)*
> 3. You would suspect _____ in a diabetic who has a viral respiratory infection and a fever. *(hypoglycemia/hyperglycemia)*

hyperglycemia A condition that results from not enough or a lack of insulin and too much sugar

hypoglycemia A condition that results from too much insulin and not enough or a lack of sugar in the blood

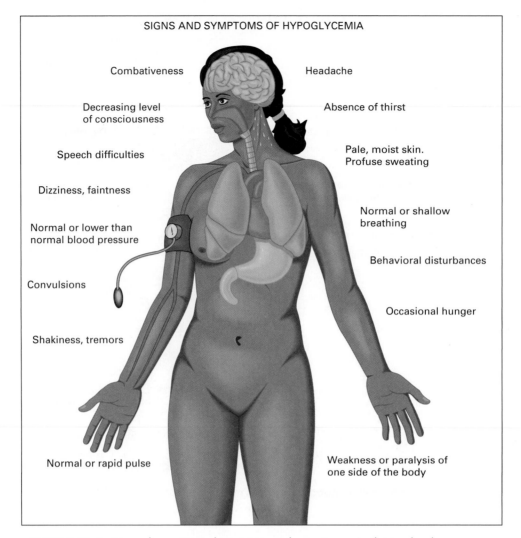

SIGNS AND SYMPTOMS OF HYPOGLYCEMIA

Combativeness

Decreasing level
of consciousness

Speech difficulties

Dizziness, faintness

Normal or lower than
normal blood pressure

Convulsions

Shakiness, tremors

Normal or rapid pulse

Headache

Absence of thirst

Pale, moist skin.
Profuse sweating

Normal or shallow
breathing

Behavioral disturbances

Occasional hunger

Weakness or paralysis of
one side of the body

FIGURE 18–2. Hypoglycemia produces signs and symptoms similar to shock.

4. You would suspect _____ in a diabetic who skipped lunch for an exercise ses-
sion, but who took prescribed insulin anyway.
(hypoglycemia/hyperglycemia)

5. Severe hyperglycemia may cause _____
breath odor. *(fruity/alcohol/no)*

6. Hypoglycemia causes _____ breath
odor. *(acetone/fruity/no)*

7. The onset of hypoglycemia is _____ .
(gradual/rapid)

18.3 First Aid Care

If you encounter a person who is unresponsive, or who
has an altered mental status, always look for signs of a
diabetic emergency—a Medic Alert tag, bracelet, or

card; signs of insulin injection (needle marks in the
thigh or abdomen); signs of oral diabetic medication
(bottles in the house); signs of poor circulation or
amputation of the toes, feet, or lower leg; or other tell-
tale signs of diabetes mellitus.

The general rule to remember about first aid care
for diabetic emergencies is simple: *When in doubt, give
sugar.* You will not harm a hyperglycemic victim by
giving sugar; the amount administered is trivial compared to what the diabetic already has in the bloodstream. However, *you may save the life of a hypoglycemic
victim by administering sugar.* Table 18-1 on page 309
compares the causes, first aid care, and signs and
symptoms of hypoglycemic and hyperglycemic emergencies. When faced with a victim who displays the
symptoms in Table 18-1, try to determine whether the
victim is diabetic by asking the victim or family members, or by looking for Medic Alert bracelets, anklets,
necklaces or cards. If you know or suspect that the victim is diabetic, and you cannot rule out hypoglycemia,

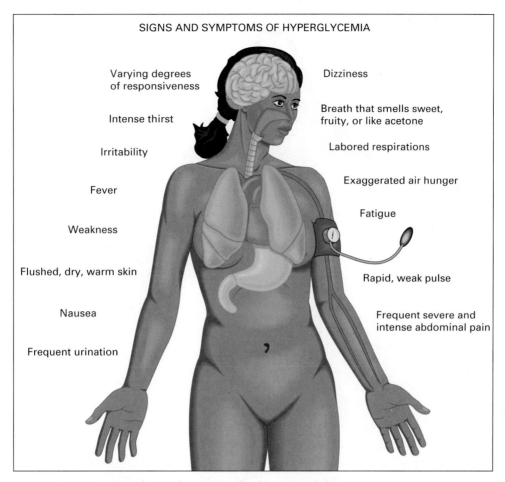

SIGNS AND SYMPTOMS OF HYPERGLYCEMIA

Varying degrees of responsiveness

Intense thirst

Irritability

Fever

Weakness

Flushed, dry, warm skin

Nausea

Frequent urination

Dizziness

Breath that smells sweet, fruity, or like acetone

Labored respirations

Exaggerated air hunger

Fatigue

Rapid, weak pulse

Frequent severe and intense abdominal pain

FIGURE 18–3. Severe hyperglycemia is also known as diabetic coma or diabetic ketoacidosis (DKA).

assume that the victim is undergoing a hypoglycemic emergency and proceed with appropriate first aid care.

Often a hypoglycemic or hyperglycemic victim may appear drunk. Always check for other underlying conditions—such as diabetic complications—when providing first aid care to someone who appears intoxicated.

First Aid Care of Severe Hyperglycemia (DKA)

Learning Objective **5** Describe and demonstrate the first aid care of a severe hyperglycemic victim.

Activate the EMS system; then:

1. Open the airway and provide artificial ventilation, if necessary.

2. Check for signs of head or neck injury that may have occurred if the victim fell when losing consciousness; if any injuries are present, administer appropriate care.

3. Be alert for vomiting; position the victim on the side with the face pointed downward to prevent aspiration and allow drainage.

4. Treat for shock; keep the victim warm.

5. Monitor the airway, breathing, and circulation vital signs every few minutes until emergency personnel arrive.

First Aid Care of Hypoglycemia

Learning Objective **6** Describe and demonstrate the first aid care of a hypoglycemic victim.

Hypoglycemia is a grave medical emergency that can cause death within a few minutes. Activate the EMS system immediately; then:

1. If the victim is able to obey commands and swallow, give orange juice, with several tablespoons of sugar mixed in it, or other drinks that contain high amounts of sugar to help increase the blood sugar

HYPERGLYCEMIA

ONSET

- Gradual, over period of days

CAUSES

Insufficient insulin and too much sugar because the victim:

- Fails to take any or enough insulin

- Eats too much food that contains or produces sugar

- Has an infection

- Is stressed

HYPOGLYCEMIA

ONSET

- Sudden, within minutes

CAUSES

Too much insulin and insufficient sugar because the victim:

- Takes too much insulin, or cannot adjust to new dosage

- Does not eat at all, or does not eat enough

- Vomits after taking insulin

- Exercises excessively

- Has been emotionally excited

FIGURE 18–4. If you cannot distinguish between severe hyperglycemia (DKA) and hypoglycemia, give sugar. You will not harm a hyperglycemic victim by doing so, and you will probably save the life of a hypoglycemic victim.

level. (See Figure 18-5.) Do not give hard candy or hard-to-swallow viscous substances because the victim may become unconscious suddenly and choke on or aspirate the object.

2. If the victim is unable to obey commands or swallow, establish an airway and administer artificial ventilation if the volume or rate of breathing is inadequate.

3. Place the victim in a lateral recumbent position.

4. Continue to monitor vital signs until emergency personnel arrive.

PROGRESS CHECK

1. For a responsive diabetic victim, when in doubt, give _____ .
   (artificial ventilation/CPR/sugar)

2. If a victim of _____ is conscious, immediately give the victim orange juice, or drinks that contain sugar.
   (hypoglycemia/hyperglycemia)

FIGURE 18–5. Administer concentrated oral glucose to a responsive diabetic victim.

TABLE 18–1	Hyperglycemia/Diabetic Ketoacidosis (DKA) and Hypoglycemia

	Hyperglycemia/Diabetic Ketoacidosis (DKA) (Diabetic Coma)	Hypoglycemia (Insulin Shock)
Causes	• The victim has not been diagnosed as diabetic and/or has not had treatment for diabetes. • The victim has not taken his/her insulin or has overeaten. • An infection has disrupted the victim's glucose/insulin balance.	• The victim has taken too much insulin or has not eaten enough. • The victim has overexercised or overexerted him/herself. • The victim has vomited after eating and taking insulin
First Aid Care	Immediately activate the EMS system, open the victim's airway, monitor vital signs, and rule out heart attack, stroke, or other emergencies.	• Responsive victim—activate the EMS system and administer sugar (granulated sugar mixed in water; orange juice; or another high-sugar-content drink) or oral glucose. • Victims with altered mental status—activate the EMS system, avoid giving liquids, turn head to side, or place in lateral recumbent position.
Symptoms and Signs	Signs and symptoms appear gradually, over a period of days. They include: • Dry mouth and intense thirst • Abdominal pain and vomiting • Gradually increasing restlessness and confusion, followed by stupor • Altered mental status, with deep, sighing respirations; weak, rapid pulse; dry, flushed warm skin; sunken eyes; normal or slightly low blood pressure. • Breath smelling of acetone (fruity odor)	Signs and symptoms appear rapidly, over a period of minutes. They include: • Dizziness and headache • Abnormal, hostile, or aggressive behavior • Fainting, convulsions, and occasionally coma • Normal blood pressure • Full, rapid pulse • Intense hunger • Pale, cold, clammy skin; profuse perspiration • Copious saliva, drooling

Summary

- Diabetes mellitus is a disease in which too little insulin is produced by the body or in which the body cannot utilize the insulin that is produced.

- Type I diabetes, or insulin-dependent diabetes mellitus, generally starts during childhood and occurs because the body produces little or no insulin. Victims need insulin injections daily.

- Type II diabetes, or non-insulin dependent diabetes mellitus, generally starts later in life. The body does not produce enough insulin or the cells do not respond to the insulin that is produced. It is usually controlled by diet, exercise, and/or medication.

- Severe hyperglycemia occurs gradually and is the result of too little insulin and too much blood sugar; it often results from infection, failure of the victim to take pre-scribed insulin, eating too much food that contains too much sugar, or stress.

- Hypoglycemia occurs rapidly and is the result of too much insulin and too little sugar; it often results when

the victim takes too much insulin, does not eat enough food, or exercises strenuously.

- A hypoglycemic victim may appear intoxicated; never automatically assume someone is drunk without ruling out hypoglycemia or hyperglycemia.

- A hypoglycemic victim may be hostile or belligerent; never make assumptions about the causes of a victim's behavior without ruling out hypoglycemia.

- Extreme hyperglycemia (DKA) causes flushed, warm, dry skin; sunken eyes; a fruity or acetone odor on the breath; extreme thirst; and lack of appetite. Hypoglycemia, on the other hand, causes pale, moist skin; dilated pupils; no unusual odor on the breath; lack of thirst; and extreme hunger.

- Both hyperglycemia and hypoglycemia represent grave, life-threatening emergencies; when in doubt, give sugar.

Key Terms

Make sure you understand the following key terms:

insulin
glucose
Type I diabetes
Type II diabetes
gestational diabetes
hyperglycemia
hypoglycemia

Critical Thinking Exercise

You are out on the bike trail when you come across a group of bikers assisting a male patient in his mid-20s sitting next to the trail. The patient is alert, but confused. He is breathing at 18 breaths per minute with good chest rise. His skin is extremely pale, cool, and clammy. His radial pulse is 124 per minute. He is unable to answer any of your questions appropriately when you attempt to gather a chief complaint and history. During your assessment, you do not note any injuries; however, you discover a medical alert tag that has inscribed "diabetic" on the back.

1. What condition do you suspect the patient is experiencing?

2. What specific signs and symptoms would lead you to that suspicion?

3. What first aid would you provide to the patient?

Chapter 18 Self-Test

Student: _____   Date: _____

Course: _____   Section #: _____

Part 1   True/False

If you believe the statement is true, circle the T. If you believe the statement is false, circle the F.

(T) F   **1.** There are two basic types of diabetes: insulin-dependent diabetes and non-insulin dependent diabetes.

(T) F   **2.** Hyperglycemia is a condition of too little insulin and too much blood sugar in the body.

T **(F)**   **3.** The hypoglycemic victim has intense abdominal pain and a rapid, weak pulse.

(T) F   **4.** The hypoglycemic victim appears extremely weak and has profuse sweating.

(T) F   **5.** If a diabetic has taken insulin but has not eaten, he or she may become hypoglycemic.

(T) F   **6.** If in doubt about whether a victim is hypoglycemic or hyperglycemic, give sugar.

Part 2   Multiple Choice

For each item, circle the correct answer or the phrase that best completes the statement.

1. A fruity odor on the breath is often a characteristic of
   a. stroke
   b. hypoglycemia
   c. severe hyperglycemia
   d. an ulcer

2. Which symptom is the characteristic clue of severe hyperglycemia?
   a. bluish lips
   b. moist, clammy skin
   c. involuntary muscular twitching
   d. fruity, sweet breath odor

3. The onset of a hyperglycemic emergency generally occurs
   a. suddenly, in 5 to 20 minutes
   b. in 1 to 2 hours
   c. in 12 to 48 hours
   d. gradually, over a period of days

4. The major first aid care for a victim who is experiencing an acute and severe hyperglycemic emergency is to
   a. monitor vital signs and rule out other possible emergencies
   b. administer insulin
   c. give a glass of orange juice
   d. try to keep the victim awake

5. A diabetic who exhibits rapid, bounding pulse; cool, clammy skin; and tremors probably is
   a. hypoglycemic
   b. hyperglycemic
   c. having a heart attack
   d. hyperventilating

6. If you cannot distinguish between hypoglycemia or hyperglycemia, you should
   a. do nothing—the wrong treatment can be deadly
   b. treat for shock and activate the EMS system
   c. give a shot of insulin or put an insulin tablet in the mouth
   d. help the victim take some kind of sugar

7. Which of the following is *not* true of severe hyperglycemia?
   a. it is the result of too little insulin or too much sugar
   b. it occurs gradually, usually over several days
   c. it is a less serious condition than hypoglycemia
   d. it can be caused by excessive exercise

8. Which of the following is *not* true of hypoglycemia?
   a. it may be caused by eating too much food
   b. it should always be treated by giving sugar
   c. it can be caused by excessive exercise
   d. it always requires immediate transport

9. Insulin
   a. absorbs excess sugar that has been eaten
   b. converts sugar into glucose in the digestive tract
   c. permits sugar to pass from the blood into body cells
   d. all of the above

10. An excess of insulin causes
    a. hyperglycemia
    b. diabetic shock
    c. insulin coma
    d. hypoglycemia

Part 3 Matching

Match the condition on the right with the description on the left.

Description

1. _A_ Too little insulin and too much blood sugar
2. _B_ A dire medical emergency
3. _B_ Hunger, headache, and muscle weakness
4. _A_ Gradual onset
5. _B_ Result of excessive exercise
6. _A_ High blood sugar
7. _B_ Rapid onset
8. _A_ Result of eating too much food that contains sugar
9. _B_ Pale, moist skin
10. _____ Labored respirations and an acetone odor on the breath
11. _B_ Need for sugar
12. _A_ Red, dry, warm skin
13. _B_ Low blood sugar

Condition

A. Hyperglycemic emergency
B. Hypoglycemia

Part 4 What Would You Do If?

1. In response to a frantic call for help from her husband, you find a middle-aged woman unconscious on her bedroom floor. The husband tells you that she has not been very responsive since the previous day and that she complained of abdominal pain. You find that she has flushed, warm, dry skin, an acetone breath odor, and a rapid, weak pulse.

2. You respond to a call of a neighbor and find a 12-year-old child who appears extremely weak. Her skin is pale and moist, she feels faint, has a headache, and is having trouble focusing her eyes. The only other person at home is her brother, who tells you that several hours ago she was fine—she had run some foot races and had not yet eaten today.

19

Acute Abdominal Distress and Related Emergencies

Learning Objectives

When you have mastered the material in this chapter, you will be able to

1 Describe the special assessment procedures used for a victim of abdominal distress

2 List the signs and symptoms of abdominal distress

3 Describe and demonstrate general first aid care for acute abdominal distress

4 List the signs and symptoms of ruptured esophageal varices

5 Describe and demonstrate the first aid care of a victim with ruptured esophageal varices

6 List the signs and symptoms of ruptured abdominal aortic aneurysm

7 Describe and demonstrate the first aid care of a victim with ruptured abdominal aortic aneurysm

John Simons was just arriving home from a company Christmas party when his neighbor ran out to the driveway. "Quick!" she cried. "Burt is inside, and he's throwing up. There's blood everywhere!"

John followed his neighbor inside to find Burt, a middle-aged man known for his heavy drinking, propping himself against the kitchen sink. He had vomited profuse amounts of bright red blood. Burt was starting to have breathing problems; he was pale, but had no pain in the stomach. The signs and symptoms, coupled with Burt's drinking history, led John to suspect ruptured esophageal varices—and he knew that seconds counted.

John called 9-1-1 and talked to a dispatcher while he positioned Burt on the floor on his left side, his face pointed downward to let the blood drain out. Burt continued to vomit blood, and John continued to maintain an open airway by letting blood and saliva drain out until paramedics arrived.

Acute abdominal distress features pain that may stem from the cardiac, gastrointestinal, genitourinary, reproductive, or other systems—or even pain that may be referred from elsewhere. According to medical reference guides, there are approximately 100 different causes of abdominal pain. In first aid, your job is generally not to identify the cause of the pain, but to give appropriate first aid care and see that the victim is taken to a medical facility for further assessment and treatment.

Abdominal distress in every victim should be considered life threatening until proven otherwise. Abdominal pain should be considered especially serious if the pain is associated with fainting, or an extremely ill appearance.

This chapter outlines appropriate assessment techniques and provides general guidelines for care regardless of the cause of the abdominal pain. It also discusses several specific conditions that are dire medical emergencies requiring rapid emergency medical attention.

19.1 Assessment

> Learning Objective **1** Describe the special assessment procedures used for a victim of abdominal distress.

Abdominal distress can be caused by a wide range of conditions, from mild to life-threatening; diagnosis must be confirmed by a physician using medical equipment. The goal of first aid is to stabilize the victim and get medical help. First aid for abdominal distress is generally the same, regardless of the cause.

In assessing a victim with acute abdominal distress, your number-one priority should be to look for signs of shock—rapid, thready pulse; restlessness; cold, clammy skin; and falling blood pressure. Irritation of the thin membrane that lines the abdomen is called **peritonitis**; in addition to causing shock, it is a grave, life-threatening condition. Shock is also common with internal bleeding or diarrhea, both of which cause substantial fluid loss.

The **abdomen** is the entire area between the nipples and the groin. For ease in assessment, the abdomen is divided into four **quadrants**, or sections (see Figure 19-1). Pain above the navel is said to be in the upper right or upper left quadrant; pain below the navel is considered in the lower right or lower left quadrant. The location, direction, and characteristics of abdominal pain are important indicators that you should note when activating the EMS system; use the quadrant name to describe where the pain occurs.

Because the abdomen may be very tender, the victim will be guarded (see Figure 19-2), and because using even slight pressure to examine the abdomen with your fingertips can aggravate existing pain, follow these general assessment guidelines:

- Determine whether the victim is restless or quiet, and whether movement causes pain.

- Look to see whether the abdomen is bloated (distended).

- Confirm the abnormal contour with the victim.

- Feel the abdomen very gently to determine whether it is tense or soft (see Figure 19-3) and whether any masses are present; never press on a pulsating abdominal mass. If you know that a specific quadrant is causing the pain or the majority of the pain, examine that quadrant last.

- Determine whether the abdomen is tender when touched and whether the victim can relax the abdominal wall upon request. Note any abdominal guarding.

- Determine the location and quadrant of the pain.

Do not waste time with extensive examination of the abdomen—it can worsen the pain and aggravate the medical condition that causes it.

Note: If the victim is a child, suspect the need for surgery if there is tenderness or guarding when you try to examine the abdomen.

PROGRESS CHECK

1. For assessment purposes, the abdomen is divided into four _____ . *(sections/quadrants/areas)*

2. In assessing a victim with abdominal distress, your number-one priority is to look for signs of _____ . *(appendicitis/internal bleeding/shock)*

3. If you know what section of the abdomen is causing pain, feel that section _____ . *(first/last/gently)*

---

peritonitis Inflammation of the lining of the abdomen

abdomen The area of the body between the nipples and the groin

quadrants Sections; the abdomen is divided into four quadrants

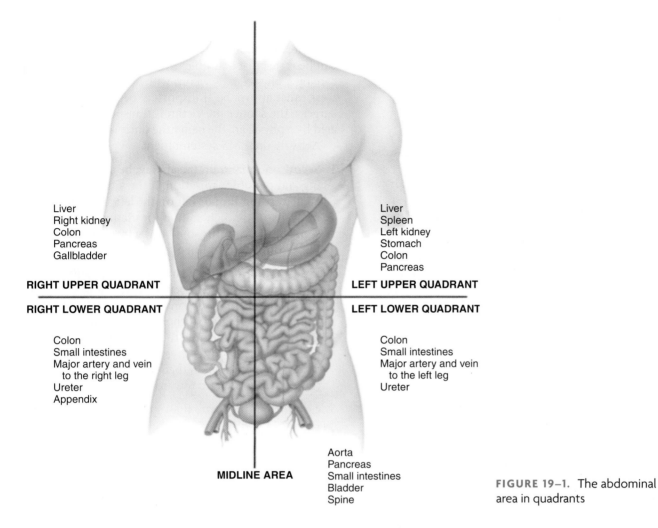

Liver
Right kidney
Colon
Pancreas
Gallbladder

Liver
Spleen
Left kidney
Stomach
Colon
Pancreas

RIGHT UPPER QUADRANT

LEFT UPPER QUADRANT

RIGHT LOWER QUADRANT

LEFT LOWER QUADRANT

Colon
Small intestines
Major artery and vein
  to the right leg
Ureter
Appendix

Colon
Small intestines
Major artery and vein
  to the left leg
Ureter

MIDLINE AREA

Aorta
Pancreas
Small intestines
Bladder
Spine

FIGURE 19–1. The abdominal area in quadrants

FIGURE 19–2. Typical guarded position for victim with acute abdominal distress

FIGURE 19–3. Gently determine if the abdomen is tense or soft.

19.2 Signs and Symptoms

> Learning Objective 2 List the signs and
> symptoms of abdominal distress.

Any severe abdominal pain should be considered an
emergency.

A victim with an acute abdomen appears very ill;
general signs and symptoms of acute abdominal distress
include:

- Abdominal pain (local or widespread)

- Cramplike pain that occurs in waves (**colicky pain**)

- Local or widespread abdominal tenderness

- Anxiety and reluctance to move

- Rapid, shallow breathing

- Rapid pulse

- Nausea and/or vomiting

- Low blood pressure

- Tense, often bloated abdomen

- Signs of shock

- Signs of internal bleeding: vomiting blood (bright
  red or the consistency of coffee-grounds) or passing
  blood in the stool (bright red or tarry black)

A victim with acute abdominal distress often lies on his
or her side with knees drawn up toward the abdomen.

> ### PROGRESS CHECK
>
> 1. Any severe abdominal pain should be
>   considered _____ . *(after the primary
>   survey/an emergency/a treatment priority)*
>
> 2. A victim of abdominal distress usually appears
>   very _____ . *(anxious/fatigued/ill)*
>
> 3. Colicky pain is a cramplike pain that occurs in
>   _____ . *(waves/infants/liver disease
>   victims)*
>
> 4. A victim of acute abdominal distress often
>   positions himself or herself on the
>   _____ . *(back/stomach/side)*

19.3 First Aid Care

> Learning Objective 3 Describe and
> demonstrate general first aid care for acute
> abdominal distress.

The goals of first aid care for acute abdominal distress are
to prevent any possible life-threatening complications
(such as hemorrhage or shock), to make the victim comfortable, and to activate the EMS system so the victim
can be transported as quickly as possible for diagnostic
care by a physician. A victim with acute abdominal distress must always be transported, because many need
surgery; the sooner the victim is transported and evaluated by a physician, the better the outcome.

Activate the EMS system; then:

1. Secure and maintain the airway; be alert for vomiting and possible aspiration. If the victim is nauseated, position him or her on the left side if it does
   not cause too much pain; if the victim vomits, save
   some of the vomitus so it can be transported with
   the victim and examined at the hospital.

2. Position the victim as comfortably as possible, and
   take steps to prevent shock. If there are signs of
   shock, place the victim on his or her back with the
   legs slightly elevated. If there are no signs of shock,
   let the victim determine the most comfortable
   position unless it interferes with first aid care. Most
   victims prefer to lie on their sides or backs with
   their knees drawn up toward the abdomen.

3. Comfort and reassure the victim (see Figure 19-4).

4. *Never give anything by mouth, and never allow the
   victim to eat or drink anything.* Never give the
   victim medications of any kind, and do not let
   the victim take medications on his or her own.
   Never give the victim an enema.

5. Record signs and symptoms, including the victim's
   description of the condition, and continue to monitor until emergency help arrives.

Figure 19-5 on page 318 illustrates several causes of
acute abdominal distress.

> ### PROGRESS CHECK
>
> 1. A goal of first aid care for acute abdominal
>   distress is to _____ . *(prevent
>   shock/predict the need for surgery/prevent
>   vomiting)*
>
> 2. Let the victim choose the most comfortable
>   position unless there are signs of
>   _____ . *(internal bleeding/
>   appendicitis/shock)*
>
> 3. If the victim is nauseated, position the victim
>   on _____ . *(the back/the left side/
>   the stomach)*

colicky pain Cramplike pain that occurs in waves

FIGURE 19–4. Reassure and monitor the victim of abdominal distress while waiting for emergency personnel to arrive.

Nausea, vomiting, and diarrhea may occur with acute abdominal distress, but they may also occur on their own—often as the result of a stomach or intestinal virus. In such a case, the nausea, vomiting, and diarrhea should clear up within a few days.

Persistent nausea and vomiting generally indicate a more serious problem (such as appendicitis or a gallstone that is blocking a bile duct), and you should seek immediate medical help. Even though nausea, vomiting, and diarrhea are not persistent and may not be signs or symptoms of a more serious problem, it's important to offer care: A victim can become seriously dehydrated if vomiting or diarrhea continue longer than several days. Some signs and symptoms of dehydration include dry, cracked lips; eyes that appear "sunken"; dry, sallow skin; extreme thirst; and dizziness or fainting when standing. Children or the elderly may become dehydrated more quickly.

Nausea and Vomiting

In addition to being caused by a virus, nausea and vomiting may also occur if a victim has had too much alcohol to drink, has motion or altitude sickness, or is extremely emotionally distressed.

To care for a victim of nausea or vomiting:

1. Encourage the victim to lie down on his or her side to help facilitate drainage and prevent breathing the vomit into the lungs in case the victim is unable to reach the bathroom.

2. If you are certain the victim is not suffering from an acute illness that will require medical attention, give him or her small amounts of clear liquids—liquids other than alcohol that do not contain caffeine. Water, clear broth, cranberry juice, apple juice, sports drinks, or flat soda can all be used.

3. If the victim is able to keep the clear liquid down for several hours, offer small amounts of carbohydrates, such as cereal, bread, rice, and pasta.

4. Do not give the victim meat or dairy products for at least 48 hours after the vomiting stops.

5. Don't allow the victim to eat regular solid foods until he or she is able to keep down fluids and carbohydrates for at least 48 hours and until a normal sensation of hunger returns.

A victim who is suffering from motion sickness should move to the middle section of the car, bus, train, boat, or plane and either close his or her eyes or focus on the distant horizon. A victim of motion sickness should not read while in a moving vehicle, should eat only light amounts of food, and should avoid looking to the side.

Regardless of the cause of vomiting, seek immediate medical attention if:

■ The victim has had a recent head injury.

■ The victim has severe projectile vomiting (the vomit shoots out of the mouth with force and in large quantity).

■ There is blood, brown grainy material, or black tarry material in the vomit.

■ The victim cannot stand without fainting or shows other signs and symptoms of dehydration.

■ The abdominal pain is constant instead of occurring just before and during vomiting.

■ The victim continues to vomit and cannot keep clear fluids down for more than 24 hours.

Diarrhea

Diarrhea is the passage of loose, watery, or unformed stools more than four times a day. The most common cause of diarrhea is an infection—bacterial, viral, or parasitic—or food poisoning. It's generally best to let diarrhea run its course because it is the body's mechanism for flushing bacteria, viruses, parasites, or contaminated food out of the body. However, dehydration can occur if the victim is not able to drink enough to replace the lost fluids. Again, some signs and symptoms of dehydration include dry, cracked lips; eyes that appear "sunken"; dry, sallow skin; extreme thirst; and dizziness or fainting when standing. As with vomiting, children and the elderly generally become dehydrated more quickly.

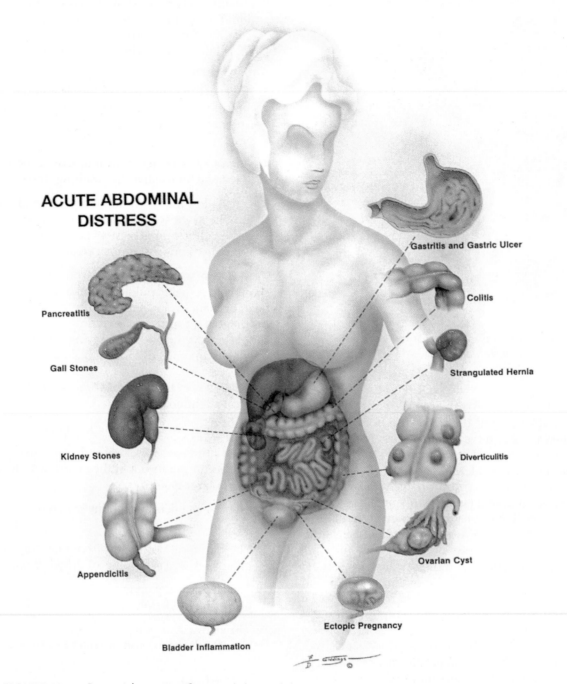

ACUTE ABDOMINAL DISTRESS

Gastritis and Gastric Ulcer

Colitis

Strangulated Hernia

Diverticulitis

Ovarian Cyst

Ectopic Pregnancy

Bladder Inflammation

Appendicitis

Kidney Stones

Gall Stones

Pancreatitis

FIGURE 19–5. Potential sources of acute abdominal distress

To care for a victim of diarrhea who is not exhibiting signs or symptoms of a potentially serious abdominal condition:

1. The single most important care for a victim of diarrhea is to have the victim drink at least 8 to 10 glasses of clear fluid per day. Water is best; you can also use clear broth, cranberry juice, apple juice, sports drinks, or flat soda. Do not give the victim alcohol or drinks containing caffeine; these increase dehydration.

2. Once the victim can tolerate clear fluids, give mild foods, such as gelatin and soup.

3. As the victim is able to tolerate mild foods, use the BRAT diet—bananas, rice, applesauce, and toast. Do not give the victim meat or dairy products until at least 48 hours after the last loose or watery stool.

As mentioned, it's best to let diarrhea run its course unless a victim becomes dehydrated. However, if a victim is in a situation where he or she must control his or her stools, you can offer over-the-counter medications that control diarrhea by tightening up the bowel. These include medications such as Kaopectate II, Pepto Diarrhea Control, Imodium A-D, or Maalox Anti-Diarrheal Caplets. Products containing bismuth (such as Pepto-Bismol and related products) should not be given to people who have aspirin sensitivity; also be aware that they may turn the tongue and/or the stools black.

Regardless of the cause of diarrhea, seek immediate medical attention if:

- The stool contains blood, which can look sticky and black (remember that bismuth products, such as Pepto-Bismol, can temporarily turn the stool black).

- The stool contains mucus.

- The victim cannot stand without fainting or shows other signs or symptoms of dehydration.

- The victim has constant, severe abdominal pain.

- The victim has a fever.

- The diarrhea does not improve within 24 hours.

19.4 Special Considerations

Ruptured Esophageal Varices

Esophageal varices are bulging, engorged, and weakened blood vessels lining the wall of the lower one-third of the esophagus. Varices can potentially develop in anyone, but they are most common in certain types of victims:

- Heavy alcohol drinkers

- Victims of liver disease (such as cirrhosis or hepatitis)

- Victims with chronic liver dysfunction

- Victims with an enlarged liver

- Victims of jaundice

Varices usually lead to painless gastrointestinal bleeding. When one or more of these varices rupture, bleeding is profuse and severe and can be fatal within minutes unless the victim has prompt treatment.

SIGNS AND SYMPTOMS

Learning Objective 4 List the signs and symptoms of ruptured esophageal varices.

Ruptured esophageal varices cause the following signs and symptoms:

- Vomiting of profuse amounts of bright red blood

- Blood welling up in the back of the throat, with or without vomiting

- Absence of pain or tenderness in the stomach

- Rapid pulse (usually more than 120 beats per minute)

- Respiratory distress

- Paleness (**pallor**)

Because esophageal varices are most common among victims with liver disease, additional signs and symptoms of ruptured varices may include those of liver disease—jaundice, an enlarged liver, or dilated veins just below the skin's surface.

FIRST AID CARE

Learning Objective 5 Describe and demonstrate the first aid care of a victim with ruptured esophageal varices.

The victim of ruptured esophageal varices needs rapid blood replacement and surgical procedures aimed at stopping the bleeding. First aid priorities are to activate the EMS system *immediately*, secure and maintain the airway, prevent the victim from inhaling blood, and treat or prevent shock.

Activate the EMS system, explaining the need for urgency; then:

1. Immediately secure an open airway.

2. Position the victim on his or her left side with the face pointed downward to allow drainage of blood and saliva. Maintaining a clear airway is critical to the victim's survival.

3. Treat for shock.

Abdominal Aortic Aneurysm

Learning Objective 6 List the signs and symptoms of ruptured abdominal aortic aneurysm.

An **abdominal aortic aneurysm** occurs when the wall of the aorta in the abdomen weakens, dilates, and eventually ruptures. One of the most lethal conditions that causes abdominal pain, it is most common in those with atherosclerosis. It is estimated that approximately 20 percent of all men over the age of 50 have abdominal aortic aneurysms.

---

esophageal varices Bulging, engorged, weakened blood vessels in the lining of the wall of the lower one-third of the esophagus

pallor Paleness

abdominal aortic aneurysm A section of the wall of the aorta in the abdomen that weakens, dilates, and eventually ruptures

SIGNS AND SYMPTOMS

The pain from a ruptured abdominal aortic aneurysm is very sudden in onset. Signs and symptoms include:

- Sudden, severe, constant pain in the abdomen or back; the pain tends to radiate to the lower back, flank, or pelvis

- Possible nausea and vomiting

- Mottled abdominal skin

- Pale legs

- Decreased or absent pulses in the groin (femoral) and foot (pedal)

If the abdomen is soft, you will be able to see a pulsating abdominal mass; if the aneurysm has burst, the abdomen will likely be hard and rigid.

FIRST AID CARE

Learning Objective **7** Describe and demonstrate the first aid care of a victim with ruptured abdominal aortic aneurysm.

Activate the EMS system without delay, explaining the need for great urgency; then:

1. Examine the abdomen very gently, if at all; pressure or firm palpation can aggravate the

emergency and cause further dissection (bursting) of the artery.

2. Treat the victim for shock and monitor vital signs until emergency personnel arrive.

PROGRESS CHECK

1. Esophageal varices are bulging, engorged _____ in the lower esophagus. *(cysts/blood vessels/ulcerated sores)*

2. Esophageal varices are most common among heavy drinkers or people with _____ . *(liver disease/heart disease/diverticulitis)*

3. The key sign of ruptured esophageal varices is vomiting of _____ blood. *(black/tarry/bright red)*

4. The first priority in treating a victim of ruptured esophageal varices is to _____ . *(maintain the airway/prevent shock/relieve pain)*

5. An abdominal aortic aneurysm that _____ represents a dire emergency. *(increases in size/ruptures/blocks the intestine)*

6. The goal in treating ruptured abdominal aortic aneurysm is to _____ . *(maintain an airway/prevent shock/relieve pain)*

Summary

- It is extremely difficult to determine which of the more than 100 possible causes of abdominal pain may be present in a given situation, so your primary goal is first aid care, not assessment.

- The special assessment procedure for acute abdominal distress is to proceed gently, determining as much as possible by sight. If you know which quadrant is the site of the victim's distress, feel that one last.

- Any severe abdominal pain should be considered an emergency. Any abdominal pain that lasts more than 6 hours, regardless of intensity, should be considered an emergency.

- The goals of first aid care for acute abdominal distress are to prevent any possible life-threatening complications (such as shock), make the victim comfortable, and arrange for transport as soon as possible.

- Unless there are signs of shock, let the victim determine the position that is most comfortable—usually on the

side or back with knees drawn up toward the abdomen. If there are signs of shock, place the victim on his or her back with legs elevated.

- When bulging, engorged, and weakened blood vessels in the esophagus rupture, the victim will vomit profuse amounts of bright red blood; your primary goal is to secure and maintain the airway and arrange for emergency transportation.

- When an abdominal aortic aneurysm ruptures, your primary goal is to prevent shock and to arrange for rapid transport.

- In cases of nausea, vomiting, or diarrhea that are caused by simple viral infections or food poisoning, you should provide supportive care to the victim and generally do not need to seek medical attention unless the victim becomes dehydrated, there is blood in the vomit or stool, or the victim is in constant abdominal pain.

Key Terms

Make sure you understand the following key terms:

peritonitis
abdomen
quadrants
colicky pain
esophageal varices
pallor
abdominal aortic aneurysm

Critical Thinking Exercise

A group of students is playing a game of pick-up basketball on an outdoor court by your college dorm. Suddenly the noise of the game stills, and it is very quiet. Curious as to the reason for the silence, you look out the window that faces the basketball court and see the players crowded around a young man who is lying on his side and holding his abdomen. His knees are in a bent position, and his face shows an expression of intense pain. You quickly leave your room and dash to the court.

1. What is the first question you would ask the victim and the bystanders?

2. What signs and symptoms would you look for to identify abdominal distress?

3. Would you direct someone to call an ambulance?

4. What first aid would you give the victim, and why?

Chapter 19 Self-Test

Student: _____ Date: _____

Course: _____ Section #: _____

Part 1 True/False

If you believe the statement is true, circle the T. If you believe the statement is false, circle the F.

T F **1.** In assessing a victim with acute abdominal distress, your number-one priority should be to assess pain.

T F **2.** The blood vomited with ruptured esophageal varices is the consistency of coffee grounds.

T F **3.** A victim with acute abdomen rarely appears ill.

T F **4.** There is usually absence of pain or tenderness in the stomach with ruptured esophageal varices.

T F **5.** If you know that the pain is originating in a certain quadrant, feel that area first.

T F **6.** Adequate assessment of an acute abdomen requires firm and steady palpation.

T F **7.** You should never give a victim of acute abdominal distress anything by mouth.

T F **8.** Severe abdominal pain should be considered an emergency.

T F **9.** The primary goal of first aid for acute abdominal distress is to make a diagnosis.

T F **10.** One primary goal in caring for a ruptured abdominal aortic aneurysm is to prevent shock.

Part 2 Multiple Choice

For each item, circle the correct answer or the phrase that best completes the statement.

1. A victim lying on one side with knees drawn up; with rapid, shallow breathing; with a rapid pulse; and who is quiet, anxious, and reluctant to move is likely to be suffering from

  a. stroke
  b. insulin shock
  c. acute abdominal distress
  d. myocardial infarction

2. Victims suffering from acute abdominal distress should be allowed to

  a. determine the most comfortable position
  b. drink liquids
  c. take personal medication
  d. all of the above

3. Pain from acute abdominal distress is often

  a. colicky
  b. shifting

  c. radiating to the shoulder or back
  d. all of the above

4. Which of the following is not appropriate first aid care for ruptured esophageal varices?

  a. position the victim to allow drainage from the mouth and throat
  b. treat the victim for shock
  c. put the victim in a supine position
  d. activate the EMS system without delay

5. Any abdominal pain that lasts longer than _____ should be considered an emergency.

  a. 30 minutes
  b. 6 hours
  c. 2 hours
  d. 24 hours

1. A victim you are assisting complains of lower abdominal pain on the right side that has increased in intensity for the last 6 hours. The victim is nauseated and nervous.

2. You are at a social gathering when a middle-aged man starts vomiting large amounts of bright red blood. The man's wife tells you that he has a history of a drinking problem. He has pale skin and a rapid and weak pulse and is experiencing some respiratory distress.

20

Seizures, Dizziness, and Fainting

When you have mastered the material in this chapter, you will be able to

1 Explain the physiology of seizures

2 List the various causes of seizures

3 List the types of seizures

4 List the signs and symptoms of generalized tonic-clonic (grand mal) seizures

5 Define status epilepticus

6 Describe assessment priorities for a seizure victim

7 Describe and demonstrate first aid care for a victim of a seizure

8 Explain the types of dizziness

9 Describe and demonstrate first aid care for a victim of fainting

On the Scene

Approaching a city transit stop on a windy day in March, Steve Broadbent saw a crowd of people gathered around a man on the ground. Walking closer, Steve saw that the man appeared to be in his late twenties and was suffering a seizure.

Steve asked a bystander to call 9-1-1 from a nearby pay phone, then asked other people in the crowd to go back to the bus loading area, hoping to protect the man's privacy. Steve quickly determined that the man had an open airway and was breathing, then removed the man's eyeglasses and loosened the first few buttons of his shirt. Steve then covered the man with his own coat to help keep him warm. A quick scan of the area showed that there were no dangerous objects in reach.

Steve continued to monitor the victim; just before emergency personnel arrived, the seizure stopped. Because it was the victim's first seizure, he was transported to the hospital for evaluation.

eurological emergencies involving a disturbance in the chemical or electrical activity of the brain are generally more frightening than life threatening. With quick recognition of the condition and vigorous airway management to prevent oxygen deprivation, you can generally prevent a major medical emergency.

Some people suffer seizures as a normal occurrence and require little or even no care. A victim who passes from one seizure to another without first regaining consciousness, however, *is* experiencing a life-threatening medical emergency.

This chapter briefly explains the physiology of seizures, explains the causes and types of seizures, outlines general first aid care for seizures, and gives guidelines for managing dizziness and fainting.

20.1 Causes and Types of Seizures

Learning Objective **1** Explain the physiology of seizures.

A **seizure** is an involuntary, sudden change in sensation, behavior, muscle activity, or level of consciousness that results from irritation or overactivity of brain cells (see Figure 20-1). In general, seizures are caused by an abnormal discharge of electrical energy in the brain; they are sudden in onset, usually occurring after only very brief warning, if any. A convulsion is the jerky muscle activity often seen in seizures. A seizure can occur without convulsions.

FIGURE 20–1. Epilepsy is one of the most common causes of seizures.

Any condition that affects the structural cells of the brain or alters its chemical metabolic balance may trigger seizures.

Causes of Seizures

Learning Objective **2** List the various causes of seizures.

A common cause of seizures is **epilepsy**, a chronic brain disorder characterized by recurrent seizures not caused by acute problems (such as head trauma, fever, or hypoglycemia). Epilepsy is a general term for many types of seizure disorders.

Seizures can also occur in anyone as a result of an acute injury to the brain or a more long-lasting condition involving the brain. Other causes include the following (see Figure 20-2):

- Acute head injury or stroke
- Low oxygen levels in the brain
- Drugs or alcohol
- Derangements in the body's chemistry
- Trauma or other injury to the brain that causes scar formation
- Reduced blood flow to the brain
- Inflammation of the brain, usually caused by bacterial, viral, or parasitic infection
- Fever, usually in children 6 months to 3 years old
- Degeneration of the central nervous system, such as from multiple sclerosis
- Congenital brain defects
- Brain tumor
- Hypoglycemia or hyperglycemia
- Severe burns
- Endocrine changes during pregnancy or menstruation

Some seizures occur spontaneously with no known cause.

seizure An involuntary, sudden change in sensation, behavior, muscle activity, or level of consciousness that results from irritation or overactivity of brain cells

epilepsy A chronic brain disorder characterized by recurrent seizures not caused by acute problems, with or without loss of consciousness

---

Causes of Seizures

Seizures can occur in anyone as a result of an acute injury to the brain, or a more long-lasting condition involving the brain.

- **Toxic**—Seizures can occur as a direct consequence of allergic reactions to drugs, using drugs or other chemicals, or withdrawal from addicting substances, especially alcohol.

- **Metabolic**—Derangements in the body's chemistry may be accompanied by a seizure.

- **Trauma**—A previous injury to the brain could result in formation of a scar, which can serve as a seizure focus.

- **Vascular**—Any condition that reduces blood flow to the brain can cause seizures.

- **Infection**—Inflammation of the brain caused by bacterial, viral, or parasitic infection.

- **Febrile**—Most commonly seen in children ages 6 months to 3 years, these seizures occur in conjunction with a fever. Fever is the most common cause of seizures in children under the age of 5; most often it is the rapid rise

in temperature, and not the degree of the fever itself, that causes the seizure.

- **Idiopathic**—By definition, this type of seizure arises spontaneously from an unknown cause.

- **Degenerative**—Disorders causing degeneration of the central nervous system, including multiple sclerosis and certain dementias, can cause seizures.

- **Congenital defects of the brain**—Particularly in infants and young children.

- **Brain tumor**—Uncommon as a cause of seizures in children. Seizures—especially local seizures—can be a first sign of brain tumor in adults.

- **Other**—Other causes of seizures include hypertension, eclampsia, severe burns, endocrine changes during pregnancy and menstruation, spurts in growth, childhood illnesses, extreme variations in sleep habits (including sleep deprivation), and swelling of brain tissue (regardless of cause).

FIGURE 20–2. The various causes of seizures (Adapted in part from Mayo Clinic Health Letter, November 1988, with permission of Mayo Foundation for Medical Education and Research, Rochester, Minnesota.)

Types of Seizures

> Learning Objective **3** List the types of seizures.

> Learning Objective **4** List the signs and symptoms of generalized tonic-clonic (grand mal) seizures.

Table 20-1 on page 328 lists the six general types of seizures and their signs and symptoms.

Status Epilepticus

> Learning Objective **5** Define status epilepticus.

Most seizures stop within 1 to 2 minutes (even though the victim may remain unresponsive for several minutes longer). In contrast, **status epilepticus** is a single seizure that lasts more than 5 minutes *or* a series of seizures that occur without the victim's regaining consciousness between them. *Status epilepticus is a dire medical emergency.* Because of the length of the prolonged or recurrent seizures, the brain is deprived of oxygen. Irreversible brain damage can result, as well as complications of the cardiac, respiratory, and renal systems.

Status epilepticus may result from a worsening of whatever caused the seizures in the first place, or it may

be the result of a new condition. It is often the result when an epilepsy victim does not take his or her medication properly.

PROGRESS CHECK

1. One of the most common causes of seizures is _____ . *(epilepsy/head injury/stroke)*

2. A seizure that causes a sudden cry or moan followed by muscle jerks and frothy saliva is a _____ seizure. *(absence/tonic-clonic/simple partial)*

3. An absence seizure is often mistaken for _____ . *(daydreaming/stroke/mental illness)*

4. Status epilepticus means the seizure has lasted _____ minutes. *(more than 5/10/more than 10)*

5. Status epilepticus represents a dire medical emergency because the brain is deprived of _____ . *(sodium/blood/oxygen)*

---

status epilepticus A severe, prolonged seizure lasting longer than five minutes or a series of seizures that occur without the victim's regaining consciousness between them

TABLE 20–1 **Seizure Symptoms**

Type of Seizure	What Happens	What It Is Often Mistaken For
Generalized tonic-clonic (grand mal)	• Sudden cry or moan • Rigidity • Muscle jerks • Frothy saliva • Shallow breathing • Bluish skin • Usually lasts 2 to 5 minutes; normal breathing then starts again	• Heart attack • Stroke
Absence (petit mal)	• Blank stare • Rapid blinking • Chewing movements • Lasts only a few seconds	• Daydreaming • Inattention • In children, deliberately ignoring adult instructions
Simple partial (jacksonian)	• Jerking in fingers and toes • Victim stays awake, aware • Jerking may progress up hand, arm, then to whole body and becomes a convulsive seizure	• Acting out • Bizarre behavior
Complex partial (psychomotor)	• Starts with blank stare, followed by chewing or other random, repetitive activity • Victim appears dazed • Mumbling • Victim picks at self, may remove clothing • Victim struggles or flails if restrained • Post-seizure confusion	• Drunkenness • Drug intoxication • Mental illness • Indecent exposure • Disorderly conduct • Shoplifting
Myoclonic	• Sudden, brief, massive muscle jerking that can involve part or all of body	• Clumsiness • Poor coordination
Atonic	• Child's legs suddenly collapse, causing child to fall • Lasts less than a minute	• Clumsiness • Lack of walking skills • Normal childhood "stage" • Normal infant movements

generalized tonic-clonic (grand mal) seizure A convulsive seizure characterized by alternating muscle rigidity and jerking, temporarily suspended breathing, and altered mental state

absence (petit mal) seizure A seizure characterized by a blank stare that lasts only a few seconds, most common in children; an absence seizure does not involve convulsions

simple partial (Jacksonian) seizure A simple, partial seizure characterized by jerking in the fingers and toes; the jerking may spread to involve the entire arm or leg, but the victim stays awake and aware. It may progress to a generalized tonic-clonic seizure.

complex partial (psychomotor) seizure A seizure that starts with a blank stare, then progresses into chewing or other random, repetitive activity; the victim seems dazed

myoclonic seizure A seizure characterized by sudden, brief, massive muscle jerks that involve part or all of the body

atonic seizure Also called a "drop attack," a seizure in which the legs of a child suddenly and temporarily collapse

20.2 Assessment and First Aid Care

Most seizures—other than status epilepticus—are self-limiting and last normally 1 to 2 minutes, although the victim may experience residual drowsiness for several hours. Seizures typically stop and start spontaneously; you cannot reduce their duration.

Generalized Tonic-Clonic Seizures

A generalized tonic-clonic seizure, previously known as a *grand mal seizure* (see Figure 20-3), occurs in stages, ranging from the warning phase to a period of recovery, and includes the following:

1. The **aura**, a peculiar "warning" sensation that lasts only a few seconds (it may be visual or auditory hallucinations, a peculiar taste in the mouth, or a painful sensation, for example)

2. The **tonic phase** lasts 15 to 20 seconds; the victim loses consciousness, there is continuous muscular contraction, and the victim stops breathing.

3. The **hypertonic phase** lasts 5 to 15 seconds; there is extreme muscular rigidity.

4. The **tonic-clonic phase** lasts 30 to 60 seconds; muscular rigidity and relaxation alternate rhythmically and in rapid succession, there is frothy saliva, and the victim may lose bowel and bladder control.

5. **Autonomic discharge** lasts for a few seconds; there is hyperventilation, salivation, and rapid heartbeat.

6. During the **postseizure phase**, the victim lapses into a coma.

7. The **postictal phase**, commonly called the recovery phase, usually lasts 5 to 30 minutes, but occasionally several hours; all muscles relax and the victim slowly becomes responsive but remains exhausted.

Assessment Considerations

> Learning Objective 6 Describe assessment priorities for a seizure victim.

Because a victim will rarely remember the seizure, you need to get a history from bystanders unless you witnessed the seizure yourself. Try to find out the following:

- What the seizure was like
- Whether the victim has a history of seizures
- Whether the victim takes medication for seizures
- How the seizure progressed
- Whether the victim has suffered a head injury
- Whether the victim uses drugs or alcohol
- Whether the victim has diabetes mellitus

In performing a physical assessment, pay particular attention to the following:

- Signs of injury to the head, tongue, or elsewhere on the body
- Signs of drug or alcohol abuse (such as alcohol on the breath or needle tracks)
- The victim's mental status
- Fever
- Presence of a Medic Alert tag or other identifying medal or bracelet

First Aid Care for Seizures

> Learning Objective 7 Describe and demonstrate first aid care for a victim of a seizure.

Although seizures are generally not life threatening, anyone who experiences a seizure for the first time should be evaluated by a physician. You should also send for medical help if the seizure lasts longer than 5 minutes; if you are uncertain of the cause; if the victim has no

> **aura** The first phase of a seizure that lasts only a few seconds and involves a peculiar sensation that may be psychic or sensory in nature
>
> **tonic phase** The early stage of a seizure during which the victim loses consciousness, and the body is completely rigid with continuous muscular contraction
>
> **hypertonic phase** The phase in a seizure that signals the end of continuous muscle contractions, characterized by extreme muscle rigidity and hypertension
>
> **tonic-clonic phase** The phase of a seizure characterized by muscular rigidity and relaxation that alternate rhythmically in rapid succession
>
> **autonomic discharge** A stage in a generalized tonic-clonic seizure that lasts for a few seconds and includes hyperventilation, salivation, and rapid heartbeat
>
> **postseizure phase** One of the final phases of a seizure, during which the victim progresses into a coma
>
> **postictal phase** The phase following a seizure, during which all muscles relax and the victim slowly becomes responsive but remains exhausted

STAGES OF GENERALIZED TONIC-CLONIC SEIZURES

A generalized tonic-clonic, or grand mal seizure is a sign of an abnormal release of impulses in the brain. It is a physical, not a psychological, disorder.

1
The victim may have an "aura" or premonition, which is part of the seizure. An aura is often described as an odd or unpleasant sensation that rises from the stomach toward the chest and throat.

For some victims the aura is always the same, such as numbness or motor activity (such as turning of head and eyes, spasm of a limb) or it may consist of a peculiar sound or taste.

2
Loss of consciousness follows the aura. The forced expulsion of air caused by contraction of the skeletal muscles may cause a high-pitched cry sound. The victim may be pale at this point with possible spasms of various muscle groups causing the tongue to be bitten.

3
Cyanosis may accompany the seizure because breathing stops during the phase of prolonged muscle contraction. Within seconds the victim will manifest an arched back and alternating contraction and relaxation of movements in all extremities (clonic convulsive movements). The attack usually lasts from about 30 seconds to 5 minutes. The victim may lose bladder and bowel control.

4
Gradually the toxic-clonic phase (convulsion) subsides. It is followed by a postictal state, characterized by a deep sleep with gradual recovery to a state of transient confusion, fatigue, muscular soreness, and headache.

FIRST AID CARE

- If the victim seems to stop breathing, monitor airway and assist ventilation if necessary. The situation becomes life-threatening if the seizure lasts for longer than 5 minutes or if the victim passes from seizure to seizure without regaining consciousness (status epilepticus). This situation requires transport and medical attention.
- The major requirements of the First Aider are the ABCDs and to protect the victim from hurting herself during a seizure.
- The victim should not be physically restrained in any way unless she is endangering her own welfare.
- Move objects, not the victim.
- Position the victim to allow for drainage and suctioning.
- Loosen tight clothing.
- If status epilepticus occurs or breathing ceases, assist breathing as necessary and transport immediately.
- Keep the victim from being a spectacle.
- Reassure and reorient the victim following the seizure.
- Allow her to rest.
- An ambulance is often called for a generalized tonic-clonic seizure, but if the victim responds normally she may not need transport. If in doubt, always transport to a medical facility.

FIGURE 20–3. Generalized tonic-clonic (grand mal) seizures

history of seizures; if the victim has more than one seizure; if the victim appears to be injured; if the victim has trouble breathing after the seizure; if the victim is a diabetic; or if the victim is an infant, child, or pregnant woman.

The general goal of first aid is to support the victim, prevent injury, and refer the victim to medical care if appropriate.

Activate the EMS system if appropriate; then:

1. Do not move the victim unless he or she is near a dangerous object that cannot be moved. Otherwise, move objects away from the victim (see Figure 20–4). Place padding under the victim's head to prevent injury.

2. Maintain an open airway.

3. Stay calm; if the victim is responsive, reassure him or her; reassure others who are with the victim.

4. Stay with the victim until the seizure has passed; if you need to get help, send someone else.

5. Never try to force anything between the victim's teeth, and never give the victim anything by mouth.

6. Remove or loosen any tight clothing, especially around the neck; remove eyeglasses.

7. Turn the victim on his or her left side with the face pointed downward (see Figure 20-5) so secretions and vomitus can drain quickly out of the mouth and so the tongue will not fall back and block the airway.

8. If the victim stops breathing, open the airway, remove anything that might impair breathing, and provide artificial ventilation.

9. Do not try to restrain the victim unless he or she is in danger from objects that cannot be moved.

10. Keep the victim from becoming a spectacle; ask bystanders to leave.

11. Following the seizure, reassure and reorient the victim; speak slowly and calmly in a normal tone of voice. Allow the victim to rest; help the victim be as comfortable as possible.

First Aid Care for Status Epilepticus

If the victim experiences status epilepticus, *you are faced with a dire medical emergency.* The number-one goal is ventilation. Activate the EMS system immediately; then:

1. Place the victim on the floor or bed, away from other furniture. Do not try to restrain the victim.

2. Clear and maintain the airway; turn the victim's head sideways to prevent aspiration.

3. Administer artificial ventilation as needed; even though it can be extremely difficult to administer artificial ventilation to a seizing person, you must do it—lack of oxygen during seizure activity is the most serious threat to life.

4. Carefully monitor vital signs until emergency personnel arrive.

PROGRESS CHECK

1. An aura may involve a _____ . (hallucination/muscle contraction/coma)

2. The period in which a seizure victim loses consciousness is the _____ phase. (clonic/tonic/hypertonic)

FIGURE 20–4. Move objects away from the seizure victim rather than trying to move the victim.

FIGURE 20–5. Position the seizure victim to allow drainage of saliva and vomit.

3. During the _____ , the victim slowly recovers. *(clonic phase/autonomic discharge/postictal stupor)*

4. During assessment of a seizure victim, pay particular attention to signs of injury to the _____ . *(throat/head/back)*

5. You should activate the EMS system if the victim has more than _____ seizure(s). *(one/two/three)*

6. The primary goal in caring for the victim of status epilepticus is _____ . *(preventing injury/maintaining airway/ maintaining oxygenation)*

20.3 Dizziness and Fainting

Two of the most common medical complaints are dizziness and syncope, or fainting. Actually, dizziness and fainting are not medical conditions at all, but are symptoms that can result from a wide variety of diseases and injuries.

Dizziness

> Learning Objective 8 Explain the types of dizziness.

Most victims are not experiencing true dizziness, or **vertigo.** Instead, they may feel woozy, light-headed, or as though they are in a dream.

True vertigo involves a hallucination of motion—the victim feels as though he or she is spinning around, or, more commonly, that the room is whirling in circles. Some feel they are being pulled to the ground; others feel the room has tilted so much that they can no longer stand up.

SIGNS AND SYMPTOMS

There are two different types of vertigo, and each causes very different signs and symptoms.

Central vertigo, the less common and most serious, signifies a dramatic medical problem involving the central nervous system and causes the following signs and symptoms:

- Dysfunction of the eye muscles
- Unequal pupil size
- Facial droop

Victims of central vertigo do not experience nausea, vomiting, hearing loss, or a whirling sensation.

Labyrinthine vertigo, which is much more common, occurs as a disturbance in the inner ear and causes the following signs and symptoms:

- Nausea
- Vomiting
- Rapid, involuntary twitching of the eyeball
- A whirling sensation
- Pale, moist skin
- Rapid heartbeat

All symptoms of labyrinthine vertigo are made worse when the victim moves; episodes can last for hours and recur over a period of many years.

First Aid Care

1. Reassure the victim; help the victim get in a comfortable position and to move as little as possible.

2. Conduct a thorough assessment to rule out any immediate life-threatening conditions.

3. Encourage the victim to see a physician.

Fainting

Fainting, or **syncope,** is a sudden and brief loss of consciousness that results when the brain is temporarily deprived of adequate oxygen. Some victims feel as though everything is going dark; then they suddenly lose consciousness. A collapse follows that puts the body in a horizontal position, which improves blood circulation to the brain. As a result, the victim rapidly becomes responsive.

Fainting itself is not a disease, but can be a symptom of a wide range of conditions and diseases—most commonly, severe emotion, fright, heat, use of certain drugs, profound pain, standing or sitting too long without moving, low blood sugar, or irregular heart rhythm.

> **vertigo** Dizziness
>
> **central vertigo** The least common type of vertigo (dizziness), which mimics a transient ischemic attack or stroke; victims do not experience nausea, vomiting, hearing loss, or a whirling sensation
>
> **labyrinthine vertigo** The most common kind of dizziness, caused by a disturbance in the inner ear and characterized by nausea, vomiting, and a whirling sensation
>
> **syncope** Fainting

SIGNS AND SYMPTOMS

Some victims have the following warning signs that they are about to faint:

- Nausea
- Light-headedness
- Weakness
- Shakiness
- Deep abdominal pain
- A pounding pain in the head

FIRST AID CARE

> Learning Objective **9** Describe and demonstrate first aid care for a victim of fainting.

If appropriate, activate the EMS system; then:

1. If the victim has not yet fainted, prevent him or her from falling by having the victim sit down (see Figure 20-6) with head between the knees or have the victim lie on the floor with legs elevated 8 to 12 inches.

2. If the victim has already fainted, keep the victim in a supine position; elevate the legs 8 to 12 inches (see Figure 20-7).

3. Monitor for possible vomiting; loosen clothing that might restrict free breathing.

4. Make a rapid assessment for any life-threatening condition that may have caused the fainting; initiate appropriate care.

5. Check for any injuries that may have occurred during the fall; treat appropriately.

6. Do not allow a person who has fainted to sit up immediately. Instead, have the victim sit up slowly and gradually.

7. Help the victim feel better by moving him or her to fresh air or by putting a cool, damp cloth on the face.

PROGRESS CHECK

1. The medical term for dizziness is _____ . (syncope/acidosis/vertigo)

2. The medical term for fainting is _____ . (syncope/acidosis/vertigo)

3. The most serious kind of vertigo, _____ vertigo, causes symptoms like those of a stroke. (central/positional/labyrinthine)

4. _____ vertigo is caused by a disturbance in the inner ear. (Central/Positional/Labyrinthine)

5. Fainting occurs when the _____ is temporarily deprived of oxygen. (heart/brain/liver)

6. You can prevent someone from fainting by placing the head _____ . (at heart level/between the knees/lower than the feet)

FIGURE 20–6. Seat the victim who feels faint. Put the head between the legs.

FIGURE 20–7. Elevate the legs of a victim who has fainted.

Summary

- A seizure is an involuntary, sudden change in sensation that is caused by irritation or overactivity of brain cells; the most common cause of seizure is epilepsy.

- In addition to epilepsy, other causes of seizures are fever, infection, head injury, brain tumor, lack of blood flow to the brain, and derangements in the body's chemistry.

- The type of seizure that involves jerking and frothing at the mouth is only one kind of seizure; others cause apparent daydreaming or erratic behavior similar to that seen with mental illness.

- You cannot lessen the duration of a seizure.

- Anyone who experiences a first-time seizure should be seen in the emergency room; you should also get medical help if the seizure lasts more than 5 minutes in an epileptic victim; if you are uncertain about the cause of the seizure; or if the victim has more than one seizure, appears to be injured, or is an infant, child, diabetic, or pregnant woman.

- To care for a seizing victim, do whatever you can to prevent the victim from injuring himself or herself.

- Status epilepticus is a prolonged seizure or a series of seizures that occur without the victim's regaining consciousness.

- The number-one goal in treating status epilepticus is oxygenation.

- Most victims of dizziness are not experiencing true vertigo, which is a hallucination of motion.

- Fainting is a loss of consciousness that occurs when the brain is temporarily deprived of enough oxygen; if placed in a supine position, the victim almost always rapidly regains consciousness.

Key Terms

Make sure you understand the following key terms:

seizure
epilepsy
status epilepticus
generalized tonic-clonic (grand mal) seizure
absence (petit mal) seizure
simple partial (Jacksonian) seizure
complex partial (psychomotor) seizure
myoclonic seizure
atonic seizure
aura
tonic phase
hypertonic phase
clonic phase
autonomic discharge
postseizure phase
postictal stupor
vertigo
central vertigo
labyrinthine vertigo
syncope

Critical Thinking Exercise

You are at a local restaurant having dinner when suddenly there is a loud commotion a few tables over. You walk over to the area and find a female patient in her later 30's on the ground, having a seizure with convulsive activity.

1. What is your first immediate action?

2. What complete first aid care would you provide for the seizing woman?

3. What history information is important to collect from family members at the scene?

4. What characteristics of the seizure would indicate a serious seizure and the need to call 9-1-1?

20 Chapter 20 Self-Test

Student: _____ Date: _____

Course: _____ Section #. _____

Part 1   True/False

If you believe the statement is true, circle the T. If you believe the statement is false, circle the F.

T **(F)**   **1.** A seizure is a voluntary, sudden change in behavior, sensation, muscular activity, and level of consciousness.

(T) F   **2.** Epilepsy is a chronic brain disorder.

T **(F)**   **3.** Seizures are always life threatening.

(T) F   **4.** Generalized tonic-clonic seizures always produce a loss of consciousness.

T F   **5.** Simple partial seizures always produce a loss of consciousness.

(T) F   **6.** Irreversible brain damage can occur from status epilepticus.

(T) F   **7.** Most seizures are self-limiting and last less than 5 minutes.

(T) F   **8.** In a postictal stupor, the victim falls into a deep sleep.

(T)(F)   **9.** Do not attempt to restrain a seizure victim unless he or she is in immediate danger.

(T) F   **10.** Dizziness and fainting are not medical conditions, but are symptoms.

(T) F   **11.** True vertigo involves a hallucination of motion.

(T) F   **12.** Fainting is a temporary loss of consciousness due to an inadequate supply of oxygen to the brain.

T **(F)**   **13.** True vertigo is an actual disturbance of the victim's sense of balance.

(T) F   **14.** The number-one goal in a status epilepticus emergency is ventilation of the patient.

Part 2   Multiple Choice

For each item, circle the correct answer or the phrase that best completes the statement.

1. A characteristic of absence seizures is

   a. convulsive movements of one part of the body
   b. brief periods where the victim appears to be daydreaming
   c. loss of consciousness
   d. repetition of inappropriate actions

2. Which of the following is *not* a stage of epilepsy?

   a. clonic phase
   b. tonic phase
   c. aura
   d. catatonic phase

3. The most serious threat in status epilepticus is

   a. lack of oxygen due to impaired breathing
   b. fractures
   c. swallowing the tongue
   d. dehydration

4. Status epilepticus in adults is

   a. a dire medical emergency
   b. a single seizure that lasts more than 5 minutes
   c. a series of seizures in an unconscious victim
   d. all of the above

5. Which of the following is *not* a first aid care procedure for seizure?

   a. stay calm and reassure the victim
   b. put a padded object between the victim's teeth
   c. do not attempt to restrain the victim unless the person is in danger
   d. stay with the victim until the seizure has passed

1. You are at a large public gathering and a person suddenly cries out, falls, becomes rigid, and has muscular jerks. He has frothy saliva on the lips and very shallow breathing. In about 5 minutes the symptoms subside, and within the next 30 minutes the symptoms reappear and subside numerous times.

2. At the same gathering, a person complains of dizziness and nausea. She is shaky, has cool skin, and tells you that she feels faint.

21

Childbirth and Related Emergencies

Learning Objectives

When you have mastered the material in this chapter, you will be able to

1 Understand basic reproductive anatomy

2 Describe the recommended first aid kit equipment for childbirth emergencies

3 List the signs and symptoms of miscarriage

4 Describe and demonstrate how to manage a seizure during pregnancy

5 Describe and demonstrate how to care for vaginal bleeding during pregnancy

6 Describe and demonstrate how to care for ectopic pregnancy

7 List the signs and symptoms of preeclampsia/eclampsia

8 Describe and demonstrate how to care for ruptured uterus

9 Explain the situations in which you would *not* try to take a pregnant woman to the hospital for delivery

10 List the signs and symptoms indicating that delivery is imminent

11 Describe how to transport a woman who is in labor to the hospital

12 Describe and demonstrate normal delivery procedures

13 Describe and demonstrate how to care for vaginal bleeding following delivery

14 Describe and demonstrate care of the newborn

15 Describe and demonstrate resuscitation of the newborn

16 Describe and demonstrate how to manage abnormal deliveries

On the Scene

Cynthia Hobbs had just pulled into her driveway after picking her children up from school when her neighbor's 9-year-old daughter ran toward the car. She had come home from school to find her mother curled up on the living room sofa in excruciating pain. Cynthia, a trained First Aider, sent her own children into the house and went to check on 36-year-old Susan Brienholt.

Susan was sitting at the end of the sofa, her arms wrapped around her knees, rocking back and forth as she moaned with pain. The pain had started about an hour earlier, she said; it was sharp and stabbing and localized on the left side. Cynthia convinced Susan to lie flat on the sofa; during a brief assessment, she noticed that Susan's pulse was rapid and that she showed other signs of shock.

Taking a quick history, Cynthia learned that Susan had missed her last two menstrual periods and suspected she was pregnant; she was about to schedule an appointment with the doctor, but had started spotting a day earlier.

Cynthia was convinced Susan had an ectopic pregnancy—a serious medical emergency. Cynthia quickly called for emergency help. She kept Susan on the sofa on her back and elevated her knees; she covered Susan with a blanket to keep her warm and slipped a pillow under her knees to keep her comfortable.

First Aiders are often called on to help pregnant women, and too often a woman is taken to a hospital in great haste because a First Aider is afraid the mother will give birth before reaching the hospital.

Although some babies *are* born at home or in vehicles, there is no need to hurry in most circumstances since the delivery will not occur in most situations for several hours. Childbirth is a normal, natural process—in only a few situations involving complications do victims need to be transported rapidly.

In order to determine whether rapid transport is necessary, you should be familiar with anatomy, the delivery process, signs, symptoms, and first aid care of both normal childbirth and obstetric complications. This chapter provides that information and outlines the care required for both normal birth and childbirth-related emergencies.

21.1 Reproductive Anatomy

Learning Objective **1** Understand basic reproductive anatomy.

The term **fetus** refers to the developing unborn baby. Other terms related to the anatomy and physiology of reproduction include the following (see Figure 21-1):

- *The uterus.* The **uterus**, the organ in which the fetus grows, is responsible for labor and expulsion of the infant. During pregnancy, the walls of the uterus become thin, and its muscle fibers stretch and thicken. The special arrangement of smooth muscle and blood vessels in the uterus allows for great expansion during pregnancy, for forcible contractions during labor and delivery, and for rapid contraction after delivery to constrict the blood vessels and prevent hemorrhage.

- *The birth canal.* The vagina and lower part of the uterus are known as the **birth canal.**

- *The placenta.* The **placenta** is a disk-shaped inner lining attached at one surface to the uterus and at the other to the umbilical cord. Rich in blood vessels, the placenta provides the fetus with nourishment and oxygen from the mother's blood and

fetus The developing unborn baby

uterus The organ in which the baby grows

birth canal The vagina and lower part of the uterus

placenta Structure on the inner lining of the uterus that provides the fetus with nourishment

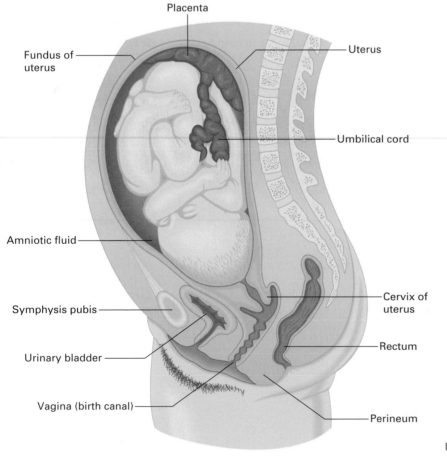

Placenta

Fundus of uterus

Uterus

Umbilical cord

Amniotic fluid

Cervix of uterus

Symphysis pubis

Rectum

Urinary bladder

Vagina (birth canal)

Perineum

FIGURE 21–1. Anatomy of pregnancy

absorbs fetal waste products into the mother's bloodstream. The exchange of nutrients and wastes occurs through a special sievelike mechanism in the placenta; the baby's and mother's blood do not mix. The placenta also produces hormones, such as estrogen and progesterone, that sustain the pregnancy.

At full term, the placenta is about 8 inches wide, 1 inch thick, and weighs about one-sixth of the baby's weight. After the birth, the placenta separates from the uterine wall and is delivered as the afterbirth.

- *The umbilical cord.* The **umbilical cord** is an extension of the placenta through which the fetus receives nourishment while in the uterus. The cord contains one vein and two arteries arranged in a spiral and enclosed in a protective, gelatinlike substance. When the baby is born, the nerveless cord resembles a sturdy rope; it is about 22 inches long and about 1 inch in diameter.

- *The amniotic sac.* Sometimes called the "bag of waters," the **amniotic sac** is filled with the amniotic fluid in which the baby floats; the sac of fluid insulates and protects the baby during pregnancy.

- *The vagina.* Extending from the neck of the uterus to the outside of the body, the **vagina** is the lower part of the birth canal and provides a passage for both menstrual flow and childbirth. The smooth muscle layer of the vagina allows it to stretch gently to accommodate the infant during delivery.

- *The perineum.* The **perineum** is the area of skin and muscle between the vagina and the anus. As the baby's head comes down the birth canal, the perineum bulges significantly—a sign of impending birth. The perineum is sometimes incised during hospital births to prevent tearing, which commonly occurs during emergency delivery.

- *Crowning.* As the head or presenting part of the baby presses against the vagina, the vagina bulges outward—a sign that delivery is imminent. **Crowning** occurs when the baby's head (or other body part) emerges at the vaginal opening.

- *"Bloody show."* During pregnancy, the opening of the **cervix** (neck of the uterus) contains a mucous plug that is discharged during labor. The expulsion of this mucous plug signals the first stage of labor and is known as the **bloody show.** The bloody show appears as pink-tinged mucus in the vaginal discharge as labor begins.

- *Presenting part.* The **presenting part** is the part of the infant that appears first from the birth canal. In a normal birth, it is the head. In some cases

(known as breech births), it may be the buttocks or both legs.

- *Miscarriage.* Expulsion of the fetus or fetal tissue prior to the 20th week of pregnancy is called a **miscarriage**. Generally, miscarriage refers to the spontaneous delivery of the fetus and placenta before the 20th week of pregnancy.

Labor

Labor—the process that begins with the first uterine contraction and ends with delivery of the baby consists of three distinct stages (see Figure 21-2 on page 340).

DILATION

During the first and longest stage, **dilation**, the cervix becomes fully dilated to allow the baby's head to pass from the uterus to the birth canal. Uterine contractions cause the cervix to stretch and thin gradually until the opening is large enough to allow the baby to pass. These contractions usually begin as an aching sensation in the small of the back; within a short time, they become cramplike pains in the lower abdomen that occur at regular intervals. At first, contractions are 10 to 20 minutes apart and are not very painful; they may even stop completely and start again later.

---

umbilical cord An extension of the placenta that resembles a sturdy rope, through which the fetus is nourished

amniotic sac A sac of fluid in which the baby floats

vagina The passage for childbirth

perineum The area of skin and muscle between the vagina and the anus

crowning The emergence of the baby's head at the vaginal opening

cervix The neck of the uterus

bloody show Pink-tinged mucus in the vaginal discharge that is evident as labor begins

presenting part The part of the baby that emerges first through the birth canal; in a normal birth it is the head.

miscarriage Loss of pregnancy before 20 weeks of gestation; also called "spontaneous abortion"

labor The process that begins with the first uterine contraction and ends with delivery of the baby and placenta

dilation The stage of labor during which the cervix dilates and contractions occur

FIRST STAGE
First uterine contraction to dilation of cervix

SECOND STAGE
Birth of baby or expulsion

THIRD STAGE
Delivery of placenta

FIGURE 21–2. Three stages of labor

The first stage of labor may last as long as 18 hours or more for a woman having her first baby; women who have had a baby before may have only 2 or 3 hours of early labor.

CROWNING AND DELIVERY

During the second stage of labor, the baby moves through the birth canal. Contractions are closer together and last longer, usually 45 to 90 seconds. As the baby moves down the birth canal, the mother experiences considerable pressure in her rectum, much like the feeling of a bowel movement. That sensation is a sign that the baby is moving down the birth canal.

As the tightening and bearing-down sensations become stronger and more frequent, the mother will have an uncontrollable urge to push down. Soon after the baby's head appears at the opening of the birth canal. Once the head is delivered, the shoulders and the rest of the body follow.

DELIVERY OF THE PLACENTA

During the third stage of labor, the placenta separates from the uterine wall, and the placenta is expelled from the uterus.

First Aid Supplies for Delivery

Learning Objective 2 Describe the recommended first aid kit equipment for childbirth emergencies.

A basic sterile obstetric pack can be included as part of a comprehensive first aid kit, although most simple first aid kits do not include these materials. Recommended equipment for an obstetric pack includes:

- Surgical scissors (for cutting the cord)
- Cord clamps
- Umbilical tape or sterilized cord
- Bulb syringe
- Five towels
- 2 × 10 gauze sponges
- Sterile gloves
- One baby receiving blanket
- Two to three sanitary napkins, individually wrapped
- Two large plastic bags
- Foil-wrapped germicidal wipes

21.2 Predelivery Emergencies

Emergencies that occur before delivery of the baby include miscarriage, seizures, vaginal bleeding not associated with the birth, ectopic pregnancy, preeclampsia, eclampsia, and ruptured uterus.

Miscarriage

Learning Objective **3** List the signs and symptoms of miscarriage.

A miscarriage (sometimes called a spontaneous abortion) occurs for any number of reasons and involves delivery of the fetus and placenta or fetal tissue before 20 weeks of pregnancy. Signs and symptoms of miscarriage (see Figure 21-3) include:

- Cramplike abdominal pain similar to labor
- Moderate to severe vaginal bleeding
- Passage of tissue
- Inability to feel the uterus
- Uterus located below the woman's navel

Activate the EMS system; then:

1. Ask the woman when her last menstrual period began. If the last period began more than 22 weeks earlier, be prepared for potential delivery of a premature baby.

2. Conduct an initial assessment; monitor vital signs.

3. Provide first aid care based on the woman's symptoms. Help control vaginal bleeding by placing

SIGNS AND SYMPTOMS OF SPONTANEOUS ABORTION

- Passage of tissue
- Heavy vaginal bleeding
- Inability to feel the uterus
- Cramplike pains in lower abdomen
- Uterus located below woman's navel

FIGURE 21–3. Diagram depicts the appropriate treatment of a victim who is cramping and bleeding, threatening miscarriage.

a sanitary napkin over the vaginal opening; never pack the vagina in an attempt to control bleeding. If the pad becomes soaked with blood, replace it.

4. Save any passed tissue or evidence of blood loss, such as bloody sheets, towels, or underwear.

5. Provide emotional support to the mother and the members of her family; intense grief is normal for both parents.

Seizure during Pregnancy

Learning Objective **4** Describe and demonstrate how to manage a seizure during pregnancy.

Seizures during pregnancy often signal eclampsia, discussed in greater detail later in this chapter. Women with certain medical conditions, such as diabetes or heart disease, are also more prone to seizures during pregnancy.

Activate the EMS system; assess as you would for any seizure victim:

1. Treat the woman based on the signs and symptoms, providing the same treatment as you would for any seizure victim. Take care to protect the woman from injuring herself.

2. Position the woman on her left side to allow for drainage of secretions or blood and to keep her tongue from blocking breathing; keep her warm, but do not overheat.

Note: Bright lights and loud noises can trigger seizures in a preeclampsia victim; dim the lights if possible and avoid making loud sounds.

Vaginal Bleeding in Late Pregnancy

Learning Objective **5** Describe and demonstrate how to care for vaginal bleeding during pregnancy.

Vaginal bleeding can sometimes occur late in the pregnancy; excessive vaginal bleeding can constitute a life-threatening emergency for either the mother or the fetus.

Possible causes of excessive bleeding late in the pregnancy include:

- **Placenta previa**, in which the placenta is positioned partially or completely over the opening of the uterus and the vagina, which leads to premature separation and bleeding

- **Abruptio placenta**, in which the normally positioned placenta prematurely separates from the uterine wall usually during the last 3 months of pregnancy

Activate the EMS system; assess the victim; then:

1. Treat the victim according to signs and symptoms, which will usually include shock. Place the victim on her left side (to prevent the baby from pressing on the woman's inferior vena cava) with her legs and feet elevated. Keep her warm, but don't overheat.

2. Place a sanitary napkin over the vaginal opening, but do not pack the vagina. Note all soaked pads and other evidence of blood loss. Save any tissue that is passed, for evaluation by a physician.

3. If the bleeding is caused by trauma, control any external bleeding with direct pressure. Care for internal bleeding as described in step 2.

Ectopic Pregnancy

Learning Objective **6** Describe and demonstrate how to care for ectopic pregnancy.

In a normal pregnancy the egg is implanted in the uterus. In an **ectopic pregnancy**, the egg is implanted outside the uterus—in the abdominal cavity, in the fallopian tube, on the outside wall of the uterus, on the ovary, or on the outside of the cervix. Approximately 90 percent of ectopic pregnancies are in the fallopian tube.

The placenta eventually invades surrounding tissue, stretching the organ and causing rupture of a blood vessel and life-threatening bleeding. Ectopic pregnancy is the leading cause of first-trimester maternal deaths and occurs in 1 of every 200 pregnancies.

Signs and symptoms of ectopic pregnancy include:

- Sudden, sharp lower abdominal pain, localized on one side
- Vaginal bleeding
- Missed menstrual period
- Pain under the diaphragm
- Pain radiating to one or both shoulders
- Tender abdomen
- A palpable mass in the abdomen (typically clotted blood)
- Lightheadedness or dizziness
- Increased pulse
- Shock

Remember: External bleeding through the vagina may be slight or heavy with ectopic pregnancy. Suspect ectopic pregnancy in any woman of childbearing age with abdominal pain, especially if any of the above-listed signs and symptoms are present.

Activate the EMS system; then place the victim on her back; keep her warm and treat for shock.

Preeclampsia/Eclampsia

Learning Objective **7** List the signs and symptoms of preeclampsia/eclampsia.

A common condition affecting about 1 in 20 pregnant women is **preeclampsia**, also known as toxemia, or "poisoning" of the blood during pregnancy. Preeclampsia occurs most frequently in the last 3 months of pregnancy and is most likely to affect women in their twenties who are pregnant for the first time.

placenta previa A condition in which the placenta is positioned abnormally

abruptio placenta A condition in which a normally positioned placenta separates from the uterine wall, usually during the last 3 months of pregnancy

ectopic pregnancy A pregnancy in which the fertilized egg is implanted outside the uterus

preeclampsia A condition in pregnancy associated with high blood pressure and swelling of the extremities; the first stage of toxemia

Preeclampsia is characterized by high blood pressure and swelling in the extremities. Any of the following signs and symptoms may occur:

- Sudden weight gain (2 pounds a week or more)

- Blurred vision or spots before the eyes

- Pronounced swelling of the face, fingers, legs, or feet (some swelling of the feet and legs is normal)

- Decreased urine output

- Severe, persistent headache

- Persistent vomiting

- Mental confusion or disorientation

- Abdominal pain

During the preeclampsia stage, a previously normal pregnant woman develops high blood pressure, swelling, headaches, and visual disturbances. During the second stage, **eclampsia**, life-threatening convulsions or coma occurs.

Activate the EMS system immediately; then:

1. Position the victim on her left side to prevent compression of the inferior vena cava, allowing better blood flow to the heart.

2. Keep the victim calm and quiet; while waiting for emergency help, keep the lights dimmed and avoid making loud noises.

3. Care for seizures or coma as you would for any other seizure or coma.

Ruptured Uterus

Learning Objective **8** Describe and demonstrate how to care for ruptured uterus.

As the uterus enlarges during pregnancy, the uterine wall becomes extremely thin, especially around the bottom. The uterus may rupture if:

- The victim has a weak uterine scar from a previous cesarean section or surgical operation

- The victim has had many previous pregnancies

- The baby is too large for the pelvic opening

- Labor is extended and forceful (extended, forceful labor may force a large baby out through the uterine wall)

As many as 20 percent of the mothers who experience it, and 50 percent of the babies involved, die from a ruptured uterus. Signs and symptoms of a ruptured uterus include:

- A tearing sensation in the abdomen

- Constant and severe pain

- Nausea

- Shock

- Minimal vaginal bleeding in most cases

- Cessation of noticeable uterine contractions (the uterus relaxes during the contraction)

- Ability to feel the baby in the abdominal cavity

Immediately activate the EMS system; treat the victim for shock, and do not allow her to have anything by mouth, because surgery will be required.

PROGRESS CHECK

1. To care for vaginal bleeding, you should _____ . *(pack the vagina/apply pressure on the abdomen/place a sanitary napkin over the opening)*

2. Seizures caused by eclampsia can be aggravated by _____ . *(bright lights/movement/ pain)*

3. The leading cause of first-trimester maternal deaths is _____ . *(ruptured uterus/abortion/ectopic pregnancy)*

4. An ectopic pregnancy is one in which the fertilized egg implants _____ . *(near the cervix/outside the uterus/at an angle)*

5. A characteristic sign of preeclampsia is _____ . *(swelling of the extremities/ cyanosis/rash)*

6. As many as _____ percent of the babies of women who suffer ruptured uterus die. *(25/50/75)*

21.3 Normal Delivery

Learning Objective **9** Explain the situations in which you would *not* try to take a pregnant woman to the hospital for delivery.

It is best to take a pregnant woman to a doctor's office, medical clinic, or hospital for delivery of the baby. As a general guideline, there are three cases in

---

eclampsia The second stage of toxemia of pregnancy, when life-threatening convulsions or coma occur which you should *not* try to transport the mother for delivery:

- When you have no suitable transportation

- When the hospital or doctor cannot be reached because of bad weather, a natural disaster, or some other kind of catastrophe

- When delivery is expected within 5 minutes

Imminent Delivery

> Learning Objective **10** List the signs and symptoms indicating that delivery is imminent.

The following signs and symptoms indicate that delivery is imminent, especially if the woman has had more than one pregnancy:

- The amniotic sac has ruptured

- Crowning occurs during contractions

- Contractions are closer than 2 minutes apart

- Contractions are intense and last from 45 to 90 seconds

- The woman feels as if she needs to have a bowel movement (a sensation caused by the baby's head in the birth canal pressing against the rectum)

- The woman's abdomen is hard

Transporting a Woman in Labor

> Learning Objective **11** Describe how to transport a woman who is in labor to the hospital.

Contact EMS to transport the woman. If a situation exists where EMS is unable to transport, follow these guidelines:

1. Keep the woman lying down during transport; remove any underclothing that could interfere with delivery.

2. Place a folded blanket, sheet, or other clean object under the woman's buttocks and lower back.

3. Have the woman bend her knees and spread her thighs apart so you can watch for the crown of the baby's head in the birth canal.

4. Never ask the woman to cross her legs or ankles; never hold the woman's legs together; and never try to delay or restrain delivery in any way—the pressure can result in permanent injury or the death of the baby.

5. If the woman vomits, turn her head to one side and clean out her mouth.

Assisting with Delivery

> Learning Objective **12** Describe and demonstrate normal delivery procedures.

If you determine that birth is imminent and EMS has not yet arrived, or that you cannot attempt transport for some other reason, you need to assist in delivery of the baby. Take the following precautions:

- If possible, use appropriate protection (protective gloves, a mask, a gown, and eye protection) against exposure to body substances.

- Do not let the woman use the bathroom, even if she feels as if she needs to move her bowels.

- Do not hold the mother's legs together or do anything else to delay delivery.

- Recognize your own limitations; contact EMS immediately upon recognition of a woman in labor whose delivery appears to be imminent.

Delivery Procedures

As you assist in delivery, stay calm; reassure the mother that you are there to help; protect the mother's modesty, and provide comfort. Try for as few distractions as possible.

If possible, use a sterile obstetrics kit packed specifically for childbirth. If your first aid kit does not have one, use materials that are as sterile or clean as possible under the circumstances.

Activate the EMS system; then:

1. If possible, take body-substance isolation precautions; exposure to blood and body fluids during delivery is usually significant. Handle blood- and body-fluid-soaked dressings, pads, and linens carefully and bag them in moisture-proof bags to prevent leakage. Wash your hands thoroughly, and wear protective gloves. If they are available, you should also wear a mask and gown.

2. Have the woman lie on a firm surface with her knees drawn up and spread apart. Her feet should be flat on the surface beneath her, and she should be positioned several feet from the edge of the bed or other surface. Place your equipment close enough to reach, but far enough from the birth canal so it will not be contaminated by a gush of blood.

3. Support the mother's head, neck, and shoulders with pillows or folded blankets so she does not feel like she is slipping "downhill."

4. Remove clothing or push it above the mother's waist. Place one sterile sheet under the woman's hips, unfolding it toward her feet, and another sheet over her abdomen and legs. Have the woman take short, quick breaths during each contraction, and long, deep breaths between contractions.

5. As the infant's head appears in the birth canal (see Figures 21-4 through 21-12), place your fingers on the bony part of the infant's skull and exert *very* gentle pressure to prevent explosive delivery. Take extra caution to avoid touching the fontanel (soft spot on the top of the baby's head). Apply gentle pressure to the perineum to reduce the risk of tearing; allowing the head to deliver between contractions can also help reduce the risk of perineal tearing.

6. If the amniotic sac has not ruptured, tear the sac with your fingers, then push it away from the baby's head and mouth as they appear.

7. As the infant's head is delivered, determine whether the umbilical cord is around the infant's neck. If it is, use two fingers to slip the cord over the baby's shoulder. If you can't move the cord, clamp and cut it as shown in Figure 21-10, then unwrap it from around the neck.

FIGURE 21–4. Crowning

FIGURE 21–5. Head delivers and turns.

FIGURE 21–6. Shoulders deliver.

FIGURE 21–7. Chest delivers.

FIGURE 21–8. Infant is fully delivered.

FIGURE 21–9. Suctioning nose and mouth

FIGURE 21–10. Cutting the cord between the two cord clamps

FIGURE 21–11. Delivery of the placenta

FIGURE 21–12. Placenta delivers.

8. When the head is delivered, support the head with one hand and suction the mouth and nostrils with a bulb syringe until they are clear. Make sure you compress the bulb syringe before you insert it into the nose or mouth. Insert the tip of the compressed bulb 1 to $1\frac{1}{2}$; inches into the baby's mouth; slowly

release the bulb to allow mucus and other fluid to be drawn into the syringe. Avoid touching the back of the mouth. Remove the syringe, then discharge the contents onto a towel. Repeat. Use the same procedure to suction the mouth and then each nostril. (Babies breathe primarily through their noses, so the nostrils must be clear.)

9. As the torso and full body are born, support the baby with both hands (see Figure 21-13). Never pull the baby from the vagina. Do not put your finger in the baby's armpit, because damage to the nerve centers there can cause paralysis. The baby will be slippery, covered with a whitish, cheeselike substance known as the **vernix caseosa**. Receive the baby in a clean or sterile towel, which will help you hold on to the baby.

10. As the feet are born, grasp the feet. Take caution not to pull on the cord as you lift or deliver the baby.

11. Continue to suction the baby's mouth and nose with the bulb syringe. The baby will probably cry almost immediately. Soon after this cry, the cord will become limp and will no longer pulsate, because the blood flow through the cord ceases at birth.

12. Dry the baby and then wrap it in a warm blanket and place it on its back. Keep the infant level with the mother's vagina until the cord is cut. If possible, assign another First Aider to monitor and care for the newborn while you finish caring for the mother.

13. Clamp, tie, and cut the umbilical cord when pulsations cease in the cord. Place two clamps or ties on the cord about 3 inches apart; the first clamp should be approximately four finger-widths from the infant. Use sterile surgical scissors to cut the cord between the two clamps. If surgical scissors and clamps are not available, try using shoelaces and a knife or scissors. Periodically check the end of the cord for bleeding, and control any bleeding that may occur by applying another clamp or tie.

14. Watch for delivery of the placenta. The placenta is usually delivered within 10 minutes—and almost always within 20 minutes—after the baby. Never pull on the cord to check whether the placenta has separated from the uterus. When the placenta appears at the vagina, grasp it gently and rotate it. Do not pull; instead, slowly and gently guide the placenta and the attached membranes from the vagina.

vernix caseosa The white, cheeselike covering on a newborn's skin

a

b

c

d

e

f

FIGURE 21–13. Normal delivery

15. When the placenta is delivered, place it in a plastic bag for transport to the hospital. A physician needs to examine the placenta and confirm that delivery was complete.

16. Place one or two sterile sanitary napkins over the vaginal opening, lower the victim's legs, and help her hold her legs together. Elevate her feet if necessary.

17. Record the time of delivery. If emergency personnel are not en route, or delayed significantly, transport the mother, infant, and placenta, keeping both the mother and the infant warm.

Vaginal Bleeding following Delivery

Learning Objective **13** Describe and demonstrate how to care for vaginal bleeding following delivery.

Vaginal loss of as much as 2 cups of blood is considered normal following delivery. If there is excessive blood loss, massage the uterus as follows:

1. Place your hand on the woman's lower abdomen above the pubis.

2. Using the palm of your hand, your fingers fully extended, the flat of your four fingers cupped around the uterus, massage in a circular motion until you feel the uterus firm up. It should feel like a hard grapefruit.

3. Have the baby suckle on the mother's breast. This releases a hormone that causes the uterus to contract.

4. If bleeding continues, check your massage technique, and continue massage.

If the mother appears to be in shock, treat for shock.

PROGRESS CHECK

1. You should not try to get a woman in labor to a hospital if _____ . *(her husband is not present/you have no suitable transportation/the mother wants a home delivery)*

2. _____ indicate(s) that delivery is imminent . *(Contractions more frequent than every 2 minutes/Severe cramplike pains/Shortness of breath)*

3. To prevent explosive delivery, exert gentle pressure on the _____ . *(pubis/vaginal opening/bony part of the baby's skull)*

4. Cut the cord _____ . *(before the baby starts breathing/as the baby starts breathing/after the cord goes limp)*

5. Before you cut the cord, it should be clamped or tied in _____ places . *(two/three/four)*

6. It is normal for a woman to lose as much as _____ of blood following birth. *(1 cup/ 2 cups/1 pint)*

21.4 Care and Resuscitation of the Newborn

Learning Objective 14 Describe and demonstrate care of the newborn.

The body surface area of an infant is proportionately greater than that of older children or adults, so infants are likely to lose more heat more quickly. Protecting newborn infants against heat loss preserves their energy and avoids the complex problem that hospitals face in trying to warm a cold infant.

A normal baby should be crying. The baby's heartbeat should be at least 100 beats per minute, and the baby's respiratory rate should be at least 40 breaths per minute.

Care of a Newborn

To care for a newborn:

1. Immediately dry the infant, paying particular attention to the head, which has a large surface area. Wrap the newborn in a blanket or a plastic bubble bag swaddle and cover the infant's head. Keep the face clear and unobstructed.

2. Repeat suctioning with the bulb syringe, making sure the infant's nostrils and mouth are clear.

3. Assess the infant, evaluating the infant's color, pulse, grimace (does the infant cry or make a facial grimace when you insert the bulb syringe?), activity, and ease of breathing. (These are the standard signs used in the Apgar scoring system, which is used to evaluate a newborn's condition.) Distress is indicated by bluish discoloration, irregular or sluggish pulse, lack of grimace, limpness, and irregular, shallow, gasping, or absent respirations.

4. Stimulate the newborn if it is not breathing or the heart rate is less than 100 beats per minute. You may simply need to encourage the infant to breathe by flicking the soles of its feet or rubbing its back in a circular motion with three fingers (see Figure 21-14).

Resuscitating a Newborn

Learning Objectives 15 Describe and demonstrate resuscitation of the newborn.

If the infant requires either rescue breathing or CPR, do the following:

1. If the infant's breathing is shallow, slow, gasping, or absent, provide artificial ventilations at the rate of one breath every 1 to $1\frac{1}{2}$ seconds. Assess again after 1 minute.

2. If the infant's heart rate is less than 100 beats per minute, provide artificial ventilations at the rate of one breath every 1 to $1\frac{1}{2}$ seconds. Reassess every 30 seconds.

3. If the infant's heart rate is less than 60 beats per minute and the infant is not responding to the artificial ventilation, start chest compression and ventilation.

PROGRESS CHECK

1. The first step in caring for the newborn is to _____ it. *(measure/dry/assess)*

2. To assess an infant, use the same factors used in the _____ scoring system. *(Apgar/Andrews/Smithson)*

FIGURE 21–14. Stimulate the newborn by rubbing the back or flicking the soles of the feet.

3. To encourage an infant to breathe, _____ the soles of its feet. *(pinch/slap/flick)*

4. To resuscitate an infant with a low heart rate, deliver artificial ventilation at the rate of _____ breaths per minute. *(30/60/100)*

5. If an infant's pulse rate is less than _____ beats per minute, deliver chest compressions. *(60/80/100)*

21.5 Abnormal Deliveries

Learning Objective **16** Describe and demonstrate how to manage abnormal deliveries.

Abnormal delivery includes prolapsed cord, breech birth, limb presentation, multiple births, presence of meconium, or premature birth.

Prolapsed Cord

A **prolapsed cord** is an umbilical cord that presents through the birth canal before delivery of the infant's head (see Figure 21-15 on page 350). Because the cord is compressed against the birth canal by the baby's head, the baby's supply of oxygenated blood is cut off, and the baby is in great danger of suffocation.

Activate the EMS system; then:

1. Position the mother with her head down or her buttocks raised, allowing gravity to reduce the pressure on the cord in the birth canal.

2. Insert a sterile, gloved hand into the vagina and push the presenting part of the fetus away from the pulsating cord. *Follow local protocol.*

3. Do not try to push the cord back into the vagina. Cover the cord with a sterile, moist towel.

4. Maintain pressure on the presenting part and monitor pulsations in the cord until emergency personnel arrive.

Breech Birth

With a **breech birth**, the buttocks or both feet of the baby are the first part presented through the birth canal. The newborn is at great risk for trauma during delivery (see Figure 21-16 on page 350), and prolapsed cord is common with breech presentation.

If the buttocks emerge first, support the emerging baby. Do *not* pull. If the head is not delivered within 10 minutes, place one hand in the vagina, your palm toward the baby's face. Form a V with two of your fingers on either side of the baby's nose, then push away the vaginal wall from the baby's nose. Maintain that position until the baby's head is delivered or EMS has arrived.

Limb Presentation

Limb presentation occurs when the infant's arm or leg protrudes first from the birth canal. The most common limb presentation is a foot. Instruct the mother not to push with the contractions. Have her pant during the contractions to prevent pushing. Activate the EMS system. Do not attempt to continue to deliver.

> **prolapsed cord** The presentation of the umbilical cord at the vaginal opening before the baby
>
> **breech birth** A situation in which the buttocks or both feet of the baby present first through the birth canal

- Activate the EMS system.

- Elevate hips and keep warm.

- Keep baby's head away from cord.

- Do not attempt to push cord back.

- Wrap cord in sterile moist towel.

FIGURE 21–15. Management of a prolapsed cord

FIGURE 21–16. Provide and maintain an airway during a breech birth if the delivery does not occur within 10 minutes after the buttocks are delivered.

Multiple Births

With nonidentical, or fraternal, twins, each twin has its own placenta; identical twins share one placenta. Even if the mother is unaware that she is carrying more than one baby, you should suspect a multiple birth if any of the following signs are present:

- The abdomen is still very large after one baby is delivered.

- Uterine contractions continue to be extremely strong.

- Uterine contractions begin again about 10 minutes after one baby has been delivered.

- The baby's size is out of proportion with the size of the mother's abdomen.

In case of multiple births, activate the EMS system; then:

1. Be prepared for complications; about one-third of second twins have a breech presentation. Expect and handle hemorrhage following the second birth. Children of multiple births tend to have low birth weights and need more resuscitation.

2. If there are no complications, deliver the second baby as you did the first.

Passage of Meconium

Meconium—the newborn's first feces—in the amniotic fluid makes the fluid greenish or brownish-yellow rather than clear. The presence of meconium indicates that the fetus has been distressed and has had a bowel movement inside the amniotic sac. If the baby breathes in any of the meconium-stained fluid, infection and aspiration pneumonia can result. Meconium passage is common in breech births.

Activate the EMS system *immediately;* then:

1. Suction the baby's nose and mouth *before* you stimulate the baby. The most critical aspect of treatment for meconium passage is to clear the nose and mouth before the baby takes its first breath.

2. Maintain the baby's airway.

Premature Birth

A **premature baby** may weigh less than $5\frac{1}{2}$ pounds and/or is born before 36 weeks of gestation. Premature babies are more susceptible to respiratory diseases and infection, and must be given special care.

You can generally tell by appearance whether a baby is premature: premature babies are thinner, smaller, have thin silky hair, no creases in the soles of the feet,

no cartilage in the outer ear, and have larger heads in proportion to their bodies.

Premature babies generally require more resuscitation. Take these additional steps to care for a premature baby:

1. Keep the baby warm; use warmed blankets or plastic bubble bag swaddle. If you take the baby to the hospital, heat your vehicle.

2. Use gentle suction with a bulb syringe to keep the baby's mouth and nose clear of fluid. Perform resuscitation if necessary.

3. Prevent bleeding from the umbilical cord; a premature infant cannot tolerate losing even minute amounts of blood.

4. Premature babies are highly susceptible to infection. Prevent contamination and do not let anyone breathe into the baby's face.

PROGRESS CHECK

1. A _____ cord is an umbilical cord that presents through the birth canal before the baby. *(pulsating/prolapsed/inverted)*

2. A _____ birth occurs when the baby's buttocks or lower extremities present first. *(breech/premature/multiple)*

3. Meconium indicates that the baby has had a _____ in the amniotic sac. *(seizure/hemorrhage/bowel movement)*

4. The primary goal if you see meconium is to _____ the baby before it takes its first breath. *(stimulate/suction/resuscitate)*

5. Suspect a multiple birth if _____ begin after delivery of a baby. *(strong contractions/fluid leaks/cyanosis)*

6. A premature baby has no _____ . *(hair/outer ear cartilage/eyebrows)*

---

meconium The feces of the newborn; greenish or brownish-yellow amniotic fluid indicates that the baby had a bowel movement in the uterus before delivery.

premature baby A baby that weighs less than $5\frac{1}{2}$ pounds and/or is born after less than 36 weeks' gestation

Summary

- Predelivery emergencies can include miscarriage, seizure, vaginal bleeding, ectopic pregnancy, preeclampsia, and ruptured uterus. Because some of these require surgery, never let the victim eat or drink.

- Do not try to take a woman who is in labor to the hospital if you have no suitable transportation, the hospital is unreachable for some reason, or you expect delivery within 5 minutes.

- When transporting a woman in labor to the hospital, allow her to lie on her back; remove her underwear and have her separate her legs so you can monitor for crowning.

- When assisting delivery, take precautions against exposure to body substances; exposure to blood and body fluids is significant during delivery.

- It is normal for a woman to lose as much as 2 cups of blood following delivery; if bleeding is significant, massage the uterus to help it contract.

- Flick the soles of a newborn's feet or massage its back gently to encourage it to take its first breath.

- Always be prepared for complications in a multiple birth.

- If the amniotic fluid is stained with meconium, suction the baby's nose and mouth before it takes its first breath.

- A premature baby is smaller than a full-term baby, lacks cartilage in the outer ear, has no creases in the soles of the feet, has fine, silky hair and has a head that is larger in proportion to the rest of its body.

- A priority in caring for a premature baby is to keep it warm.

Key Terms

Make sure you understand the following key terms:

fetus	labor
uterus	dilation
birth canal	placenta previa
placenta	abruptio placenta
umbilical cord	ectopic pregnancy
amniotic sac	preeclampsia
vagina	eclampsia
perineum	vernix caseosa
crowning	prolapsed cord
cervix	breech birth
bloody show	meconium
presenting part	premature baby
miscarriage	

Critical Thinking Exercise

You are working in the first aid tent at the local fair when a pregnant woman is brought in by her husband. She tells you that she has been having abdominal discomfort for the last day; however, she began to experience severe pain with contractions about one hour ago. The contractions are much more intense, lasting longer, and occurring much more frequently. Her due date is five days from today.

1. What do the characteristics of the contractions indicate?

2. What signs and symptoms would indicate an imminent delivery?

3. If delivery is imminent, how would you proceed?

Student: _____   Date: _____

Course: _____   Section #: _____

Part 1   True/False

If you believe the statement is true, circle the T. If you believe the statement is false, circle the F.

T F   **1.** Emergency childbirth is just that—measures that should be taken when it is impossible for the mother to reach a hospital or physician.

T F   **2.** If you are close to a medical facility and the birth begins, tell the mother to clamp her legs tightly together and try to keep the baby's head inside the birth canal.

T F   **3.** It is important to take the placenta to the hospital with the mother and the baby.

T F   **4.** A gentle pull on the baby as it is being born will give a more efficient delivery.

T F   **5.** An umbilical cord that is wrapped around the baby's neck must be quickly, but gently, removed.

T F   **6.** After delivery, gentle massage of the uterus helps control the mother's bleeding.

T F   **7.** You should always try to reach a hospital, no matter how soon delivery is likely to be.

T F   **8.** When taking a mother in labor to the hospital, keep her seated with a seatbelt on; keeping her seated discourages the birth.

T F   **9.** It is normal for a woman to lose as much as 2 cups of blood following birth.

T F   **10.** In case of prolapsed cord, grasp the cord and tuck it back into the vagina.

Part 2   Multiple Choice

For each item, circle the correct answer or the phrase that best completes the statement.

1. If the baby's head emerges from the birth canal and the amniotic sac is still unbroken, you should
   a. wait for the baby to emerge completely
   b. tear the bag with your fingers so the fluid can drain
   c. carefully puncture the bag
   d. wait for EMS team to arrive

2. Be prepared to deliver when the pregnant woman's labor contractions are
   a. 5 minutes apart
   b. 3 minutes apart
   c. 2 minutes or less apart
   d. 10 minutes apart

3. To decide whether to transport the mother by car or call EMS
   a. ask the mother if she is having her first baby
   b. examine the mother for signs of crowning
   c. ask the mother if she needs to move her bowels
   d. all of the above

4. As the baby's head emerges, you should
   a. push gently on the bony part of the head
   b. pull gently on the top of the head

   c. apply downward pressure
   d. grasp under the arms

5. If the baby does not begin to breathe by itself, you should
   a. immediately stimulate and reassess
   b. hyperextend its neck
   c. use the Holgar-Nielson method of resuscitation
   d. turn the baby upside down and gently shake it

6. The longest stage of labor will probably be
   a. the dilation stage
   b. the expulsion stage
   c. the placental stage
   d. none of the above; all stages are about equal in length

7. The developing baby is attached by the umbilical cord to the
   a. cervix
   b. placenta
   c. amniotic sac
   d. perineum

8. If you think you have time to transport the mother to the hospital, *do not*

   a. keep the mother lying down
   b. allow the mother to go to the toilet immediately before you leave
   c. keep the mother relaxed
   d. have the mother bend her knees and spread her thighs apart so you can watch for crowning

9. Crowning is when

   a. the position of the baby is incorrect for delivery
   b. the baby's head can be seen at the opening of the birth canal
   c. the bag of waters is not broken
   d. the baby is suffering a lack of oxygen

10. Ectopic pregnancy occurs when

    a. more than one egg is fertilized
    b. the fertilized egg implants outside the uterus
    c. the placenta separates from the uterus
    d. the uterus ruptures

11. Victims of ectopic pregnancy and ruptured uterus require immediate

    a. CPR
    b. transport to the hospital

12. To help control bleeding after delivery

    a. massage the uterus
    b. pack the vagina with sterile pads
    c. place sterile pads over the vaginal opening
    d. apply direct pressure to the abdomen

13. Encourage a baby to breathe following delivery by

    a. slapping the soles of its feet
    b. flicking the soles of its feet
    c. pinching the soles of its feet
    d. spanking it

14. You should suspect a multiple birth if

    a. the size of the baby does not correspond to the size of the mother's abdomen
    b. strong contractions begin after the baby is born
    c. uterine contractions continue after the baby is born
    d. all of the above

15. Meconium in the amniotic sac means the baby was distressed and is described as

    a. blood in the amniotic fluid
    b. greenish-brown, dark, tarry material in the amniotic fluid
    c. red fluid
    d. clear fluid

Also in question 8:

   c. placement in the prone position
   d. neurological assessment

Part 3   Matching

Match each stage of childbirth with its description.

Description

1. _____ The placenta is delivered.
2. _____ Contractions occur and the "bag of waters" breaks.
3. _____ The baby is born.

Stage of Labor

A. Dilation
B. Expulsion
C. Placental

Part 4   What Would You Do If?

You are at a neighboring apartment where a woman is in labor. The hospital is 30 minutes away. She suddenly says, "The baby's coming—*now*!" This is her sixth child. What questions would you ask the mother? What preparations would you make for childbirth? How would you assist the childbirth?

22

Pediatric and Geriatric Emergencies

On the Scene

Shortly after settling four of the children she cared for down for story time, day-care provider Becky Christensen noticed that 6-year-old Chelsea Weist had stayed on a chair in the family room instead of joining the others. As she approached the little girl, Becky saw that she was obviously quite ill.

Chelsea was sitting awkwardly in the overstuffed chair, leaning forward, breathing through her mouth. Though Chelsea was not struggling to breathe, Becky noticed a short wheeze as she exhaled. Chelsea was drooling profusely.

When Becky began asking Chelsea questions, the child had a very difficult time answering. Alarmed, Becky immediately suspected asthma, a condition Chelsea's mother had warned her about.

Becky quietly excused herself, called for an ambulance, then returned to Chelsea with the inhaler Chelsea's mother left at the day care. She kept the little girl sitting up in the chair and knelt next to her, reassuring and calming her gently. Becky helped Chelsea use her inhaler until paramedics arrived a few minutes later. As they prepared Chelsea for transport, Becky called the child's mother so they could meet at the emergency room. Becky's calmness and reassuring manner, combined with the inhaler, helped prevent Chelsea from making her asthma attack worse.

As a First Aider, you will often have to care for people at two extremes of the age spectrum—children (infants, children between 1 and 12, and adolescents) and the elderly (those over 65). Each group presents special physical and emotional challenges that need to be considered each time you give care.

This chapter explains the special assessment considerations you need to make, summarizes special emergency situations for each age group, and outlines first aid care for those emergency situations.

22.1 Assessing the Child

Children are not simply small adults; rather, there are important psychological and physical differences between adults and children (see Figure 22-1). Although a breathing problem is always a breathing problem, and a bleeding wound is always a bleeding wound, the way you approach them in a 5-year-old child can differ from the way you approach them in an adult.

That is not all: When you deal with a child in distress, you also deal with parents or caregivers in distress. It is natural for parents to be upset, to cry, to blame themselves, or to blame someone else. Let parents feel they are participants in their child's care; calm and cooperative parents will help reassure the child.

Special Assessment Techniques

Learning Objective 1 Explain special assessment techniques to use with children.

It is difficult to assess pain in children because they lack both the body awareness to describe the exact location of the pain and the vocabulary to describe it.

During your first look at the child, ask yourself these questions:

- Does the child look sick?
- Is the child in shock?

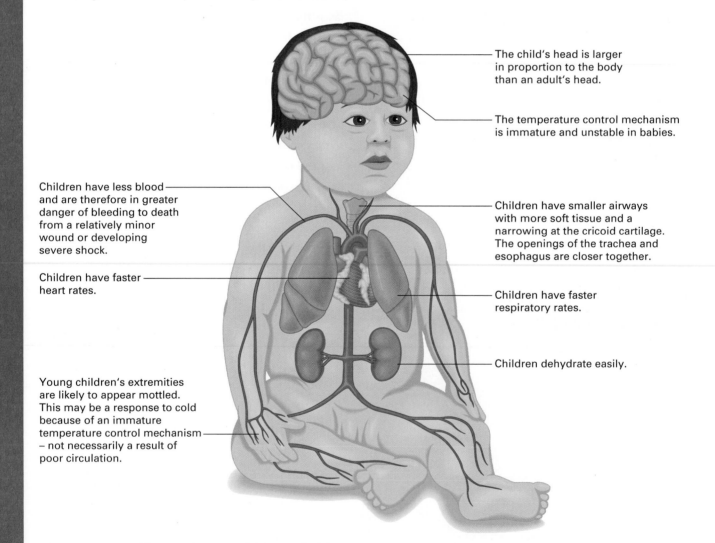

The child's head is larger in proportion to the body than an adult's head.

The temperature control mechanism is immature and unstable in babies.

Children have less blood and are therefore in greater danger of bleeding to death from a relatively minor wound or developing severe shock.

Children have faster heart rates.

Children have smaller airways with more soft tissue and a narrowing at the cricoid cartilage. The openings of the trachea and esophagus are closer together.

Children have faster respiratory rates.

Children dehydrate easily.

Young children's extremities are likely to appear mottled. This may be a response to cold because of an immature temperature control mechanism – not necessarily a result of poor circulation.

FIGURE 22–1. Differences between children and adults

- Is the child in extreme pain?

- How is the child breathing?

Regardless of the child's age, follow these general procedures when assessing a child (see Figure 22-2):

- Prepare yourself psychologically so you can radiate confidence, competence, and friendliness.

- If you are a stranger to the child, remember that children between age 1 and 6 seldom like strangers, especially if their parents are not there.

- Get as close to the child's eye level as possible.

- Explain what you are doing in terms the child can understand; speak in a calm, quiet voice and avoid "baby talk."

- Save the most painful parts of the assessment for last.

- Involve the parents as much as possible.

- Be honest. "It will hurt when I touch your leg, but it will only last a minute. If you feel like crying, that's okay."

- Be gentle; do everything you can to reduce the child's pain, and use restraint only when absolutely necessary—and then use minimal restraint.

Obtaining a History

If the situation is life threatening, take the primary survey quickly and manage serious conditions promptly.

FIGURE 22–2. Establish gentle contact and examine the child visually.

If you have more time, use the following guidelines in obtaining a history:

- Do not let upset parents and a screaming child unnerve you; take the time you need to get the information you need.

- Get information from parents or other witnesses, not the child.

- Ask when symptoms developed, how they progressed, and what care has already been given.

- If there was an accident, determine the details of the accident, the mechanism of injury, and what first aid care has already been given.

Taking Vital Signs

> Learning Objective **2** Explain how children's vital signs differ from those of adults.

You need to check a child's vital signs more frequently than you would an adult's. Your overall impressions of how the child looks and acts are more important and can tell you more about the child's status than any one vital sign.

Keep these considerations in mind:

- *Respirations.* Children breathe faster than adults—the average for an infant is 40 breaths per minute, and for an 8-year-old it is 25 breaths per minute. Take respiratory rates frequently by placing your hand on the child's stomach; increases are significant, as is the quality of breathing (inadequate, noisy, and so on).

- *Pulse.* To take a pulse quickly, use the radial pulse in a child, the brachial pulse in an infant. Rapid pulse can be normal in a scared or overly excited child, but a slow pulse is a worrisome sign that can be caused by a serious lack of oxygen, pressure in the skull, depressant drugs, or several comparatively rare medical conditions.

- *Temperature.* A child's temperature is a much more important warning sign than an adult's because it can change so quickly; young children can develop high fevers rapidly, so monitor the temperature frequently.

- *Neurological assessment.* Assessing possible neurological damage in a child is similar to assessment of an adult, but the stimuli must be more simple. For example, in testing response to painful stimuli, pinch the skin between the child's thumb and forefinger. Watch for other simple things, such as the child's ability to recognize familiar objects and people and the ability to move the arms and legs purposely.

1. When assessing a child, you should position yourself _____ . *(above the child/below the child/at the child's eye level)*

2. During assessment, check the most painful part _____ . *(quickly/last/first)*

3. You should check a child's vital signs more _____ than you do an adult's. *(frequently/thoroughly/quickly)*

4. A child breathes _____ than an adult. *(slower/faster/more deeply)*

5. Check a child's respiratory rate by placing your hand on the child's _____ . *(chest/stomach/back)*

6. Take an infant's pulse at the _____ pulse. *(carotid/radial/brachial)*

22.2 Emergencies Involving Children

Most emergencies involving children are managed in the same way as those involving adults. However, the different size and psychological development of a child means that you must treat some emergencies differently. Use the following considerations:

- Because the head of an infant or small child is large in proportion to the body, head injury is more likely. Assume cervical spine injury if the child has any injury above the clavicles or is unconscious.

- Because the liver, spleen, and kidneys of children are not as well protected as those of adults, and because they constitute a larger proportion of the abdominal cavity, they are more susceptible to blunt trauma.

- Because a child's skin surface is large compared to body mass, children are more susceptible to hypothermia, hyperthermia, and dehydration.

- Injuries of the extremities can also damage the growth plates.

- Infants have proportionally large tongues, and a relaxed tongue can block the airway.

- Most children involved in trauma will have enlarged stomachs, which can press against the diaphragm and make breathing difficult.

- It is especially important to stop bleeding in a child quickly; what is comparatively minor blood loss in an adult can constitute major bleeding in a child.

Common Emergencies in Children

Learning Objective 3 List special emergency situations involving children.

Some of the most common emergencies in children involve respiratory distress or obstructed airway (see Figure 22-3). Children are more susceptible than adults to respiratory distress because they have smaller air passages and less reserve air capacity.

Learning Objective 4 Describe the signs and symptoms of the following respiratory conditions: croup, epiglottitis, and asthma.

Two emergencies that may be difficult to distinguish are infectious **croup** and **epiglottitis** (see Figure 22-4). Use the guidelines in Table 22-1 to distinguish the two.

Most children are vaccinated against epiglottitis. Fortunately, it is now relatively rare to see epiglottitis in children.

Asthma is very common in children, especially among those with allergies. It can cause wheezing, an overly inflated chest, increasingly impaired breathing, exhaustion, sleepiness, rapid pulse, and cyanosis.

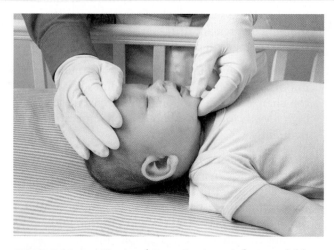

FIGURE 22–3. Airway obstruction in an infant or child may be relieved by keeping the head in a neutral or slightly extended position.

croup A viral infection that causes swelling beneath the glottis and progressive narrowing of the airway

epiglottitis A bacterial infection that causes swelling of the epiglottis and blocking of the airway

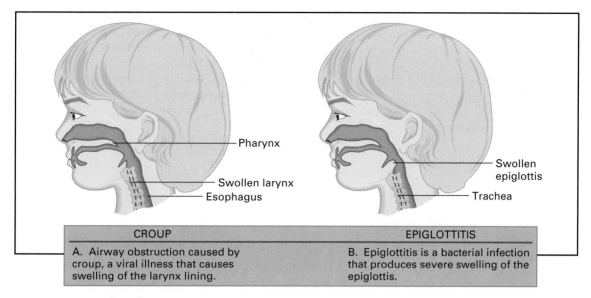

	CROUP	EPIGLOTTITIS
	A. Airway obstruction caused by croup, a viral illness that causes swelling of the larynx lining.	B. Epiglottitis is a bacterial infection that produces severe swelling of the epiglottis.

FIGURE 22–4. Croup and epiglottitis

TABLE 22–1	**Croup and Epiglottitis**	
	Croup	**Epiglottitis**
Cause	Viral infection of the upper airway	Bacterial infection
Physiology	Swelling beneath the glottis that progressively narrows the airway	Inflammation and swelling of the epiglottis
Signs and Symptoms	Peculiar whooping sound; high-pitched squeaking sounds; hoarseness; coughing with a harsh "seal bark" *Severe attacks are dangerous*	Pain on swallowing; high fever; drooling; difficulty speaking, but no hoarseness; mouth breathing; insistence on sitting up and leaning forward with chin thrust outward
First Aid Care	Keep the child in a comfortable position, usually propped up; activate the EMS system or take the child to the hospital	*Epiglottitis is life threatening.* Keep the child calm and relaxed; *do not let the child lie down*; do not examine the child's throat; activate the EMS system

Asthma should be regarded as a serious medical emergency.

Asthma care guidelines:

1. Allow the child to assume the position of greatest comfort—almost always sitting or semisitting. Additionally, give an asthma victim plenty of fluids, which help loosen and thin mucus in the air passages.

2. Be calm and reassuring.

3. Activate the EMS system or take the child to a medical facility.

4. If allowed as part of your training, assist the patient with his or her inhaler. Even retrieving an inhaler and bringing it to the patient is valuable.

> Learning Objective **5** Discuss other common emergencies among children.

Cardiac Arrest

Most of the cardiac arrests in children result from airway obstruction and/or respiratory arrest; the remaining cases are caused by shock. As when treating an adult, the goal is to keep the brain oxygenated and to begin care rapidly.

The signs and symptoms of cardiac arrest in a child (see Figure 22-5) include:

- Unresponsiveness
- Seizure (early in onset of arrest due to hypoxia)
- Gasping or absent respiratory sounds
- Absence of chest movement
- Pale or blue skin
- Absent pulse

For guidelines on CPR in infants and children, see Chapter 6.

Seizures

Seizures in a child can be caused by any condition that would cause them in adults—head injury, meningitis, oxygen deficiency, drug overdose, and hypoglycemia, among others. While adults rarely have seizures caused by fever, children under the age of 6 do.

To treat a seizure in a child, activate the EMS system; then:

1. Turn the child onto his or her side to prevent the tongue from relaxing and shifting backward, blocking the air passage.
2. Do not hold the child down, but place the child where he or she will not fall or strike something. A rug on the floor is excellent; so is a crib with padded sides.
3. Loosen tight or restrictive clothing.
4. Sponge a feverish child with lukewarm water.

Shock

The major causes of shock in children are blood loss, acute infection, and heart failure. Loss of body heat will cause newborns to go into shock, because they cannot shiver or warm themselves by moving around and because their surface area is large in relation to their body weight.

The signs and symptoms of shock in a child (see Figure 22-6) include:

- Paleness
- Cold, moist skin
- Low blood pressure
- A rapid, thready pulse
- Lack of vitality
- Extreme anxiety
- Unconsciousness

To care for shock, activate the EMS system, have the child lie flat, keep the child warm and as calm as possible, and monitor vital signs frequently.

PROGRESS CHECK

1. Injuries of the extremities in a child can also damage the _____ . (bone marrow/growth plates/large ball-and-socket joints)
2. An infant has a proportionally large _____, which can block the airway. (tongue/epiglottis/larynx)
3. Most children involved in trauma have an enlarged _____, which can interfere with breathing. (tongue/larynx/stomach)
4. A characteristic "seal bark" cough is a sign of _____ . (asthma/croup/epiglottis)

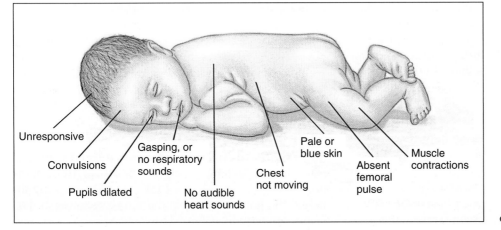

FIGURE 22–5. Signs of cardiac arrest in a child

Unresponsive · Convulsions · Pupils dilated · Gasping, or no respiratory sounds · No audible heart sounds · Chest not moving · Pale or blue skin · Absent femoral pulse · Muscle contractions

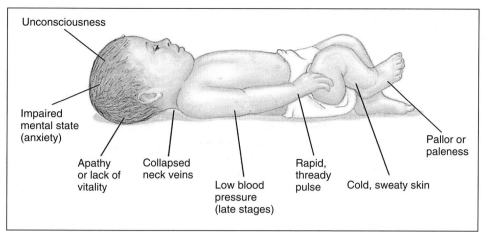

Unconsciousness

Impaired mental state (anxiety)

Apathy or lack of vitality

Collapsed neck veins

Low blood pressure (late stages)

Rapid, threadly pulse

Cold, sweaty skin

Pallor or paleness

FIGURE 22–6. Signs of shock in a child

5. A child who is drooling, having difficulty speaking, and having difficulty swallowing probably has _____. *(asthma/croup/epiglottitis)*

6. Seizures in a child can be caused by _____, which rarely causes seizures in an adult. *(head injury/oxygen deficiency/fever)*

7. _____, which does not usually cause shock in older victims, can cause shock in an infant. *(Blood loss/Loss of body heat/Major trauma)*

22.3 Sudden Infant Death Syndrome and Child Abuse

Sudden Infant Death Syndrome

Learning Objective 6 Describe how to manage a case of sudden infant death syndrome.

Sudden infant death syndrome (SIDS), more commonly known as "crib death," is the number-one cause of death among infants between 1 month and 1 year of age. It cannot be predicted or prevented, and almost always occurs while the baby is sleeping.

The typical SIDS case involves an apparently healthy infant, frequently born prematurely, and usually between the ages of 4 weeks and 7 months, who suddenly dies in his or her crib. There is usually no indication of a struggle, though some infants have obviously changed position at the time of death. A red blotchiness of the skin is usually apparent.

While researchers are not sure of the cause, recent studies indicate that inadequate amounts of oxygen in the blood may occur several weeks before a sudden death. Other causes may be alterations in brain activity, alterations of respiratory control and cardiac rhythm, and apnea followed by hyperventilation.

The guidelines for managing a SIDS case vary by location; *follow local protocol*, keeping these general guidelines in mind:

1. *Even if the child is obviously dead, have someone activate the EMS system and immediately begin infant CPR.*

2. Be aware of the parents' extreme distress; the best first aid is to make them feel that everything possible has been done for their child. Leave no room for "ifs" and "maybes." Parents will often feel guilt. Be careful not to make judgmental statements that add to guilt.

3. After the ambulance arrives, encourage the parents to accompany their baby in the ambulance and arrange for someone to stay with other children at the home.

Child Abuse and Neglect

Learning Objective 7 Explain how to identify child abuse and neglect.

Thousands of cases of child abuse and neglect are reported annually in the United States—and because they occur chiefly in the privacy of the home, no one knows how many more cases go unreported.

IDENTIFYING ABUSE

The abuser—usually a parent, stepparent, or boyfriend or girlfriend of the child's parent—often behaves in an evasive manner when confronted, volunteering little information or giving contradictory versions of what happened to the child. An abusing adult may show outright hostility toward the child, and rarely shows any guilt.

sudden infant death syndrome (SIDS) Sudden death of an apparently healthy infant, usually while asleep

Type of Abuse/ Neglect	Physical Indicators	Behavioral Indicators
Physical Abuse	Unexplained bruises and welts • on face, lips, mouth • on torso, back, buttocks, thighs • in various stages of healing • clustered, forming regular patterns • reflecting shape of article used to inflict them (electric cord, belt buckle) • on several different surface areas • regularly appear after absence, weekend, or vacation • especially about the trunk and buttocks Be particularly suspicious if there are old bruises in addition to fresh ones Unexplained burns • cigar, cigarette burns, especially on soles, palms, back, or buttocks • immersion burns (occur when a child is immersed in scalding water; when hands are immersed, burns look like reddened gloves; when feet are immersed, burns look like socks. Doughnut-shaped burns may appear on buttocks and genitalia.) • showing the pattern of electric stove burner, iron, etc. • rope burns on arms, legs, neck, or torso Unexplained fractures (particularly if multiple) • to skull, nose, facial structures • in various stages of healing • multiple or spiral fractures Unexplained lacerations or abrasions • to mouth, lips, gums, eyes • to external genitalia	Wary of adult contacts Apprehensive when other children cry Behavioral extremes: • aggressiveness • withdrawal Frightened of parents Afraid to go home Reports injury by parents The child is apathetic and *may not* cry despite his or her injuries The child has been seen by emergency personnel recently for related complaints The child's injury occurred several days before you were called
Sexual Abuse	Difficulty in walking or sitting Torn, stained, or bloody underclothing Pain or itching in genital area Bruises or bleeding in external genitalia, vaginal or anal areas Venereal disease, especially in preteens Pregnancy	Unwilling to change for gym or participate in physical education classes Withdrawal, fantasizing, or infantile behavior Bizarre, sophisticated, or unusual sexual behavior or knowledge Poor peer relationships Delinquent or run-away Reports sexual assault by caretaker
Emotional Abuse	Speech disorders Lags in physical development Failure to thrive	Habit disorders (sucking thumb, biting, rocking, etc.) Conduct disorders (antisocial, destructive, etc.) Neurotic traits (sleep disorders, inhibition of play) Psychoneurotic reactions (hysteria, obsession, compulsion, phobias, hypochondria) Behavioral extremes: • complaisant, passive • aggressive, demanding Overly adaptive behavior: • inappropriately adult • inappropriately infantile Developmental lags (mental, emotional) Attempted suicide
Neglect	Consistent hunger, poor hygiene, inappropriate dress Consistent lack of supervision, especially in dangerous activities or for long periods Physical problems or medical needs that indicate lack of a caregiver Abandonment	Begging, stealing food Extended stays at school (early arrival and late departure) Constant fatigue, listlessness, or falling asleep in class Alcohol or drug use Delinquency (e.g., thefts) States there is no caretaker

FIGURE 22–7. Physical and behavioral indicators of child abuse and neglect. (*Note:* Much of the above will not be obvious in the field—but the information can help you understand what may have precipitated the emergency.)

Abuse can be physical, emotional, or sexual, or may fall into the category of neglect. Each type of abuse has distinct characteristics that may allow you to identify the child as an abuse victim (see Figure 22-7) in general, look for the following signs (see Figures 22-8 through 22-13):

■ The child is fretful, frightened of parents, afraid to go home, wary of adults, or apathetic (a child who does not cry, despite injuries)

■ Abrasions, lacerations, incisions, bruises, broken bones, or multiple injuries in various stages of healing

■ Injuries on both the front and the back or on both sides

■ Unusual wounds, such as circular burns

■ Injuries to the head, back, and abdomen, including the genitals

■ Pain, itching, bruises, or bleeding in the genital, vaginal, or anal areas

■ Injuries that do not match the mechanisms of injury described by the parents or caregivers

FIGURE 22–8. Signs of physical abuse

FIGURE 22–9. Signs of physical abuse—fractured humerus as a result of being shaken by the arm

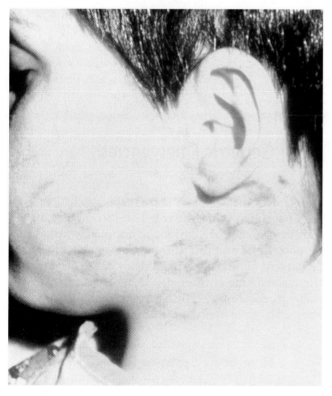

FIGURE 22–10. Signs of physical abuse—hand bruise on the face

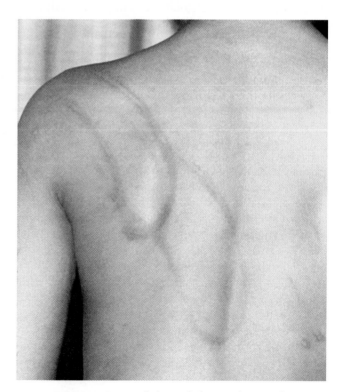

FIGURE 22–11. Signs of physical abuse—bruises from an electrical cord

FIGURE 22–12. Signs of physical abuse—restraining by tying

FIGURE 22–13. Signs of physical abuse—burns from foot held on an electric stove

FIRST AID CARE

1. Calm the parents; let them know by your actions that you are there to help and render first aid care. Speak in a low, firm voice.

2. Focus attention on the child; speak softly to the child, using the first name. Never ask the child to re-create the situation while in the crisis environment or with the suspected abuser still present.

3. Conduct a thorough, head-to-toe exam; care for injuries appropriately.

4. It is not your responsibility to confront any adult with the charge of child abuse; be supportive and nonjudgmental while at the scene.

5. *Always* report your suspicions of child abuse to the proper authorities, and maintain total confidentiality with others regarding the incident.

PROGRESS CHECK

1. Sudden infant death syndrome occurs when an apparently _____ infant dies while sleeping. *(distressed/healthy/ill)*

2. Even if a victim of SIDS is obviously dead, you should _____. *(begin infant CPR/treat for shock/do a primary survey)*

3. An abuser often shows _____ toward the child. *(compassion/guilt/hostility)*

4. Suspect child abuse if the child is _____. *(frightened of parents/clinging to parents/affectionate to parents)*

5. If you suspect child abuse, you should _____. *(confront the parents at the scene/report your suspicions to authorities/ask the child to confirm your suspicions)*

Caring for Yourself

Almost half of the children in the United States who die from accidents are pronounced dead either at the scene or as they arrive at the hospital. The sudden and/or violent death of a child, either before you arrive or while you are giving first aid, is emotionally wrenching. The possibility of child abuse or neglect can be especially difficult to deal with emotionally.

If you are faced with such a situation, control your emotions while at the scene so you can render the best possible care and so you can support other victims. After the case is over, however, it is important to talk about your feelings and sort through your emotions. If you do not, you may well develop worry about your own children or disturbing nightmares. If necessary, seek professional help or participate in stress debriefing.

22.4 Geriatric Emergencies

People over the age of 65 present special challenges to the First Aider. While the elderly represent a small but rapidly growing percent of the population, they take 30 percent of all prescription drugs and account for 25 percent of all fatal injuries. They have an average of three coexisting chronic diseases, take three times as many medications as the general population, and are affected by the physiology of aging.

How Body Systems Change with Age

Learning Objective **8** Explain how body systems change with age.

Body systems change with age (see Figure 22-14), affecting the signs and symptoms manifested in common medical emergencies. To complicate matters, many elderly people suffer from malnutrition and have a combination of different disease processes in varying stages of development. To give effective first aid, you need to recognize these changes (see Table 22-2 on page 366).

Differing Signs and Symptoms

While many medical problems present a standard set of signs and symptoms in the general population, the changes involved in the aging process can cause the following altered signs and symptoms in the elderly.

In myocardial infarction:

- Pain is less common.

- Aching shoulders and indigestion are common.

- The most common symptoms are shortness of breath, fatigue, and anxiety.

In congestive heart failure:

- Little or no dyspnea is present.

In pneumonia:

- Fever is usually absent (it is a classic sign of pneumonia in other age groups).

Neurological System
• Brain changes come with age.
• Clinical depression is common.
• Altered LOC is common.

Cardiovascular System
• Hypertension is common.
• There are changes in heart rate and rhythm.

Gastrointestinal System
• Constipation is common.
• Deterioration of structures in mouth is common.
• There is general decline in efficiency of liver.
• Swallowing is impaired.
• Malnutrition is result of deterioration of small intestine.

Musculoskeletal System
• Osteoporosis is common.
• Osteoarthritis is common.

Respiratory System
• Cough power is diminished.
• There is increased tendency for infection.
• There is less air and less exchange of gases due to general decline.

Renal System
• Drug toxicity problems are common.
• General decline in efficiency.

Skin
• Perspires less.
• Tears more easily.
• Heals slowly.

Immune System
• Fever is often absent.
• There is lessened ability to fight disease.

FIGURE 22–14. Physical changes in the elderly

TABLE 22-2	Physical Changes in the Elderly	
The System	**How It Changes**	**What the Changes Mean**
Cardiovascular	Calcium is deposited in areas of wear and tear; fibrous tissue thickens; vessels lose elasticity; the heart pumps less volume	Blood pressure increases; the heart rate may not increase, even with infection, shock, or stress
Musculoskeletal	Osteoporosis makes bones less dense	Susceptibility to fractures; delayed healing
Immune	Changes in the components of the immune system, weakening	Little or no fever in response to infection, recurrence of disease
Neurological	Conditions that accompany aging can aggravate dementia	Confusion; lack of accurate victim history
Gastrointestinal	Reduced salivary flow, deterioration of mouth structures	Susceptibility to various medical conditions and malnutrition
Renal	Kidneys become smaller; arteries that supply them become hard and brittle	Susceptibility to infection and disease
Skin	Becomes thin, tears easily; less attachment between layers; cells are produced less rapidly; less perspiration; dulled sense of touch	Susceptibility to injury; delayed healing; loss of protective barrier; inability to describe pain accurately
Respiratory	Calcium deposits in rib cage make it difficult for lungs to expand; less air enters lungs; less gas exchange; tissues degenerate; lungs lose elasticity; cilia are no longer as mobile	Susceptibility to infection; delayed recovery

- Chest pain is much less common.

- Cough is much less common.

Special Assessment Considerations

> Learning Objective 9 Explain special issues to consider in assessing the elderly.

Assessment of the elderly victim can be difficult; the following factors can complicate evaluation (see Figure 22-15):

- The elderly become debilitated much more rapidly; a minor problem can become major within a few hours.

- The victim may be taking a number of medications.

- As many as one in four elderly have psychiatric disorders, which can be the cause of some symptoms (such as clouding of consciousness).

- It can be difficult to separate the effects of aging from the consequences of disease.

- The victim's chief complaint may seem trivial.

- The victim may fail to report important symptoms.

- The geriatric victim is likely to suffer from more than one disease at a time.

- Aging may change the victim's response to illness and injury, causing you to underestimate the severity of the victim's condition.

FIGURE 22–15. It is often necessary to consider special issues when assessing an elderly victim.

- The elderly person's temperature-regulating mechanism may be depressed, leading to absence of fever even with severe infection.

- Communication problems are common because the senses diminish, especially sight and hearing.

- Common complaints of geriatric victims that may not be specific to any one disorder include fatigue and weakness, dizziness/vertigo/syncope, falls, headache, insomnia, loss of appetite, inability to void, and constipation/diarrhea.

Special Examination Considerations

Be alert to the following when examining an elderly victim:

- The victim may be fatigued easily.

- The victim may be wearing several layers of clothing.

- You need to explain actions clearly before assessing the elderly victim.

- The victim may minimize or deny symptoms out of fear of being bedridden or institutionalized or of losing a sense of self-sufficiency.

Special Trauma Considerations

Learning Objective **10** Discuss special issues to consider in caring for trauma in the elderly.

Situations that would call for basic care with victims in other age groups call for aggressive care in the elderly, and the elderly are at greater risk for sustaining traumatic injury because of the following factors:

- They may have slower reflexes, failing eyesight and hearing, arthritis, less elastic blood vessels, and fragile tissues and bones.

- They are at higher risk for trauma from criminal assault.

- They are prone to head injury, even from relatively minor trauma; signs and symptoms of brain compression develop more slowly, sometimes over days or weeks.

- They often have a significant degree of degenerative disease of the cervical vertebrae, which can gradually compress the roots of nerves to the arms or possibly to the spinal cord itself. Sudden neck movement, with or without fracture, can cause spinal cord injury.

PROGRESS CHECK

1. _____ is less common in elderly victims of myocardial infarction. *(Pain/Indigestion/Shortness of breath)*

2. There is usually little or no _____ in elderly victims of congestive heart failure. *(edema/cyanosis/dyspnea)*

3. _____, a classic sign of pneumonia, is usually absent in the elderly. *(Weakness/Pain/Fever)*

4. Signs or symptoms may be masked in elderly victims because they usually _____ . *(take multiple medications/are immobile/have failing eyesight)*

Summary

- When assessing a child, try to stay at the child's eye level, speak in a calm and quiet voice, avoid "baby talk," involve the parents, and save the most painful part of the assessment for last.

- Check a child's vital signs more frequently than you would an adult's; remember, too, that your overall impression of how the child looks and acts can be more important than any one vital sign.

- Children are more susceptible to head injury; blunt trauma of the liver, spleen, and kidneys; hypothermia, hyperthermia, and dehydration; and blocking of the airway by a relaxed tongue.

- A comparatively small blood loss in an adult can constitute major bleeding in a child.

- Respiratory problems—such as croup, epiglottitis, and asthma, are serious medical emergencies in children. Epiglottitis can cause death if untreated.

- Always initiate infant CPR in cases of sudden infant death syndrome, even when the baby is obviously dead.

- Never confront parents about child abuse at the scene; always report your suspicions to appropriate authorities later.

- The physiological changes of aging can make the elderly more susceptible to disease and can alter usual signs and symptoms as well.

- When assessing the elderly, remember that they often fail to report important symptoms, often take a combination of medications, and often have several coexisting chronic diseases.

Key Terms

Make sure you understand the following key terms:

croup
epiglottitis

sudden infant death syndrome (SIDS)

At a motor-vehicle accident, one of the victims is a 3-year-old in a safety seat. He is screaming at the top of his lungs, and he has a shallow gash in his thigh from which blood is oozing. His older sister has been thrown from the car and is unconscious. The driver is staggering up and down the road sobbing.

1. Who would you attend to first, and why?

2. How would you approach the child in the car seat for a physical assessment?

3. What would you do to try to calm the child in the car seat?

22 Chapter 22 Self-Test

Student: _____ Date: _____

Course: _____ Section #: _____

Part 1   True/False

If you believe the statement is true, circle the T. If you believe the statement is false, circle the F.

T   F   **1.** Do not allow a child victim to have any contact with his or her parents.

T   F   **2.** Get as close as you can to the child's eye level during assessment.

T   F   **3.** Children between the ages of 1 and 6 enjoy strangers and are usually easy to assess.

T   F   **4.** Never tell a child the truth about his or her pain.

T   F   **5.** Children are more susceptible than adults to respiratory problems.

T   F   **6.** The special needs of elderly people may require some modification of first aid techniques.

T   F   **7.** Elderly victims have more pain with myocardial infarction than younger victims.

T   F   **8.** The elderly are often taking several regular medications, which can mask signs and symptoms.

Part 2   Multiple Choice

For each item, circle the correct answer or the phrase that best completes the statement.

1. When assessing children, you should
   a. avoid "baby talk"
   b. perform the most painful part of the assessment first
   c. stay above the child's eye level
   d. keep the child and parents separated

2. In assessing infants or small children, you will be less effective if you
   a. are gentle
   b. talk quietly and calmly
   c. separate the child and parent
   d. allow the child to remain with a parent

3. In caring for a suspected victim of child abuse, you should *not*
   a. focus attention on the child while you give first aid care
   b. question the child about abuse in front of the parents
   c. make efforts to calm the parents
   d. report your suspicions of child abuse to proper authorities

4. When managing a SIDS situation, you should *not*
   a. immediately initiate infant CPR
   b. encourage parents to accompany their baby in the ambulance
   c. discuss a SIDS case with colleagues
   d. talk out your feelings after a SIDS emergency

5. In children up to age 2, seizures are often due to
   a. epilepsy
   b. fever
   c. hyperglycemia
   d. drowning

6. The major causes of shock in children are
   a. blood loss, fever, head injury
   b. near-drowning, respiratory distress, seizures
   c. blood loss, acute infection, heart failure
   d. fever, head injury, epiglottitis

7. SIDS most often occurs
   a. among twins or triplets
   b. in low-income families
   c. among very sick children
   d. while the baby is sleeping

8. Which of the following is not true of child abuse and neglect?
   a. abuse may be physical, emotional, or sexual
   b. the adult who abuses a child typically shows remorse
   c. signs of child abuse include abrasions, lacerations, and broken bones
   d. we do not really know how many children are abused

9. What changes take place in the immune system of the elderly as a result of infection?
   a. stress on the immune system is more likely to lead to fever
   b. the salivary glands degenerate
   c. the white cell count does not increase normally
   d. the cilia lose mobility

10. Which of the following factors tend to make assessment of the elderly more difficult?
   a. they may have multiple disorders
   b. they rarely take medications
   c. they usually report symptoms
   d. all of the above

23

Bites and Stings

Learning Objectives

When you have mastered the material in this chapter, you will be able to

1 Distinguish between poisonous and nonpoisonous snakes

2 List the factors that determine the severity of pit viper bite

3 List the signs and symptoms of a pit viper bite

4 List the signs and symptoms of a coral snake bite

5 Determine when medical help is needed for insect bite

6 List the signs and symptoms of black widow spider bite

7 Explain why the bite of the brown recluse spider is so serious

8 List the signs and symptoms of scorpion sting

9 List the signs and symptoms of anaphylactic shock

10 Identify the two important differences between the bites and stings of marine animals and those of land animals

11 Describe and demonstrate first aid care for bites and stings

12 Describe and demonstrate first aid care for marine life poisoning

13 Describe and demonstrate how to remove a tick

On the Scene

On a late October afternoon, 28-year-old Andrew Wyatt was clearing out a corner of his garage to make room for firewood. As he reached into a dark area behind some tools, he felt a definite pinprick on the back of his hand. Jerking his hand into the light, he examined it closely; he could not tell whether he had been bitten or had merely brushed his hand against the sharp edge of a tool. Dismissing the incident, Andrew went back to work.

Within about half an hour, Andrew realized his hand was aching. He also started having intense pain and spasms in his shoulders, back, and abdomen—far greater than the mild muscle stress he should have felt from the work he was doing. Alarmed, he walked next door and described his symptoms to Nate Ford, a trained First Aider and Scoutmaster.

Andrew was grimacing and his face was flushed. Placing the back of his hand against Andrew's skin, Nate found that Andrew was feverish. By then, Andrew was also complaining of headache and nausea. Nate suspected the bite of a black widow spider—a suspicion that was confirmed when the two of them returned to Andrew's garage and carefully moved a few tools in the corner to reveal the spider.

Nate reassured Andrew, then got him into the car. Nate draped his jacket over Andrew's chest to help preserve body warmth and placed a cold compress on his hand over the bite site. Nate then drove Andrew the 6 miles to a local medical center, where physicians took over caring for the bite.

nsect bites and stings are common, and most are considered minor. It is only when the insect is poisonous or when the victim has an allergic reaction and runs the risk of developing anaphylactic shock that the situation becomes an emergency.

Proper first aid care for insect bites and stings and for snakebite can save lives and prevent permanent tissue damage. This chapter outlines the kinds of bites and stings that are of special concern, lists signs and symptoms, and provides basic guidelines for first aid care.

23.1 Snakebite

Learning Objective **1** Distinguish between poisonous and nonpoisonous snakes.

Approximately 50,000 people are bitten by snakes every year in the United States; of those, 8,000 are bitten by poisonous snakes; fewer than five of those die. There are only four kinds of poisonous snakes native to the United States: rattlesnakes, coral snakes, water moccasins (also known as cottonmouths), and copperheads (Figures 23-1 through 23-4). Rarely, a victim may be bitten by a poisonous exotic snake that has been smuggled or imported into the United States. Fewer than 12 people die each year in the United States from snakebite, almost all from rattlesnake bite. (Though coral snakes are actually more poisonous, their teeth are small and slanted backward, making it difficult for them to inject very much venom.) Most who die from snakebite do so because of an allergic reaction or because of existing poor health.

Nonpoisonous snakebites are not considered serious and are generally treated as minor wounds; only poisonous snakebites are considered medical emergencies. Symptoms generally occur immediately, but only occur in about one-third of all poisonous snakebites; the majority of people do not have symptoms, usually because no venom was injected into the victim.

Most poisonous snakes have the following characteristics:

- Large fangs; nonpoisonous snakes have small teeth. The exception is the **coral snake**, a poisonous snake that has small teeth rather than fangs.

- Vertical slits for pupils, much like those of a cat, (**elliptical pupils**); nonvenomous snakes have round pupils.

- A heat-sensitive pit between the eye and the nostril on each side of the head. This identifies the snake as a **pit viper**. (It's not important to distinguish what species a pit viper is, since the same antivenin is used to treat all pit viper bites in North America.)

- A variety of differently shaped blotches on a background of pink, yellow, olive, tan, gray, or brown skin. The exception is the coral snake, which is ringed with red, yellow, and black.

- The triangular head is larger than the neck.

FIGURE 23–1. Western diamondback rattlesnake

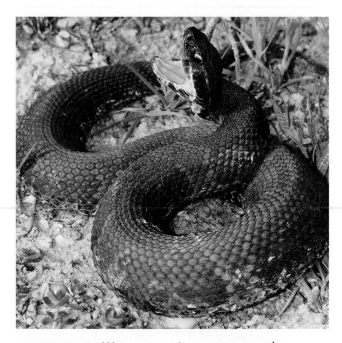

FIGURE 23–2. Water moccasin or cottonmouth

coral snake A type of poisonous snake that does not have a pit or fang

elliptical pupils Pupils that are vertical slits, like those of a cat

pit viper A type of poisonous snake, such as a rattlesnake, characterized by a pit between the eyes and nostril

FIGURE 23–3. Coral snake

FIGURE 23–4. Copperhead

Be aware that pit vipers can still bite for a time after they are dead (usually about 20 minutes).

Severity of Snakebite

Learning Objective 2 List the factors that determine the severity of a pit viper bite.

The severity of a pit viper bite is gauged by how rapidly symptoms develop, which depends on how much poison was injected. Adult snakes inject more venom, but the venom of young snakes is three times more poisonous. Other factors that determine the severity of a snakebite include the following:

- The location of the bite (fatty tissue absorbs the venom more slowly than muscle tissue)

- Whether disease-causing organisms are in the venom

- The size and weight of the victim

- The general health and condition of the victim

- How much physical activity the victim engaged in immediately following the bite (physical activity helps spread venom)

A nonpoisonous snake leaves a horseshoe-shaped bite pattern. Be aware, however, that some nonpoisonous snakes do have venom that can cause discomfort. As a general rule, you can safely assume that the victim has not been poisoned if the burning pain characteristic of pit viper bite does not develop within 1 hour of the bite.

Signs and Symptoms of Snakebite

Learning Objective 3 List the signs and symptoms of a pit viper bite.

The signs and symptoms of pit viper bite (see Figures 23-5 through 23-7) include

- Two distinct fang marks about half an inch apart at the bite site, which may or may not bleed (in some cases there may be only one fang mark)

FIGURE 23–5. Snakebite to the hand

FIGURE 23–6. Rattlesnake bite

MOTION OF STRIKE:
Shallow, slanting penetration is typical of snakebite, since snakes tend to hold the head level when striking. Wound depth and venom deposit vary with the species, the length of the fangs, and the snake's excitement. Even if the 1¼ inch fangs of the Eastern diamondback rattlesnake penetrate almost their full length, the slanting wound may be no more than ¼ inch from the skin surface.

Fang

Pit

Bite pattern:

Elliptical pupil

Poison gland

- Immediate burning pain
- Swelling, discoloration
- Distinct puncture wound
- Blood oozing from wound

FIGURE 23–7. Poisonous snakebites

- Immediate and severe burning pain and swelling around the fang marks, usually within 5 minutes but sometimes taking as long as 4 hours to develop (swelling may affect the entire arm or leg)
- Purplish discoloration and blood-filled blisters around the bite, usually within 2 to 10 hours
- Numbness around the bite

In cases of severe reaction, the victim may experience:

- Nausea and vomiting
- Rapid heartbeat
- Low blood pressure
- Weakness and fainting
- Numbness and tingling of the tongue and mouth
- Excessive sweating
- Fever and chills
- Muscular twitching
- Convulsions
- Dimmed vision
- Headache
- A minty, metallic, or rubbery taste in the month

> **Learning Objective 4** List the signs and symptoms of coral snake bite.

The signs and symptoms of coral snake bite include:

- One or more tiny scratch marks in the area of the bite (a coral snake "chews" its victim), usually in a semicircle pattern
- A minty, metallic, or rubbery taste in the mouth
- Little or no pain and swelling
- Little or no discoloration
- Blurred vision and drooping eyelids
- Slurred speech
- Increased salivation and sweating
- Drowsiness
- Difficulty in breathing
- Nausea and vomiting
- Shock
- Paralysis
- Coma

The signs and symptoms of a pit viper bite generally occur immediately; those of a coral snake bite are usually delayed by at least 1 and as many as 8 hours. Treatment for snakebite is discussed later in this chapter.

23.2 Insect Bites and Stings

For most people, insect bites and stings are uncomfortable or even painful, but not life threatening, and first aid care is aimed at reducing pain and discomfort. Specific insects inflict bites or stings that cause specific signs and symptoms; for example, the bite of a black widow spider results in signs and symptoms different from the bite of a fire ant or a tick. However, some general signs and symptoms apply to all insect bites and stings:

- A mark from the bite or sting
- Pain or tenderness at and surrounding the bite or sting
- Redness at and surrounding the bite or sting
- Swelling around the bite or sting
- A venom sac, stinger, tentacle, or other remnant of the insect at the bite or sting

Various factors affect how serious the signs and symptoms are. The victim's age, size, and weight impact his or her reaction to a bite or sting; reactions are generally more severe in infants and the elderly. Other factors include the location of the bite or sting (most serious are bites and stings on the face), how much poison was injected with the bite or sting, and how much time has elapsed since the bite or sting occurred.

Allergic reactions to insect bites and stings cause more pronounced signs and symptoms. Approximately 1 of every 200 Americans have severe allergy to the stings of bees, wasps, hornets, and yellow jackets. *Severe allergic reactions result in a life-threatening condition called anaphylactic shock*, which will be discussed later in this chapter. As part of first aid care, you should always monitor the victim for signs of developing allergic reaction and be prepared to get medical help immediately should that occur.

Learning Objective **5** Determine when medical help is needed for insect bite.

Most insect bites are treated like any other wound. Generally, medical help is necessary only if any of these conditions are present:

- Itching lasts longer than 2 days.
- Signs of infection develop.
- Signs of an allergic reaction develop.
- The insect is poisonous, most often black widow or brown recluse spiders (which can be fatal).

General first aid care for insect bites and stings is found later in this chapter.

Black Widow Spider

Learning Objective **6** List the signs and symptoms of black widow spider bite.

The **black widow spider** (see Figure 23-8 on page 376) is generally characterized by a shiny black body, thin legs, and a crimson red marking on its abdomen underside, usually in the shape of an hourglass or two triangles. *Note:* Of the five species in the United States, only three are black (the others are brown and gray), and not all have the characteristic red marking. Black widow spiders are usually found in dry, secluded, dimly lit areas; they have extremely strong, funnel-shaped webs. They are found throughout the United States.

Black widow spider bites are the most painful type of spider bite and are the leading cause of death from spider bites in the United States. Those at highest risk

black widow spider A poisonous spider identified by a red mark shaped like an hourglass on its underside

FIGURE 23–8. Black widow spider

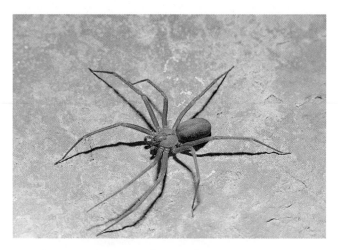

FIGURE 23–9. Brown recluse spider

FIGURE 23–10. Brown recluse spider bite

for developing severe reactions to bites are children under the age of 16, adults over the age of 60, people with chronic illness, and anyone with chronic high blood pressure. Get medical help; an antivenin is available for black widow spider bites.

In addition to the general signs and symptoms of bites and stings, black widow spider bites cause:

- Sharp pinprick pain at the site, followed by dull pain in the area of the bite (pain peaks in 2 to 3 hours and lasts 12 to 48 hours)

- Small red fang marks

- Severe muscle spasms and rigidity, especially in the shoulders, back, chest, and abdomen, starting within 1 to 4 hours of the bite

- Fever and chills

- Profuse sweating

- Headache and dizziness

- Restlessness

- Anxiety

- Nausea and vomiting

- Weakness

- Drooping eyelids

Brown Recluse Spider

> Learning Objective **7** Explain why the bite of the brown recluse spider is so serious.

The **brown recluse spider** (see Figure 23-9) is generally brown but can range in color from yellow to dark chocolate brown, with darker legs. The characteristic marking is a brown, violin-shaped marking on the upper back. In the United States, brown recluse spiders are found mostly in the southern and midwestern states; there are none in the Pacific northwest.

The bite of the brown recluse spider creates a serious medical condition: the bite does not heal, and requires surgical repair (see Figure 23-10).

The brown recluse spider bites only when it is trapped against the skin. Unfortunately, most victims are unaware that they have been bitten, because the bite is often painless at first. Initial signs and symptoms include redness with moderate itching and swelling at the site of the bite. Several hours after the bite, the site becomes bluish and a blood-filled blister appears beneath the skin; the blister may be surrounded by a white periphery or a red halo in a bull's-eye pattern. Within 7 to 10 days, the bite becomes a large ulcer. It continues to scab over; then the scab falls off to reveal an even larger ulcer (sometimes called a *volcano lesion*). This cycle continues until the victim receives surgery and skin grafting.

> **brown recluse spider** A brown poisonous spider identified by a violin-shaped mark on its back; brown recluse spider bites do not heal and require surgical grafting

Several other spiders can cause unusual irritation, but are not fatal. The "hobo" spider (the common aggressive house spider) is common in the Pacific Northwest. Its bites cause signs and symptoms similar to bites of the brown recluse spider. Tarantulas, when threatened, flick hairs onto the victim's skin that can cause hives for as long as three weeks. Although they look menacing, they usually bite only if they are extremely provoked.

Scorpion

> Learning Objective **8** List the signs and symptoms of scorpion sting.

Other than the black widow and brown recluse spiders, the other most potentially dangerous arachnids are scorpions. Scorpions are found throughout most of Mexico; in the United States, scorpions (Figure 23-11) are found in the desert Southwest and in dry areas of Utah and Nevada. Of the three species of scorpion in the United States that sting and inject poisonous venom, only the venom of one is generally fatal. The severity of the sting depends on the amount of venom injected. Ninety percent of all scorpion stings occur on the hands.

Though scorpions have a pair of crablike pincers, the stinger that injects the venom is actually at the end of the tail. Most stings occur at night, when scorpions are the most active.

In addition to the general signs and symptoms of bites and stings, scorpion stings cause sharp pain at the sting site that is followed by numbness or tingling. Other signs and symptoms may include swelling (swelling does not always occur), a blister or lesion at the site of the bite, profuse sweating or salivation, abdominal pain, muscle cramping, nausea and vomiting, difficulty breathing or swallowing, and irregular heartbeat. In cases of severe reaction, the victim will experience drooling, poor coordination, incontinence, and seizures. Death from scorpion sting is rare.

Because it is difficult to tell which scorpions are poisonous, you should treat any scorpion sting as an emergency and seek immediate medical help. Antivenin is available for scorpion venom.

Fire Ants

Most common in the southeastern United States, fire ants get their name not from their color (which may range from red to black), but from the intense, fiery, burning pain their bite causes.

Fire ants bite down into the skin, then pivot, using their tail stingers repeatedly; the result is a characteristic circular pattern of stings (see Figure 23-12). Fire ant stings produce extremely painful blisters that are filled with fluid. At first the fluid is clear; later it becomes cloudy. Fire ant stings can also cause a large local reaction, characterized by swelling, pain, and redness that affect the entire area. Fire ant stings can cause anaphylactic shock, though that is not common. Deaths are rare.

Ticks

Tick bites are serious because ticks can carry and transmit to humans tick fever, Rocky Mountain spotted fever, and other bacterial diseases. The deer tick can also transmit Lyme disease, which can cause long-term neurologic complications.

FIGURE 23–11. Scorpion

FIGURE 23–12. Fire ant bites

Rocky Mountain spotted fever occurs throughout North and South America, and is not more common in the Rocky Mountain area—though that is where it was first identified. It gets its name in part from the spotted rash that appears soon after the victim is infected; the rash often starts on the wrists or ankles, but it spreads fairly rapidly to other areas of the body. Other signs and symptoms of Rocky Mountain spotted fever include severe headache, muscle aches, joint aches, and fever and chills. Without early medical intervention, the infection becomes extremely dangerous; untreated, victims die from kidney failure or shock.

Once somewhat isolated, Lyme disease has now been identified in more than 40 states. Deer ticks are found on beaches as well as in grassy and wooded areas. Because they are extremely small (about the size of a poppy seed), many people are unaware that they have been bitten. The majority of Lyme disease cases occur in May and June. The disease begins with a rash, which may look like a black-and-blue bruise, then develops slowly into flu-like symptoms. Over a period of years, if left untreated, it causes memory loss, vision disturbances, and arthritis.

Ticks (see Figure 23-13) are visible after they have attached themselves to the skin and have become engorged with blood; they often choose warm, moist areas, such as the scalp, other hairy areas such as the armpits or the groin, and skin creases. Tick bites are generally painless; many victims are unaware that they have been bitten and do not even see the tick at first. As the tick becomes engorged with blood, it can become as much as 50 times larger.

The only appropriate first aid care for tick bite is prompt removal of the tick, which can help prevent infection. Never pluck an embedded tick out of the skin; you may force infected blood into the victim. For information about safe tick removal, see "Removing a Tick" later in this chapter.

Centipedes

Various species of centipedes are found throughout the world. The only centipede in the United States whose bite is dangerous to humans is the giant desert centipede, which can be as long as 8 inches. Contrary to myth, they do not sting with their feet; they bite, injecting venom with fangs. In addition to causing redness and swelling, the bite of a centipede can cause swollen lymph glands. Symptoms may last for as long as three weeks.

Insect Stings

The stinging insects include the honeybee, bumblebee, wasp, hornet, and yellow jacket. Most are aggressive only when their hives or nests are disturbed, or when they feel threatened, though one fairly new breed of "Africanized" bees, or "killer" bees, (a cross between African bees and more placid European bees) are much more aggressive. Though swarms are rare, any of the stinging insects may sting in swarms. Honeybees and bumblebees leave the stinger and venom sac behind, embedded in the skin, so they can sting only once; hornets and wasps do not lose their stingers, so they can sting repeatedly. Figure 23-14 shows the wasps, bees, and fire ants that commonly attack humans.

The normal reaction to an insect sting is a sharp, stinging pain followed by an itchy, swollen, painful wheal. Redness, tenderness, and swelling at or around the sting site—even if severe—is considered to be a local reaction in the absence of other symptoms. Local reactions are rarely serious or life threatening. Stings on the face, especially the mouth or eyes, are considered more serious, even if the reaction is local. Most serious are stings inside the mouth or throat, which usually occur when the insect is accidentally swallowed.

Anaphylactic Shock

Learning Objective **9** List the signs and symptoms of anaphylactic shock.

Almost 2 million Americans are severely allergic to the venom of bees, wasps, hornets, and yellow jackets. Allergic reactions, which cause anaphylactic shock, are much more serious than local reactions. For people with allergies, a single sting may cause death—on the average, within 10 minutes of the sting, but almost always within the first hour, making it critical to get

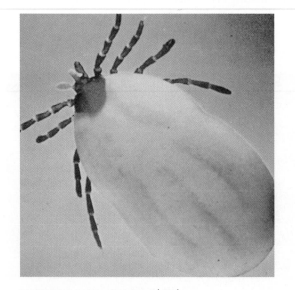

FIGURE 23-13. Engorged tick

The following members of this group can attack humans, causing local pain, redness, swelling, and subsequent itching. Always consider the possibility of anaphylaxis.

HONEYBEE: Found throughout the United States at any time of the year, except in colder temperatures when they remain in their hives. In the Northeast and Midwest, they are the insects most likely to cause sting reactions. Hives are usually found in hollowed out areas such as dead tree trunks. Honeybees principally ingest nectar of plants, so they are often seen in the vicinity of flowers. The honeybee loses its barbed stinger after a sting, leaving the venom sac and stinger in place in the wound.

YELLOW JACKET: A principal insect causing sting reactions in the Northeast and Midwest. Yellow jackets tend to be prevalent in late summer and fall. Nests are located in the ground. Often seen in picnic areas and garbage cans, yellow jackets are ill-tempered and aggressive and can deliver multiple stings at one time. They often sting without being provoked.

WASPS: The most likely insect to cause sting reactions in the Southeast and Southwest. Wasps tend to nest in small numbers under the eaves of houses and buildings. They are carnivores that are found in picnic areas, garbage cans, and food stands. Can deliver multiple stings at one time.

YELLOW HORNET AND WHITE-FACED OR BALD-FACED HORNET: Seen mainly in the spring and early summer. Nests usually found in branches and bushes above ground. They are carnivores that are seen in picnic areas, garbage cans, and food stands. Can deliver multiple stings at one time.

FIRE ANT: Fire ants can range from red to black and live in loose dirt mounds. They are found throughout the southern states as far west as New Mexico. Fire ants may cause serious illness and/or anaphylaxis. The ant attaches itself to the skin with its strong jaws and swivels its tail stinger about, inflicting repeated stings.

FIGURE 23–14. Wasps, bees, and fire ants
Adapted with permission from: John W. Georgitis. "Insect Stings—Responding to the Gamut of Allergic Reactions," *Modern Medicine*.

immediate medical help. It is also critical to remove an embedded stinger within 20 to 30 seconds to reduce the amount of residual venom that is injected. The sooner the symptoms occur, the more serious the reaction and the greater the threat of death. More than a hundred people in the United States are killed every year by insect stings; most deaths (approximately 80 percent) are caused when swelling of the airway obstructs the breathing.

Many people who are allergic to insect stings don't know it; only 15 percent have had previous allergic reactions to stings. The range of signs and symptoms of allergic reaction and anaphylactic shock include:

- Nausea and vomiting
- Itching of the throat
- Faintness
- Dizziness
- Generalized itching
- Hives
- Redness of the skin
- Generalized swelling, including the eyelids, lips, and tongue
- Upper airway obstruction
- Difficulty swallowing
- Shortness of breath, wheezing, or stridor
- Drippy nose
- Labored breathing
- Abdominal cramps
- Confusion
- Loss of consciousness
- Convulsions
- Low blood pressure

Victims of anaphylactic shock need rapid medical care. Activate the EMS system immediately. If the victim has a sting kit, help him use it. Monitor airway, breathing, and circulation until emergency personnel arrive.

PROGRESS CHECK

1. In addition to general signs of insect bite, a sign of black widow bite is _____ . *(cramps/ulcerated skin/fluid-filled blisters)*

2. A brown recluse spider bite is especially serious because it _____ . *(causes neurological damage/does not heal/goes unnoticed)*

3. Fire ants sting in a characteristic _____ pattern. *(circular/parallel/random)*

4. Ticks can cause a serious problem because they carry _____ . *(meningitis/encephalitis/Rocky Mountain spotted fever)*

5. Anaphylactic shock is a severe _____ that can cause death within a few minutes. *(sting/allergic reaction/venom)*

6. _____ leave the stinger behind, so they can sting only once. *(Wasps/Hornets/Bees)*

23.3 Marine Life Bites and Stings

Learning Objective **10** Identify the two important differences between the bites and stings of marine animals and those of land animals.

There are approximately 2,000 poisonous marine animals. While most live in temperate or tropical waters, they can be found in virtually all waters. Most are not aggressive; in fact, most marine life poisoning occurs when a victim swims into or steps on an animal. Bites and stings, when they do occur, are not only painful, but can cause serious illness. Allergic reactions to the venom can cause breathing problems, heart problems, and paralysis.

Some marine animals—such as eels or sharks—inflict injury by biting or ripping the soft tissues. Shark bites are considered the most devastating of all animal bites, and cause injury much like that of a chainsaw. Others—such as the stingray—cause puncture wounds with their spines. And still other marine animals—including the coral, anemone, and jellyfish, among others—sting their victims.

There are two important differences between the bites and stings of marine animals and those of land animals. First, the venom of marine life may cause more extensive tissue damage than that of land animals. Second, venoms of marine organisms are destroyed by heat, so heat—not ice—should be applied to marine bites and stings.

In cases of bites and stings by marine life, try to identify the animal—some very effective antivenins are available. Figures 23-15 through 23-25 illustrate several types of marine life. Figures 23-26 and 23-27 show the stings of jellyfish and stingray.

First aid care for marine animal bites and stings is discussed later in this chapter.

FIGURE 23–15. Jellyfish

FIGURE 23–16. Southern stingray

FIGURE 23–17. Tentacles of the Portuguese man-of-war

FIGURE 23–18. Lionfish

FIGURE 23–19. Feather hydroid

FIGURE 23–20. Sea anemone and clownfish

FIGURE 23–21. Fire coral

FIGURE 23–22. Crown-of-thorns starfish

FIGURE 23–23. Sea urchin

FIGURE 23–24. Scorpion fish

FIGURE 23–25. Moray eel

FIGURE 23–26. Jellyfish sting

FIGURE 23-27. Stingray sting

FIGURE 23-28. Scraping a honeybee stinger away with the edge of a credit card

PROGRESS CHECK

1. Poisonous forms of marine life are found in _____ waters. *(temperate/tropical/all)*

2. The venom of marine animals causes _____ tissue damage than that of poisonous land animals. *(less extensive/more extensive/more varied)*

3. The venom of marine animals is destroyed by _____ *(cold/heat/antiseptics)*

23.4 First Aid for Bites and Stings

Learning Objective 11 Describe and demonstrate first aid care for bites and stings.

General First Aid Care

In any case of a bite or sting, monitor the victim continuously for signs or symptoms of an allergic reaction. For general first aid care, activate the EMS system if the victim's condition warrants it; then:

1. If the stinger is still present, remove it by gently scraping against it with the edge of a credit card (see Figure 23-28), the edge of a knife, or your fingernail. Be careful not to squeeze the stinger with tweezers, forceps, or your fingers; doing so can force additional venom from the venom sac into the wound. (Make sure you remove the venom sac—it can continue to secrete venom even though the stinger is detached from the insect.)

2. Wash the area around the bite or sting gently with a soap solution; if necessary, irrigate the area with a large amount of clean water. Never scrub the area; venom makes the tissues fragile. Make sure that the liquids flow away from the body to prevent further contamination.

3. Remove any jewelry or other constricting objects as soon as possible—ideally, before any swelling begins.

4. Lower the site of the bite or sting slightly below the level of the victim's heart.

5. Apply a cold compress to the site of an insect bite or scorpion sting to relieve pain and swelling. Do not apply cold to snakebites; apply heat to injuries inflicted by marine animals.

6. Apply a paste of baking soda and water to relieve the pain of bee sting. Use vinegar or lemon juice to relieve the pain of a wasp sting. You can also take aspirin (for adults only) or acetaminophen to relieve the pain of insect stings.

7. Observe the victim carefully for at least 30 minutes to determine whether he or she is developing the signs and symptoms of an allergic reaction (see Figure 23-29); treat as needed. For guidelines on the treatment of anaphylactic shock, see Chapter 6.

8. Keep the victim calm, limit physical activity, and keep the victim warm; arrange for transport as soon as possible. If the victim shows any signs of allergic reaction, the victim needs to be transported immediately.

9. Help a victim who carries an insect sting kit to use the kit as he/she has been instructed to do (see Figures 23-30 and 23-31).

First Aid Care for Snakebite

Specific treatment for snakebite varies, depending on the kind of snake involved. The most important thing you can do for a victim of poisonous snakebite is to get

FIRST AID CARE:

Place ice pack over sting site.

Assist patient with medication from in-sect sting kit (if a kit is available and state and local protocols allow you to do so).

Carefully scrape stinger and venom sac away.

Immediate care and transport to a medical facility are necessary to prevent death.

ALLERGIC MANIFESTATIONS:

Mild symptoms may be itching of eyes, mouth, or ears, flushing of skin, widespread hives, and a dry cough.

A moderate reaction can include abdominal pain, nausea and vomiting, constricted feeling in the throat and chest, or wheezing.

A severe reaction can include all symptoms listed above, plus confusion, anxiety, hoarseness, dyspnea, or weakness.

Maintain an open airway and monitor vital signs throughout. If patient is cyanotic, adminis-ter oxygen. Be prepared to manage respiratory arrest.

FIGURE 23–29. Allergic reaction to insect venom

FIGURE 23–30. Assist the victim who has a history of allergic reactions to insect stings and carries a sting kit.

FIGURE 23–31. Administering an EpiPen for anaphylactic shock caused by insect sting

immediate medical treatment. Antivenin must be given within four hours.

Standards for first aid care have changed signifi-cantly over the years amid considerable controversy. Regardless of the type of snakebite, never

- Cut the skin, which can cause infection
- Use a tourniquet, which can result in loss of a limb
- Apply ice, which causes more rapid absorption of the venom
- Use electric shock, which can cause severe injury

Instead, do the following:

1. Treat a *nonpoisonous snakebite* as you would any minor wound; clean with soap and water, cover with a dry sterile dressing, and seek medical advice.

2. For *pit viper bite*, move the victim away from the snake (they will bite more than once, and can strike half their body length). Keep the victim calm and quiet; if possible, the victim should not walk. Clean the bite with soap and water, then splint the affected extremity. Seek medical attention *immediately*; antivenin is available only in hospitals (partly because of its short shelf life) and must be administered within 4 hours.

3. For *coral snake bite*, gently wash the bite with soap and water and wrap the entire extremity with several elastic bandages, exerting moderate pressure to slow the spread of venom. Use overlapping turns to keep the pressure from the bandage firm, beginning at the end of the limb farthest from the heart; gently stretch the bandage as you wrap. Use figure-eight turns around the knee or elbow. When you have finished, the bandage should be firm, but you should be able to slip your finger under the bandage. Leave the toes or fingers exposed so you can check for any kind of discoloration, which would indicate that the bandage is wrapped too tightly; the victim should also stay alert for numbness or tingling in the fingers or toes, which also indicate that the bandage is too tight. Seek medical attention immediately: An effective antivenin is available.

If you are more than an hour from medical care and *if* you are trained to use the Extractor™ (commercial suction device), use it to suction the wound. Never cut the skin; suction for 30 minutes. You must still get medical help, since the Extractor™ removes at most 30 percent of the venom.

First Aid Care for Marine Life Poisoning

Learning Objective 12 Describe and demonstrate first aid care of marine life poisoning.

In general, bites and stings inflicted by marine life should be treated the same as soft-tissue injuries. However, follow these specific guidelines as needed:

- If the injury occurred in the water, move the victim to a dry area as quickly as possible.

- If the victim was stung by a stingray, spiny fish, or sea urchin, flush the site with water (you can use sea water), immobilize the site, and soak it in hot water for 30 minutes; the water should be as hot as the victim can stand, without being hot enough to scald the skin. Then clean and cover the wound.

- If the victim was stung by a jellyfish, Portuguese man-of-war, coral, hydra, or anemone, carefully remove dried tentacles; do not rub the tentacles or touch them with your bare hands. Pour vinegar on the affected area or soak the affected area in vinegar to denature the toxin. If you don't have vinegar, use rubbing alcohol or a baking soda paste. Never rinse the site with ammonia or fresh water; fresh water can cause the stinging mechanism to fire. Do not use meat tenderizer—the active ingredient that helped reduce pain is no longer an ingredient in most brands of meat tenderizer.

- If the victim was stung by a sponge or bristleworm, apply white woodworking glue to the sting; allow it to dry, peel it off, and apply cortisone cream.

- If the victim was stung by an octopus, cone shell, or sea snake, use the Extractor™ to suction the wound for 30 minutes, then wrap the entire extremity with several elastic bandages to achieve compression.

- Use tweezers to remove any material that sticks to the sting site on the surface of the flesh, then irrigate the wound with hot water.

- Never try to remove spines that are embedded in joints, deeply embedded in skin, or embedded in areas richly supplied by nerves or blood vessels.

- Apply heat or soak the affected area in hot water for at least 30 minutes.

- Have the victim check with a doctor to see if a tetanus shot is needed.

Activate the EMS system immediately if:

- The victim does not know what stung him or her

- The victim is having trouble breathing

- The sting is on the face or neck

- The victim has had allergic reactions to previous marine animal stings

- The victim is bleeding heavily

Removing a Tick

Learning Objective 13 Describe and demonstrate how to remove a tick.

A tick's mouth has a barb that helps it attach to its victim. *You should never try to remove a tick that is embedded in the skin.* If the tick's head is attached to the skin but the tick's body is not embedded in the skin, you should wear gloves and use a pair of tweezers to remove the tick. Use fine-tipped, pointed tweezers that are not rasped or etched. In an emergency, if you do not have gloves, protect your fingers from contacting the tick by using tissue, plastic wrap, or paper wrapped around your fingers. To remove a tick that is not embedded in the skin:

1. Using fine-tipped tweezers, grasp the tick as close as possible to the point where it is attached to the skin. If you do not have tweezers, use your fingers, making sure to avoid direct contact with the tick.

2. Pull slowly, firmly, and steadily until the tick is dislodged. Do not twist or jerk the tick, because that may result in incomplete removal. Avoid squashing an engorged tick during removal, because infected blood may spread contamination.

3. Wash the bite area thoroughly with soap and water and apply an antiseptic or antibiotic ointment to the area.

4. Apply a cold pack or use Calamine lotion to relieve any pain and swelling.

5. Encourage the victim to report the tick bite to a doctor. Redness at the site is not serious, but a rash or flu-like symptoms that develop later could indicate disease.

Never use a hot match, gasoline, rubbing alcohol, petroleum jelly, or fingernail polish to remove a tick. All have been shown to be ineffective and using them could injure the victim.

Seek medical help if:

- You cannot remove the tick
- Part of the tick remains in the skin after you have removed it
- The tick is embedded in the skin

PROGRESS CHECK

1. To remove a stinger, _____ it. (squeeze/twist/scrape)

2. Apply _____ to all bites except snakebite and those of marine animals. (antiseptic/heat/cold)

3. Monitor the victim continuously for signs of_____ . (anaphylactic shock/dyspnea/rapid pulse)

4. Pour _____ on marine life stings to denature the toxin. (rubbing alcohol /vinegar /hydrogen peroxide)

5. Remove the barbs of marine life unless they are embedded in _____ . (the chest/a joint/the abdomen)

6. When you remove a tick, be careful not to _____ it. (squeeze/break/twist)

Summary

- Most poisonous snakes have large fangs, elliptical pupils, and a characteristic pit between the eye and the nostril on each side of the head. The exception is the coral snake, which has small teeth and round pupils.

- The signs and symptoms of pit viper bite occur almost immediately; those of coral snake bite may be delayed by as long as 8 hours.

- Pit viper bites cause severe, burning pain and marked swelling; coral snake bites cause little or no pain or swelling.

- Generally, medical help is not needed for insect bites unless itching persists for longer than 2 days, infection develops, there are signs of allergic reaction, or the insect is poisonous. Otherwise, insect bites are cared for the same as other wounds.

- The bite of a black widow spider causes pain and spasms in the shoulders, back, chest, and abdomen and a rigid, boardlike abdomen.

- The bite of the brown recluse spider is especially serious because it does not heal; surgical grafting is necessary.

- Tick bites are especially serious because ticks carry disease, such as Lyme disease and Rocky Mountain spotted fever.

- Marine life venom causes more widespread tissue damage than venom from land animals, and it is destroyed by heat rather than cold.

Key Terms

Make sure you understand the following key terms:

coral snake
elliptical pupils
pit viper

black widow spider
brown recluse spider

Critical Thinking Exercise

It is a beautiful fall day in southern Utah, and you are hiking in Zion National Park. You are enjoying the spectacular views of fortress-like red rock splashed with the green of juniper trees. Suddenly a hiker approximately 50 feet behind you screams. As you quickly turn to ascertain what caused the scream, you see the crying victim holding her lower right leg and just barely catch the image of a tan/rust colored snake slithering into the underbrush. You immediately move to the victim.

1. What immediate first action would you take?

2. If the victim confirms your suspicion of snakebite, what signs and symptoms would you look for?

3. What would cause you to suspect a rattlesnake bite?

4. If you suspect a pit viper bite, what first aid would you administer?

Chapter 23 Self-Test

Student: _____   Date: _____

Course: _____   Section #:_____

Part 1   True/False

If you believe the statement is true, circle the T. If you believe the statement is false, circle the F.

T   F   **1.** Two of the most common signs and symptoms of pit viper bite are immediate and severe burning pain and swelling.

T   F   **2.** Ice should be applied to pit viper bites.

T   F   **3.** Coral snake bites leave the same distinct fang marks as a pit viper bite.

T   F   **4.** Venoms of marine animals are destroyed by heat.

T   F   **5.** Tentacle stings from a jellyfish should be cleansed with rubbing alcohol.

Part 2   Multiple Choice

For each item, circle the correct answer or the phrase that best completes the statement.

1. Most poisonous snakes have
   a. multicolored rings around the body
   b. elliptical pupils
   c. small teeth
   d. flat heads

2. Venoms of aquatic organisms
   a. may cause severe vomiting
   b. can cause anaphylactic shock
   c. are destroyed by heat
   d. are activated by cold

3. Which of the following is *not* a symptom of coral snake bite?
   a. blurred vision
   b. paralysis
   c. black and blue discoloration
   d. drowsiness and slurred speech

4. Coral snakes inject poison through
   a. long fangs in the forward part of the upper jaw
   b. long fangs in both the upper and lower jaw
   c. a chewing motion
   d. long fangs in the lower jaw

5. The first step in providing first aid care for a honeybee sting is to
   a. grasp the stinger with a pair of tweezers and gently pull it out
   b. apply wet mud to the sting area; let it dry
   c. apply baking soda to the affected area
   d. remove the stinger by scraping it gently

6. Which of the following is recommended in the care of marine life poisoning?
   a. apply heat
   b. carefully remove tentacles or other material on the surface of the skin
   c. irrigate the wound with water
   d. all of the above

7. Which of the following is *not* a sign or symptom of a poisonous snakebite?
   a. severe pain and burning
   b. swelling of the wound
   c. discoloration of the wound
   d. a series of small, shallow puncture wounds

8. Characteristics of the majority of poisonous snakes include
   a. irregularly shaped blotches on the skin
   b. fangs
   c. elliptical pupils
   d. all of the above

Part 3   Matching

Match each characteristic with the type of snake.

Characteristic   **Snake**

1. _____ Bite is a series of small, shallow puncture wounds   **A.** Poisonous
2. _____ Wound begins to swell and discolor   **B.** Nonpoisonous
3. _____ Differently shaped blotches on background of pink, yellow, olive, tan, gray, or brown skin
4. _____ Elliptical pupils
5. _____ Large, triangular head
6. _____ Round pupils
7. _____ Large, hollow fangs
8. _____ Immediate pain and burning from a bite
9. _____ Pit between the eye and nostril

Part 4   What Would You Do If?

1. You are hiking in the foothills just outside your community, about 20 minutes from town. You find a teenage boy in shorts who has been bitten by a snake on the lower leg. There are two distinct puncture wounds. The boy is experiencing severe pain and burning; is nauseated and sweating; and feels weak. His heartbeat is rapid.

2. A young woman who was just stung by a bee is dizzy, is short of breath, has difficulty swallowing, and has generalized itching and swelling.

24

Burn Emergencies

Learning Objectives

When you have mastered the material in this chapter, you will be able to

1 Understand the various burn classifications and how they relate to the anatomy of the skin

2 Identify the characteristics of superficial (first-degree), partial-thickness (second-degree), and full-thickness (third-degree) burns

3 Calculate the extent of burns using the Rule of Nines

4 Explain how to assess the severity of burns

5 Describe appropriate burn management for thermal and radiant burns

6 Identify the signs and symptoms of inhalation injuries

7 Describe appropriate first aid care for inhalation injuries

8 Describe appropriate first aid care for chemical burns

9 Understand how electrical energy and lightning can injure the body

10 Describe appropriate first aid care for electrical shock

11 Describe appropriate first aid care for injuries inflicted by lightning

On the Scene

Eleven-year-old Kevin Thompson took a can of lighter fluid from his family's garage to a friend's house, where he and three other children planned to make a "fire ball" to settle a neighborhood quarrel. Huddled at the side of the house, Jonathan Parker crumpled up a section of the morning newspaper, and Kevin doused the wad with fluid. Quinn Merritt struck a large wooden kitchen match and dropped it on the damp papers. Flames exploded from the paper. Neighbor Steve Harding, hearing their screams, ran to the boys. Jonathan's shirt was ablaze; his left hand was blistered, his right hand and forearm charred. Steve ripped off his jacket and used it to smother first the shirt, then the burning newspapers. Steve noticed that Jonathan's nasal hair was singed, but knew from his screams that he was still breathing. Steve sent Kevin into the house to call 9-1-1 and told him to bring a clean sheet from the linen closet. Steve then helped Jonathan lie down on the grass, covered Jonathan's arms and chest with the sheet Kevin had found, and continued to watch the boy's breathing while waiting for the ambulance to arrive. Steve's quick action helped confine the injury and prevent contamination and infection.

ore than two million burn accidents occur each year in the United States. Most burns occur at home, and most deaths from burns are a result of house fires. Of those who are burned—in fires, by chemicals, by the sun, in automobile accidents, or in other kinds of accidents—more than 12,000 die as a result of their burns and almost one million require long-term hospitalization. Burns are a leading cause of accidental death in the United States; the number of productive years lost to burns is greater than those lost to cancer, heart disease, and strokes.

Burns can be complex injuries. In addition to the damage to tissues caused by the burn itself, a burn injury can impair the body's normal fluid/electrolyte balance, temperature, thermal regulation, joint function, manual dexterity, and physical appearance. There is also often associated trauma—most often internal injury, blunt trauma, head injury, multiple fractures, and serious lacerations.

This chapter teaches how to determine the seriousness of a burn, gives guidelines for the management of a burn, and discusses the care of victims who have sustained inhalation injuries, chemical burns, and electrical and lightning injuries.

Assessment of Burns

The seriousness of a burn is determined by the following factors:

- Depth of the burn
- Percentage of the body burned
- Severity of the burn
- Location of the burn
- Accompanying complications (such as preexisting physical or mental conditions)
- Age of the victim

Figure 24-1 illustrates how burns affect the body.

Degree of the Burn

Learning Objective **1** Understand the various burn classifications and how they relate to the anatomy of the skin.

HOW BURNS AFFECT THE BODY

Fluids accumulate in upper airways

Proteins clot, enzymes break down

Heart rate increases, then plunges

Bones soften

Hormones are disrupted

Fluids accumulate in body

Red blood cells die (causing anemia)

Platelets destroyed (blood can't clot)

Muscles degenerate

Body cells die

Arteries dilate

Liver swells

Kidney function disrupted Urinary output decreases

Fluid leaks from capillaries

Epidermis
Dermis
Blister
Plasma oozes out
Plasma flows away

Blood vessel in skin
NORMAL SKIN

Dilated porous vessel
BURNED SKIN

SKIN SURFACE
DESTROYED

FIGURE 24–1. Burns may cause shock by damaging surface tissue and disrupting and dilating underlying blood vessels, which may lead to extensive loss of plasma.

Burns are classified according to the depth of the burn and the damage to the skin (Table 24-1). A **superficial burn**, also known as a **first-degree burn**, involves only the outermost layer of the skin, known as the epidermis. The burned area appears red and dry and is painful. A **partial-thickness burn**, also classified as a **second-degree burn**, is typically very red or white, very painful, and moist, and it may produce blisters. A partial-thickness burn affects both the epidermis and the dermis. A **full-thickness**, or **third-degree, burn** damages all of the layers of the skin and may affect the subcutaneous tissue, muscle, and bone. This is the most severe type of burn. The skin appears dry, leathery, charred, or white. There is no pain in the full-thickness burned area since the nerves have been completely destroyed; however, the area surrounding the full-thickness burn may be painful. Superficial and partial-thickness burns typically surround the full-thickness burn, causing the victim to experience some pain associated with the burn (see Figures 24-2 through 24-11 on pages 392–393).

> Learning Objective **2** Identify the characteristics of superficial (first-degree), partial-thickness (second-degree), and full-thickness (third-degree) burns.

As a very rough rule, use the following guide to guess the depth of a burn:

- If the burn is a scald on bare skin and the victim is an adolescent or adult, the burn is probably superficial or partial-thickness, involving only the outer layer of skin, because the heat from such a burn dissipates rapidly. If the victim is an infant or an elderly person (see Figure 24-12 on page 393), the burn may be deeper.

- A thermal burn (a burn caused by flames) is usually partial- or full-thickness.

- Hot grease can produce a full-thickness burn. Grease cools slowly and is difficult to remove; therefore, it may cause extensive damage before it can be removed.

- Burns caused by electricity or chemicals are almost always critical burns because of the extensive, unseen damage that accompanies even apparently minor skin injuries. Victims with such burns are almost always hospitalized so physicians can monitor vital signs and functioning of major organs.

Percentage of Body Burned

> Learning Objective **3** Calculate the extent of burns using the Rule of Nines.

superficial (first-degree) burn A burn that involves only the epidermis, or outer layer of skin, characterized by pain and redness

partial-thickness (second-degree) burn A burn that involves both the epidermal and dermal layers of the skin, characterized by blistering, swelling, and pain

full-thickness (third-degree) burn A burn involving all layers of the skin as well as fat, muscle, and bone; a third-degree burn is characterized by dry, leathery, charred skin

TABLE 24–1	**Classifications of Burns**		
	Superficial (First-Degree)	**Partial-Thickness (Second-Degree)**	**Full-Thickness (Third-Degree)**
Causes	Flash of electricity, flame, scald, the sun	Contact with hot liquids or solids, flash of electricity, flame, chemicals, the sun	Contact with hot liquids or solids, flame, chemicals, or electricity
Layers of Skin Affected	Epidermal layer only	Epidermis and dermis	Epidermis, dermis, subcutaneous tissues, muscle, bone
Appearance	Skin surface is dry and reddened; no blisters or swelling	Skin is moist and mottled, ranging from white to cherry red; blistered	Skin is dry and leathery; charred blood vessels are often visible; skin is a mixture of white, dark, and charred
Symptoms	Extremely painful	Extremely painful	Victim may feel no pain in the immediate full-thickness burn area because nerve endings have been destroyed
Healing Time	2 to 5 days	5 to 21 days	Weeks to years
Prognosis	No scarring; temporary discoloration	Some scarring	Usually requires surgery and Skin grafting

FIGURE 24–2. Contact burn from a steam iron

FIGURE 24–3. Partial- and full-thickness burns

FIGURE 24–4. Full-thickness burns

FIGURE 24–5. Partial- and full-thickness burns

FIGURE 24–6. Partial- and full-thickness burns

FIGURE 24–7. Partial-thickness burns

FIGURE 24–8. Partial- and full-thickness burns

FIGURE 24–9. Partial-thickness burns

FIGURE 24–10. Partial-thickness burns

FIGURE 24–12. Scalds are the most common causes of burns in children under 8 years old.

There are two methods you can use to determine quickly the percentage of the body that has been burned: the **Rule of Nines** and the **palmar surface method**.

The Rule of Nines (see Figure 24-13 on page 394) divides the body into regions: head and neck (9 percent), posterior trunk (18 percent), anterior trunk (18 percent), each upper extremity (9 percent), each lower extremity (18 percent), and external genitalia (1 percent). In an infant, the head and neck are considered to be 18 percent and the lower extremities are each considered to be 14 percent of the body surface. An alternative method is the palmar surface method. The palm of the victim's hand is equal to approximately 1 percent of the body surface, regardless of the

victim's age. You can estimate the burned surface by comparing its size to the size of the victim's palm.

> **Rule of Nines** A method of estimating how much body surface was burned by mentally dividing the body into regions, each representing 9 percent (or a multiple of 9 percent) of the body surface
>
> **palmar surface method** A method of using the size of the victim's palm to estimate the percentage of body surface that has been burned

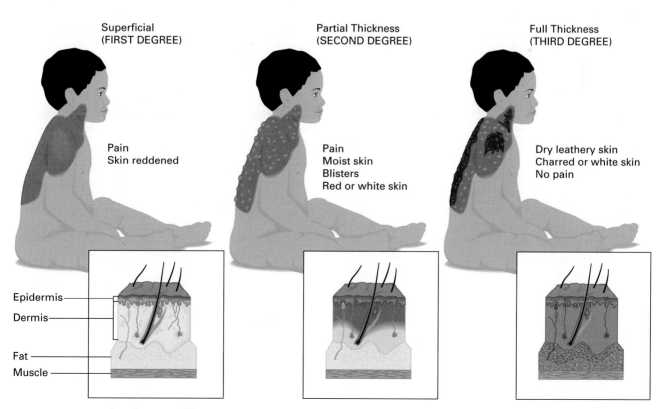

Superficial
(FIRST DEGREE)

Pain
Skin reddened

Partial Thickness
(SECOND DEGREE)

Pain
Moist skin
Blisters
Red or white skin

Full Thickness
(THIRD DEGREE)

Dry leathery skin
Charred or white skin
No pain

Epidermis
Dermis

Fat
Muscle

FIGURE 24–11. Classification of burns by depth

THE RULE OF NINES

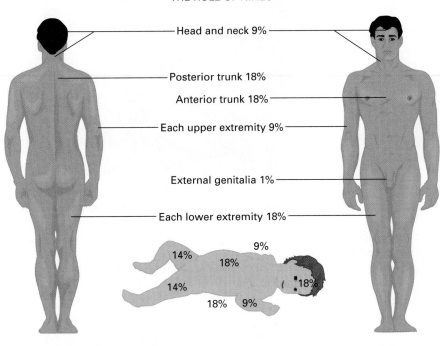

Head and neck 9%

Posterior trunk 18%

Anterior trunk 18%

Each upper extremity 9%

External genitalia 1%

Each lower extremity 18%

9%
14%
18%
14%
18%
18%   9%

FIGURE 24–13. The Rule of Nines is a quick method of estimating how much body surface is burned.

Severity of the Burn

> Learning Objective 4 Explain how to assess the severity of burns.

The severity of the burn is based on the depth of the burn, the extent (percentage of body surface area burned), and the location of the burn. The burn severity is classified as minor, moderate, or critical (Table 24-2 and Figure 24-14). Any time a burn involves the hands, feet, face, airway, or genitalia, it is considered to be critical due to possible loss of function.

Location of the Burn

Certain areas of the body are more critically damaged by burns than others. Burns on the face or neck are extremely dangerous because of possible injury to the eyes or possible airway and respiratory complications.

Other locations that are particularly critical in burn injuries are the hands, feet, and external genitalia. Any burn that completely burns the circumference of an extremity, the neck, or chest is very serious. These burns can act like a tourniquet and cut off blood supply to the lower extremity, strangulate the victim, or keep the chest from expanding. Victims with burns in any of these areas should be taken to a hospital or burn center immediately.

Accompanying Complications and Age of the Victim

People who have major diseases, such as heart disease or diabetes, or who have other injuries will always react more severely to a burn, even a minor one.

The age of the victim may also be a complicating factor. Children under the age of 5 and adults over the age of 55 tolerate burns very poorly. Because the elderly and the young have extremely thin skin, they will sustain much deeper burns from a much less severe source. The young and elderly also have a disproportionate fluid-to-surface-area ratio, so even a small fluid loss can result in serious problems. Also, the immune system is incompletely developed in the young child and is usually compromised in the elderly.

PROGRESS CHECK

1. In a superficial burn, the skin is _____ and extremely painful. *(mottled/reddened/ moist)*

2. A partial-thickness burn affects both the epidermal and dermal layers of skin and is characterized by _____ . *(blistering/dryness/ charring)*

3. A full-thickness burn can extend to the bone and may cause the victim little or no pain because _____ . *(the victim is in shock/the nerve endings are destroyed/the victim is usually unconscious)*

4. You can quickly assess the amount of body surface involved by using the Rule of Nines, which divides the body into _____ . *(regions that each represent 9 percent of the body surface/nine regions/nine areas most critical if burned)*

TABLE 24–2	**Severity of Burns**		
	Critical Burn	**Moderate Burn**	**Minor Burn**
Superficial (First Degree)	More than 75% of an adult's body surface	50–75% of an adult's body surface	Less than 20% of an adult's or child's body surface
Partial-Thickness (Second Degree)	More than 30% of body surface in adults, more than 20% in a child	15–30% of body surface in adults, 10–20% in a child	Less than 15% of body surface in adults, less than 10% in a child
Full-Thickness (Third Degree)	More than 10% of the body surface in adults, more than 2–3% in a child	2–10% of the body surface, excluding the face, hands, feet, and genital area	Less than 2% of the body surface
Other Types	Burns that involve the face, hands, feet, or genital area; burns complicated by respiratory tract injuries, other major injuries, or fractures; burns of any degree in victims with serious underlying medical conditions; most chemical burns; all electrical burns		

5. The most serious burn in an adult is
_____ . *(a full-thickness burn covering 10 percent of the body/a partial-thickness burn covering 30 percent of the body/an electrical burn)*

6. Burns on the face are considered especially serious because of possible _____ .
(disfigurement/injury to the mouth/airway closure)

Critical burns include:

• All inhalation injuries

• Electrical burns

• Deep acid burns

• Burns in patients with underlying physical or medical conditions

• Superficial burns that cover more than 75% of the body surface

• Partial-thickness burns covering more than 30% of the body-surface in an adult, 20% or more in a child

• Full-thickness burns covering more than 10% of body surface in an adult and 2% to 3% in a child

• Partial-thickness or full-thickness burns involving the face, eyes, ears, hands, feet, or genitalia

FIGURE 24–14. Critical burns are burns complicated by respiratory tract injury and other major injuries.

24.2 Burn Management

The first priority in first aid care is to prevent further injury. The problems most often associated with burns are:

- Airway or respiratory difficulties
- Toxic inhalation
- Related musculoskeletal injuries
- Loss of body fluids, contributing to shock
- Pain, contributing to shock
- Anxiety, contributing to shock
- Swelling
- Infection due to destruction of skin tissue

General Care of Thermal and Radiant Burns

The most common burns are thermal burns (caused by flame) and radiant burns (caused by radiant heat, such as the sun). Fatalities resulting from a fire are typically due to airway closure associated with a burn to the upper airway, inhalation of toxic smoke, or other trauma. It is unlikely that the victim will die from the burn itself. Complications such as severe infection and fluid loss will occur several hours after the burn. Therefore, immediately following a burn, it is critical to focus on assessing and managing the airway, breathing, and any other life-threatening injuries to the victim. Afterward, determine the extent and severity of the burns and gather a complete history. Ask when the burn occurred, what has been done to care for the burn, whether the victim was trapped in an area with steam or smoke, whether the victim lost consciousness, what caused the burn, and whether the victim has any history of significant heart disease, diabetes, or other serious illness.

First Aid Care

Learning Objective **5** Describe appropriate burn management for thermal and radiant burns.

Care of a thermal or radiant burn must start immediately—preferably at the moment of burning. Remember: A First Aider does not *treat* a burn, but merely cares for the burn until the victim can be transported to a hospital or burn center for thorough treatment.

Your first priority is to prevent further injury to the victim or injury to others and *to stop the burning*. Your second priority is to manage the airway and breathing, then care for the burn injury. Specific guidelines for the care of other types of burns are listed later in this chapter; regardless of the type of burn, follow these general guidelines:

1. Remove the victim from the source of the burn. Move the victim far enough away from a fire so no smoke is inhaled; remove the victim from the source of a chemical spill; if the victim was struck by lightning, move to shelter.

2. Eliminate the cause of the burn—put out the fire, wash away the chemicals, and so on. Immerse scald or grease burns in cold water to stop the burning (see Figure 24-15); if the victim's clothes are on fire, douse the victim with water and remove all clothing, jewelry, and shoes that are not sticking to the skin. Roll the victim on the ground to extinguish flames only as a last resort; the potential for wound contamination is great, and infection is a major killer of burn victims.

3. Assess ABCDs, and manage respiratory and cardiac complications. Continually assess the airway and breathing status if the victim:

   - Wheezes or coughs while breathing
   - Has a sooty or smoky smell on the breath
   - Has particles of soot in the saliva
   - Has burned mucous membranes in the mouth or nose

Inhalation of superheated air, steam, or flames may burn the lining of the upper airway, causing severe

FIGURE 24–15. Cooling a burn by submerging the burned area in cold running water

swelling. This might create a partial or complete airway obstruction. Also, inhalation of toxic smoke can make breathing ineffective.

4. Activate the EMS system as soon as possible.

5. Continue to assess the victim's vital signs until medical help arrives.

6. Stop the burning process by applying cool water to the burn. Never break any blisters that have formed on the skin. This will increase the incidence of infection by breaking the skin barrier. Apply dry sterile dressings to the burned area. It is very important to keep the burned area as clean and uncontaminated as possible and to use sterile dressings to reduce the chance of infection. If less than 10 percent of the body is burned, wet sterile dressings can be used (follow local protocol). Sterile water should be used to wet the dressing. Wet dressings provide some pain relief. A sterile burn kit contains dressings and other items to manage the burn (see Figure 24-16). Do not use plastic or other nonbreathable, nonsterile materials to dress the burn, as these will encourage bacteria growth.

Never apply butter, grease, or fat to a burn. Do not use burn gels or salves on any partial-thickness or full-thickness burns. Do not apply ice or an ice pack to a burn; if less than 10 percent of the body surface area is involved, you can apply a cool compress. For a superficial burn only you can apply an aloe vera gel or a nonscented moisturizer to keep the skin moist. A victim with a partial-thickness burn greater than 10 percent of the body surface area or any full-thickness burn should be transported to a medical facility for further care. Figure 24-17 through 24-24 illustrate care of burns.

FIGURE 24-17. Cover burn with dry sterile dressing.

FIGURE 24-18. Cover burn and treat victim for shock.

FIGURE 24-19. Separate burned fingers with sterile gauze.

FIGURE 24-20. Separate burned toes with sterile gauze.

FIGURE 24-16. Burn-care kit

PROGRESS CHECK

1. One of the most common types of burn is _____ . *(chemical/thermal/electrical)*

2. The first priority in burn care is _____ . *(preventing further injury/removing the source of the burn/moving the victim away from the source of the burn)*

FIGURE 24–21. Apply moist, sterile pads to burned eyes.

FIGURE 24–22. Remoistening a burn dressing

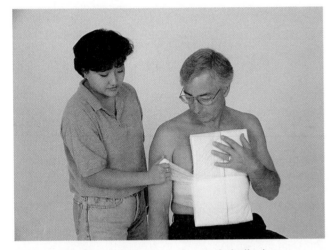

FIGURE 24–23. Application of a sterile bulky burn dressing for moderate and critical burns

FIGURE 24–24. Cover moderate and critical burns with a thick, clean, dry, sterile, dressing and loosely bandage in place.

3. You should always check for _____ complications immediately. *(burn/shock/airway and respiratory)*

4. If less than 10 percent of the body surface is burned, cover the burned area with _____ . *(ice packs/adherent gauze/wet sterile dressings)*

24.3 Inhalation Injuries

More than half of all fire-related deaths are caused by smoke inhalation. Most of those who die in residential fires do so because they have inhaled heated air, smoke, or other toxic gases—not because they have been burned to death. Suspect **inhalation injury** in any victim of thermal burn, especially if the victim was confined in an enclosed space at any time during the fire.

There are three causes of inhalation injuries that accompany burns:

- Heat inhalation
- Inhalation of toxic chemicals or smoke
- Inhalation of carbon monoxide (the most common burn-associated inhalation injury)

When heat is inhaled, mucous membranes and linings get scorched, and swelling partially blocks the airway. Because edema (swelling) and other damage can be

inhalation injury An injury caused by breathing in heat, toxic chemicals, smoke, or carbon monoxide progressive, the inhalation injury may appear to be mild at first, but may become more severe. Depending on what was burned, how completely the materials were burned, how long the victim was exposed to the smoke, and whether the victim was in a confined space, the symptoms may occur within a few minutes, but may not appear for many hours.

Signs and Symptoms

> Learning Objective **6** Identify the signs and symptoms of inhalation injuries.

Specific signs and symptoms of inhalation injury (see Figures 24-25 and 24-26) are:

- Facial burns
- Singed nasal hairs
- Burned specks of carbon in the saliva
- A sooty or smoky smell on the breath
- Respiratory distress, accompanied by
  - Restriction of chest-wall movement
  - Restlessness

FIGURE 24–26. Facial inhalation burns

- Chest tightness
- Difficulty in swallowing
- Hoarseness
- Coughing
- Cyanosis
- Noisy breathing
- Actual burns of the mucous membranes in the mouth or nose

Assume respiratory injury if in doubt, especially if facial burns are present.

Inhalation of Toxic Fumes

The most common respiratory emergency results from the inhalation of noxious chemicals, **carbon monoxide** fumes, or smoke. **Toxic** fumes can result from the burning of a number of ordinary household objects, such as carpets, draperies, wall coverings, floor coverings, upholstery, and lacquered wood veneer on furniture. There are almost three hundred toxic substances that result from the burning of wood alone.

When toxic fumes are inhaled, mucosa in the lungs swell and break, leaking fluid into the nearby alveolar spaces and damaging the cilia. Mucus builds up and plugs the air passages. The final result is reduced oxygen exchange, which can eventually cause death if left untreated.

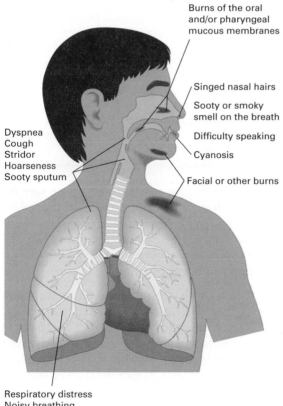

Burns of the oral and/or pharyngeal mucous membranes

Singed nasal hairs

Sooty or smoky smell on the breath

Difficulty speaking

Cyanosis

Facial or other burns

Dyspnea
Cough
Stridor
Hoarseness
Sooty sputum

Respiratory distress
Noisy breathing
Restricted chest movement

FIGURE 24–25. Signs and symptoms of inhalation burns

> **carbon monoxide** An odorless, colorless, tasteless, poisonous gas resulting from incomplete combustion of anything containing carbon
>
> **toxic** Poisonous

Carbon Monoxide

Carbon monoxide is released during the combustion of most things, especially cellulose materials, such as wood, paper, and cotton. Carbon monoxide poisoning is the major cause of death at the scene of a fire. Because carbon monoxide is colorless, odorless, and tasteless, it is extremely difficult to detect.

Because burns usually do not alter levels of consciousness, assume that any burn victim who is unconscious is suffering from carbon monoxide poisoning. Other signs and symptoms include:

- Headache
- Weakness
- Nausea and/or vomiting
- Loss of manual dexterity
- Confusion, lethargy, irrational or reckless behavior

Do not wait for the traditional sign of cherry-red skin—it is a very late sign, and might not even occur until after death.

First Aid Care

Learning Objective 7 Describe appropriate first aid care for inhalation injuries.

To prevent further respiratory complications:

1. Activate the EMS system immediately.

2. Remove the victim as far as possible from the source of the toxic fumes, especially if it is a fire; try to situate the victim in fresh air.

3. Clear the airway and provide artificial ventilation if breathing is absent or ineffective.

4. Place the victim in an upright position to allow for easier breathing unless injuries contraindicate it.

5. Remove any clothing that may restrict chest movement, including neckties and necklaces, if they are not sticking to the skin.

6. If respiratory distress occurs, maintain an adequate airway.

PROGRESS CHECK

1. Suspect inhalation injury in any victim of thermal burn, especially if the victim was _____ . *(in contact with chemicals/in an enclosed space/lying down when burned)*

2. The most common cause of an upper airway burn is _____ . *(smoke/heat/carbon monoxide)*

3. The signs and symptoms of inhalation injury may be delayed because the _____ associated with it is progressive. *(shock/swelling/infection)*

4. Always assume respiratory injury if the _____ is (are) burned. *(face/chest/upper extremities)*

5. Always assume that any burn victim who is _____ is suffering from carbon monoxide poisoning. *(in a confined space/burned on the face/unconscious)*

 24.4 ## Chemical Burns

It is extremely difficult to assess the depth and severity of chemical burns (see Figure 24-27) in a first aid setting; therefore, the general guideline is to *treat all chemical burns aggressively.* Chemicals continue to burn as long as they are in contact with the skin, and chemical burns are considered to be critical burns.

Every victim of chemical burns needs to be transported to a hospital. Speed is essential: The more quickly you are able to remove the source of the burn and initiate care, the less severe the burn will be.

First Aid Care

Learning Objective 8 Describe appropriate first aid care for chemical burns.

Before beginning first aid care, make sure it is safe to approach the victim; if not, wait for trained rescue personnel to arrive. During each step of rescue, make sure to protect yourself from contamination. If possible, put on protective gloves to guard yourself from injury before you start caring for the victim.

1. Brush any dry powder off the skin, then flush the burned area vigorously in a steady stream of water; a shower or garden hose is ideal. (The pressure should not be too great; high pressure will drive chemicals into the pores of the skin.) Irrigate the area continuously for at least 20 minutes under a steady stream of water. *There are three important exceptions to this rule:*

- Lime powder creates a corrosive when mixed with water; make sure that all traces have been removed from not only the skin, but the clothing before flushing with water (see Figures 24-28 through 24-30).

FIGURE 24–27. Chemical burn

FIGURE 24–28. Lime powder should be brushed off the skin before flushing with water.

FIGURE 24–29. After brushing off lime powder, flush the skin with water—if possible, with copious amounts of water, as with a garden hose.

- Phenol (carbolic acid) should be washed off with alcohol; the burn area should then be irrigated with water.

- Concentrated sulfuric acid produces heat when mixed with water and may cause greater burn injuries unless flushed vigorously with a hose or in a shower. *Follow local protocol.*

2. While flushing the burn area, remove the victim's clothing, shoes, stockings, and jewelry.

3. If the victim is able, have him or her wash with soap and water, then rinse thoroughly, after you have finished irrigating the burn.

4. If any chemicals splash into the victim's eyes, use a faucet or hose on low pressure to irrigate the eyes for at least 20 minutes (see Figure 24-31); make sure contact lenses are removed. You can also use a

FIGURE 24–30. A chemical burn victim flushing himself off under an emergency wash/shower system at the worksite

pan, bucket, cup, or bottle; make sure to irrigate well underneath the lids.

5. When you have finished flushing, cover the burned area with a dry sterile dressing.

6. Activate the EMS system as soon as possible. If you can, get the name of the chemical, or send the container to the hospital with the victim.

Note: Never try to use an antidote, and do not try to neutralize a burned area with alkali or acid solutions; you may intensify the injury.

FIGURE 24–31. Flushing a chemical burn of the eye

1. Because it is so difficult to determine the depth and severity of a chemical burn in a first aid setting, the general guideline is to treat all chemical burns _____ . *(with dry dressings/aggressively/as minor)*

2. Before beginning first aid care for a chemical burn, you must _____ . *(activate the EMS system/find the chemical container/make sure it is safe to approach the victim)*

3. Immediately treat a chemical burn by irrigating the area for at least _____ minutes. *(20/30/40)*

4. After you remove the victim's clothing, continue irrigating the area for at least _____ minutes. *(20/30/40)*

5. The most essential part of caring for chemical burns is _____ . *(speed/accuracy/timing)*

24.5 Electrical Burns

Understanding electrical burns is critical; it will not only enable you to help a victim, but may also save your own life.

Protecting Yourself and the Victim

If you feel a tingling sensation in your legs as you approach the victim, *stop*—that sensation indicates that the ground is energized and that you are at risk of electrocution. When approaching any accident that involves downed power lines or other electrical hazards, follow these procedures:

- Look for downed wires whenever a vehicle has struck a power pole. If it is dark, use a flashlight to inspect the poles and the surrounding area.

- *Never attempt to move downed wires!* Notify the power company and request an emergency crew.

- If a downed power line is lying across a wrecked vehicle, *do not touch the vehicle,* even if the victims inside are seriously injured. If you touch the vehicle, you will likely be electrocuted. If the victims in the car are conscious, warn them not to leave the vehicle.
  If the car begins to burn, instruct victims in the car to open the door and jump as far away as they can from the car. If they touch the car and the ground at the same time, they will likely be electrocuted.

- If a victim is holding a power tool, look for cords; the tool does not have to be on to present an electrical hazard.

- If a victim is in a pool, turn off all power at the main switch before entering the water.

- If a victim is found in a bathtub with an electrical appliance that has energized the water, *pull the plug of the appliance before you touch the victim.*

Types of Electrical Burns

There are three general kinds of electrical burns:

- **Thermal burns**, caused when electricity causes flames that then burn the skin; with thermal burns, electricity does not actually pass through the body.

- **Contact burns**, which occur where the current is most intense, at the points where electrical current enters and exits the body (see Figures 24-32).

- **Arcing injuries** (or **flash burns**), caused when a current jumps from one surface to another, burning nearby skin, electricity does not actually pass through the body.

Severity of Electrical Shock

The severity of electrical shock is determined by the following factors:

- Voltage and amperage of the current

thermal burn A burn caused by flames

contact burn A burn caused by touching either a hot surface or a live electrical circuit

arcing injury (flash burn) An injury caused when an electrical current jumps from one surface to another; nearby skin is burned, but electricity does not actually pass through the skin

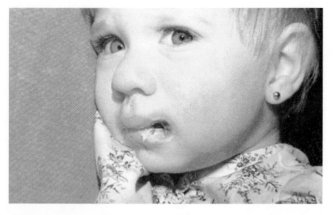

FIGURE 24–32. Electrical contact burn caused by chewing on an electrical cord

- Amount of time the victim was exposed to the shock
- Amount of moisture on the victim
- Amount of the victim's body surface that is in contact with water
- Amount of insulation worn by the victim
- Area of the body through which the current passes
- Type of current (AC or DC)

Signs and Symptoms of Electrocution

Learning Objective **9** Understand how electrical energy and lightning can injure the body.

If you are unsure whether a person has experienced an electrical shock, examine the victim for the following signs and symptoms (see Figures 24-33 and 24-34):

- Dazed and confused condition
- Obvious and severe burns on the skin surface
- Unconsciousness
- Weak, irregular, or absent pulse
- Shallow, irregular, or absent breathing
- Possibility of multiple severe fractures due to intense muscular contractions

First Aid Care for Electrical Shock

Learning Objective **10** Describe appropriate first aid care for electrical shock.

To care for a victim of electrical shock, activate EMS immediately.

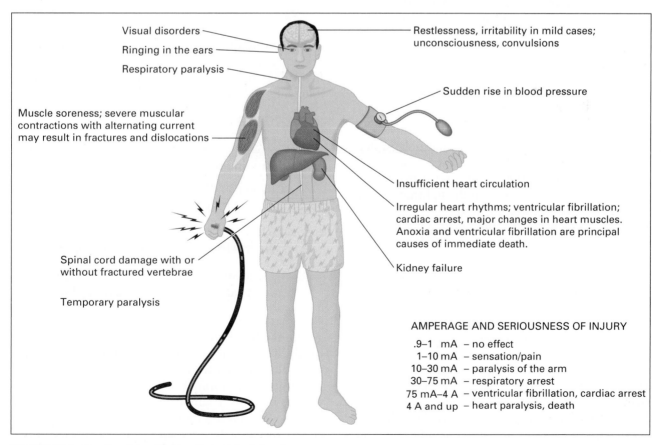

Visual disorders

Ringing in the ears

Respiratory paralysis

Muscle soreness; severe muscular contractions with alternating current may result in fractures and dislocations

Spinal cord damage with or without fractured vertebrae

Temporary paralysis

Restlessness, irritability in mild cases; unconsciousness, convulsions

Sudden rise in blood pressure

Insufficient heart circulation

Irregular heart rhythms; ventricular fibrillation; cardiac arrest, major changes in heart muscles. Anoxia and ventricular fibrillation are principal causes of immediate death.

Kidney failure

AMPERAGE AND SERIOUSNESS OF INJURY

.9–1 mA – no effect
1–10 mA – sensation/pain
10–30 mA – paralysis of the arm
30–75 mA – respiratory arrest
75 mA–4 A – ventricular fibrillation, cardiac arrest
4 A and up – heart paralysis, death

FIGURE 24–33. Possible effects of electrical shock

FIGURE 24-34. Deep full-thickness electrical burn

1. Your first priority is to protect yourself; follow the guidelines outlined on page 402. Do not approach the victim unless you can do so safely.

2. Check the victim's breathing and pulse; immediately start CPR and apply the AED if available, even if you are unsure about the extent of injury.

3. If the victim fell or was thrown, treat for spinal injuries.

4. If the victim is conscious and his or her condition is not urgent, provide basic burn care for source and ground wounds (see Figure 24-35), and splint fractures.

5. Treat the victim for shock.

Lightning Injuries

Lightning kills approximately 300 people each year in the United States, more than any other natural disaster. The most common cause of death is cardiac arrest. Of the people struck by lightning who survive, many have some kind of residual effect from the lightning strike (such as some vision or hearing loss).

Although some people are injured by a direct lightning strike, more often the injury is caused when electric current travels down a nearby object (such as a building or a tree) and "splashes" onto the victim. For that reason, people who are caught in storms should stay away from solid objects such as trees and fences. Occasionally, victims are also injured by holding onto an object that is struck by lightning or from currents that travel along the ground.

Always assume that a victim of lightning strike has sustained multiple injuries; most are knocked down or thrown, so also assume spinal injury and other possible trauma. A person who has been struck by lightning does *not* hold a charge, so it is safe to handle and treat the victim.

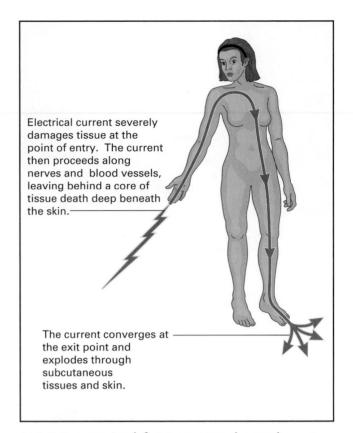

Electrical current severely damages tissue at the point of entry. The current then proceeds along nerves and blood vessels, leaving behind a core of tissue death deep beneath the skin.

The current converges at the exit point and explodes through subcutaneous tissues and skin.

FIGURE 24-35. Look for two separate burns when electricity is the cause of injury.
(Adapted from *Hospital Medicine*, May 1989, page 85.)

Burns due to lightning are usually minor and are not a primary concern (see Figures 24-36 and 24-37). Lightning strike victims usually sustain injury to the following body systems:

- The nervous system
- The skin
- The heart and the vascular system

See Chapter 27 for information about how to prevent a lightning injury.

First Aid Care of Lightning Injuries

Learning Objective 11 Describe appropriate first aid care for injuries inflicted by lightning.

The goal of first aid for lightning victims is to oxygenate the heart and the brain until the heart regains its ability to function. You should always continue resuscitation (artificial ventilation and chest compressions) of lightning victims longer than you would victims of other trauma—even if the victim appears lifeless. Victims of lightning strike have a greater chance of resuscitation than victims of cardiac or respiratory arrest due to other causes. The heart has a

FIGURE 24–36. Lightning burn

FIGURE 24–37. Lightning burn

natural tendency to start beating on its own without any intervention.

If the strike occurred in an open area, quickly move the victim to a protected area to reduce the chance of a second strike. If a group has been struck, care for those in cardiac or respiratory arrest first. Those who display vital signs will probably recover spontaneously.

To care for lightning strike victims:

1. Activate the EMS system immediately.

2. Survey the scene, assess what happened, and make sure the victim is safe from further injury. Remove debris that has fallen on the victim, and move the victim away from any source of electricity.

3. Assess breathing and pulse; if appropriate, begin artificial ventilation or CPR. Apply an AED if the victim is pulseless. *The key to survival is early, vigorous, prolonged resuscitation efforts.* Hold the head in a neutral position and bring the jaw forward gently in case of spinal injury.

4. Stabilize the victim's neck to prevent aggravating a possible cervical spine injury. If possible, move the victim to dry ground after stabilizing the neck.

5. If the victim is conscious, check movement in all extremities; determine the victim's reaction to pain.

6. While waiting for medical help to arrive, assess the victim for open wounds or fractures, and provide appropriate care.

PROGRESS CHECK

1. If a downed power line is lying across a vehicle, _____ . *(have occupants of the car get out/use a wooden pole to move the line/do not touch the vehicle)*

2. If a victim is found in the bathtub with an appliance that has energized the water, _____ . *(unplug the appliance/drain the bathtub)*

3. An arcing injury occurs when _____ . *(an extremity is struck by lightning/a current enters the body/a current jumps from one surface to another)*

4. Your first priority in treating an electrical shock victim is to _____ . *(remove the source of electricity/ protect yourself/get the victim away from the electrical source)*

5. Always assume a victim of lightning strike has sustained _____ . *(multiple injuries/cardiac arrest/internal burns)*

6. Victims of lightning strike have a greater chance of resuscitation than victims of arrest from other causes because _____ . *(the heart may restart on its own/body temperature is slightly elevated)*

7. The goal of first aid for lightning victims is to _____ . *(prevent further injury/oxygenate the heart and brain/restore circulation)*

Summary

- Burns are classified by the depth of the burn and the damage to the skin and underlying tissues. First-degree burns are superficial burns, second-degree burns are partial-thickness burns (they burn through only part of the skin's layers), while a third-degree burn is a full-thickness burn (involving all layers of the skin).

- You can quickly assess how much of a victim's body surface is burned by using either the Rule of Nines or the palmar surface method.

- Burns of the face, hands, feet, or genitals are always considered critical.

- The first priority in first aid care for burns is to prevent further injury. To treat, begin by removing the victim from the source of the burn and by eliminating the cause of the burn.

- Inhalation injuries cause the majority of deaths from fire; the most common burn-associated inhalation injury is carbon monoxide poisoning. Always assume that an unconscious burn victim has inhaled carbon monoxide fumes.

- Always assume inhalation injury has occurred with any thermal burn, whenever the face is burned, or whenever a victim was confined in an enclosed space.

- The key to treating chemical burns is aggressive, vigorous, prolonged irrigation; the more quickly you initiate care, the less severe the burn will be. Begin by irrigating for at least 20 minutes.

- Before you approach any victim of electrical injury, make sure it is safe to do so.

- The goal of first aid treatment for a victim of lightning strike is to oxygenate the heart and brain until the body resumes circulation on its own.

Key Terms

Make sure you understand the following key terms:

superficial (first-degree) burn
partial-thickness (second-degree) burn
full-thickness (third-degree) burn
Rule of Nines
palmar surface method
inhalation injury
carbon monoxide
toxic
thermal burn
contact burns
arcing injury (flash burn)

Critical Thinking Exercise

You are at a local park when a family at the pavilion begins to yell and scream for help. You run over and see a man in his mid-forties lying in a puddle of water next to the electric cooler. A family member indicates that the man went to plug in the cooler when a loud pop was heard and a large spark was seen. The man is not moving. You note a burn to the hand with the cord in it and burns to both bare feet.

1. What would be your immediate action?

2. If the patient is pulseless and not breathing, how would you proceed?

3. What would you suspect the extent of the burns to be?

Chapter 24 Self-Test

Student: _____ Date: _____

Course: _____ Section #: _____

Part 1 True/False

If you believe the statement is true, circle the T. If you believe the statement is false, circle the F.

T F **1.** More than half of all fire-related deaths are caused by smoke inhalation.

T F **2.** With an inhalation injury, most of the damage done to the upper airway is a result of inhalation of carbon monoxide.

T F **3.** Common signs and symptoms of upper-airway injury from inhalation include burned specks of carbon in the sputum, hoarseness, coughing, and cyanosis.

T F **4.** Carbon monoxide poisoning is the major cause of death at the scenes of most fires.

T F **5.** Superficial (first-degree) thermal burns should be immersed in cool water.

T F **6.** All partial-thickness (second-degree) burns should not be immersed in cool water.

T F **7.** Chemical burns should be continuously irrigated for at least 20 minutes.

T F **8.** A lime powder burn should be treated like any other chemical burn.

T F **9.** Lightning causes more deaths than any other type of electrical burn.

T F **10.** Smoke-inhalation victims may have facial burns.

T F **11.** Victims of lightning strikes have greater chances of resuscitation and survival following cardiac arrest than victims of cardiac arrest due to other causes.

T F **12.** If a group has been struck by lightning, care for those in cardiac arrest first.

T F **13.** While approximately two-thirds of all those struck by lightning die as a result, approximately one-third can be revived.

T F **14.** Always assume that a victim of a lightning strike has sustained multiple injuries.

Part 2 Multiple Choice

For each item, circle the correct answer or the phrase that best completes the statement.

1. The First Aider's first action at a burn accident should be to
   a. remove the victim from the source of the burn
   b. examine the victim for respiratory or cardiac complications
   c. determine the severity of the burn
   d. open and maintain the victim's airway

2. The first step in caring for a small superficial burn is usually to
   a. transport the victim to a medical facility as soon as possible
   b. cover the area with a moist, bulky dressing
   c. apply grease or petroleum jelly to the area
   d. submerge the burned area in cold water

3. Covering a partial-thickness thermal burn of less than 10% of body surface area with a wet, sterile dressing can
   a. reduce swelling
   b. relieve pain

   c. prevent infection
   d. a and b are correct

4. First aid care for a chemical burn caused by dry lime is to
   a. flush the lime with running water
   b. apply a neutralizer to the lime
   c. first brush the dry lime from the victim's skin, hair, and clothing
   d. apply an occlusive bandage

5. What should be done to care for most chemical burns?
   a. neutralize the area with alkali or acid solutions
   b. remove clothing while flushing the area with water
   c. locate an antidote before treating; water may intensify the reaction
   d. cover the area with a dry, sterile gauze

6. Immediate care in the case of a lightning victim should consist of
  a. determining the victim's reaction to pain
  b. treating for shock
  c. getting the victim under cover
  d. restoring and maintaining breathing and heartbeat

7. According to the Rule of Nines, which of the following areas is estimated to be 9 percent of the body area?
  a. one leg
  b. back of trunk
  c. front of trunk
  d. one arm

8. In a serious burn case, pain is best relieved by protecting the burn from air through the application of a
  a. burn spray
  b. thick, clean, dry dressing
  c. thick, petroleum-based burn ointment
  d. soybean-oil-based burn ointment

9. Which of the following causes the most damage in upper-airway inhalation injury accompanying burns?
  a. heat
  b. toxic chemicals
  c. carbon monoxide
  d. smoke

10. What care should be given if clothing or debris is sticking to a burn that is severe?
  a. remove it carefully
  b. soak the involved area in cool salt water
  c. leave it alone
  d. scrub the involved area with a soft brush and water

11. Which of the following comes first in first aid care of an electrical burn victim?
  a. separating the victim carefully from the electrical source
  b. initiating CPR
  c. opening the airway
  d. locating entrance and exit wounds

12. According to the Rule of Nines, the infant's head area represents what percent of the total body area?
  a. $4\frac{1}{2}$ percent
  b. 9 percent
  c. 15 percent
  d. 18 percent

13. What should a First Aider do if he or she comes across a downed power line lying across a wrecked vehicle?
  a. instruct conscious victims to attempt to jump from the vehicle
  b. tell conscious victims to stay inside the vehicle and wait for a power company crew
  c. tell victims to turn on the ignition and move the vehicle
  d. throw a blanket or jacket over the line, and instruct conscious victims to leave the vehicle

14. Possible effects of electric shock include
  a. ringing in the ears
  b. visual disorders
  c. kidney failure
  d. all of the above

Part 3 Matching

Match each description with a severity level.

1. _____ Full-thickness burns between 2 and 10 percent of the body of an adult excluding face, hands, and feet)

2. _____ Burns complicated by respiratory tract injury and/or fractures

3. _____ Superficial burns that cover more than 75 percent of the body surface

4. _____ Partial-thickness burns covering between 15 and 30 percent of an adult's body surface

5. _____ Partial-thickness burns over less than 15 percent of an adult's body surface

6. _____ Full-thickness burns involving more than 10 percent of an adult's body surface

7. _____ Partial-thickness burns covering more than 30 percent of an adult's body surface

8. _____ Full-thickness burns that cover more than 2 to 3 percent of a child's body surface

9. _____ Full-thickness burns that involve face, hands, feet, or genital area

10. _____ Superficial burns covering 50 to 75 percent of an adult's body surface

11. _____ Partial-thickness burns covering less than 10 percent of a child's body surface

A. Critical
B. Moderate
C. Minor

1. A 10-year-old boy was playing with gasoline and received burns on his abdomen and lower extremities.

2. An industrial worker has dry lime powder spilled over his whole body.

3. A teenage boy is hit by lightning on a golf course. He is not breathing and has no detectable carotid pulse.

25

Heat and Cold Emergencies

Learning Objectives

When you have mastered the material in this chapter, you will be able to

1 Explain how the body attempts to maintain normal body temperature

2 Explain how the body loses heat

3 Describe and demonstrate appropriate first aid care for heatstroke

4 Describe and demonstrate appropriate first aid care for heat exhaustion

5 Describe and demonstrate appropriate first aid care for heat cramps

6 Identify the signs and symptoms of hypothermia

7 Describe and demonstrate appropriate first aid care for hypothermia

8 Identify the signs and symptoms of frostbite

9 Describe and demonstrate appropriate first aid care for frostbite

On the Scene

Sixteen-year-old Daniel Stringham and four of his friends were running along a stretch of highway in a rural area of the county, training for an upcoming marathon race. Daniel, a stocky teenager who had not kept up the training schedule of the others for the past few months, was struggling to keep up.

As the rest of the boys rounded a curve in the road, Daniel collapsed. Daniel's skin was dry and red; though he felt extremely hot, he was not sweating. He was breathing rapidly and sounded as if he was snoring. As the boys gathered around him, it was obvious that he was confused—he did not know where he was and seemed very anxious.

Parker Merritt sent one of the runners to a nearby home to call 9-1-1. With the help of the others, Parker moved Daniel into the shade of a tree. The boys removed Daniel's shirt, shorts, socks, and shoes; two of them brought water in their cupped hands from a nearby irrigation ditch and splashed it over Daniel's chest, arms, and legs while Parker fanned him briskly with his running shorts. By the time EMTs arrived on the scene, Daniel's temperature was starting to decrease. Parker's quick action had prevented serious complications.

Heat and cold can lead to a number of different injuries—some minor, some life threatening. Critical to your ability to care for those injuries is a basic understanding of the way the body maintains its temperature and how it adjusts physiologically to extremes in heat and cold.

25.1 Temperature Regulation

> **Learning Objective 1** Explain how the body attempts to maintain normal body temperature.

The human body stubbornly defends its constant core temperature of 98.6°F. If that temperature is to be maintained, heat loss must equal heat production. The body maintains equilibrium by varying blood flow to the outer part of the body. When the core temperature rises, vessels near the skin dilate, and the blood brings increased heat to the skin. If the outside environment is cooler than the skin, the heat is dissipated by radiation and convection; if the environment is hot, heat is also dissipated by evaporation of sweat. Temperature moves from a warmer surface or body to a cooler surface or body.

How the Body Loses Heat

> **Learning Objective 2** Explain how the body loses heat.

The body loses heat in the following five ways (see Figure 25-1):

1. **Radiation**, whereby heat is transferred from the surface of one object to the surface of another without actual contact; radiation is the primary way the body loses heat.

2. **Conduction**, whereby heat is transferred from the surface of one object to the surface of another through direct contact; heat loss through conduction can be 25 times greater in cold air than in cold water.

3. **Convection**, whereby cold air in immediate contact with the skin is warmed by the skin; heated molecules move away, cooler ones take their place, and the cycle repeats itself.

> **radiation** The loss of body heat to the surface of another object without physical contact
>
> **conduction** The loss of body heat to nearby objects through direct physical touch
>
> **convection** The loss of body heat to surrounding air, which becomes warmer, rises, and is replaced with cooler air

MECHANISMS OF HEAT LOSS

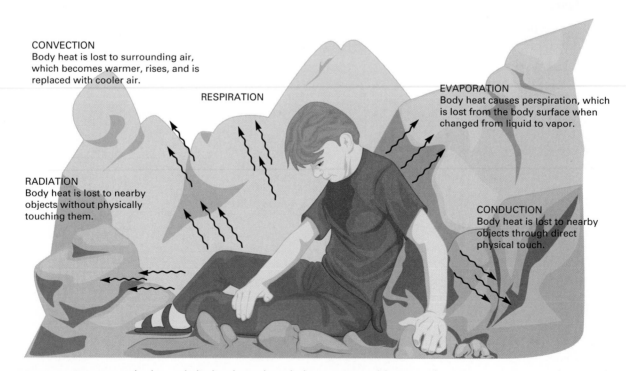

CONVECTION
Body heat is lost to surrounding air, which becomes warmer, rises, and is replaced with cooler air.

RESPIRATION

EVAPORATION
Body heat causes perspiration, which is lost from the body surface when changed from liquid to vapor.

RADIATION
Body heat is lost to nearby objects without physically touching them.

CONDUCTION
Body heat is lost to nearby objects through direct physical touch.

FIGURE 25–1. A wet, poorly dressed climber has taken shelter among cold, wet rocks.

4. **Evaporation**, whereby body heat causes perspiration, which is lost from the body surface when it is changed to vapor; two-thirds of evaporative loss is through perspiration.

5. **Respiration**, whereby body heat loses through breathing; one-third of evaporative loss is through respiration.

If the body gets overheated, blood flow is increased to the skin. Vessels at the skin surface dilate, the heat in the blood is taken to the skin surface, and the heat is then lost through radiation, convection, and evaporation (perspiration).

The phenomenon of convection has been incorporated into the concept of windchill. A unit of windchill is defined as the amount of heat that would be lost in an hour from a square meter of exposed skin surface with a normal temperature of 91.4°F. In essence, the windchill factor combines the effects of the speed of the wind and the temperature of the environment into a number that indicates the danger of exposure. Windchill, through the associated convections, will cause the body to cool at a much greater rate.

How the Body Conserves Heat

The body conserves heat in three ways:

1. Blood vessels constrict, keeping the warm blood in the core of the body

2. Hairs stand erect, trapping warm air immediately next to the skin

3. Little or no perspiration is released to the skin surface for evaporation

How Clothing Affects Thermal Equilibrium

Clothing provides thermal resistance to heat loss, insulating the skin by trapping air between its fibers. Unfortunately, most people do not understand how to use clothes to their best advantage in regulating body temperature.

Heat loss needs to be increased when the body is active and decreased when it is inactive. But the way most people wear clothes in cold weather defeats both purposes—they wear too many layers while they are working, and too few layers while they are resting.

Consider what happens when you perspire. In hot weather, clothes act as a barrier to evaporation of perspiration, reducing the effectiveness of the cooling system of the body. In cold weather, a person who wears too many layers of clothing perspires heavily, and the layer of clothing next to the skin stays wet. As a result, the person loses heat 240 times faster than if the clothing remains dry.

PROGRESS CHECK

1. Heat loss through radiation involves the transfer of heat from the body to another surface without _____. *(interference/direct contact/evaporation)*

2. Convection, central to the concept of windchill, occurs when air molecules surrounding the skin get _____, rise, and are replaced by cooler air. *(moved by the wind/caught in a draft/warmed by the skin)*

3. Heat loss through conduction involves the transfer of heat from one surface to another through _____. *(direct contact/indirect contact/clothing fibers)*

4. Through evaporation, perspiration is changed from liquid to _____ and carries heat away with it. *(gas/solid/vapor)*

25.2 Heat-Related Injuries (Hyperthermia)

Heat-related injuries (**hyperthermia**) fall into three major categories: heatstroke, heat exhaustion, and heat cramps. They are most common when the temperature and humidity are high and there is little or no breeze. When the ambient temperature reaches 90°F, the ability to lose heat through radiation is ineffective. At a relative humidity of 75 percent or greater, heat loss through evaporation becomes ineffective. Most susceptible are:

- Athletes
- Workers near furnaces or ovens
- Those in poor physical condition
- Alcoholics
- The obese
- The chronically ill
- Those who have not adjusted to the environment
- Those with heart disease

evaporation The loss of body heat when perspiration is changed from liquid to vapor

respiration The loss of body heat through normal breathing

hyperthermia Greatly increased body temperature

- People using certain drugs (such as diuretics)
- Burn victims
- The elderly
- Children

Heatstroke

Heatstroke—sometimes called *sunstroke*—is a true life-threatening emergency that occurs when the body's heat-regulating mechanisms fail to effectively cool the body. The body becomes overheated, body temperature rises dangerously high, and about half of all victims do not sweat.

Because no cooling takes place, the body stores increasing amounts of heat, the heat-producing mechanisms speed up, and eventually brain cells are damaged, causing permanent disability or death. Untreated victims die.

There are two kinds of heatstroke: *classic,* in which people lose the ability to sweat (generally affecting the elderly or chronically ill); and *exertional,* in which victims involved in physical exertion and muscle stress retain the ability to sweat (see Figure 25-2). However, these victims may dehydrate, thereby losing the ability to cool through evaporation.

SIGNS AND SYMPTOMS

Heatstroke (see Figure 25-3) is indicated by:

- Body temperature of 105°F or more
- Hot, red skin that is moist or dry

heatstroke A life-threatening emergency caused by a disturbance in the body's temperature regulation mechanism, characterized by extreme fever, hot and dry or moist skin, delirium, or coma

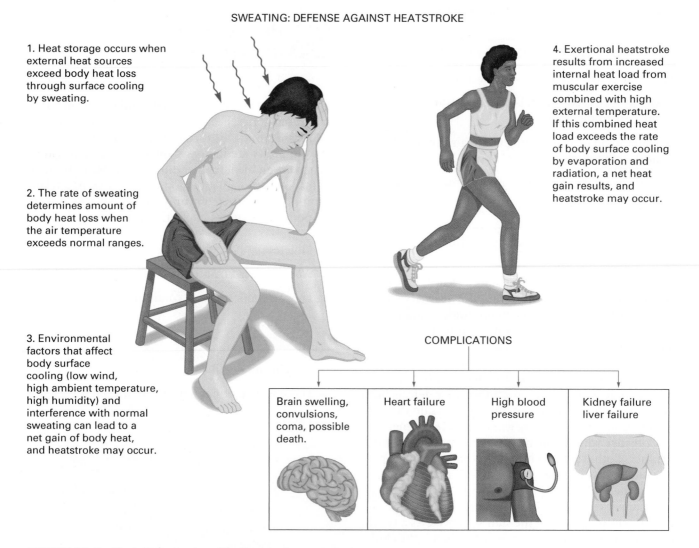

SWEATING: DEFENSE AGAINST HEATSTROKE

1. Heat storage occurs when external heat sources exceed body heat loss through surface cooling by sweating.

2. The rate of sweating determines amount of body heat loss when the air temperature exceeds normal ranges.

3. Environmental factors that affect body surface cooling (low wind, high ambient temperature, high humidity) and interference with normal sweating can lead to a net gain of body heat, and heatstroke may occur.

4. Exertional heatstroke results from increased internal heat load from muscular exercise combined with high external temperature. If this combined heat load exceeds the rate of body surface cooling by evaporation and radiation, a net heat gain results, and heatstroke may occur.

COMPLICATIONS

Brain swelling, convulsions, coma, possible death.

Heart failure

High blood pressure

Kidney failure liver failure

FIGURE 25–2. Heatstroke is a true life-threatening emergency.

Initial deep, rapid, snore-like breathing that becomes shallow and weak

Increasing dizziness and weakness

Hot, red skin

Nausea and/or vomiting
Loss of appetite

Muscular twitching
Convulsions

Possible loss of consciousness
Coma

Headache

Dilated pupils

Dry mouth

Mental confusion and anxiety
Possible hysteria and combativeness
Delirium

Rapid, strong pulse →

Temperature 105°–110°F →

Decreased blood pressure →

FIGURE 25–3. Signs and symptoms of heatstroke

- Initially rapid, strong pulse
- Later rapid, weak pulse
- Initially constricted pupils
- Later dilated pupils
- Tremors
- Mental confusion or anxiety
- Irritability or aggression
- Initially deep, rapid breathing
- Later shallow, weak breathing
- Headache
- Dry mouth
- Shortness of breath
- Loss of appetite
- Nausea and vomiting
- Dizziness and weakness
- Seizures or sudden collapse

Heatstroke victims usually have compromised levels of consciousness, ranging from disorientation to coma.

FIRST AID CARE

> Learning Objective **3** Describe and demonstrate appropriate first aid care for heatstroke.

Heatstroke is a true medical emergency; every minute counts. First aid care of heatstroke is aimed at *immediate* cooling of the body. Activate the EMS system; then take these steps:

1. Establish an airway and, when possible, remove the victim from the source of heat.

2. Remove as much of the victim's clothing as possible, down to his or her underwear; then use a combination of these methods to cool the victim until his or her mental status returns to normal:

   - Pour cool water over the victim's body, or spray the victim with cool water. Fan the patient vigorously.
   - If the victim begins to shiver, slow the cooling method (shivering produces heat).
   - *Never* use isopropyl alcohol to cool the skin; the skin absorbs the alcohol, which can be toxic.

3. Never give the victim stimulants or hot drinks.

4. As the body cools, seizures or vomiting may occur. Position the victim to allow for easy drainage.

5. Monitor the victim's temperature while you wait for emergency personnel to arrive. If the temperature starts to climb, start cooling procedures again. (The temperature must drop below 102°F and must stay that low before the danger has passed.)

Heat Exhaustion

The most common heat injury, **heat exhaustion** occurs in an otherwise fit person who engages in extreme physical exertion in a hot, humid environment. It is actually a mild form of shock brought on by the pooling of blood in the vessels just below the skin, causing blood to flow away from the major organs of the body.

As a result of prolonged and profuse sweating, the body loses large amounts of salt and water. When the water is not replaced, blood circulation diminishes, affecting brain, heart, and lung functions. The most critical problem in heat exhaustion is dehydration.

SIGNS AND SYMPTOMS

The primary signs and symptoms of heat exhaustion are:

- Headache
- Weakness
- Fatigue
- Nausea and/or vomiting
- Diarrhea
- Loss of appetite

- Dizziness and faintness
- Profuse sweating
- Pale, cool, ashen skin
- Normal-to-slightly elevated temperature
- Dilated pupils
- Weak, rapid pulse
- Thirst
- Difficulty walking
- Collapse or brief period of unconsciousness
- Possible muscle cramps

See Figure 25-4 for a comparison of the signs and symptoms of heat exhaustion and heatstroke. The two most distinct differences between heatstroke and heat exhaustion are the condition of the skin and the body temperature (see Table 25-1).

FIRST AID CARE

> Learning Objective **4** Describe and demonstrate appropriate first aid care for heat exhaustion.

To treat heat exhaustion

1. Move the victim to a cool place, remove as much of the victim's clothing as possible and fan the victim lightly. Make sure the victim does not get chilled or begin to shiver.

> **heat exhaustion** A heat-related emergency caused by excessive loss of water and salt through sweating, characterized by cool, clammy skin and a weak, rapid pulse

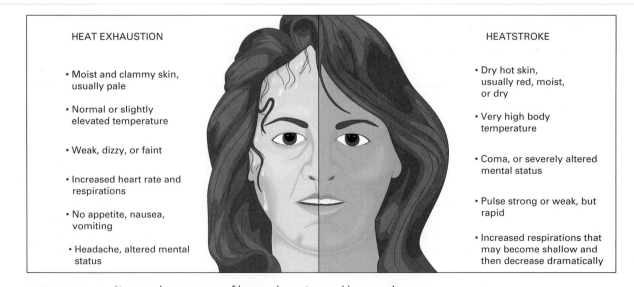

HEAT EXHAUSTION

- Moist and clammy skin, usually pale
- Normal or slightly elevated temperature
- Weak, dizzy, or faint
- Increased heart rate and respirations
- No appetite, nausea, vomiting
- Headache, altered mental status

HEATSTROKE

- Dry hot skin, usually red, moist, or dry
- Very high body temperature
- Coma, or severely altered mental status
- Pulse strong or weak, but rapid
- Increased respirations that may become shallow and then decrease dramatically

FIGURE 25–4. Signs and symptoms of heat exhaustion and heatstroke

TABLE 25-1	**Heatstroke and Heat Exhaustion**	
Condition	Skin Condition	Body Temperature
Heatstroke	Flushed, hot to the touch, wet or dry	High—usually 105° to 106°F
Heat exhaustion	Cool, pale, clammy	Normal or slightly elevated

FIGURE 25-5. The victim with heat exhaustion should be kept supine with feet elevated.

FIGURE 25-6. If the victim with heat exhaustion is fully conscious, give him or her cool water.

2. Have the victim lie down, raise the feet 8 to 12 inches (see Figure 25-5).

3. If the victim is fully conscious, give him or her cool water or a commercial sports drink to drink at the rate of half a glass every 10 minutes for 1 hour (see Figure 25-6). *Never give the victim salt tablets.* If the victim is nauseated or vomits, stop giving fluids and activate the EMS system immediately.

4. If the victim is unconscious, immediately activate EMS, and manage the airway and ventilation.

5. Take the victim's temperature every 10 to 15 minutes. If the temperature is above 101°F or is rising,

or if the victim is unable to drink fluids or vomits after drinking fluids, or the victim does not improve, immediately activate the EMS system.

Heat Cramps

The least common and least serious heat injury, **heat cramps** are muscle spasms that occur when

- The body loses too much salt and other electrolytes during profuse sweating
- Calcium levels are low
- Too much water and not enough electrolytes are consumed

Muscles rely on a strict balance of water, calcium, and sodium; whenever that balance is disrupted, heat cramps can result. In essence, the cramp occurs because the muscle contracts but does not relax.

Hot weather is not a prerequisite—a person who exercises strenuously in cold weather and perspires can develop heat cramps if he or she drinks water but does not replace salt.

SIGNS AND SYMPTOMS

Heat cramps can range from mild to extremely painful muscular cramps and pain, and are most common in the legs, calves, and abdomen. Other signs and symptoms include (see Figure 25-7 on page 418):

- Rapid heartbeat
- Sweaty skin
- Normal body temperature
- Faintness and dizziness
- Exhaustion or fatigue

> **heat cramps** Muscle spasms caused by a disturbance in the electrolyte balance of the muscles; generally seen when the body loses too much salt and other electrolytes during profuse sweating

SIGNS AND SYMPTOMS OF HEAT CRAMPS

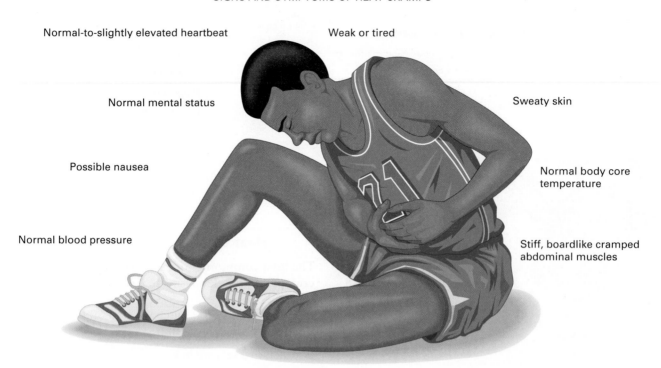

Normal-to-slightly elevated heartbeat

Weak or tired

Normal mental status

Sweaty skin

Possible nausea

Normal body core temperature

Normal blood pressure

Stiff, boardlike cramped abdominal muscles

Severe muscular cramps and pain, especially of the arms, fingers, legs, calves, and abdomen

FIGURE 25–7. Heat cramps are the most common but least serious heat injury.

- Stiff, boardlike abdomen
- Possible nausea and vomiting
- Normal consciousness level

FIRST AID CARE

Learning Objective 5 Describe and demonstrate appropriate first aid care for heat cramps.

1. If the victim is in a hot environment, remove him or her from the heat immediately; have the victim rest in a cool place.

2. Administer sips of water or a sports drink at the rate of half a glass every 15 minutes. *Do not use salt tablets.*

3. Apply moist towels to the victim's forehead and over the cramping muscles. To relieve pain, try gently stretching the involved muscle groups.

4. Explain to the victim what happened and why so the victim can avoid a recurrence; the victim should avoid exertion of any kind for at least 12 hours, or heat cramps will recur. Activate the EMS system if the victim has other illnesses or injuries, if other symptoms develop, or if the victim's condition worsens or does not respond to care.

PROGRESS CHECK

1. _____ is a life-threatening condition; untreated, all victims die. *(Heatstroke/Heat exhaustion/Heat cramps)*

2. The two most reliable and distinct differences between heatstroke and heat exhaustion are body temperature and _____ . *(level of consciousness/condition of the skin/pattern of breathing)*

3. In heatstroke, the skin is hot, red, and _____ . *(wet/dry/either wet or dry)*

4. The top priority in treatment of heatstroke is _____ . *(monitoring pulse/immediate cooling of the body/monitoring body temperature)*

5. If the victim's temperature starts rising again after you have started treatment for heatstroke, you should _____ . *(activate the EMS system immediately/submerge the victim in cool water/begin cooling procedures again)*

6. Heat exhaustion results from _____ . *(elevated body temperature/loss of fluid and electrolytes/vessel dilation)*

7. The most critical problem in heat exhaustion is _____ . *(dehydration/overheating/circulatory disturbance)*

8. Heat cramps occur because of disruption in the muscle's balance of calcium, water, and
_____ . (*sodium/potassium/phosphorus*)

9. To treat heat cramps, give the victim sips of
_____ . (*hot water/cold water/salt water*)

25.3 Cold-Related Injuries (Hypothermia)

Major injuries related to extreme cold temperature are general hypothermia, immersion hypothermia, and frostbite. Cold-related injury can occur at any time of year if a person is exposed to the elements for an extended period, is sweating heavily and exposed to wind, or is a victim of near-drowning. *Remember:* A number of conditions other than cold weather can affect the body's ability to regulate its own temperature.

General Hypothermia

The most life-threatening cold injury, general **hypothermia** affects the entire body with severe generalized cooling. (see Table 25-2). In general, thermal control is lost once the body temperature is lowered to 95°F; coma occurs when the body's core temperature reaches approximately 79°F.

Factors contributing to hypothermia, even in the absence of cold environment, include

- Certain drugs (i.e., central nervous system depressants)
- Surgery
- Water activities
- Existing disease
- Trauma
- Massive blood loss
- Extremes of age (very young or very old)
- Immobility

Basically, hypothermia occurs when the body loses more heat than it produces; death can occur within hours of the first signs and symptoms depending on the rate of cooling. (see Figure 25-8 on page 420).

hypothermia Greatly decreased body temperature

TABLE 25–2	Summary of General Hypothermia			
Predisposing Factors	**Signs Others See**	**Symptoms Victims Feel**	**Prevention**	**First Aid Care**
• Poor physical condition	• Loss of coordination; slow, stumbling pace	• Violent shivering (early)	• Rest and eat before exertion	• MINIMIZE HEAT LOSS; protect victim from cold
• Failure to eat and drink enough	• Speech distortion	• Fatigue	• Nibble on high-energy food continuously while outdoors	• Place insulting pad between victim and the ground
• Little body fat	• Forgetfulness	• Feeling of extreme cold or numbness		
• Inadequate clothing	• Lack of judgment; irrational ambition	• Loss of coordination: stumbling, thick speech, disorientation	• Wear windproof outer clothing	• Wrap victim in dry clothing and/or blankets
• Lack of shelter from snow, rain, wind	• Overactive imagination; possible hallucinations		• Carry emergency protective equipment	• Keep victim dry; remove wet clothing
• Wetness (from perspiration, precipitation, or immersion)	• Pale, cold skin	• Rigidity of muscles after shivering stops	• If outdoors in wilderness, make camp immediately if storm arises, injury occurs, or you get lost	• ADD HEAT; have victim get into sleeping bag with another person
• Exhaustion	• Dilated pupils	• Pale, cold skin		
	• Slow, shallow breathing (late)	• Pulse slow, irregular, or weak (late)		• Give warm liquids
	• Confusion, stupor, possible unconsciousness		• Keep moving; this keeps the body producing heat; if camped, use shelter and isometric exercises	• Keep victim in physical contact with others for body heat

STAGES OF HYPOTHERMIA (Cold-Related Injury)

Stage 1: **Shivering** is a response by the body to generate heat. It typically does not occur below a body temperature of 90°F.

Stage 2: **Apathy and decreased muscle function.** First fine motor function is affected, then gross motor functions.

Stage 3: **Decreased level of consciousness** is accompanied by a glassy stare and possible freezing of the extremities.

Stage 4: **Decreased vital signs,** including slow pulse and slow respiration rate.

Stage 5: **Death.**

FIGURE 25–8. Hypothermia is an acute medical emergency requiring immediate attention.

However, treatment should always be attempted—cases ave been documented in which victims have survived core temperature as low as 64.4°F.

SIGNS AND SYMPTOMS

Learning Objective **6** Identify the signs and symptoms of hypothermia.

Because it is extremely difficult to measure core body temperature in the field, when you suspect hypothermia you should rely instead on signs and symptoms (see Figures 25-9 and 25-10).

- Skin that is cold to the touch (To test, place the back of your hand against the skin of the victim's abdomen.)

- Uncontrollable shivering

- Vague, slurred, thick speech

- Amnesia and incoherence

- Disorientation, confusion

- Poor judgment

- Staggering gait

- Dizziness

- Pale, cold waxen skin

- Stiff and hard muscles

- Sluggish pupils

- Increased heart and respiratory rates (early)

- Decreased heart and respiratory rates (late)

- Dehydration

- Drowsiness and/or stupor

- Apparent exhaustion

- Unconsciousness

FIRST AID CARE

Learning Objective **7** Describe and demonstrate appropriate first aid are for hypothermia.

The basic principles of first aid care for hypothermia include preventing heat loss, possibly rewarming the victim as quickly and safely as possible, and remaining

FIGURE 25-9. Signs and symptoms of hypothermia

FIGURE 25-10. Hypothermia victims with a core temperature lower than 90°F require extreme care in handling and rapid transport to the hospital.

alert for complications. Immediately get the victim out of the cold. After activating the EMS system:

1. Check the victim's vital signs. Measure for 1 full minute, because vital signs are slowed and weak in hypothermia. (A hypothermic victim may breathe only three or four times per minute and have a pulse of only 5 to 10 beats per minute.) If there is no pulse, open the airway and begin CPR. If an AED is available, deliver only one shock. If that does not correct the rhythm, continue CPR and do not deliver any additional shocks.

   Note: According to American Heart Association guidelines, you should attempt CPR on a hypothermia victim in cases when you ordinarily would not attempt CPR—even in the presence of fixed and dilated pupils. Do not attempt CPR if there are other obviously lethal injuries, if cold has made the chest wall too rigid to perform CPR, if the victim was submerged in water for more than 60 minutes, or if transport for gradual rewarming will be drastically delayed.

2. Handle the victim *very* gently. Don't let the victim walk around or move much on his or her own.

3. Keep the victim in a supine position to prevent shock and increase blood flow to the brain. *Do not elevate the legs;* doing so causes cold blood to flow to the heart.

4. Prevent further heat loss:

   - Move the victim to a warm, sheltered place.
   - Insulate the head and body, especially the core.
   - Do not allow the victim's skin to be exposed to wind, cold air, or water spray.
   - Remove wet clothing, then layer dry clothing and coverings on top of the victim.
   - If the victim is wearing a coat, place the victim's arms next to his or her body instead of in the sleeves of the coat.
   - Insulate the victim from the ground with blankets, plastic sheets, newspapers, plastic air-bubble packing material, or a sleeping bag.

5. Never rub or manipulate the arms or legs; you could force cold blood from the viens into the core circulation and heart, causing abnormal heart rhythm or cardiac arrest.

6. Never give the victim tobacco, coffee, or alcohol. Give warm fluids only after uncontrollable shivering stops and the victim is completely conscious (the victim must be able to swallow and cough).

FIRST AID CARE FOR SEVERE HYPOTHERMIA

Severe hypothermia makes the victim appear dead—the victim may be in a coma, be cold to the touch, have fixed and dilated pupils, be in shock, have slow or no reflexes, breathe only once or twice per minute, be stiff, or assume a fetal position. The key in hypothermia is that *a person is not dead until he or she is warm and exhibits no signs of life. Always assume the victim is still alive,* and provide the following care:

1. *Never* try to rewarm a severely hypothermic victim. Insulate the victim against further heat loss, but do not apply any source of heat. Handle the victim *extremely* gently.

2. Assess vital signs over a 1-minute period; if there is no heartbeat during the 1 minute, start CPR.

3. If the victim is not breathing, administer gentle mouth-to-mouth or mouth-to-mask/barrier device at a rate of 10 to 12 breaths per minute in an adult, or 12 to 20 breaths per minute in an infant or child.

4. Maintain airway, breathing, and circulation until EMTs arrive.

Immersion Hypothermia

Immersion hypothermia—lowering of the body temperature that occurs as a result of immersion in cold water—should be considered in all cases of accidental immersion.

Body temperature drops to equal water temperature within 10 minutes; when the water is 50°F or lower, death can occur within a few minutes.

A number of factors cause more rapid cooling when the body is immersed in the water. They include:

- Water temperature (colder water speeds body cooling)
- Body size (small, thin people cool more quickly)
- Clothing (clothing helps insulate the body and slows cooling)
- Physical activity (trying to swim or tread water makes the victim cool off faster due to the principle of convection)
- Alcohol (alcohol dilates surface blood vessels and promotes rapid cooling)

FIRST AID CARE

The immediate priority in immersion hypothermia is to remove the victim from the water. Do not allow the victim to move rapidly in the water. Lift the victim from the water in a horizontal position. Once the victim is out of the water

1. Activate the EMS system immediately.

2. Maintain the victim's airway, breathing, and circulation.

3. Keep the victim still and quiet; the coldest blood is in the extremities, and it will circulate rapidly to the heart with movement.

4. Follow insulating and rewarming guidelines as for general hypothermia, remembering to handle the victim *very* gently.

If a victim in the water cannot be rescued immediately, instruct the victim to exert as little effort as possible, keep head and face out of the water, cross legs under the water, and do as little as possible to stay afloat. If there is more than one victim in the water, have them form a tight circle with their chests together to maintain heat (see Figure 25-11).

Frostbite

Frostbite, the freezing of body tissue, and **frostnip**, freezing of the skin surface, often accompany hypothermia. In those cases, care of the hypothermia always takes precedence.

Frostbite, which most commonly affects the hands, feet, ears, nose, and cheeks, occurs when ice crystals form between the cells of the skin and then grow by extracting fluid from the cells (see Figure 25-12 on page 424). The temperature of the skin must be below freezing—usually at about 28°F or lower—before tissues of the body will freeze. Circulation is obstructed, causing additional damage to the tissue.

The likelihood of frostbite is increased by:

- Any kind of trauma
- Loss of blood
- Extremes of age
- Tight or tightly laced footwear
- Use of alcohol during exposure to cold
- Wet clothing

> **frostbite** Damage to the tissues resulting from prolonged exposure to extreme cold
>
> **frostnip** Freezing of the skin surface

HELP OR HUDDLE

A person wearing a flotation device can minimize heat loss and increase chances of survival by assuming the Heat Escape Lessening Position, or HELP (above), in which the knees are pulled up to the chest and the arms crossed. Groups of three or more can conserve heat by wrapping their arms around one another and pulling into a tight circle.

FIGURE 25–11. Conserving body heat to help prevent immersion hypothermia
(Reprinted with permission of Publisher from James R. Blackman, "Caught in Cold Water," *Emergency Medicine,* January 30, 1985, Copyright © 1985 by Quadrant HealthCom Inc.)

1. FIRST DEGREE (Frost Nip)
   Affects tips of ears, nose, cheeks, fingers, toes, chin—skin blanched white, painless

FROSTBITE is localized cooling of the body

- 70% of the body is composed of water.

- When the body is subjected to excessive cold, the water in the cells can freeze; resulting ice crystals may even destroy the cell.

- Never rub the skin of a victim with frostbite; rubbing can result in permanent tissue damage.

2. SECOND DEGREE
   Affects skin and tissue just beneath skin; skin is firm and waxy, tissue beneath is soft, numb, then turns purple during thawing.

3. THIRD DEGREE
   Affects entire tissue depth; tissue beneath skin is solid, waxy white with purplish tinge.

1. **First Aid Care for First-Degree Frostbite:**
   The skin can be warmed by applying firm pressure with a hand (no rubbing) or other warm body part, by blowing warm breath on the spot, or by submerging in warm water bath.

2. **First Aid Care for Second-Degree Frostbite:**
   Treatment includes submerging in warm water bath.

3. **First Aid Care for Third-Degree Frostbite:**
   This victim needs immediate hospital care. Dry clothing over the frostbite will help prevent further injury. Submerging in warm water can help thaw. Rewarm by immersion in water heated to 100°–110° F, and maintain body core temperature. The frostbitten part should not be rubbed or chafed in any way. The part should not be thawed if the victim must walk on it to get to the medical facility or if it will be re-exposed to the cold with the potential of refreezing. Do not delay activating the EMS system for rewarming.
   Follow local protocol.

FIGURE 25–12. The three stages of frostbite

TABLE 25-3	Stages of Frostbite		
Extent of Injury	Appearance of Frozen Skin	Appearance of Skin after Rewarming
First degree (layers of skin only)	White, plaquelike	Red, hot, and dry, with itching, burning, swelling, and pain
Second degree (skin and the layer just beneath the skin)	White with blisters filled with clear fluid	Blisters filled with straw-colored fluid; swelling and intense burning and pain
Third degree (skin and the layers beneath the skin)	Discolored, fails to blanch with pressure, deep small blisters filled with dark fluid	Blisters filled with bloody fluid; severe swelling, with some tissue death and pain
Fourth degree (skin, muscle, and bone)	White to deep purple skin; no pain, swelling, or blisters; full-thickness freeze	Numbness; significant death of the skin, muscle, and bone

- High altitudes
- Race (Blacks are three times more likely than Whites to experience frostbite.)

SIGNS AND SYMPTOMS

> Learning Objective **8** Identify the signs and symptoms of frostbite.

It is very difficult to assess frostbite; while frozen, even severely frostbitten tissue can appear almost normal. In general, the appearance of the skin varies depending on the extent of injury (see Table 25-3).

Figures 25-13 and 25-14 illustrate third- and second-degree frostbite.

The signs and symptoms of frostnip include skin that is reddened, swollen, and painful.

FIRST AID CARE

> Learning Objective **9** Describe and demonstrate appropriate first aid care for frostbite.

To care for frostnip, gently rewarm the affected skin by placing it against warm skin (the skin of the abdomen,

or in the armpit or groin) or immerse it in a warm water bath. Never rub the skin. It will tingle when it is warm.

To care for frostbite, activate the EMS system immediately; then take these steps:

1. Immediately remove the victim from the cold environment.

2. Keep the tissue frozen until you can initiate care; *never thaw tissue if there is any chance of its refreezing.* If the tissue refreezes, the ice crystals will be larger and will do greater damage to the tissues.

3. Protect the injured tissue from friction or pressure; never poke or squeeze the tissue. Remove constricting clothing or jewelry that is not sticking to the skin.

4. Thaw frostbitten tissue in a water bath (see Figure 25-15 on page 426). Fully immerse the frozen extremity without allowing it to touch the sides or bottom of the container; check the water temperature with a thermometer, and keep it between 100° and 110°F by adding warm water. Never use any kind of flame or electric heat, and

FIGURE 25–13. Third-degree frostbite

FIGURE 25–14. Second-degree frostbite

FIGURE 25–15. Thaw the frostbitten part rapidly in water just above normal body temperature (100°–110°F).

never use dry heat. *Never* rub or massage frostbitten skin or rub it with snow or alcohol. Never break any blisters caused by frostbite.

5. Keep rewarming until the skin color no longer improves (rewarming to this point may take as long as 40 minutes).

6. Cover the thawed parts with loose, dry, sterile dressings and elevate the extremities. Place sterile gauze between the fingers and toes to reduce the risk of increased injury.

7. While waiting for emergency personnel to arrive, monitor vital signs and keep the victim warm. Do not let the victim walk if the feet are involved, and do not let the victim smoke. Do not re-expose the the thawed part to the cold.

PROGRESS CHECK

1. Because taking core temperature is difficult in the field, you should rely on _____ to identify hypothermia. *(skin temperature/ signs and symptoms/what the victim tells you)*

2. The priority in treating hypothermia is to _____ . *(start rewarming right away/remove the victim from the cold environment/rewarm rapidly)*

3. The priority in treating immersion hypothermia is _____ . *(getting the victim out of the water/preventing drowning/drying the victim)*

4. You should never thaw frostbitten tissue if there is any danger of _____ . *(refreezing/delayed transport/increased injury)*

5. Frostbitten tissue should be thawed using _____ . *(steam/dry heat/warm water)*

Summary

- The body maintains its temperature by variations in the blood flow.

- Body heat can be lost through radiation, conduction, convection, evaporation, and respiration.

- There are three kinds of heat-related injury, or hyperthermia—heatstroke, heat exhaustion, and heat cramps.

- Heatstroke is a life-threatening emergency; untreated victims die.

- Heatstroke occurs when the temperature-regulating mechanisms of the body fail and the body can no longer cool itself.

- Heat exhaustion is a mild state of shock that occurs when profuse sweating results in severe loss of salt, other electrolytes and water.

- Heat cramps occur when the balance of water, salt, and calcium in the muscles is disrupted.

- A victim of general hypothermia can appear to be dead, but you should give first aid care unless there are other obviously lethal injuries. A victim should never be considered dead until he or she exhibits no signs of life.

- The key in treating immersion hypothermia is to get the victim out of the water.

- Frostbite is freezing of body tissues; never warm or thaw frostbitten tissue if there is any danger of its refreezing.

Key Terms

Make sure you understand the following key terms:

radiation	heatstroke
conduction	heat exhaustion
convection	heat cramps
evaporation	hypothermia
respiration	frostbite
hyperthermia	frostnip

Critical Thinking Exercise

You are out for an early spring morning jog in the local park when you come across a man in his mid-forties lying on a park bench who appears to be unresponsive. As you approach him, you notice his skin is extremely pale with cyanosis to his face and neck, and his breathing is extremely shallow and slow. He does not respond when you shout at him. He is dressed lightly in a tee shirt and cotton pants with shoes and no socks. You also find a bottle of wine next to the bench. The overnight temperature was in the high 50s. His radial pulse is very weak and slow. His skin is very cold and stiff to the touch.

1. What condition do you suspect the victim is experiencing?

2. What signs and symptoms would make you suspect the condition?

3. What first aid would you provide to the victim?

Student: _____ Date: _____

Course: _____ Section #: _____

Part 1 True/False

If you believe the statement is true, circle the T. If you believe the statement is false, circle the F.

T F **1.** Heatstroke commonly occurs under conditions of high temperature, high humidity, and low wind velocity.

T F **2.** First aid care of heatstroke is aimed at immediate cooling of the body.

T F **3.** To treat heatstroke, remove the victim's clothing, moisten the skin with cool water, and direct a fan at the skin.

T F **4.** Heat exhaustion is the most common heat injury.

T F **5.** The most critical problem in heat exhaustion is dehydration.

T F **6.** In heat exhaustion, the skin is flushed and hot; in heatstroke, the skin is cool and pale.

T F **7.** Do not give a heat exhaustion victim fluids by mouth.

T F **8.** Heat cramps are the least common and least serious heat injury.

T F **9.** Heat cramps occur only in hot weather.

T F **10.** Death can occur within 2 hours of the first signs and symptoms of hypothermia.

T F **11.** Hypothermia can occur even in warm weather (65°F).

T F **12.** Whenever possible, keep a hypothermia victim in a sitting position.

T F **13.** If a hypothermia victim is not shivering, do not try to rewarm the victim.

T F **14.** Active rewarming of a hypothermia victim should always be attempted before transporting the person to a hospital.

T F **15.** Never try to completely actively rewarm a severely hypothermic victim.

T F **16.** A victim of immersion hypothermia should be encouraged to increase physical activity.

T F **17.** Always thaw a frostbitten part.

T F **18.** Frostbite should be thawed gradually.

T F **19.** If possible, use dry heat to thaw frostbitten parts.

Part 2 Multiple Choice

For each item, circle the correct answer or the phrase that best completes the statement.

1. Which of the following is *not* a means for the body to lose heat?
a. evaporation
b. osmosis
c. convection
d. radiation

2. The phenomenon of convection has been incorporated into the concept of
a. windchill
b. evaporation
c. perspiration
d. hyperthermia

3. The most important characteristic of heatstroke is

    a. profuse perspiration
    b. dizziness
    c. very hot skin
    d. painful muscle cramps or spasms

4. The most important first aid care procedure for victims of heatstroke is to

    a. treat for shock
    b. replace lost body fluids
    c. cool the body in any way possible
    d. give the victim salt-and-sugar water

5. The two most distinct differences between heatstroke and heat exhaustion are

    a. pulse rate and presence of perspiration
    b. skin condition and pupil reaction
    c. body temperature and presence of perspiration
    d. body temperature and skin temperature

6. The victim suffering from heat exhaustion can be identified by

    a. hot, dry, flushed skin
    b. cool, moist skin and rapid breathing
    c. cool, dry skin; dizziness; and headache
    d. hot, moist skin; labored breathing; and slow pulse

7. The most serious heat-related emergency is

    a. heat exhaustion
    b. heatstroke
    c. heat cramps
    d. all are equally serious

8. Which of the following is *not* a procedure for care of a victim of immersion hypothermia?

    a. handle the victim gently
    b. encourage the victim to walk around to increase circulation
    c. layer dry clothing over the victim's wet clothing
    d. protect the victim from the wind

9. For which of the following reasons should a frostbitten part be left frozen?

    a. assessment has not been confirmed
    b. pain becomes severe as thawing takes place
    c. there is a possibility of refreezing
    d. acclimatization needs to be increased

10. A frostbitten part should be rewarmed

    a. by rubbing
    b. with water between 100° and 110°F
    c. with heat from a fire or stove
    d. with water between 75° and 85°F

Part 3   Matching

Match the type of emergency with the appropriate signs/symptoms and first aid care.

Signs/Symptoms and Care

1. _____ Pale, clammy skin
2. _____ Firm, waxy, white skin
3. _____ Hot, flushed, dry skin
4. _____ Painful abdomen
5. _____ Body temperature of 106°F
6. _____ Do not rub or chafe
7. _____ Give sips of cool salt water
8. _____ Slow, slurred speech
9. _____ Apply cool water and fan aggressively.
10. _____ Sweating mechanisms fail

Type of Emergency

A. Heatstroke
B. Heat exhaustion
C. Heat cramps
D. Frostbite
E. Hypothermia

Part 4   What Would You Do If?

1. A middle-aged man who is playing baseball on a hot and humid day becomes dizzy and weak. He has moist, pale, clammy skin; complains of a headache; and is nauseous.

2. You arrive at a winter campout area and find a victim who is confused and disoriented. She has a stumbling gait, and her face appears bloated and cyanotic. She also seems irrational, and her speech is thick and slurred.

26

Water Emergencies

Learning Objectives

When you have mastered the material in this chapter, you will be able to

1 Explain the difference between drowning and near-drowning

2 Explain the difference between "wet" and "dry" drowning

3 Explain why you should always try to resuscitate someone who has had an accident in cold water

4 Explain how to safely reach someone in trouble in the water

5 Describe and demonstrate how to protect a victim in the water if you suspect spinal injury

6 Describe and demonstrate first aid care for a near-drowning victim

7 Describe the various kinds of diving emergencies

8 List the signs and symptoms of air embolism and decompression sickness

9 Describe and demonstrate first aid care for a victim of air embolism or decompression sickness

10 Describe and demonstrate first aid care for a victim of barotrauma

On the Scene

On a late-July afternoon, Daniel Martin and his two young children were enjoying relief from the searing summer heat at a mountain lake 30 miles outside of town. As his youngest child grasped a rope swing for a turn over the water, Daniel saw a teenage girl struggling to stay afloat about 15 feet from shore.

Daniel knew the water that far from shore was too deep for him to touch bottom, and he had limited confidence in his own swimming skills. Acting quickly, he tied a large thermos jug to the long tow rope from his car trunk. Positioning himself solidly against a tree at the lake's edge, he threw the object out to 13-year-old Karen Francis. When she grasped it and clung to it for buoyancy, Daniel pulled Karen to shore.

She was weak and shaken. Daniel had her lie down on a grassy area at the lake's edge. She seemed to be breathing well and had a pulse; a quick primary survey revealed no bleeding or suspected fractures. Using his two sons' beach towels, Daniel covered Karen to help preserve her body heat. Following Karen's directions, Daniel sent a nearby woman to find Karen's parents, who gently helped her into their motor home and took her into town for evaluation at an emergency room.

Nearly 9,000 people die each year in the United States from water accidents, and drowning is the fourth common cause of death from unintentional injury. While the nation's approximately 5,000 drownings each year are most commonly associated with water emergencies, drownings actually cause only a fraction of the nation's water-related deaths. The rest are mostly caused by accidents suffered while diving or during deep-water exploration, boating, and water skiing. Water-related deaths may also result from motor vehicle accidents. In addition to drowning and near-drowning, water-related accidents can cause bleeding, soft-tissue injuries, and fractures.

This chapter details water-safety techniques to protect you as a First Aider, outlines first aid procedures to use with drowning and near-drowning victims, and explains appropriate first aid care for victims of diving accidents.

Note: Unless a water emergency occurs in open, shallow water that has a stable, uniform bottom, never go out into the water unless you are

- a good swimmer;

- specially trained;

- wearing a personal flotation device; and

- accompanied by other rescuers.

26.1 Drowning and Near-Drowning

Learning Objective 1 Explain the difference between drowning and near-drowning.

The most frequent drowning victims are young adults between the ages of 15 and 24, and children under the age of 5. Most children drown in home swimming pools, and the vast majority of home swimming pool drownings involve toddlers. Children also often drown in irrigation ditches and drainage canals.

Drownings and near-drownings do not always occur in large bodies of water: an adult can drown in just a few inches of water, and an infant in even less. Recent studies indicate that one-fourth of all infants who drown do so in 5-gallon buckets; others drown in bathtubs and toilets.

Be aware that anyone, even a good swimmer, can get into trouble in the water. Be alert for signs that an emergency is developing; pay attention to any swimmer who is behaving oddly, and watch for these signs:

- Sudden splashing

- Screams

- Calls for help

- A swimmer who is thrashing

Remember, a swimmer who is floating and appears to be fine might actually be a distressed swimmer—one who is able to stay afloat, but who is actually too tired to get to the side of the pool or to the shore of a lake. A distressed swimmer might be trying to swim, but will be making little or no forward progress; he or she might be treading water, clinging to some kind of support, or calling for help. A distressed swimmer may not seem to be in imminent danger, but is actually at great risk for drowning if not rescued quickly.

Remember, too, that there may be more than one drowning victim at a scene.

Near-drowning is defined as at least temporarily surviving near suffocation due to submersion. **Drowning** is death from suffocation due to submersion.

Learning Objective 2 Explain the difference between "wet" and "dry" drowning.

"Wet" drowning occurs when a victim aspirates fluid (water or vomit) or a foreign body into the lungs. **"Dry" drowning** occurs when a severe muscle spasm of the larynx cuts off respiration but does not allow aspiration of a significant amount of fluid into the lungs (see Figure 26-1). It is estimated that approximately 10 to 15 percent of all drownings are "dry"—and autopsies reveal that only about 15 percent of all drowning victims aspirate enough water to cause death directly. Panic can often contribute to the death of the person who loses self-control in a water accident (see Figure 26-2 on page 434). In **secondary drowning**, the victim is resuscitated but dies within 96 hours from the incident, usually as a result of breathing water into the lungs and developing aspiration pneumonia. Pneumonia generally does not develop for 48 to 72 hours after the incident, which is why all near-drowning victims should have follow-up medical care.

---

near-drowning Survival, at least temporarily, of near suffocation due to submersion

drowning Death from suffocation due to submersion

"wet" drowning Drowning in which water enters the lungs

"dry" drowning Drowning in which little or no water enters the lungs

secondary drowning Death from aspiration pneumonia following resuscitation after a water accident

Drowning can be the result of cold, fatigue, injury, disorientation, intoxication, or limited swimming abilities.	The drowning victim struggles to inhale air as long as possible. Eventually the victim inhales water or a muscle spasm of the larynx closes the airway.	Loss of consciousness, convulsions, cardiac arrest, and death may follow.

FIGURE 26–1. Drowning

There are two basic types of drowning: **active drowning** and **passive drowning**. An active drowning victim is vertical in the water, is not kicking, is still breathing, and is usually moving his or her arms in an effort to bob out of the water and get a breath of air. The swimmer can't call for help, because all energy is expended on the effort to breathe. You have less time to rescue a passive drowning victim who is not moving, not breathing, and who is face-down in the water, either submerged or near the surface.

Prognosis for near-drowning is best when victims are submerged for fewer than 5 minutes and when CPR is started within 10 minutes of submersion.

Among victims of water-related accidents, those with the poorest prognosis are older victims, those who struggle in the water, those who suffer associated injuries, those who are submerged for a long time, and those who are in warm, dirty, or brackish water. Standard water-safety precautions can be taken to prevent near-drowning accidents, such as:

- Children should be under constant supervision if a lake, pool, or pail of water of any size is nearby.

- Water sports and alcohol never mix.

- Life preservers or life jackets should always be worn when boating.

- Swimmers should always go into the water feet-first *unless* the area has been clearly marked for diving and there are no visible obstructions.

- Swimmers should find out all they can about the area in which they are swimming and about any potential hazards, such as currents and sudden changes in the depth of the water. Swimmers should know where it is safe to enter and exit the water, where obstructions exist, and where the deep and shallow areas are.

- Generally, swimmers should not swim if extreme conditions exist—it is too hot, too cold, too far away from safety, the swimmer is too tired, or the swim would require too much strenuous activity.

- Swimmers should obey all posted signs, stay out of restricted areas, and swim only in those areas supervised by a lifeguard.

- Swimmers should always swim with a buddy—never alone.

active drowning Drowning in which the victim is struggling in the water and is still breathing

passive drowning Drowning in which the victim is not breathing and is face-down in the water

FIGURE 26–2. In water accidents, panic can often contribute to the death of the person who loses self-control.

Resuscitating Cold-Water Submersion Victims

> Learning Objective **3** Explain why you should always try to resuscitate someone who has had an accident in cold water.

There is a significant difference between warm-water and cold-water drownings: When a person dives into cold water (below 68°F), the **mammalian diving reflex** can prevent death, even after prolonged submersion.

Here is how it seems to work: When the face is submerged in cold water, breathing is inhibited, the heart rate slows, and the blood vessels throughout most of the body constrict. However, blood flow to the heart and brain is maintained. In this way, oxygen is sent and used only where it is needed immediately to sustain life.

The colder the water, the more oxygen is diverted to the heart and brain. The diving reflex is more pronounced, and cooling is more rapid, in the young. In water at or below 68°F, the body's metabolic requirements are only about half of normal.

Note that the notion of the mammalian diving reflex is somewhat controversial. Recent research suggests that the mammalian reflex occurs in a number of marine mammals—such as whales, porpoises, seals, and walruses—but does not occur in humans. Some researchers suggest that cold-water survival is due not to the diving reflex but to hypothermia, which slows the metabolism and reduces the body's need for oxygen.

Generally, you can resuscitate victims who have been submerged in cold water even after 30 minutes or longer in cardiac arrest. As a guideline, any pulseless, nonbreathing victim who has been submerged in cold water should be resuscitated.

Some experts advise providing resuscitation to every drowning victim, regardless of water temperature—even those who have been in the water for a prolonged period. *Follow local protocol.*

Ensuring Your Own Safety

> Learning Objective **4** Explain how to safely reach someone in trouble in the water.

In cases where a lifeguard or other trained professional is present, you can try to reach the victim with a reaching assist. *You must always attempt a reaching assist with*

> **mammalian diving reflex** A reflex that prevents death after submersion in cold water

utmost concern for your own safety; if you neglect your own safety, you could become an additional victim.

Never enter anything but very shallow water with a stable, uniform bottom unless:

- You know how to swim

- You have been trained in water-rescue techniques

- You are not injured

- You are sure you can comfortably handle the victim considering your and the victim's height and weight

- You are wearing a personal flotation device

- You are accompanied by other rescuers

If you go into the water, try to hold on to a secure object (such as a piling, pool ladder, or overflow trough) with one hand as you reach out to the victim with your other hand.

A victim in shallow water may be able to stand and walk out of the water with assistance. To help such a victim, grasp the wrist nearest you and drape the victim's arm across your shoulders. Wrap your free arm around the victim's waist, maintain a firm grasp, and walk the person out of the water.

You may also be able to drag a victim out of shallow water. Standing behind the victim, support the neck with your forearms as you grasp under the victim's arms. Walking backward, drag the victim out of the water.

If the victim is conscious and close to shore:

- Make sure you have firm, solid footing and cannot slip into the water.

- Keep your body low, and lean backward as you pull the victim to reduce your risk of being pulled into the water.

- Hold out an object for the victim to grab; the best thing to use is a rope. You can also use an oar, branch, fishing pole, towel, shirt, belt, or other strong object that will not break. Equipment for reaching swimmers is often kept at the side of commercial swimming pools. Look for a fiberglass or aluminum pole with a large hook on one end (a *shepherd's crook*).

- Once the victim has grabbed the object, pull the victim to shore. If you are using a shepherd's crook and the swimmer is unable to reach it, hook it around the swimmer's body and pull the swimmer in. You can also use a shepherd's crook to reach a swimmer on the bottom of a pool.

If the victim is conscious but too far away to reach, you can try a throwing assist by throwing something that will help the victim stay afloat or reach the shore. A number of throwing devices can be used:

- **Ring buoy**—a floatable ring made of buoyant material attached to a lightweight tow line or rope

- **Heaving line**—a floatable, buoyant line that is usually kept coiled; the line or rope should be a bright, easily visible color (such as yellow or white)

- **Throw bag**—a nylon bag that contains 50 to 70 feet of coiled floating line; this is a commercial device commonly found on boats, and contains a foam disk to preserve its shape and keep it from sinking

- **Heaving jug**—a homemade device made of a gallon-sized plastic container filled with a half-inch of sand or water and tied to a floating line

Take these steps in a throwing assist:

1. Make sure you have firm, solid footing and that you cannot slip into the water. Assume a stride position in which the leg opposite your throwing arm is positioned forward, a stance that will help you keep your balance. Keep your feet apart and your knees bent.

2. Step on the end of the floatable line with your forward foot. Make sure you do not step on the coiled part of the line with your other foot.

3. Shout at the victim to get his or her attention, explain that you are going to throw an object, and instruct the victim to grab the object.

4. Aiming slightly beyond where the victim is in the water, bend your knees and throw the object using a swinging underhand motion; keep a good length of coiled rope or line in your other hand.

5. If the object doesn't reach the victim, rapidly pull the line back and repeat the throw, aiming beyond where the victim is in the water. Don't try to recoil the rope or line before you throw it a second time.

6. Once the victim has grabbed the object, rope, or line, keep your knees bent and lean back—away from the water—as you slowly and steadily pull the victim to safety.

If the victim is unconscious or too far to reach with a line, you will need to go to the victim. If at all possible, use a boat. Otherwise, never try to go to the victim unless you meet the safety criteria listed above.

Once you reach the victim, carefully turn him or her faceup, following the precautions listed in the next section.

Head or Spinal Injury

Learning Objective **5** Describe and demonstrate how to protect a victim in the water if you suspect spinal injury.

If the victim might have been involved in a diving accident, you should suspect head and/or spinal injury. You should also suspect spinal injury in any swimmer who is unconscious (especially one in shallow, warm water). Approximately 1,000 neck and back injuries occur during water activities each year in the United States. Permanent paralysis can result. Most of these injuries occur in shallow water.

In the case of possible spinal injury, the goal is to support the back and stabilize the head and neck as other care is given. It is important to stabilize the victim in the water properly, then to remove the person carefully from the water. The American National Red Cross suggests that the victim not be removed from the water until a backboard or other rigid support can be used as a splint. Always check to see whether a professional lifeguard is available before you attempt to move a victim with suspected spinal injury.

There are two basic immobilization techniques you can use to stabilize a victim's head, neck, and back in the water, regardless of whether the victim is face-up or face-down—the head splint and the hip/shoulder support.

HEAD SPLINT

The head splint provides better stabilization than hip/shoulder support, and should be used when the victim is face-down and is at or near the surface of the water and keeps the victim's head, neck, and back stable while you turn the victim over in the water (see figure 26-3). Follow these steps:

1. Stand at the victim's side.

2. Firmly grasp the victim's arms midway between the shoulder and elbow; grasp the victim's right arm with your right hand and the victim's left arm with your left hand.

3. Gently move the victim's arms up alongside his or her head, trying not to cause any movement of the head, neck, or back as you do so.

4. Squeeze the victim's arms against his or her head, keeping the head aligned with the body.

5. Bend your knees until the water reaches your shoulders, then slowly and carefully glide the victim forward in the water.

6. As you continue to slowly glide the victim forward, slowly rotate the victim until he or she is face-up. To rotate the victim, push the arm closest to you under the water while you pull the arm farthest from you across the surface of the water.

7. Keeping the head aligned with the body, cradle the victim's head in the crook of your arm.

8. Maintain the victim in this position until additional rescue help arrives.

HIP/SHOULDER SUPPORT

If the victim is face-up in the water, use the hip/shoulder support to limit movement of the victim's head, neck, and back. Follow these steps:

1. Stand at the victim's side.

2. Bend your knees until the water reaches your chest.

3. Slide one arm under the victim's hips and the other under the victim's shoulders, keeping the victim's body horizontal.

4. Don't lift the victim's body, but provide enough support to keep the victim's face out of the water.

5. Maintain support, keeping the victim's body as straight as possible, until help arrives.

If you are not specially trained in water rescue:

- Do not remove the victim from the water.

- Keep the victim afloat on his or her back.

- Always support the head and neck level with the back.

- Maintain the airway and support ventilation in the water.

- Wait for help.

PROGRESS CHECK

1. _____ is death from suffocation due to submersion. *(Near-drowning/Drowning/Asphyxia)*

2. Victims submerged in _____ water have the poorest prognosis. *(cold/warm/deep)*

3. "Dry" drowning occurs when a severe spasm of the _____ cuts off respiration, but water does not enter the lungs. *(trachea/bronchioles/larynx)*

4. The _____ reflex helps victims submerged in cold water survive longer. *(mammalian/Freudian/subdiaphragmatic)*

5. Never go in the water unless you can swim and have been trained, and are _____ . *(in good health/prepared to perform rescue breathing/wearing a flotation device)*

26.2 First Aid Care for Near-Drowning

Learning Objective 6 Describe and demonstrate the first aid care for a near-drowning victim.

To care for near-drowning victims, activate the EMS system; then take these steps:

1. Remove the victim from the water as quickly and safely as you can. If you suspect that the victim has spinal injury:

   - Minimize movement of the victim's head, neck, and back.

   - Keep the victim's head in line with the body.

   - Never pull on the victim's head.

   - Position the victim face-up as quickly as you safely can, as described below.

   - Support the victim at the shoulders and hips to help keep the victim's face out of the water.

   - Maintain in-line immobilization and secure the victim to a backboard before removing the person from the water.

   - If you find the victim facedown, splint the victim's head and neck with your arms or the victim's arms (see Figure 26-3), then roll the victim over, supporting the back and stabilizing the head and neck. Keeping the head and neck in line with the back, slide a backboard under the victim; secure the victim to the backboard (see Figure 26-4 on page 438).

   - If possible, apply a rigid cervical collar or place padding at the sides of the victim's head to keep it from moving.

   - Float the board to shore or poolside and lift the victim from the water.

2. If you do not suspect spinal injury, place the victim on the left side so that water, vomitus, and secretions can drain from the upper airway.

3. Assess for breathing and pulse.

HEAD SPLINT TECHNIQUE

a. Extend the victim's arms. Press them against the head to create a splint.

b. Move the victim forward to a horizontal position. Begin to rotate the victim.

c. Lower yourself until the water is at shoulder level and the victim is faceup.

d. Bring the victim's head to rest in the crook of your arm until help arrives.

FIGURE 26–3. The head splint technique immobilizes the head and neck while the victim is being turned in the water. (Adapted from Pat Samples, "Spinal Cord Injuries: The High Cost of Careless Diving," *The Physician and Sportsmedicine*, July 1989.)

A Splint head and neck with arms.

B Roll victim over.

C Ensure airway and breathing.

• Victim not breathing. Begin rescue breathing (at your own risk), and rescue from water as soon as possible.

• Victim breathing. Slide backboard under victim.

D Apply a rigid extrication collar.

E Float board to poolside.

F Remove victim from water.

FIGURE 26–4. Immobilize suspected diving accident victim, using a backboard or firm, flat object, such as a door. Follow local protocols.

4. If there is no breathing, establish an airway as rapidly as you can and begin ventilations.
Note: Water in the airway can cause resistance to ventilations. Once you have determined that there are no foreign objects in the airway, apply ventilations with more force until you see the victim's chest rise and fall.

5. If there is no pulse, begin chest compressions and perform CPR, as described in Chapter 5. Continue resuscitation until emergency personnel arrive.

A near-drowning victim needs to be taken to a hospital or medical facility, even if you think the danger has passed. A near-drowning victim can develop complications and die as long as three or four days after the incident. (Approximately 15 percent of all drowning deaths are due to secondary complications.)

Ice Rescues

If a person falls through ice into water, never attempt a rescue by walking onto the ice. Standing on solid ground, extend a secure object (such as a limb, pole, ladder, branch, or life jacket) for the victim to grasp. If you can do so safely, pull the victim to you. If not, have the victim hold onto the object to stay afloat until help arrives.

Never go even near the edge of broken ice unless there is someone to support you.

PROGRESS CHECK

1. If you suspect spinal injury, stabilize the neck and spine _____ you remove the victim from the water. *(before/after/while)*

2. If you suspect spinal injury, apply a cervical collar and secure the victim to a _____ . *(buoyant device/stable object/spine board)*

3. _____ can cause resistance to ventilations. *(Spasms/Swelling of the airway/Water in the airway)*

4. Near-drowning victims should always be taken to the hospital; 15 percent of all drowning deaths are due to _____ . *(aspiration/laryngeal spasm/secondary complications)*

26.3 Diving Emergencies

Learning Objective 7 Describe the various kinds of diving emergencies.

Diving emergencies can result either from diving into a pool or other relatively shallow body of water or from the sport of diving in deep water with scuba gear.

Diving in Shallow Water

Injuries to the head and neck and fractures of the arms, legs, and ribs can be sustained when diving into shallow water from a diving board, shore, poolside, boat, or dock. Neck and spinal injuries can also occur in deeper water if a diver hits an object either before or after entering the water.

You should always assume that someone who dives into shallow water has sustained neck and spinal injuries, even if the diver is still conscious. If the victim is still in the water, provide care as you would for a near-drowning, stabilizing the neck and spine as described in the previous section. If the victim has left the water, provide care as you would for any other victim with suspected neck and spinal injuries.

Deep-Water Diving

A major complication of deep-water diving emergencies is coma, which may result from asphyxiation, head injury, heart attack, air tank contamination, intoxication, or aspiration. It can also result from air embolism or decompression sickness, two emergencies that require recompression.

Air Embolism

Air embolism generally occurs when a diver holds his or her breath during a dive. The deeper the diver descends, the less pressure is exerted against the body; as a result, the air in the lungs expands rapidly, rupturing the alveoli and damaging adjacent blood vessels. Air bubbles then enter the bloodstream, making it difficult for the blood to carry oxygen and nutrients to body tissues. The onset of air embolism is rapid.

Decompression Sickness

Decompression sickness (often called *the bends*) usually occurs when a diver comes up too quickly from a deep, prolonged dive. Gases (usually nitrogen) breathed by the diver are absorbed into the bloodstream; as the diver comes up, the nitrogen is transformed into tiny bubbles, which lodge in body tissues and enter the bloodstream. Decompression sickness is gradual in onset, and symptoms usually occur 12 to 24 hours after the dive.

air embolism A diving injury in which air bubbles enter the bloodstream

decompression sickness A diving injury in which gases (usually nitrogen) enter the bloodstream

SIGNS AND SYMPTOMS

> Learning Objective 8 List the signs and symptoms of air embolism and decompression sickness.

The following signs and symptoms are common to both air embolism and decompression sickness:

- Itchy, blotchy, or mottled skin
- Difficulty breathing
- Dizziness
- Chest pain
- Severe, deep aching pain in the muscles, joints, and tendons
- Blurred or distorted vision
- Partial deafness, distortion of senses
- Nausea and vomiting
- Numbness or paralysis
- Staggering gait or lack of coordination

In addition, air embolism can cause:

- Frothy blood in the nose and mouth
- Swelling and a grating sound (crepitus) in the neck
- Loss or distortion of memory
- Cardiac or respiratory arrest
- Behavioral changes (sometimes the only sign)

In addition, decompression sickness can cause:

- Swelling of the extremities
- A migrainelike headache
- Choking or coughing
- Inability to empty the bladder
- Hallucinations

FIRST AID CARE

> Learning Objective 9 Describe and demonstrate first aid care for a victim of air embolism or decompression sickness.

To care for a victim of air embolism or decompression sickness, activate the EMS system. Then:

1. If there is no sign of neck or spine injury, position the victim on the left side; slant the entire body 15 degrees with the head down to force air or gas bubbles to stay in the abdomen.

2. Provide basic life support; administer ventilations and initiate CPR if needed. Life support is critical in these cases because oxygen reduces the size of nitrogen bubbles and improves circulation.

3. Monitor the victim continuously until emergency personnel arrive. The victim needs to be taken to a recompression chamber for treatment.

Barotrauma

> Learning Objective 10 Describe and demonstrate first aid care for a victim of barotrauma.

Sometimes called *the squeeze,* **barotrauma** occurs during ascent or descent when air pressure in the body's air cavities (such as the sinuses or middle ear) becomes too great. As a result, tissue in the air cavities is injured; for example, the eardrum or sinus may rupture.

Barotrauma is marked by mild to severe pain in the affected area, possible discharge from the nose or ears, extreme dizziness, nausea, and disorientation.

Victims of barotrauma must be cared for at a medical facility immediately to prevent permanent blindness, deafness, residual dizziness, or the inability to dive in the future. Provide the same care as you would for air embolism or decompression sickness and send for medical help immediately.

PROGRESS CHECK

1. Always assume that someone who dived in shallow water has sustained _____ . *(respiratory injury/abdominal injury/spinal injury)*

2. A major complication of deep-water diving emergencies is _____ . *(coma/head injury/spine injury)*

3. Decompression sickness is sometimes called _____ . *(the squeeze/the bends)*

4. Victims of air embolism or decompression sickness need treatment in a _____ . *(recompression chamber/iron lung/resonance imager)*

---

barotrauma A diving emergency in which body cavities are subjected to extreme pressure

Summary

- Drowning is death from suffocation due to asphyxiation; near-drowning is survival, at least temporarily, from near suffocation due to submersion.

- In 10 to 15 percent of all drownings, water did not enter the lungs; instead, the victim died because a spasm of the larynx cut off respiration.

- Among victims of water accidents, those with the poorest prognosis include older victims, those who struggle in the water, those who suffer associated injuries, those who have prolonged submersion time, and those who are in warm, dirty, or brackish water.

- The mammalian diving reflex may enable victims in cold water to survive far longer than those in warm water.

- Never go into water to rescue a swimmer unless you can swim, have been trained in water-rescue techniques, are wearing a personal flotation device, and are accompanied by other rescuers.

- If you suspect that a near-drowning victim has sustained spinal injuries, immobilize the spine before you remove the victim from the water.

- If you can, immobilize the spine before you perform other rescue operations, such as giving rescue breathing in the water.

- A near-drowning victim should always be taken to a hospital; complications can occur as many as 3 or 4 days later and are the cause of 15 percent of all drowning deaths.

- Always assume that a victim of a diving accident has sustained neck and spinal injuries, even if the diver is still conscious.

- A major complication of deep-water diving emergencies is coma.

- Victims of deep-water diving emergencies need rapid transportation to a medical center; many need treatment in a recompression chamber.

Key Terms

Make sure you understand the following key terms:

near-drowning	passive drowning
drowning	mammalian diving reflex
"wet" drowning	air embolism
"dry" drowning	decompression sickness
secondary drowning	barotrauma
active drowning	

Critical Thinking Exercise

It is the "Dog Days" of August—hot and muggy. You have joined your college colleagues for a trip to a favorite high mountain lake to escape the valley heat.

Just as you are setting up camp on the shore of the lake, you hear panicked screams for help out in the water. You quickly locate the source of the screaming—a teenage girl floundering in the cold mountain lake about 30 feet offshore. She is definitely in trouble and trying to keep her head above water.

1. What considerations must you quickly decide upon in order to rescue her?

2. How would you rescue her?

3. Once you have her on shore, what first aid measures would you take?

26 Chapter 26 Self-Test

Student: _____ Date: _____

Course: _____ Section #: _____

Part 1 True/False

If you believe the statement is true, circle the T. If you believe the statement is false, circle the F.

T F **1.** Drowning always results from inhaling water, and a drowning victim's lungs always contain water.

T F **2.** Warm-water drowning and cold-water drowning are virtually the same.

T F **3.** If you suspect that a victim of a water accident has sustained a back or neck injury, you should *not* move him or her from the water before strapping to a backboard.

T F **4.** A near-drowning victim may still die up to 2 days following successful resuscitation.

T F **5.** If a victim is in trouble near a deck or the pool's edge, it is always best to rescue the person by getting into the water yourself.

T F **6.** A spinal injury victim who is in the water should be removed from the water immediately, then splinted on shore.

T F **7.** The diving reflex causes blood to be shunted from the body core into the extremities.

T F **8.** An estimated 10 to 40 percent of all drownings are "dry."

T F **9.** A near-drowning victim should always be transported to a hospital, even if the victim appears to have recovered.

T F **10.** Fifteen percent of all drowning deaths are the result of secondary complications.

Part 2 What Would You Do If?

You are at a mountain lake and see a child floating facedown, 20 to 30 feet offshore.

27

Wilderness Emergencies

Learning Objectives

When you have mastered the material in this chapter, you will be able to

1 List the specific information you should have about the wilderness area you will visit before you leave home

2 Explain what kinds of information the first aid leader should have about each member of the group

3 Outline basic survival techniques for cold weather

4 Discuss special ways of handling food and water while in the wilderness

5 List the signs and symptoms of the major altitude-related emergencies

6 Discuss special assessment techniques to use in a wilderness setting

7 Discuss special considerations for managing shock in a wilderness setting

8 Discuss special considerations for performing CPR in a wilderness setting

9 Discuss special considerations for management of soft tissue and musculoskeletal injuries in a wilderness setting

10 Discuss special considerations in immobilizing a victim in a wilderness setting

11 Discuss rescue techniques for the victim of an avalanche

12 Discuss the options for wilderness evacuations and the factors affecting the decision to evacuate a victim

One June morning, four college students set out before dawn to climb to the summit of Mount Timpanogos, the highest peak of the Wasatch Range of the Rocky Mountains. The hike to the 12,000-foot summit, though rigorous, was frequently completed by climbers in a single day.

The group made good time throughout the morning, stopping only occasionally to eat a piece of fruit or adjust their gear. When the four stopped at about noon to eat lunch, 21-year-old Brock Miller, who had been lagging behind, complained of a severe headache. When the other three suggested that he might have low blood sugar from not eating much all morning, he said he felt nauseated and did not want to eat. Brock leaned against an outcropping of granite while the others ate a hearty lunch.

When it was time to go, Brock resisted. He felt too fatigued, he said. On closer observation, Brock's friend Curtis Carson noticed that, even though Brock had been resting for almost an hour, he was having difficulty breathing. His headache and nausea had both intensified.

Curtis recognized Brock's signs and symptoms as those of acute mountain sickness that had progressed into high-altitude pulmonary edema, and he knew that Brock's condition could deteriorate rapidly unless he was taken to a lower altitude immediately. Curtis took Brock's gear, and all three hikers assisted him several miles to the nearest ranger station, where a Forest Service employee drove him to an area hospital for treatment that reversed the potentially fatal condition.

This chapter was written by Chad N. Smith.

onfronting any medical emergency can be challenging, but it can be especially difficult in a wilderness setting. *Wilderness* is defined by the Wilderness Medical Society as a "remote geographical location more than one hour from definitive medical care." By this definition, you could be in a "wilderness" setting not only while fishing, camping, or hiking in the mountains, but while at home if you live in a remote town or are on a farm, ranch, or at a vacation home. *Wilderness* could even describe a large city where medical facilities have been overwhelmed by a disaster, effectively putting a victim more than an hour from medical care.

First aid in the wilderness requires a specialized focus for a number of reasons. To begin with, in a wilderness setting you might have to deal with injuries or illnesses that you would not commonly encounter in a more traditional setting—such as frostbite, wild animal attacks, or altitude sickness. You might have to provide more advanced care than would normally be required of a First Aider, such as cleaning a wound or reducing a dislocation.

In a traditional wilderness setting you are generally at increased risk for injury, are far from the comfort and safety of the 9-1-1 system, and are in potentially hostile environments. You may have to deal with extremes in temperature or with exposure to adverse weather conditions. You might have very limited resources for dealing with any medical emergencies.

Besides coping with limited equipment or supplies, you may be 8 to 12 hours away from the nearest phone or radio and may not have any transportation. Even if you can quickly call for emergency help, it might take hours for the help to reach you, and it might be extremely difficult to describe exactly where the emergency scene is in terms that will help personnel find you without delay. In many cases, you will be the only help the victim has for hours—or, possibly, days. Depending on the extent of the injury, you might need to provide some advanced medical care as well.

Specific things can be done to prevent medical emergencies in the wilderness—but despite precautions, injuries and sudden illnesses do happen. As a result, it is important to be prepared and to understand the special implications of first aid in the wilderness. You might be forced to make difficult decisions without access to the emergency medical system. Finally, you might have to render care for an extended period of time instead of the brief or limited first aid care you are accustomed to; in fact, you might need to stay with an injured victim for several days. This chapter explains the importance of working to prevent problems in the wilderness, reviews basic survival techniques, discusses common outdoor first aid problems, and outlines special considerations for first aid treatment in the wilderness.

27.1 Prevention of Wilderness Emergencies

> **Learning Objective 1** List the specific information you should have about the wilderness area you will visit before you leave home.

Most wilderness emergencies are preventable, and the impact of most medical emergencies in the wilderness can be reduced through proper planning and preparation.

Proper preparation includes being properly equipped—not only with first aid supplies, but with food, water, appropriate clothing, extra clothing, and materials for constructing shelter. Always be prepared for a change in the weather. Always check with rangers or other officials to determine existing and expected conditions. And always travel with at least one other person (ideally, three or more), let people at home know exactly where you are going, and give an estimated time of return.

Never enter a wilderness area without at least one leader who has been to the area before, who knows the way, and who has information on these factors:

- What terrain can be expected
- What special equipment is needed for planned activities
- What weather conditions are likely
- How long the trip will take
- What hazards may be encountered and what level of risk is involved in the anticipated activities
- What resources will be available in case of emergency and how to send for help
- Maximum anticipated delay in getting medical help to the area

This leader should have final say about the equipment, route, camp, daily goals, and so on.

> **Learning Objective 2** Explain what kinds of information the first aid leader should have about each member of the group.

A *first aid leader* (who might be the same person as the group leader) should consider these factors when planning a trip:

- Determine what first aid supplies are needed for the specific area.
- Ensure that adequate and appropriate first aid supplies are available

- Know how to use supplies and equipment that will be carried (such as two-way radios or flares).

- Know the previous experience and pertinent medical history of each member of the party, including preexisting medical conditions, prescribed medications, and allergies.

- Ensure that any required medications or appropriate supplies are taken into the wilderness (though he or she does not necessarily need to carry those supplies).

- Understand appropriate wilderness first aid procedures and have training and experience in using them; ideally, more than one person in the group should be trained in first aid.

Part of the planning for any trip into a wilderness area should include deciding how the group will handle a serious medical emergency. Wilderness first aid kits should be carefully stocked to handle the *long-term care* of potential victims, because you may be hours from medical help when emergencies occur. Ideally, First Aiders in the wilderness setting should have a thorough understanding of human anatomy and physiology as well as knowledge of some basic nursing principles.

PROGRESS CHECK

1. Before entering a wilderness area, you should specifically plan how you will handle _____ . *(animal attacks/food shortages/serious medical emergencies)*

2. The first aid leader should know the _____ of each member of the party. *(medical history/name/next of kin)*

3. First aid in wilderness settings often involves _____ care. *(advanced/long-term/specialized)*

4. A wilderness first aid kit should be packed to allow the group to handle a _____ . *(trauma/serious medical emergency/disaster)*

27.2 Basic Survival

Learning Objective 3 Outline basic survival techniques for cold weather.

Physiologically, the human body requires shelter, water, and food, in that order. Severe weather conditions can incapacitate—and possibly kill—a person in about 3 hours. Without water, a person will die in 3 days. A normally healthy individual can survive for about 3 weeks without food.

In the wilderness, you need to remember the **Rule of Threes**—when a person faces a combination of all three conditions—severe weather, no water, and no food—survival time is considerably reduced.

Shelter

Ideally, shelter should do just that: *shelter* you from heat, wind, cold, and/or moisture. As you seek shelter in the wilderness, remember the principles of how the body loses heat that were discussed in Chapter 25. To begin with, dress appropriately; use layers of clothing to maximize your ability to stay warm, and to increase your flexibility in changing weather. Wear synthetic long underwear; cotton, although absorbent, loses the ability to insulate as soon as it gets damp. Use natural-fiber pants, sweaters, and jackets to insulate. As an outer layer, wear fabric that is breathable, windproof, and waterproof. Wear a synthetic liner under fleece socks, and use water-repellent footwear with good traction. Use windproof and waterproof mittens and a wool hat that covers your entire head, including your ears. Insulate yourself from the ground using blankets, towels, clothing, a sleeping bag, or dry leaves. If the ground is wet, put something waterproof (such as a raincoat, poncho, or tarp) between the ground and the insulation.

Various kinds of shelter will work to keep you warm as long as you:

- Stay out of the bottom of valleys or canyons; heat rises, and the lowest area will also be the coldest.

- Avoid setting up a shelter on a ridge or the top of a mountain where you would be exposed to wind.

- Place your shelter downwind of some sort of windbreak, such as a large rock, mound of dirt, or bank of trees or bushes.

You can seek shelter in a natural cave or overhang, or you can construct your own shelter from tree branches, canvas and rope, or snow. A snow cave or snow trench can keep you warm, as can plastic garbage bags. A tent is ideal *if* it is located out of the wind. If a tent is placed in a windy area, it will actually increase heat loss by convection through a process called "**billowing**." Body heat

---

Rule of Threes A rule stating that survival time is considerably reduced if a victim is without all three factors required for survival: shelter, water, and food

billowing Loss of heat inside a tent when the wind flaps the sides of the tent and warm air is replaced with cold air warms the inside of the tent; as the wind flaps the sides of the tent, the warm air gets blown away and is replaced by cold air.

If you seek shelter in a vehicle, protect yourself from carbon monoxide poisoning:

- Run the heater and engine for no longer than 15 minutes each hour.
- Open the window a crack while the engine is running.
- Check periodically to make sure the exhaust pipe is not blocked with snow, ice, or other debris.

> Learning Objective 4 Discuss special ways of handling food and water while in the wilderness.

Water

Plan for water purification before you enter a wilderness area. The best method is to strain the water for large particles, then bring it to a full boil for 2 to 8 minutes, depending on the altitude. The higher the altitude, the longer you need to boil the water to destroy all microorganisms effectively.

The second best method of purifying water is with a commercially manufactured filter. Ideally, choose one that filters out organisms as small as 2 microns in size, which will eliminate *Giardia lamblia*, a cause of profuse diarrhea. Carefully follow manufacturer's instructions for use.

If you are forced to use snow as a water source, melt it before purifying and drinking it. While it seems a simple way to add water to the body, eating snow carries a high price in terms of heat loss. You can melt snow with a stove, over a campfire, or with a candle.

Food

Before entering the wilderness, plan for plenty of nutritious food for each member of your party. Pack the correct kinds of food in adequate amounts, then protect it as if your life depends on it. It does.

Eating is one way the body produces energy, which also produces heat. Make sure there is enough food for each member of your party to eat three nutritious meals each day, as well as for each person to have several high-energy snacks. If you are likely to face uncertain weather or terrain conditions that could delay your party by even 1 day, allow for extra food.

Improper handling and storage of food in a wilderness setting can have both simple consequences (you could lose your food) and dangerous results (you could be attacked and severely injured by animals foraging for your food). Wilderness animals that commonly steal food range from the nonthreatening (pack rats, squirrels, birds, and weasels) to the dangerous (bears, wolves, and coyotes).

To keep your food safe and protect yourself from injury, follow these procedures:

- Store food supplies some distance from your campsite.
- Store food supplies off the ground; hanging food in stuff sacks is advised.
- Avoid cooking foods with especially strong odors, such as bacon.
- Remember that food refuse also will attract wildlife; burn as much as you can, then keep remaining garbage a safe distance from your campsite and off the ground.

PROGRESS CHECK

1. A person can survive for approximately _____ days without water. *(2/3/4)*

2. The most important factor for survival in cold weather is _____ . *(food/water/shelter)*

3. When a victim faces a combined lack of shelter, water, and food, the "Rule of _____" goes into effect. *(Survival/Threes/Convection)*

4. Always try to construct a shelter _____ . *(in the bottom of a canyon/downwind of a windbreak/on top of a ridge)*

5. Tents do not provide any _____ . *(moisture resistance/security/insulation)*

6. The best method of purifying water in the wilderness is _____ . *(purification tablets/filtration/boiling)*

7. The higher the altitude, the _____ you should boil water to kill organisms. *(longer/less time)*

8. To protect yourself from predators, _____ your food away from your campsite. *(bury/hang/cover)*

27.3 Altitude-Related Problems in the Wilderness

> Learning Objective 5 List the signs and symptoms of the major altitude-related emergencies.

Altitude-related illness generally occurs at altitudes of more than 8,000 feet, although it has been recorded at altitudes of 6,000 feet. Altitude-related problems vary in severity with the rate of ascent and the altitude attained: the most severe problems occur with rapid ascent to high altitudes. Altitude-related illness is not uncommon, affecting one-fourth of people from lower elevations who visit areas higher than 6,000 feet, such as ski resorts and hiking areas. The risk of developing altitude-related illness increases if the altitude is ascended more quickly. It is caused by a lack of oxygen: There is plenty of oxygen in the air, but the lower atmospheric pressure at higher elevations does not provide as much pressure to drive oxygen into the body. Simply, the body struggles to maintain necessary levels of oxygen.

Anyone at a high enough altitude can get altitude sickness, but different people can respond very differently to altitude—even high altitude. The following factors help determine the risk of falling victim to altitude sickness:

- Genetic influences and other individual differences that determine how a person responds to altitude.

- The person's general state of health; a number of illnesses can increase the risk of getting altitude sickness, as can factors like fatigue, dehydration, and malnutrition.

- The altitude the person reaches—the higher the altitude, the greater the risk of altitude sickness.

- The rate of ascent—the more quickly the victim ascends, the greater the risk of altitude sickness. Slow, gradual ascents are generally safer.

It *is* possible to acclimate to higher elevations. Over time, the body produces more red blood cells and increases the chemicals that allow oxygen to transfer to the body cells. The body also develops more blood vessels, especially in muscle tissue. In the meantime, respiratory and heart rates and volumes increase. It takes approximately 6 weeks for the acclimatization process to occur. Most victims of altitude-related illness ascended too high, too quickly. Dehydration aggravates altitude-related illness, too, as do factors such as general health, fatigue, malnutrition, or the presence of any illness or injury. Certain prescription medications, such as acetazolamide (Diamox), can help prevent altitude-related illness.

Generally, altitude-related illness develops within the first 12 hours that the victim is at the higher altitude. Regardless of the specific illness, the most common symptom is headache. Altitude-related illness is often mistaken as a common cold or the flu (or even an alcohol-induced hangover), because the symptoms are similar.

Although it is not common, several types of altitude-related illness can be fatal. Seek medical help immediately if the victim develops any of the following:

- Noisy breathing

- Persistent cough

- Shortness of breath while resting

- Vomiting

- Loss of balance

- Confusion or disorientation

Acute Mountain Sickness

The mildest form of altitude sickness is **acute mountain sickness**, which mimics a severe hangover. Signs and symptoms include:

- Headache that develops during the night and is present when the victim wakes up in the morning

- Swollen face and puffiness under the eyes

- Nausea and loss of appetite

- Fatigue that is out of proportion with the amount of exertion

- Sore throat (caused by dry air)

- Shortness of breath with even mild exertion

Mild acute mountain sickness generally occurs at altitudes above 8,000 feet among those who have climbed too quickly. Acute mountain sickness occurs more often when the weather is cold and windy, when hikers are fatigued or anxious, or when hikers are dehydrated or have upper respiratory infections.

To treat acute mountain sickness:

1. *Stop climbing immediately;* rest and see whether symptoms improve.

2. If symptoms do not improve within a day or two, descend 2,000 to 3,000 feet as quickly as possible.

3. Prevent or correct dehydration by drinking at least 4 quarts of fluid every day; eat a high-carbohydrate, high-calorie diet while climbing.

4. Use aspirin to treat mild headache.

High Altitude Pulmonary Edema

In **high altitude pulmonary edema (HAPE)**, fluid from the body is slowly transferred to the lungs; the body's

acute mountain sickness An altitude-related illness that resembles a severe hangover

high altitude pulmonary edema (HAPE) An altitude-related illness that causes fluid to go into the lungs from body cells ability to take on oxygen is diminished. HAPE is caused by reaching a new altitude too quickly, and although it can occur at lower altitudes, it generally starts at about 10,000 feet. Unlike acute mountain sickness, which usually causes symptoms within a few hours, the signs and symptoms of HAPE do not develop until as long as 72 hours after reaching the new altitude. Untreated, HAPE can cause death in fewer than 12 hours after symptoms begin.

The signs and symptoms of HAPE include:

- Severe shortness of breath, even when resting

- Cyanosis (bluish discoloration of the lips, fingernails, and mucous membranes lining the mouth)

- "Moist" breathing that produces rattling and crackling

- Cough that produces pink, frothy sputum

A victim of HAPE needs *immediate* medical treatment in a compression chamber. *The most important thing you can do is descend immediately* and seek medical help for the victim.

High Altitude Cerebral Edema

High altitude cerebral edema (HACE) causes a dangerous buildup of fluid levels in the brain, resulting in swelling of the brain tissue and increased pressure inside the skull. The brain has nowhere to expand other than downward, through the **foramen magnum**—the hole at the base of the skull that houses the brain stem. Pressure on the brain stem affects cardiac function, respiratory function, and blood pressure; associated pressure on the cerebellum affects balance and motor dexterity.

Signs and symptoms include the following:

- Severe headache

- Severe nausea and vomiting

- **Ataxia** (inability to maintain balance)

- Dizziness

- Extreme fatigue, progressing to coma

Untreated, HACE can cause death within a few hours after the onset of symptoms. It is critical to get the victim to a lower altitude as quickly as possible.

First Aid for Altitude-Related Illness

To care for victims of altitude-related illness, *get the victim to a lower elevation as quickly as possible.* If the victim cannot walk, the victim must be carried or transported on an improvised stretcher. Encourage the victim to drink as much water as possible.

Once the victim is at a lower altitude and symptoms have eased, keep the victim at rest for 12 to 24 hours.

PROGRESS CHECK

1. Altitude-related illness is caused by a lack of _____ . *(oxygen/fluids/nutrients)*

2. Acute mountain sickness causes symptoms much like those of a severe _____ . *(cold/hangover/migraine headache)*

3. High altitude pulmonary edema is characterized by _____ , even after rest. *(fatigue/muscle soreness/difficulty breathing)*

4. High altitude cerebral edema is characterized by _____ . *(ataxia/muscle cramping/ double vision)*

5. Regardless of the illness, treat altitude problems by getting the victim to _____ . *(rest /lie down/a lower altitude)*

27.4 Special Wilderness Considerations

Almost any accident or illness that can occur under regular conditions can occur in the wilderness. Although the same general principles of assessment and care should be used in the wilderness, some special considerations apply.

Assessing the Scene

In order to determine what happened and in order to safely assist the victim, you need to assess the entire scene. Generally, it is best not to move a victim until you have finished first aid and you know that the victim has been stabilized. However, conditions at the scene might pose enough of a danger to both you and the victim that it is not safe or wise for you to care for the victim there. For example, there might be a risk of falling rocks or unstable tree limbs, or the victim might be in standing water or might be threatened by a stream of kerosene, gasoline, or some other harmful chemical. You might also determine that you need to move the victim away from the threat of a snake or

---

high altitude cerebral edema (HACE) An altitude-related illness that causes swelling of the brain and increased pressure inside the skull

foramen magnum The opening at the base of the skull that houses the brain stem

ataxia Inability to keep balance

wild animal, or you might need to move the victim to shelter and out of adverse weather conditions.

Certain basic stabilization for specific injuries, such as spinal injuries, must be done before moving a victim, but in most cases you can safely move the victim to a better spot before you provide first aid care.

Assessing the scene can also help you determine the probable mechanism of injury, especially if there are no bystanders or witnesses who can tell you what happened. Look for the most likely cause of the accident and imagine yourself in the victim's place as a hint about how the victim got hurt and what injuries he or she might have.

Assessing the Victim

> Learning Objective **6** Discuss special assessment techniques to use in a wilderness setting.

The primary difference between assessment in the wilderness and elsewhere is time; the primary survey should be the same, but you should spend more time doing a detailed secondary survey in a wilderness setting.

Under normal circumstances, the role of a First Aider is to identify and stabilize the most serious injuries while activating the EMS system. In such situations you generally do not have to worry about cleaning wounds, changing dressings, or adjusting splints, for example. In the wilderness, on the other hand, you will probably have to assume responsibility for the victim for a longer period of time, and the treatment you give based on the secondary survey might be the only treatment the victim receives for 12 hours or longer (see Figure 27-1).

Your assessment is especially vital in getting the right kind of help for the victim: First responders may have

to carry the appropriate equipment over miles of rough terrain to treat the victim; you want to make sure it is done right the first time. Your assessment should include detailed and accurate information about the mechanism of injury, the victim's wounds, what is being done for the victim, and—most important— where you are. Always send at least two people for help; if possible, identify your location on a spare map that you send along.

One of the most essential parts of assessment in the wilderness is *charting*—accurate documentation of:

- The mechanism of injury or illness

- The victim's vital signs, taken periodically the entire time the victim is under your care

- Your observation of the victim's condition, given periodically

- Your treatment plan and how it was carried out

This kind of information is vital to medical personnel, who will use it to establish *their* treatment plan. If you cannot provide a record of the victim's condition from the time of injury or illness until the victim arrives at the hospital, then the victim's *baseline* vital signs may be hours—or possibly days—old.

To determine the type of records you should keep, remember the mnemonic, C-H-A-R-T:

C Chief complaint (What did the victim tell you?)

H History (What happened?)

A Assessment (What signs and symptoms did you find?)

R$_x$ Treatment (What did you do for the victim?)

T Transport and disposition (After you cared for the victim, where did the victim go? Did the victim leave? Was it on foot, in a car, in an ambulance, in a helicopter?)

Finally, assessment in the wilderness setting is important because it allows you to determine whether the injury or illness is serious enough to abandon the trip. Some injuries or illnesses may cause discomfort but can safely be treated at the site; others call for aggressive action aimed at evacuating the victim and transporting the person to a hospital. Adequate assessment lets you know the difference.

Determining a Plan

After assessing the scene, assessing the victim, and providing first aid care, you need to determine your plan: Do you need to call for help, do you need to evacuate

FIGURE 27-1. Assessing a victim in a wilderness setting

the victim, and, if either of these apply, how will you proceed?

There are basically four options for getting help in a wilderness situation:

1. You can treat the victim where you are until the victim has recovered enough to walk out on his or her own or with minimal assistance.

2. You can carry the victim to help, either on an improvised litter or with any of a series of carries.

3. You can send a pair of people to get help—or, in a critical enough situation, you can leave the victim alone while you go to get help.

4. You can stay with the victim and call for help by cellular phone, radio, or signal; talking to emergency medical personnel by phone or two-way radio can be an excellent source of information as you work to care for the victim as well as plan for evacuation.

The option you choose will obviously depend on a number of factors. First is the condition of the victim: Is advanced medical care urgently required to save the victim's life or to dramatically improve the victim's chance of successful recovery? If you are not able to call for help with a cell phone or two-way radio, is it possible to signal for help? In general, it is not a good idea to leave a victim alone while you go for help; do that only as a last resort. Any victim you leave should be stabilized, should have adequate clothing and shelter, and should be able to reach enough food and drink to provide for him or her until help arrives. Give the victim a clear idea of when to expect help, and explain the route you are going to take. If the victim is unconscious, place him or her on the left side with the face pointing downward to facilitate drainage of fluids and prevent choking, and make sure the victim is warm and protected.

Regardless of who goes for help, make sure that person marks the route. Use masking tape, duct tape, surveyor's tape, or strips of cloth tied on tree branches to clearly mark the way you are traveling. If nothing else is available, break the branches of trees or shrubs to indicate your path. It can be extremely easy to get lost in wilderness areas, and you might reach help only to discover that you're unable to find your way back to the victim. Before you decide whether to evacuate, consider the distance, terrain, weather conditions, and risk. You might determine that it is safer to stay where you are than to try to evacuate a victim through risky conditions over steep and hazardous terrain. But if you are being threatened by dropping temperatures or an impending storm, you might decide it is best to try to evacuate.

See the end of the chapter for specific information about evacuation.

First Aid for Shock

Learning Objective 7 Discuss special considerations for managing shock in a wilderness setting.

Shock may not initially be present, but may develop while you are waiting for help. Make sure you take measures to prevent shock, and watch for signs of developing shock each time you check the victim. There are two goals of shock management:

1. Increase and maintain the effective circulating volume of blood.

2. Reduce the oxygen debt being incurred by the body.

You need to place the victim in the correct position, maintain a normal body temperature, and replace lost fluids.

Management of shock is detailed in Chapter 6. Special considerations in the wilderness setting include the following:

- **Maintaining temperature**—If you have placed the victim on the cold ground, you must provide insulation; place a blanket, coat, layers of pine needles, or other material between the victim and the ground (see Figure 27-2). If you are in a hot climate, shade the victim from the sun.

- **Replacing fluids**—If you have access to the EMS system, you should never try to replace fluids; if you are in a wilderness setting hours from medical help and shock is progressing, give the victim small sips of water *if the victim is fully conscious*. Monitor closely for nausea, and be prepared to turn the victim on his or her side if vomiting occurs.

FIGURE 27–2. First Aider in wilderness area, treating a victim for shock and maintaining temperature

Cardiopulmonary Resuscitation

Learning Objective 8 Discuss special considerations for performing CPR in a wilderness setting.

The most daunting aspect of performing CPR in a wilderness setting is the fact that advanced cardiac life support is *not* simply a phone call away. Because victim survival depends on immediate defibrillation, advanced life support, medications, and rapid transport, the prognosis for a victim of cardiac arrest in the wilderness is grim. That is especially true if the victim has suffered significant blood loss or has sustained a severe injury, such as spinal injury or massive head or chest injury. There is another factor as well: It is very difficult to perform CPR on a victim while he or she is being evacuated from the wilderness.

Regardless of that fact, begin CPR as soon as assessment indicates it, and continue aggressive and *prolonged* CPR, especially in cases of cold-water drowning or lightning strikes; spontaneous resuscitation can often occur in these cases. Chest compressions cannot support circulation for very long, but you can successfully continue rescue breathing for hours with a victim who has a pulse.

Standards for performing CPR necessarily differ in a wilderness setting from a normal setting, where medical help is available within minutes. The standards also vary depending on the condition of the victim. It can be extremely difficult to decide when to stop resuscitation efforts, and if help does not arrive, you will have to make the decision on your own. The National Association of Emergency Medical Services Physicians (NAEMSP) has issued sets of guidelines that help wilderness First Aiders know when to start CPR and how long to continue resuscitation efforts. If the victim has a normal body temperature or has only mild hypothermia, and is not breathing, begin rescue breathing immediately; if you cannot detect a pulse, start chest compressions as well. Generally, you should stop chest compressions if the pulse does not start after 30 minutes of CPR, *unless:*

- The victim has hypothermia.
- The victim has been submerged in *cold* water for less than one hour.
- The victim was buried in an avalanche (these victims generally die from either suffocation or blunt-force trauma).
- The victim was struck by lightning.

In cases of hypothermia, the metabolism slows, and it is possible for the victim to survive longer without oxygen. Because chest compressions can cause a specific type of heart attack called ventricular fibrillation, you should make absolutely certain there is no pulse before you start CPR for a hypothermic victim. Since the pulse can be very slow with hypothermia, feel for the pulse for a full 30 to 45 seconds. Victims of avalanche or lightning strikes often take longer to resuscitate, but can often be successfully resuscitated after an hour or more.

According to the NAEMSP, you should *not* begin CPR if:

- The victim has been in cardiac arrest for more than 30 minutes, and there have been no efforts to resuscitate him or her.
- The victim has an injury that is obviously fatal.
- The victim's chest is frozen.
- The victim's core temperature is lower than 60°F.
- The victim has been submerged in water for longer than 60 minutes.
- Proceeding with CPR will place the rescuer at risk.

Lightning Deaths and Injuries

Because people in wilderness settings are often in open or high-altitude areas and may be unable to find suitable shelter in case of a sudden storm, they are more prone to being struck by lightning. In addition, storms are more likely to occur over high mountain areas, where hikers and campers are exposed. Nationally, most lightning strikes occur in June, July, and August, possibly because more people are outside during the summer months. Most happen between noon and 6 P.M.—again, possibly because more people are outside during daylight hours—and most involve only a single victim. The most common cause of death from lightning strike is cardiopulmonary arrest; the second most common is central nervous system damage. Most victims of lightning strike suffer only minor burns.

PREVENTING LIGHTNING INJURY

The best way to prevent lightning injury is to be aware of weather forecasts before you go into a wilderness area. If a sudden storm does occur, estimate your distance from the lightning by counting the seconds between a lightning flash and the associated thunderclap, then divide by five; the result is the number of miles between you and the lightning.

The second line of defense against lightning strikes is to *get away from objects that tend to conduct electricity.* Immediately get out of and away from water; get off of and away from metal farm equipment, golf carts, bicycles, scooters, and motorcycles. Put down golf clubs and fishing rods. Stay away from anything that is metal, including ladders, pipes, rails, fences, and clotheslines. A group of people should spread out, leaving several yards between each person to minimize the chance of conducting electricity from one person to another.

Finally, *seek shelter.* Your goal is to avoid being the highest point in the area, as you would be if you were standing on top of a hill, in an open field, or in a boat. Instead, move into a valley or ravine. Don't stand under anything that is the highest point in the area, such as an isolated tall tree. Don't seek shelter in a small, isolated structure that stands in an open area (such as an equipment shed or ranger hut). If you are in a wooded area, seek shelter under a dense group of low trees. If you are in a hard-top car, stay inside.

If you feel your hair stand on end, a lightning strike is imminent. *Do not lie flat on the ground;* as little of your body as possible should touch the ground. Crouch as you would to catch a baseball and cup your hands over your ears to minimize the risk of your eardrums rupturing.

FIRST AID CARE FOR LIGHTNING STRIKES

Chapter 24 provides detailed information on the care of a lightning strike victim. Essentially, you should assess the victim as quickly as possible and begin CPR if the victim is in cardiac arrest. Spinal injuries are common when victims are thrown to the ground, so stabilize the victim before beginning CPR. If more than one person has been struck by lightning, begin assessment with the one who is quiet and motionless.

First Aid for Soft-Tissue Injuries

Learning Objective 9 Discuss special considerations for management of soft-tissue and musculoskeletal injuries in a wilderness setting.

Use direct pressure to control external bleeding. Maintain pressure for 10 minutes after bleeding has stopped to make sure a clot has formed.

If the victim has been burned, take immediate measures to cool the burn; using cool water is best. Cover the burn with a sterile burn dressing or a clean, dry cloth after applying a thin layer of antibiotic ointment to the burn. Elevate the burned area, prevent the victim from getting chilled, and give fully conscious victims plenty of water or clear juice to drink.

If a laceration, incision, avulsion, puncture, or abrasion is large enough or dirty enough to overwhelm the body's immune system, you will have to deal with the threat of infection—and what you do during the first few hours is critical. To prevent infection:

1. Irrigate the wound immediately to flush out as much bacteria, dirt, and debris as possible. Use boiled water or saline; ideally, squirt the water or solution from a squeeze bottle to provide some pressure, which will help remove dirt and debris

from the wound. *Do not use hydrogen peroxide, alcohol, or povidone-iodine directly on the wound.*

2. If tissue has been completely avulsed, wipe or scrub it away with a gauze pad and sterile water or saline; if an avulsion is only partial, clean the tissue thoroughly and place it in its normal anatomical position.

3. Bring the edges of the wound together as closely as you can to the position they were in before the skin was separated. Use commercially prepared tapes, strips, or pieces of adhesive tape to hold the edges of the wound together.

4. Dress and bandage the wound.

5. If dressings get soaked with blood, remove the blood-soaked dressings, locate the bleeding vessel, and apply direct pressure to stop the bleeding.

If you are a day or more away from medical care, you will need to inspect the wound periodically for signs and symptoms of infection and change the dressing. Follow these guidelines:

- Always wash your hands thoroughly before removing the dressing.
- Keep all dressing materials sterile.
- If necessary, reclean the wound.
- If signs of infection are present (an expanded area of redness, red streaks, heat, pulsating localized pain, pus, or a foul odor), apply a warm, moist compress to the wound for 20 minutes. Remove the compress for 20 minutes; repeat. If there are signs of infection, you should inspect the wound every 4 hours.
- Apply a sterile dressing, then bandage.

ATTACKS BY WILD ANIMALS

Wild animal attacks are much more common outside the United States because there are few large wild animals in areas with significant population. However, the United States is home to alligators, crocodiles, cougars, bears, moose, elk, and bison, and these animals can cause great harm if they attack. Smaller wild animals, such as raccoons and badgers, may also attack and cause injury, especially if cornered.

The priorities in caring for soft-tissue injuries due to wild animal attacks are the same as for other soft-tissue injuries: control bleeding and prevent infection. Larger animals can cause extensive tissue damage, and resulting injuries may bleed profusely. If the animal is still in the area, it is essential that you protect yourself and the victim from further injury.

If you encounter a wild animal, slowly and quietly back away from the animal. Many animals will attack if they feel threatened—and running can cause them to become predatory. Most experts advise that you fight back aggressively if attacked—pound the animal with your fists, kick the animal, or strike the animal with anything you can use as a weapon, such as a flashlight. *Important exceptions are the grizzly bear or a black bear with cubs;* in these cases, lie down and play dead.

An important part of preventing wild animal attacks is awareness of which animals inhabit the area where you are. Signs are posted in many recreational areas, especially those in state and national parks. Ask rangers or other officials about recent animal sightings, and ask about prevention techniques. Above all, use common sense; keep food in sealed containers, avoid cooking foods with strong aromas (such as bacon), and keep garbage in metal containers with tight-fitting lids.

First Aid Care for Musculoskeletal Injuries

DISLOCATIONS

Although a First Aider does not normally try to correct a dislocation when medical help is available, it is sometimes necessary to reduce, or align, a dislocated joint in the wilderness, where medical help will be delayed. Reducing a dislocation is generally much easier immediately following the injury, before swelling occurs, and can:

- Stabilize and protect the joint

- Significantly reduce pain

- Protect blood circulation to the involved arm or leg

- Make it easier to move or evacuate the victim

You should never try to correct a dislocation involving the elbow or hip. Dislocations of these joints resemble fractures, and attempts at reducing them can compromise circulation and cause further injury. You can, however, try to align the front of the shoulder, the kneecap, or a finger in a wilderness setting. *Stop efforts to reduce the dislocation if you feel resistance in the joint or if you increase the victim's pain.*

SHOULDER DISLOCATION

Almost all dislocations of the shoulder involve the anterior (front) joint. A victim with a dislocated anterior shoulder joint will not be able to hold the upper arm next to the body, will not be able to touch the opposite shoulder with the hand on the injured side, and the shoulder will not have its characteristic rounded shape. It's usually easy to see the dislocation if you compare the injured shoulder to the uninjured one.

It is fairly easy to correct the dislocation of an anterior shoulder joint, and it can be critical if blood circulation or nerve function to the hand is affected. To determine whether circulation or nervous function are intact, check the hand for warmth, pulses, sensation, and movement. If the hand is cool, tingling, or numb, or if pulse is absent or the victim cannot move the hand, you need to act quickly to align the shoulder joint.

There are two ways to align the shoulder joint. The first uses simple traction:

1. Have the victim lie flat, face-down, on a picnic table or other object that is high enough so the victim's arm can hang over the side without touching the ground.

2. Place a folded towel or other soft object in the victim's armpit to cushion the arm.

3. With the victim's palm facing inward, secure a 10- to 15-pound weight to the arm between the elbow and wrist. Cushion the weight and strap it to the arm with a rope or belt, making sure you do not slow circulation.

4. The joint will pop back into place when the muscles become tired enough to completely relax; this may take an hour or longer.

5. Once the joint is reduced, protect the injured side with a sling and swathe.

The second method requires two First Aiders:

1. Have an assistant loop a belt, strap, shirt, sleeping bag, towel, or other object under the armpit and around the victim's chest.

2. While you gently but steadily pull the injured arm out to the victim's side, have your assistant pull gently but steadily in the opposite direction, using the object to provide countertraction against the chest.

3. As you pull, slowly rotate the arm until it is in a baseball-throwing position; hold that position until the muscles tire enough to allow the joint to pop back into place. This generally takes 10 to 15 minutes.

4. Once the joint is reduced, protect the injured side with a sling and swathe.

Never try to align a shoulder joint by placing your foot in the victim's armpit while you pull on the injured arm.

KNEECAP DISLOCATION

A dislocated kneecap will generally turn to the outside; the deformity will be obvious, and the victim will be most comfortable with the knee bent. If medical help will be delayed, you can usually correct a dislocated kneecap by simply straightening the leg; you may need to gently push the kneecap back into place as you straighten the leg.

Once the kneecap is in the correct position, splint the leg to stabilize it. If possible, use ice to relieve swelling and pain. With the leg in a splint, most victims can walk with only minimal assistance (such as using a branch as a walking stick).

All victims of kneecap dislocation should see a doctor, even if the dislocation was successfully corrected in the wilderness.

FINGER DISLOCATION

A dislocated finger will look deformed, and the victim will not be able to use it. Often, the victim will be able to correct the dislocation; otherwise, you should try to correct it only once. *Never try to correct a dislocation at the base of the thumb or the base of the index finger;* these dislocations require surgical correction.

To correct a finger dislocation, hold the finger in a slightly flexed position. Pull the fingertip gently outward as you push the joint back into place. Even if you are able to reduce the dislocation, immobilize the hand with the fingers in cupping shape, as if the victim were holding a ball.

SPLINTING A FRACTURE

Splinting a fracture in a wilderness setting (see Figure 27-3) requires more than the usual amount of care and consideration: The victim may be in the splint for several days. Follow these guidelines:

- If you do not have access to a splint, improvise with tree limbs, smaller branches lashed together, camp shovels, paddles, oars, skis, ski poles, walking sticks, tent poles, or similar objects.

- Victim comfort is essential, because medical help may be delayed. Make sure you pad the splint well.

- It is vital that you check often for signs of impaired circulation or nerve function.

- While you should *not* normally try to realign an angulated fracture, you may have to do so in a

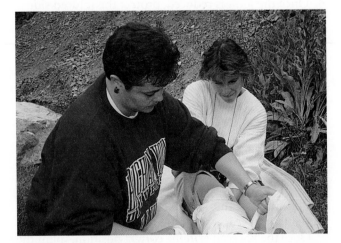

FIGURE 27–3. Splinting a leg fracture in the wilderness

wilderness setting—splinting a severely angulated fracture in the position found and leaving it that way for many hours or even days will almost certainly result in permanent loss of function. Realign as soon after the injury as you can; do not try to "set" the bone, but make sure the normal circulation and nerve function are intact.

- If you are fewer than 3 hours from a hospital, cover the wound from an open fracture with a dry, sterile dressing and splint the fracture. If you are more than 3 hours from a hospital, gently clean the wound and exposed bone ends with a sterile dressing soaked with sterile water. *Do not irrigate the wound.* Cover with a dry, sterile dressing, then splint. All open fractures require immediate medical attention, so arrange to evacuate the victim.

Spinal Injuries

Learning Objective **10** Discuss special considerations in immobilizing a victim in a wilderness setting.

It can be difficult even for a physician using an X-ray to properly diagnose a spinal injury, so it is extremely difficult in the wilderness to determine whether an accident victim has sustained injury to the spine. However, it is always best to err on the safe side: If the victim of a spinal injury is not properly treated, permanent damage (including paralysis or even death) can result.

SIGNS AND SYMPTOMS

While assessment can be difficult, spinal injuries cause at least one of the following:

- Tenderness or pain running up the center of the back side of the neck

- A painful injury somewhere other than the back or neck

- Weakness, tingling, or numbness in the feet, legs, hands, or arms

- Altered mental status, ranging from disorientation or confusion to coma

Someone who is struck by lightning almost always suffers some degree of spinal injury when thrown to the ground. Hikers who fall can also suffer spinal injury, as can victims of skiing, water-skiing, or boating accidents. Those who are using drugs or alcohol are at significantly increased risk of sustaining spinal injuries in accidents.

Generally, you can assume that spinal injury has *not* occurred if the victim:

- Is fully alert
- Has no other injuries that might distract from pain in the back or neck
- Does not complain of neck or back pain
- Can move the fingers and toes
- Has a normal sense of touch in the fingers and toes
- Is not intoxicated by drugs or alcohol

In these cases you do not need to immobilize the victim.

Chapter 13 provides more information on the signs and symptoms of spinal injury, and the proper assessment of a victim for spinal injury.

IMMOBILIZING A VICTIM

If you determine that spinal injury may exist, you need to immobilize the victim to prevent permanent injury. Since commercial backboards and cervical collars are often not available in the wilderness, you will probably need to improvise. Because it is not always possible to fully immobilize a victim, do the best you can with the materials you have available.

You can usually move the head to its normal position, with the eyes forward, before immobilizing the victim; that is the most stable position for the spine. *Do not try to move the head if the victim complains of pain or if you feel resistance.* In such a case, splint the spine in the position in which you found the victim.

To immobilize a victim in a wilderness setting without a commercial backboard:

- Remember that the victim may have to be secured to your improvised backboard for many hours, or even days. You will have to make allowances for eliminating waste (leave a strategically placed hole or space), sliding the victim into a sleeping bag, and feeding the victim.

- Improvise a backboard by lashing together tree branches, walking sticks, the external frames of backpacks, or other similar objects.

- Use a rolled-up blanket to immobilize the neck. Place the blanket behind the victim's head, allowing both long ends to fall across the victim's chest; cross the ends on the chest; applying gentle tension on both long ends, pass them under the victim's opposite arms; attach the ends securely to the backboard.

- Make sure you pad thoroughly to keep the victim comfortable. Provide plenty of padding over bony prominences and under the buttocks. Do not tie the legs absolutely flat; place a small amount of

padding under the knees. Unless absolutely necessary, do not tie down the hands.

Avalanche Rescue

Learning Objective 11 Discuss rescue techniques for the victim of an avalanche.

The increasing popularity of backcountry winter mountain sports—such as cross-country skiing, snowmobiling, snow boarding, and mountaineering—has caused a rapid increase in deaths from avalanche over the past three decades in both the United States and Canada.

An avalanche is a rapidly moving or falling mass of snow; the snow usually contains rocks, soil, ice, and other debris that is picked up along its path (such as tree branches). Once the avalanche stops moving, the snow sets up rapidly and becomes solid, making it almost impossible for someone who is buried under even a foot of snow to dig himself or herself out.

Avalanches kill in two ways: by suffocation and by blunt-force trauma. In the first way, the victim is buried in snow, and snow can often enter the nose and mouth, making it impossible for the victim to breathe. Even if the airway is clear, the pressure from several feet of snow can make it impossible for the chest to expand, which in turn makes it impossible for the victim to breathe. Even when neither of these factors exists, burial in snow eventually causes suffocation. An estimated two-thirds of avalanche victims die as a result of suffocation.

About one-third of all avalanche victims die from blunt-force trauma—especially to the head and neck—as they are swept along the path of the avalanche. Victims may be smashed into trees or rocks, sustaining fatal injuries, or swept off of cliffs and killed in the subsequent fall.

A victim who has not been fatally injured can be rescued from an avalanche if

- there is some kind of air pocket surrounding the victim.
- rescuers act with great speed.
- there has not been a fatal blunt-force injury.
- the victim is not buried too deeply (there has never been a successful rescue of a victim buried under more than 6 feet of snow).

During the first 15 minutes of burial, the victim's chances of being found alive are good. After 15 to 30 minutes of burial, about half of all victims can be successfully rescued. A victim who has been buried for more than 30 minutes has a poor chance of survival.

Remember: the conditions that cause an avalanche to occur—most often a heavy snowfall after unusually warm temperatures, which cause an unstable foundation—often contribute to a series of avalanches. In determining the rescue of an avalanche victim, it is essential to make sure that the danger of avalanche has passed and that rescuers will not be at risk of being caught themselves.

The greatest success for the victim of an avalanche occurs if he or she has a rescue transceiver or beacon; these are the best methods for locating victims. Probe lines and search dogs are effective, but generally find victims only after they are dead.

SURVIVING AN AVALANCHE

If you survive an avalanche, take the following steps to help rescue other victims:

1. If you are the only rescuer, do a quick search as described in the following steps before sending for help. If there are additional rescuers, immediately send someone for help. If you are in a remote back-country area where you cannot reach the ski patrol or other help, all survivors should remain in the area and search until there is no longer any hope of survival for those who are buried (generally longer than an hour).

2. Mark the spot where you last saw the victim; you can use a piece of clothing, a piece of equipment, a tree branch, or anything else that contrasts with the snow.

3. Move to the area below where you last saw the victim, and quickly search for any clues of the victim. Use a tree branch, ski pole, or ski to probe the snow in likely burial spots.

4. If you and the victims have beacons, immediately switch your beacon to the receive mode and listen for the beeping sounds from a buried beacon.

5. If there is the chance of a second avalanche, get to safety immediately. If there is more than one survivor, have one person stand in a safe place and shout to other rescuers, warning them to get to safety.

RESCUING A VICTIM

Before you try to rescue the victim of an avalanche, it is critical that you be as certain as possible that there is no danger of another avalanche. If you are sure there is no further danger and you have found a victim, take these steps:

1. Immediately clear the snow away from the victim's head, chest, and stomach.

2. If there is a second rescuer, immediately send that rescuer for help.

3. Clear the victim's airway, and check for breathing and circulation.

4. If the victim has a pulse but is not breathing, start rescue breathing; if the victim does not have a pulse, start CPR.

5. Once the victim is breathing and has a pulse, check for severe bleeding; apply direct pressure to control any bleeding.

6. Examine the victim for possible spinal injury; if you suspect that the neck or spine may have been injured, stabilize the victim's head, neck, and back.

7. Keep the victim as warm as possible until help arrives and you are able to completely get the victim out of the snow.

Wilderness Evacuation

> **Learning Objective 12** Discuss the options for wilderness evacuations and the factors affecting the decision to evacuate a victim.

Once you have provided first aid care for a victim, you need to decide when and how to call for help or get the victim out of the wilderness and to a hospital or physician's office. Sometimes medical assistance will come to you at the scene; several factors have to be considered, however, and unless you are dealing with a life-threatening injury, it is generally better to try to evacuate the victim instead of requesting that medical rescuers come to you.

CALLING OR SENDING FOR HELP

In some wilderness situations, you will have a way to quickly call for help—usually by means of a cell phone or two-way radio. Two important factors will increase the efficiency of the help you receive: accurately describing your location and providing complete information about the situation.

First, unless you are certain of your location and its distance from roads or other clear points, don't try to approximate mileage. If you don't know exactly where you are, describe prominent landmarks that will help rescuers pinpoint your location—if you can, choose landmarks that are visible both in daylight and in the dark. If there are no prominent landmarks and there are other rescuers on hand, you may want to consider sending someone to meet EMS personnel at an easy-to-identify landmark or at a main road.

If you are trained to use flares, you can use them to mark your location if you are not in a heavily wooded area or in a dry area that could easily ignite. Follow local protocol in the use of flares.

Second, gather all the information you can about the situation, and prepare to give it when you call for help. Include information about the victim's condition, the extent of injuries, the treatment you have already provided, and the general environment and terrain. Giving this kind of information will enable EMS personnel to be more effective in developing a plan and preparing for the most appropriate kind of treatment.

If you have no way to call for help, you need to improvise a way to send a distress signal to potential rescuers. A widely used technique is to send a signal in sets or series of three—three shouts; three flashes of light from a flashlight, lamp, or mirror; three smoky fires; three blasts of a whistle; three shots; and so on. If you use fires, build them in a triangle pattern at least 50 yards apart so they can be clearly distinguished as separate fires. Take extreme caution with fire: keep dirt or water on hand to extinguish the fire quickly, and never leave a fire unattended.

If there are multiple rescuers, you might consider sending for help. Make sure that enough people are available to stay with the victim; they should be the people who are best equipped to treat the victim. Whenever possible, send at least two people together to go for help, minimizing the risk of danger or injury to the rescuers. If going for help will involve challenges or potential hazards, send only those who are equipped to handle the potential problems.

The rescuers who go for help should take a written description of the victim's injury, a map indicating where the victim is located, the names of everyone who stays behind with the victim, and a description of the terrain and access routes (if known). This information should be in writing in case something happens to the rescuers. Rescuers who go for help should mark their way at frequent intervals so that they can find their way back. It's important that they look back at the area they just traveled at regular intervals—the area may look different from that perspective.

If you are the only rescuer, have no way to signal for help, are reasonably sure no one will come by, and are unable to evacuate the victim, you may need to leave the victim alone and go for help. Carefully plan the route you will take, and make sure you can lead rescuers back to the victim.

Before you leave, make sure the victim is stable, and that you have provided for the victim's care during the time you will be gone—make sure the victim has easy access to water, food, and a container that can be used as a urinal. Check any dressings or bandages to make sure they have not slipped and that they are not too tight. Make sure, too, that the victim has enough clothing to stay warm, has shelter from the elements (including the sun), and is protected from the ground. Clearly explain that you are going for help, and give the victim some time estimate in which he or she can expect you to return. Write down the route you will be taking, what time you are leaving, and what time you expect to return; leave that written information with the victim.

As you travel, mark your path frequently and regularly. Look back at frequent intervals to make sure you can recognize your path from that perspective.

DECIDING TO EVACUATE

Not all victims need to be evacuated. Those with minor illnesses or injuries are often fine after being treated and given the chance to rest for a day or two. Other victims, however, will need to be evacuated from the wilderness so they can receive advanced medical help.

Your decision to evacuate will depend on the severity of the victim's injuries, the first aid skills of the rescuers at the scene, the psychological condition of both the victim and the rescuers, how much equipment is available, how long it will take to evacuate the victim, and how much it will cost to evacuate the victim.

Some situations require immediate evacuation. You should rapidly evacuate a victim who has:

- Spinal injuries, with no movement/sensation in the fingers or toes
- Severe hypothermia
- Bleeding that is uncontrolled or difficult to control
- An injury on the foot or hand that requires stitches
- An open fracture
- An injury to an arm or leg in which there is no pulse in the injured extremity
- An injury to the head or trunk that requires stitches calls for evacuation within 24 hours

Although you do not need to use rapid evacuation, you should generally consider evacuation as soon as is reasonably possible if the victim has these symptoms:

- Chest pain that is not due to injury of the ribs
- Severe, debilitating pain
- Signs and symptoms of serious altitude-related illness
- An infection that is getting worse
- Blood passing from the mouth or rectum (other than that caused by a minor and obvious condition)
- Significant psychological distress

Generally, you should work toward evacuating any victim who is not improving, whose signs or symptoms are getting worse, or whose injury or illness makes it impossible for the victim to travel at a reasonable pace on his or her own. Do not evacuate a victim of mild hypothermia who has normal mental status.

DECIDING HOW TO EVACUATE

There are a number of ways to evacuate an injured or ill victim. Simplest is to accompany the victim while he or she walks out of the wilderness; even people with leg, ankle, or foot injuries may be able to walk with assistance (e.g., using a tree branch or ski pole as a walking stick) once the injury has been treated and stabilized. A victim who is walking out should be accompanied by at least two rescuers; ideally, two rescuers should be sent ahead to notify authorities.

A second option is to carry the victim out; this can be done on an improvised litter or with any number of carries. Unfortunately, carrying a single victim out of a wilderness situation can require as many as 16 rescuers who have to battle rough or steep terrain, difficult conditions, adverse weather, and fatigue. At least six people should be carrying the litter at all times over smooth terrain; they should rest and rotate with six other rescuers every 15 minutes. If the terrain is rough, at least eight people should carry the litter at all times, and they should rest and rotate at least every 100 yards.

In remote areas, victims can sometimes be evacuated by helicopter. This type of rescue is costly and requires trained personnel who may be placed at risk during the rescue. A helicopter rescue should be used only if the pilot believes conditions are safe enough, the victim's life will be saved, the victim will have a dramatically better chance for recovery, or ground evacuation is too dangerous, will be unusually prolonged, or is impossible.

In deciding how to evacuate a victim, you need to take the following into consideration:

- How severely ill or injured is the victim? Is the victim's condition life threatening?

- What kind of psychological condition is the victim in?

- How much time would it take to evacuate the victim by each method, considering the distance, terrain, weather conditions, and other factors?

- What kinds of medical and rescue skills do the rescuers have?

- What type of equipment is available to the rescuers?

- What is the psychological condition of the rescuers?

- How much risk do the rescuers face?

- How much will the rescue cost?

Obviously, preserving the life of the victim is a more important consideration than the cost: If an expensive helicopter rescue is necessary to save a life, and there are no other feasible alternatives, the cost is not the major consideration.

If a helicopter is used in the rescue, make sure all people at the scene follow safety guidelines. Never approach a helicopter until one of the pilots signals that it is safe to do so. Protect your eyes against flying dirt as you approach the helicopter. Never approach a helicopter in a standing position or from the uphill side; stay as low as possible in a crouching position, and approach from a downhill side when possible. Never approach from the rear; the tail rotors spin so rapidly that they can be invisible.

If you need to signal the helicopter to indicate your location, use flares or hold a mirror toward the sun and flash it as much as possible directly toward the helicopter. If you do not have flares or a mirror:

- In daylight, use tree branches, logs, strips of tent material, toilet paper, or strips of clothing to mark an X on the ground. Make the sign as large as you possibly can to make it easier to see from the air. If there is snow, you can trample the sign into the snow. Remember: there are few straight lines or right angles in nature. So you will increase the odds of being seen if you use those in your signal.

- In daylight, build a campfire and use smoke to signal the helicopter. Rags soaked in engine oil or shards of rubber will create a heavy, black smoke

- In darkness, build a campfire and use the flames to signal the helicopter.

Death of a Victim

If a victim dies in the wilderness, you will have to manage a situation that First Aiders in urban areas are unlikely to face. Follow these guidelines:

- Immediately following the death, provide emotional and psychological care to survivors, who will undoubtedly be disturbed by the death. See Chapter 28 for information on psychological emergencies.

- Depending on the religious beliefs of others in the group, some sort of ceremony may be appropriate and comforting. Improvise; if possible, do not remove religious jewelry from the body.

- Note the time, cause, and location of the death. If you can, note the place on a map; if you have to transport the body across county or state lines, you may need to notify authorities in each jurisdiction later.

- Protect the body from predators and from the elements until you can transport it or until authorities arrive. *Do not encase a body in a sleeping bag;* the goal is to cool the body as rapidly as possible. Wrap the body in a tarp, groundcloth, or tent; if someone cannot stay with the body to protect it, hang it from a sturdy tree or over a ledge, or cover it with large stones.

- Notify authorities as quickly as possible. If they can, they should come to you. Packing a body out can be extremely difficult: search and rescue handbooks advise that, depending on terrain, it requires *at least* eight healthy people to carry a body 1 mile. Those eight must then rest while eight *additional* rescuers carry the body the next mile.

PROGRESS CHECK

1. When assessing a victim in the wilderness, spend more time on the _____ survey than you otherwise would. *(initial/primary/secondary)*

2. To manage a shock victim, insulate the victim from _____ . *(the air/the ground/moisture)*

3. Replace fluids in a shock victim by giving the victim _____ of water. *(small sips/one glass/large amounts)*

4. Wound management in the wilderness involves cleaning the wound and _____ . *(removing dead tissue/suturing the wound/changing the dressings)*

5. Whenever you splint a fracture or immobilize a victim to a backboard, pay special attention to _____ . *(strapping/padding/lashing)*

6. If a victim dies in the wilderness, it's easiest to _____ . *(have authorities come to the scene/carry the victim out)*

Summary

- Never enter the wilderness without a leader who has been to the area before and who can predict probable terrain, weather conditions, and hazards.

- Before entering a wilderness area, make a specific plan about how you will handle serious medical emergencies.

- Most wilderness emergencies are preventable. Protect yourself and others from the elements by setting up camp downwind from a windbreak. Avoid setting up camp in the bottom of a canyon or on a ledge.

- Plan for plenty of food and water for every member of your party; purify water by boiling it or filtering it, and keep food well secured and at a distance from your campsite.

- Altitude-related illness can occur at altitudes as low as 6,000 feet; the key to treatment is to get the victim to a lower altitude quickly.

- Because you are likely to be many hours—or even days—from medical help, you need to take special considerations in the assessment and treatment of victims in a wilderness setting. Examples include conducting a more detailed assessment; replacing fluids for shock victims; cleaning wounds; reducing fractures; and taking responsibility for the body of someone who has died.

Key Terms

Make sure you understand the following key terms:

Rule of Threes
billowing
acute mountain sickness
high altitude pulmonary edema (HAPE)
high altitude cerebral edema (HACE)
foramen magnum
ataxia

Critical Thinking Exercise

It is a beautiful spring day in May. The "cabin fever" of winter semester has motivated you and several friends to go rock-climbing in the nearby mountain range.

Soon you are testing your muscles and skills against the rigors of the rocky cliff high up the side of a very challenging mountain. Your adrenaline is flowing. Suddenly a cold wind whips the cliff and you hang on tightly as the wind pushes you in a pendulum fashion. Dark clouds come rolling in, and cold rain commences.

As you quickly glance over and down to check out the rest of your party you see a colleague who seems to be frozen with fear on the face of the cliff. He screams, then suddenly free-falls to crash on the rocks 30 feet below. You carefully but quickly belay down the cliff to the victim of the fall. Two other colleagues reach him at the same time as you.

1. In what order of priority would you pursue lifesaving measures?

2. Would you move the victim or keep him where he is?

3. After emergency care is provided, what would you do to stabilize the victim and attempt to prevent shock and hypothermia?

4. Would you evacuate the victim or bring help to him? How?

Chapter 27 Self-Test

Student: _____ Date: _____

Course: _____ Section #: _____

Part 1   True/False

If you believe the statement is true, circle the T. If you believe the statement is false, circle the F.

T   F   **1.** When entering the wilderness, you should always go with someone who has been to the area before.

T   F   **2.** You will get the most effective shelter if you set up camp in the bottom of a canyon.

T   F   **3.** Tents provide adequate shelter from moisture and insulation from wind.

T   F   **4.** People can get altitude-related illness at altitudes as low as 6,000 feet, though it is more common at altitudes of 8,000 feet and higher.

T   F   **5.** The best treatment for a victim of altitude-related illness is to stop for a day; the victim will "acclimate" and recover in that period.

T   F   **6.** When conducting victim assessment in the wilderness, spend more time on the secondary survey than you normally would.

T   F   **7.** Do not even attempt CPR in a wilderness setting; because paramedics are so far away, the victim probably will not survive anyway.

T   F   **8.** Even if you are several days from help, do not give fluids to a shock victim.

T   F   **9.** Help prevent wound infection by irrigating the wound with sterile water.

T   F   **10.** Make a victim on a backboard more comfortable by strapping the legs down flat.

Part 2   Multiple Choice

For each item, circle the correct answer or the phrase that best completes the statement.

1. If you are more than 3 hours away from medical help, treat an open fracture by
   a. irrigating the wound
   b. gently cleaning the wound and bone ends
   c. setting the bone
   d. placing the limb in traction

2. All but which of the following indicate wound infection?
   a. pus
   b. red streaks
   c. confined area of redness
   d. pulsating localized pain

3. If a wound develops signs of infection
   a. irrigate the wound with a disinfectant, such as hydrogen peroxide
   b. apply a topical antibiotic salve to the wound
   c. apply a warm, moist compress to the wound
   d. cut away any decaying tissue

4. CPR in a wilderness setting should be aggressive and prolonged, especially in cases of
   a. warm-water drownings
   b. falls
   c. lightning strikes
   d. animal attacks

5. An essential part of assessment in the wilderness setting is
   a. charting
   b. billowing
   c. testing reflexes
   d. determining the level of consciousness

6. Before entering a wilderness area, a first aid leader should
   a. purchase a commercial wilderness first aid kit
   b. review a good first aid text
   c. make specific plans about how he or she will handle a serious medical emergency
   d. map out the terrain

7. Because tents do not provide adequate insulation against the wind, you should pitch your tent
   a. in the bottom of a canyon
   b. at the top of a ridge
   c. downwind from a windbreak
   d. with extra-long stakes

8. The preferred method of purifying water in a wilderness setting according to the text, is
   a. boiling it
   b. using water purification tablets
   c. filtering it
   d. using household bleach

9. High altitude cerebral edema causes
   a. stroke
   b. increased pressure inside the skull
   c. impaired circulation
   d. double vision

10. High altitude pulmonary edema results when fluid is forced from body cells into the
    a. bloodstream
    b. brain
    c. heart
    d. lungs

11. A characteristic sign of high altitude pulmonary edema is
    a. coughing
    b. frothy sputum

    c. difficulty breathing, even at rest
    d. chest pain

12. High altitude cerebral edema, which can cause death within a few hours, forces the brain through the foramen magnum, affecting functions regulated by the
    a. cerebrum
    b. temporal lobe
    c. brain stem
    d. meninges

13. The most crucial treatment for any altitude-related illness is
    a. rapidly getting the victim to a lower altitude
    b. encouraging the victim to drink plenty of fluids
    c. keeping the victim at rest
    d. keeping the victim at the current altitude so he or she can become acclimated

14. When immobilizing a victim to a backboard in a wilderness setting, you must plan and allow for
    a. elimination of wastes
    b. rapid evacuation
    c. improvised strapping
    d. intravenous lines

15. If a victim dies in a wilderness setting, you should
    a. allow the body to cool as quickly as possible
    b. encase the body in a sleeping bag
    c. bury the body
    d. tag the body, then go for help

Part 3   What Would You Do If?

1. While hiking in a wilderness area, a member of your party falls and lacerates her arm on the jagged edge of a rock. The 2-inch wound is contaminated with dirt and small pieces of bark; it is bleeding moderately.

2. On the third day of a week-long trip into a remote mountainous area, one of your hiking companions sustains an open fracture of the lower leg. You are at least a day and a half from medical help.

28

Psychological Emergencies and Disasters

On the Scene

Twenty-one-year-old Jeffrey Huntington was called to a neighbor's apartment; a middle-aged man sat quietly at the far end of the living room. Fearing that her husband was extremely ill, his wife asked Jeffrey for help in determining what was wrong.

Jeffrey did a quick primary survey that turned up no evidence of life-threatening problems. He then did a secondary survey while he obtained a history from 52-year-old Helen Canterbury. Her husband's symptoms had developed fairly slowly, she said. He was "hearing voices," though he was oriented to time and place, and his pupils were even and responded to light.

With a calm and direct manner, Jeffrey started talking to Clifton Canterbury. Jeffrey expressed confidence in Clifton's ability to maintain control of his situation, and together they discussed the symptoms that were bothering Clifton. Through keen observation and knowledge of behavioral emergencies, Jeffrey was able to accurately assess Clifton as a victim of a psychological—not a physical—emergency.

Working with Helen, Jeffrey was able to convince Clifton that he needed to see a physician about the symptoms that were bothering him. While Helen called for an ambulance, Jeffrey waited with Clifton, listened to his story, and empathized with his situation. When paramedics arrived, Clifton was calm enough to be transported without resistance or restraint.

Physical first aid is tangible—it involves bandaging wounds, splinting bones, or restoring breathing. You perform physical care, and you can immediately see the results of your efforts.

Caring for psychological emergencies is different. You cannot readily see the comfort that you provide to someone who is panicked or agitated. It is hard to gauge immediately the results of caring for someone who is depressed and suicidal. But in terms of victim care, psychological support is often as important and life saving as is first aid for physical trauma.

This chapter outlines the goals and basic principles of psychological care, teaches how to distinguish between physical and psychological emergencies, discusses important assessment considerations, details legal considerations, and details methods of care. It also gives important information about mass-casualty situations and teaches how to perform triage.

28.1 Goals and Basic Principles

A psychological emergency is a situation in which a person exhibits "abnormal" behavior—behavior that is unacceptable or intolerable to the victim, the family, or the community. The abnormal behavior may be due to a psychological condition (such as a mental illness), to extremes of emotion, or even to a physical condition (such as a lack of oxygen or low blood sugar).

Goals of Psychological Care

Learning Objective 1 Discuss the goals of psychological first aid care.

Psychological first aid care should be planned and developed with four goals in mind:

1. To help the person begin functioning normally again as soon as possible

2. When the victim cannot be returned to normal quickly, to minimize as much as possible the victim's psychological disability

3. To decrease the intensity of the victim's emotional reaction until professional help is available

4. To keep the victim from hurting self or others

Figure 28-1 lists signs and symptoms that may indicate a psychological emergency.

Basic Principles of Care

Learning Objective 2 Outline the basic principles of psychological first aid care.

Providing care in psychological emergencies requires that you understand the following basic principles:

- Every person has limitations. In a psychological emergency, every person there—including you—is susceptible to emotional injury.

SIGNS AND SYMPTOMS OF
PSYCHOLOGICAL EMERGENCIES

Fear

Mania

Anxiety

Depression

Confusion

Withdrawal

Behavioral deviance

Loss of contact
with reality

Anger

FIGURE 28–1. One or more of the signs and symptoms listed above may indicate a psychological emergency.

- Each person has a right to his or her feelings. A person who is emotionally or mentally disturbed does not want to feel that way, but at that particular time, those feelings are valid and real.

- Each person has more ability to cope with crisis than he or she might think. For every manifestation of crazed emotion, the victim no doubt has some strength left within.

- Everyone feels some emotional disturbance when involved in a disaster or when injured. A particular physical injury might be especially devastating to a certain person—for example, a relatively minor hand injury may seem of little consequence, but it could ruin the career of a concert violinist.

- Emotional injury is just as real as physical injury. Unfortunately, physical injury is more visible, so it is more often accepted as being "real."

- People who have been through a crisis do not just "get better." Do not expect automatic results; you are first on the scene, and your role is to provide a positive beginning to a long, difficult healing process.

- You will encounter people of all races and cultural backgrounds (see Figure 28-2). Come to terms with your own feelings as you approach a situation, and take the time to understand the victim's perspective.

The main consideration in giving psychological first aid care is to develop confidence and rapport with the victim. Keep these guidelines in mind:

- Identify yourself.
- Express your desire to help.
- Use understandable language.
- Maintain eye contact.
- Listen intently and be empathetic.
- Act interested and concerned.
- Give calm and warm reassurance.
- Do not invade the victim's "space" until the person feels comfortable.
- Never use any physical force unless the victim is a threat to self or others.
- Never lie to or mislead the victim.
- Do not engender false hope.
- Do not judge, criticize, argue, or be overly sympathetic.
- Explain the situation to the victim and your plan of action; let the person know that you are in control.
- Avoid stock phrases such as "Everything will be OK."

Victims with Special Communication Needs

Geriatric	Pediatric	Deaf	Blind

• Do not assume senility or lack of understanding.
• Use victim's name.
• Check for hearing deficiency.
• Allow extra time for response.
• Ask victim what makes him or her most comfortable.
	• Victim may be frightened.
	• Victim may be modest.
	• Move slowly.
	• Explain procedures.
	• Use simple terms.
	• Allow child to keep toy, blanket, etc.
	• Be honest about pain caused by procedure.
	• Dolls may be useful to demonstrate procedure.
	• Parents and siblings may be useful to help calm and explain.
		• Determine if victim can read lips.
		• Position yourself properly.
		• Use interpreter if necessary and possible.
		• Use universally understood signs:
		   sick
		   hurt
		   help
		   etc.
		• Use written messages.
			• Determine if victim has hearing impairment.
			• Do not shout.
			• Explain incident and procedures in detail.
			• Lead victim if ambulatory, alerting the person to obstacles.

Non–English Speaking	Confused and/or Developmentally Disabled
• Use interpreter if possible. • Use gestures. • Refer to illustrated charts.	• Determine level of understanding. • Speak at appropriate level. • Wait for delayed response. • Evaluate understanding and explain again if necessary. • Listen carefully.

FIGURE 28–2. Victims of psychological emergencies may have special communication needs.

PROGRESS CHECK

1. A goal of psychological first aid care is to minimize _____ . *(pain/life-threatening conditions/psychological disability)*

2. Psychological first aid care is aimed at decreasing the intensity of the victim's _____ . *(pain/emotional reaction/fear)*

3. In an emergency involving a psychological crisis, every person—including you—is susceptible to _____ injury. *(emotional/physical/sudden)*

4. Emotional injury is just as _____ as physical injury. *(frequent/real/deviant)*

28.2 Psychological Crises

Learning Objective **3** List the factors that cause psychological changes.

A number of factors can cause a change in a person's behavior, among them situational stresses, medical illnesses, psychiatric problems, alcohol, or drugs. Some of the most common reasons behavior may change are:

- Low blood sugar in a diabetic, which can cause delirium, confusion, and even hallucinations

- Lack of oxygen

- Inadequate blood flow to the brain

- Head trauma

- Mind-altering substances, such as alcohol, depressants, stimulants, psychedelics, and narcotics

- Psychogenic substances, which can cause psychotic thinking, depression, or panic

- Excessive cold

- Excessive heat

Distinguishing between Physical and Psychological Causes

Learning Objective **4** Distinguish between psychological and physical emergencies.

As obvious as it sounds, you need to be sure you are dealing with a psychological, and not a physical, emergency. For example, you might detect what smells like alcohol on a victim's breath, but do not assume the vic-

tim is simply intoxicated. Diabetic coma can cause an odor on the breath that smells like alcohol. Antabuse, a drug used by alcoholics to decrease alcohol dependency, can also cause a breath odor similar to that of alcohol.

Remember that psychological changes and crises often follow (or are a result of) physical trauma or illness. Even if all the clues point to strictly a psychological problem, assess adequately to rule out a physical cause.

Specific Crises

Learning Objective **5** Discuss common psychological emergencies, including panic, agitation, and bizarre thinking and behavior.

Specific crises you may be confronted with as a First Aider include panic, agitation, bizarre thinking and behavior, victims who pose a danger to themselves (such as those who are suicidal), and victims who pose a danger to others (such as those who are violent). See Table 28-1 for a comparison of these emergencies.

PROGRESS CHECK

1. Low blood sugar in a diabetic can cause delirium, confusion, and _____. *(hallucinations/memory loss/hyperactivity)*

2. Alcohol, depressants, stimulants, psychedelics, and narcotics are all examples of _____. *(medication/mind-altering substances/situational stresses)*

3. Psychological emergencies are _____ physical emergencies. *(the same as/distinct from)*

28.3 Suicide

Suicide is any willful act designed to end one's own life. Suicide is now the eighth leading cause of death in the United States among all ages and the third leading cause of death among college-age students. Three

suicide Any willful act designed to end one's own life

	TABLE 28–1	**Common Psychological Emergencies**	

Disorder	Description	Manifestations
Panic	A response to stress that results in overwhelming feelings of helplessness; victims fear losing control	Intense fear, tension, restlessness, dizziness, hyperventilation, tingling around the mouth and fingers, spasms of the hands and feet, feelings of choking or smothering, irregular heartbeat
Agitation	Response to a situation that causes uneasiness or upset	Resentment, suspicion, impatience, irritability, anxiety, anger directed at an inappropriate source
Bizarre thinking and behavior	Thought or behavior patterns that are inappropriate	Highly exaggerated mistrust, hostility, elaborate delusions, coldness, antagonism, debilitating distortions of speech and thought, bizarre delusions, social withdrawal, lack of emotional expression
Danger to self	Depression causes the desire to harm self	Sad appearance, crying spells, listlessness, withdrawal, despondence, severe restlessness, feelings of worthlessness, helplessness, and hopelessness
Danger to others	Violence precipitated in an attempt to gain security or control	Nervous pacing, shouting, threatening, cursing, throwing objects, clenched teeth or fists

times more women than men *attempt* suicide, but three times more men are successful. Our geriatric population has significant depression and elevated rates of suicide. Suicide peaks in the spring and again in the fall, and is lowest during the month of December. Many believe that suicide is vastly underreported because of the stigma that still surrounds it.

Many suicide victims make last-minute attempts to communicate their intentions; most do not really want to die, but use the suicide attempt as a way to get attention, receive help, or punish someone. Every suicidal act or gesture should be taken seriously, and the victim should be transported for evaluation (see Figure 28-3 on page 470).

Risk Factors

Learning Objective **6** Discuss the risk factors for suicide.

The risk factors for suicide include the following:

- Being a male over 40 and being single, widowed, or divorced; men account for 70 percent of all suicides, and suicide is five times higher among people who are widowed or divorced.

- Alcoholism or drug abuse

- Depression; suicide is more common among people who are severely depressed.

- Suicidal gestures; approximately 80 percent of people who succeed in committing suicide made previous attempts.

- A plan; at highest risk are victims who have formulated a highly lethal plan and told others about it.

- An unusual gathering of articles that could be used to commit suicide (such as a gun or a large quantity of pills) or immediate access to a device that could be used to commit suicide

- A previous history of self-destructive behavior, even if that behavior was not overtly suicidal

- A recent diagnosis of serious illness, especially an illness that signals a loss of independence (suicide is especially high among those who are HIVpositive and among the elderly who have been diagnosed with chronic disease).

- The recent loss of a loved one; suicides also occur when a person's close emotional attachments are perceived to be in danger.

- An arrest, imprisonment, or the loss of a job (general signs that the victim has lost control or is unable to manage life).

During assessment, you may notice that:

- The victim is in an unsafe environment or is holding a dangerous object (such as a gun, knife, or rope).

- The victim displays self-destructive behavior, either before you arrived or during your assessment.

First Aid Care

Learning Objective **7** Describe how to manage a suicidal person.

Suicide Emergencies

Misconception	Fact
People who talk about suicide don't commit suicide.	Eight out of ten people who commit suicide have given definite warnings of their intentions. Almost no one commits suicide without first letting others know how he or she feels.
You can't stop a person who's suicidal—he or she is fully intent on dying.	Most people who are suicidal can't decide whether to live or die. Neither wish is necessarily stronger.
Once a person is suicidal, he or she is suicidal forever.	People who want to kill themselves are only suicidal for a limited time. If they're saved from feelings of self-destruction, they can often go on to lead normal lives.
Improvement after severe depression means that the suicidal risk is over.	Most persons commit suicide within about 3 months of the beginning of "improvement," when they have the energy to carry out suicidal intentions. They can also show signs of apparent improvement because their ambivalence is gone—they've made the decision to kill themselves.
If a person has attempted suicide, he or she won't do it again.	Many of those who commit suicide have previously attempted to do so.

Assessing Lethality
Age and Sex
• Incidence of suicide is highest in adolescents (ages 15 to 24) and in persons age 40 and over.
• Men succeed at suicide more often than women.
• Geriatric (older) patients frequently experience depression and have elevated rates of suicide.

Plan: Remember these points:
• Does the victim have a plan? Is it well thought out?
• Is it easy to carry out (successfully)?
• Are the means available? (For example, does the victim have pills collected, or a gun?)
• A detailed plan and available means carries maximum potential for lethality.

Symptoms
• What is the victim thinking and feeling?
• Is the person in control of his or her behavior? (Being out of control carries higher risk.)
• Alcoholics and psychotics are at higher risk.
• Depressed people are most at risk at the onset and at decline of depression.

Relationships with Significant Others
• Does the person have any support? Family, friends, therapist?
• Has the person suffered any recent losses?
• Is the person still in contact with people?
• Is the person telling family he or she has made a will?
• Is the person giving away prized possessions?

Medical History
People with chronic illnesses are more likely to commit suicide than those with terminal illnesses. Incidence of suicide rises whenever a victim's body image is severely threatened—for example, after surgery or childbirth.

The goal is to shift the intensity of a suicidal act from a desire to commit suicide to conflict over the need to commit suicide. The following guidelines can help:

• Specifically talk to the person about his or her intent.
• Ask the person how serious he or she is about killing himself or herself.
• Ask what concerns the person has about taking his or her life. The person will probably have some conflict.
• Ask the person why suicide is the answer to his or her problems.
• Ask what other alternatives the person has considered and what problems block the choice of other alternatives.
• Ask what hope the person has—even if it seems remote or blocked.
• By this time you may have helped decrease the intensity of the person's need to commit suicide, even though this change may be temporary.
• Always get professional help.
• A suicidal person should be transported to the hospital for evaluation even if he or she says everything is okay. Police assistance may be necessary.

FIGURE 28–3. Suicide emergencies

To manage a suicide emergency, activate the EMS system; then:

1. Make sure you are safe—your safety is of utmost importance. If you cannot guarantee your own safety, call the police and wait for them to arrive. Once the scene is safe for you, quickly survey for instruments the person might use to cause self-injury; discreetly remove any dangerous articles.

2. Assess the person for physical injury; first aid treatment for physical injury has priority.

3. Assess the seriousness of the person's thoughts and feelings. Do not be afraid to ask the person directly about suicidal thoughts. Always take a suicide threat seriously; if the person has a plan, the problem is more serious than it would be with someone who has considered suicide but has not figured out how.

4. Calm the person and stay with him or her. Never leave a suicidal person alone.

5. If it is necessary to protect the person from self-harm, use restraints. Never use restraints as a substitute for observation, and never use metal handcuffs.

As you deal with a suicidal person (see Figure 28-4), follow these guidelines:

- Listen carefully.

- Accept all the person's complaints and feelings; do not underestimate what the person may be feeling.

- Do not trust "rapid recoveries." The person needs to be taken to the hospital even if he or she seems to be "better."

- Be specific in your actions; do something tangible for the person, such as arranging for a clergyman to meet the person at the hospital.

- Never show disgust or horror when you care for the person.

- Never try to shock a person out of a suicidal act. Never argue or challenge the person to go ahead.

PROGRESS CHECK

1. _____ are at highest risk for suicide. *(Married men/Divorced men/Single women)*

2. You should consider a suicide threat to be especially serious if the person has a _____ . *(gun/knife/plan)*

3. The best strategy for managing a suicidal person is to _____ . *(give the person space/never leave the person alone/always use restraints)*

4. The first step in managing a suicide emergency is to _____ . *(restrain the person/protect your own safety/ask about the person's plan)*

28.4 Assessment

Learning Objective 8 Discuss the principles of assessment for psychological emergencies.

When assessing victims of a psychological emergency, follow these guidelines:

1. Identify yourself and let the victim know you are there to help. Show through your actions that you have confidence in the victim's ability to maintain self-control and control of the situation (see Figure 28-5 on page 472).

2. Tell the victim what you are doing; be honest, but do not frighten the victim.

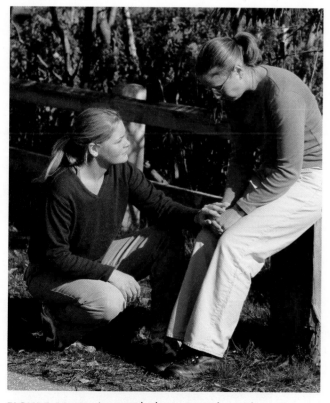

FIGURE 28-4. Approach the potential suicide victim with empathy and concern.

3. Ask questions in a calm, reassuring voice. Be polite, use good manners, show respect, and make no assumptions or judgments.

4. Allow the victim to tell you what happened. If you can, interview the victim in a quiet room where the victim has privacy. Show you are listening by rephrasing or repeating part of what the victim says.

5. Acknowledge the victim's feelings. Use phrases such as, "I can see that you are very depressed," or "I understand that you must feel frightened."

6. Assess the victim's mental status by asking specific questions that will help you measure the victim's level of consciousness, orientation, and contact with reality.

Assessing the Potential for Violence

Violence is generally an attempt to gain security or control. Anger or violence may be a response to illness or the victim's way of coping with feelings of helplessness. It can also be precipitated by victim mismanagement (real or perceived), psychosis, alcohol or drug intoxication, fear, panic, or head injury.

To determine the potential for violence (see Figure 28-6):

■ Size up the scene. Locate the victim visually before you approach. Determine whether the victim is disoriented, whether drugs or alcohol are involved, whether the victim has a gun or other weapon, whether the situation involves a hostage, and whether others are involved.

■ Early in the assessment—before you physically approach the victim—determine whether you can handle the situation alone. Even a small person who is sufficiently agitated can be very difficult to handle. If you doubt that you can handle the victim alone, call the police and wait for them to arrive.

■ Take a history. Ask bystanders what has been going on. Has the victim been violent or threatened violence? Does the victim have a history of violence, aggression, or combativeness?

■ Anticipate violence if the victim is standing or sitting in a way that threatens self or others, if the victim's fists are clenched, or if the victim is holding anything that could be used as a weapon.

■ Anticipate violence if the victim is yelling, cursing, arguing, or verbally threatening to hurt self or others.

■ Monitor the victim's physical activity. Signs of potential violence include moving toward the caregiver, carrying a heavy or threatening object, using quick or irregular movements, and having muscle tension.

FIGURE 28-5. When dealing with a psychological emergency, be calm and show through your actions that you have confidence in the victim's ability to maintain self-control.

PROGRESS CHECK

1. When you approach the victim, you should _____ . *(tell the victim what you are doing/try to take the victim by surprise/divert the victim's attention)*

2. A good assessment strategy is to _____ the victim's feelings. *(deny/try to change/acknowledge)*

3. A risk factor for violence is a history of _____ . *(head injury/arrest/aggression)*

4. Anticipate violence if the victim has _____ . *(head injury/clenched fists/run away)*

5. Anticipate violence if the victim is _____ . *(cursing/disoriented/hallucinating)*

6. A person with quick, _____ moves is at risk for becoming violent. *(dramatic/sweeping/irregular)*

Disruptive and Aggressive Victims: Assessment Guidelines

Any behavior that presents a danger to the victim or others or that delays or prevents appropriate care is disruptive and may precipitate a psychological emergency. Common causes of disruptive behavior include stress-induced hysteria; aggression; alcohol or drug problems; neurological trauma; metabolic imbalances; organic brain syndromes; psychological disorders.

Assessing the Situation

- What information do you have from the situation—what happened?
- Is the environment (emotional, social, and/or physical) dangerous to you and/or others?
- Does the victim seem agitated, elated, depressed, or restless?
- Has the person already demonstrated aggressive or violent behavior?
- Does the person talk loudly and in sarcastic terms?
- Does the person use vulgar language?
- Is the person easily provoked to anger?
- Does the person have a limited attention span?
- Does the person seem to be out of control or disoriented?
- Does the person seem to be afraid or panicky?
- Does the person have a weapon?
- Is there evidence of alcohol or drug abuse?
- Is a domestic disturbance involved?
- Has criminal activity occurred?

If you answer **yes** to several or most of the above questions, use extreme caution. If possible, try not to control or suppress the victim's behavior. Rather, allow the person to express feelings. *Remember*—the most effective way to deal with a victim who exhibits aggressive and/or violent behavior is to reduce the crisis and prevent further disruptive behavior. The safest thing to do in these situations is to call the police.

FIGURE 28–6. Assessing disruptive and aggressive victims

28.5 Legal Considerations

Learning Objective **9** Discuss the legal considerations involved in managing psychological emergencies.

Every time you respond as a First Aider, you have a chance of encountering the legal system. That chance becomes greater when you are responding to victims with psychological problems. To reduce your legal liability, follow these guidelines:

- *When possible, get consent.* Simply stated, consent is permission to treat. In most states, you could be charged with assault and battery if you force a person to have treatment against his or her will. Review the consent information in Chapter 1.

- *If a victim refuses care,* carefully document what has happened. If the victim threatens to hurt self or others and you can demonstrate reason to believe that the victim's threats are real, the victim can be transported by EMTs or law enforcement without consent. Remember—you must be able to document your belief that the victim is a threat.

- *Avoid unreasonable force.* If it is necessary to restrain a victim, use **reasonable force**—only the amount of force required to keep the victim from injuring self or others. The amount of force considered reasonable depends on the victim's size and strength, behavior, and mental state and the method of restraint (soft restraints or straps are usually considered reasonable; metal cuffs are not).

In most areas, you need police authorization to use reasonable force in restraining a victim without consent. In most areas, First Aiders can use reasonable force to defend against an attack by an emotionally disturbed victim without fearing legal consequences. The basic guideline is to avoid any act or physical force that may injure the victim during restraint.

- *Seek police direction.* It is always a good idea to involve law enforcement if there is any threat of violence. Police officers serve a twofold purpose in cases such as this: They provide protection from injury, and they serve as credible witnesses if a victim later tries to sue you.

- *Protect yourself against false accusations.* Carefully and completely document everything that happens during the situation; include details of the victim's abnormal behavior. In most jurisdictions, anything documented at the scene is considered legally admissible evidence, and anything not documented is hearsay.

reasonable force The amount of force required to keep a person from injuring self or others

■ *Manage a crime scene.* You may find, when called to the scene of a psychological emergency, that the person has either committed or been the victim of a crime or harmed himself or herself. If you help at the scene of a criminal act, your first concern is to care for the injured victims.

■ Always cooperate with local law enforcement.

■ Disrupt or touch evidence as little as possible.

■ If the victim is moved, mark the original body position.

■ Provide reassurance and emotional support. Common victim responses include outrage, disbelief, withdrawal, hysteria, and depression.

■ Make victim care a priority. Never choose evidence collection over victim care. Both can be done simultaneously.

To avoid disturbing crucial evidence that is needed by law enforcement in investigating the crime, follow these guidelines:

■ Do not allow bystanders into the area.

■ Where appropriate, assist police in collecting and recording anything on the victim, such as blood, hair, seminal fluid, gunpowder residue, or clothing fibers.

■ Take extreme care not to disturb any evidence that is not on the victim's body (footprints, soil, broken glass, tire tracks, and so on).

■ Never touch or move suspected weapons unless it is absolutely necessary in treating the victim's injuries.

■ If you need to tear or cut away clothing to expose a wound, do not cut through a bullet hole or knife slash in the clothing.

■ If the victim was strangled and still has the rope or cord around the neck, cut it instead of untying it— the knot can be used as evidence and may identify the perpetrator.

■ Document in writing who is at the crime scene when you arrive.

■ If the victim is obviously dead when you arrive, do nothing and disturb nothing. Call the police and wait for them to arrive.

PROGRESS CHECK

1. Whenever possible, get _____ before you care for a victim. *(help/protection/consent)*

2. Use _____ only to restrain a victim. *(metal cuffs/ropes/reasonable force)*

3. The amount of force that is reasonable to restrain a victim depends in part on the victim's _____ . *(history/size/illness)*

4. If you have to restrain a victim, try to involve the _____ . *(police/victim's family/bystanders)*

5. To protect yourself against false accusations, _____ everything that happens while you are at the scene. *(photograph/document/think about)*

6. If a victim was involved in a crime, take extra care not to disturb _____ . *(the police investigation/the evidence/the next of kin)*

28.6 First Aid Care for Psychological Emergencies

Managing a Violent Victim

Learning Objective 10 Describe how to manage a violent victim.

Your first priority is to protect yourself. Never go into a potentially violent situation by yourself. To keep yourself safe and protect the victim (see Figure 28-7), do the following:

■ If you are outdoors and can do so, walk on the grass, not the sidewalk.

■ If you are using a flashlight, hold it beside—not in front of—your body.

■ If you are walking with someone else, walk single file; only the first person in line should carry a flashlight.

■ As you approach the scene, make a mental map of all possible places for **concealment** (objects that will hide you, such as shrubbery) and **cover** (objects that will both hide you and stop bullets, such as trees). Keep scanning the area for movement.

■ Stand to the side of a door when you knock on it; never stand in front of it.

■ As soon as the door is open, assess the situation before you decide whether to retreat and call for help.

concealment A place or an object that will hide you, such as shrubbery

cover An object that will both hide you and stop bullets, such as a tree

Disruptive and Aggressive Victims: Management Guidelines

Don'ts	Do's
• Don't put yourself in a position of danger. • Don't attempt to diagnose, judge, label, or criticize the victim. • Don't isolate yourself from other helpers. • Don't isolate yourself with a victim who has a record of potential violence. • Don't disturb a victim with first aid care or taking vital signs any more than is necessary. • Don't turn your back on the victim. • Don't position yourself between the victim and the only doorway. • Don't forget that a disturbed victim's moods can fluctuate rapidly. • Don't reject any of the victim's complaints—acknowledge them. • Don't threaten, lie, bluff, or deceive the victim. • Don't take insults personally. • Don't rush into action. • Don't show hostility toward the victim's words or actions. • Don't appear aggressive or defensive. • Don't be overly friendly. • Don't sound authoritarian or demanding when you speak to the victim. • Don't attempt to restrain a victim unless you have adequate assistance to do so safely. It is best to call the police.	• If danger exists, create a safe zone and wait for assistance (police and/or emergency units). • Keep bystanders outside of safe zone. • Remove any person or object from the environment that seems to be triggering the victim's aggression. • Convey a sense of helpfulness rather than hostility or frustration. • Establish voice control by asking bystanders what the problem is loud enough so that the victim can hear you. • Identify yourself. • Let the victim know what you expect. • Present a comfortable, confident, and professional manner. • Ask the victim his or her name and what the problem is. • Listen to, but do not respond to insults and abusive language or take them personally. • Be honest. • Speak in short sentences with simple ideas and explanations. • Remain relaxed and confident. • Adjust your physical distance from the victim to a safe range—at first no closer than approximately 10 or 15 feet. Move closer only after adequate assessment reveals that it's safe to do so. • Respect the victim's difficulty in maintaining self-control. Tell the person that you are aware of the problem, and acknowledge her or his attempt to deal with it. • Acknowledge the victim's complaints—you do not have to agree, but acknowledge that the person has a reason to be upset. • Use gestures and other nonverbal messages carefully. They might communicate the opposite of what you intend. A disturbed victim might interpret friendliness and smiling as an attempt at trickery. • If your preventive actions fail to reduce hostile, violent, and combative behavior, the victim is in control and it may be necessary to restrain the victim to protect self and others. • Assess the victim's strengths. • Make certain that you have a plan and sufficient help to prevent injury to the victim and yourself.

FIGURE 28-7. Managing disruptive and aggressive victims

- Negotiate with the victim from a safe distance (at least 6 feet away) and position (facing the victim). Never turn your back on the victim.

- Keep the door to the room open, and identify as many exits as possible. Regardless of the situation, make absolutely sure you have at least one certain route of escape.

- Always follow a victim down a hallway or stairway. Never lead the way.

- Never ignore or disregard a weapon. In a calm and nonconfrontational way, tell the victim that you want to help, but you cannot do so until the weapon is released. Ask the victim to put the weapon in a neutral place.

How to Calm Psychological Emergency Victims

Learning Objective 11 Describe and demonstrate methods of calming a person undergoing a psychological emergency.

Because psychological emergencies are difficult, you may need to use techniques you would not consider with victims of other kinds of emergencies. Following are some techniques to use in addition to the typical techniques used during assessment:

1. Maintain a comfortable distance from the victim; many victims are threatened by physical contact.

2. Do not make any quick movements. Act quietly and slowly; let the victim see that you are not going to make any sudden moves (a fear that can precipitate violence).

3. Respond honestly to the victim's questions, but do not foster unrealistic expectations. Instead of saying, "You have nothing to worry about," say something like, "Despite all the problems you've had, you seem to have lots of people around you who really care about you." Reassure the victim that visual or auditory disturbances are temporary and will clear up with treatment. Always tell the truth.

4. Never threaten, challenge, or argue with disturbed victims. Many psychologically disturbed victims will be adept at picking out your weaknesses; remain kind and calm.

5. When you can, involve trusted family members or friends.

6. Never leave the victim alone; psychological emergency victims are escape risks. Once you have responded to the emergency, the victim's safety is legally your responsibility.

7. Maintain good eye contact with the victim, for two reasons: First, direct eye contact communicates your control and confidence. Second, the victim's eyes can reflect emotions and tell you whether the victim is terrified, confused, struggling, in pain, or dying.

8. Do not force the victim to make decisions, because the victim has probably lost the ability to cope effectively.

9. If the victim has attracted a crowd, do what you can to disperse it so you can deal with the victim on a one-to-one basis.:

Restraining a Victim

> Learning Objective 12 Describe and demonstrate how to restrain a violent victim.

A difficult situation arises when a victim is out of control. If you believe the victim may be dangerous to self or others, you must notify the police. Never leave a violent victim alone; watch the victim constantly, and stay alert.

Restraint should be avoided unless the victim is a danger to self and others. Use of restraints may require police authorization; if you are not authorized by state law to use restraints, wait for someone with authority.

A violent physical struggle is usually brief, because most people cannot sustain the intensity needed; however, if you still feel the need for restraints:

1. Gather enough people to overpower the victim clearly before you attempt restraint.

2. Plan what you are going to do before you attempt restraint. Everyone involved should know what is going to happen.

3. Use only as much force as needed for restraint; never inflict pain or use unwarranted force in restraining a victim.

4. Estimate the range of motion of the victim's arms and legs, and stay beyond that range until you actually are ready to begin restraint.

5. Once you have made the decision to restrain, act quickly. Part of restraint involves taking the victim by surprise; your delay or indecision could allow the victim to get the upper hand.

6. Approach the victim with at least four people, one assigned to each limb, at the same time. Secure the victim's limbs together with restraints of soft leather or cloth.

7. The victim should be placed faceup (supine). Monitor the victim carefully. Restrained victims have been known to stop breathing (positional asphyxia) and have other medical problems due to exertion and preexisting conditions.

Once you have applied restraints, do not remove them. Reassess the victim's circulation frequently to make sure the restraints are not binding. Document the reason you felt it necessary to restrain the victim, and thoroughly document the technique you used for the restraint.

PROGRESS CHECK

1. After you have knocked on the door at a site where there is a potential for violence, stand _____ . (in front of the door/away from the door/to the side of the door)

2. When dealing with a violent person, _____ . (use a gentle touch on the arm/hold the arm firmly/avoid physical contact)

3. Use soft leather or _____ to restrain a victim. (cloth/wire/metal cuffs)

4. At least _____ people should be involved in restraining a victim. (two/three/four)

28.7 Mass Casualties and Disasters

When the situation involves more than one casualty, people may become dazed, disorganized, or overwhelmed. The American Psychiatric Association has identified five possible types of reactions (see Figure 28-8) in such situations:

1. Normal

2. Blind panic

3. Depression

4. Overreacting

5. Conversion hysteria

Emotional Reactions in Mass Casualties and Disasters

Reactions	Signs and Symptoms	Do's	Don'ts
Normal	Fear and anxiety Muscular tension followed by trembling and weakness Confusion Profuse perspiration Nausea, vomiting Mild diarrhea Frequent urination Shortness of breath Pounding heart These reactions usually dissipate with activity as the person gains self-control.	Normal reactions usually require little emergency care. Calm reassurance may be all that is necessary to help a person pull himself together. Watch to see that the individual is gaining composure, not losing it. Provide meaningful activity. Talk with the person.	Don't show extreme sympathy.
Panic (blind flight of hysteria)	Unreasoning attempt to flee Loss of judgment—blindness to reality Uncontrolled weeping or hysteria often to the point of exhaustion Aimless running about with little regard for safety Panic is contagious when not controlled. Normally calm persons may become panicked by others during moments when they are temporarily disorganized.	Begin with firmness. Give something warm to eat or drink. Firmly, but gently, isolate the person from the group. Get help if necessary. Show empathy and encourage the person to talk. Monitor your own feelings. Keep calm and know your limitations.	Don't brutally restrain the person. Don't strike the person. Don't douse the person with water. Don't give sedatives.
Overactive	Explodes into flurry of senseless activity Argumentative Overconfident of abilities Talks rapidly—will not listen Tells silly jokes Makes endless suggestions Demanding of others Does more harm than good by interfering with organized leadership Like panic, overactivity is contagious if not controlled.	Let the person talk and ventilate feelings. Assign and supervise a job that requires physical activity. Give something warm to eat or drink.	Don't tell the person he is acting abnormally. Don't give sedatives. Don't argue with the person. Don't tell the person he or she shouldn't act or feel this way.
Underactive (daze, shock, depression)	Cannot recover from original shock and numbness Stands or sits without talking or moving Vacant expression Emotionless "Don't care" attitude Helpless, unaware of surroundings Moves aimlessly, slowly Little or no response to questioning Pulls within self to protect from further stress Puzzled, confused This victim cannot take responsibility without supervision.	Gently establish contact and rapport. Get the person to ventilate feelings and let you know what happened. Show empathy. Be aware of feelings of resentment in yourself and others Give the person warm food or drink. Give and supervise a simple, routine job.	Don't tell the person to "snap out of it." Don't show extreme pity. Don't give sedatives. Don't show resentment.
Severe physical reaction (conversion hysteria)	Severe nausea Conversion hysteria—the victim converts anxiety into a strong belief that a part of his body is not functioning (paralysis, loss of sight, etc.). The disability is just as real as if the person had been physically injured.	Show interest. Find a small job for the person to do to take his or her mind off the injury. Make the person comfortable and summon medical aid. Monitor your own feelings.	Don't say, "There's nothing wrong with you" or, "It's all in your head." Don't blame or ridicule. Don't call undue attention to the injury. Don't openly ignore the injury.

FIGURE 28–8. Emotional reactions in mass casualties and disasters

Source: American Psychiatric Association

With **conversion hysteria**, the victim's mood may shift rapidly from extreme anxiety to relative calmness; the victim may then convert anxiety to a physical dysfunction, such as hysterical blindness, deafness, or paralysis.

Managing Mass Casualty or Disaster Situations

Learning Objective **13** Discuss how to manage mass casualties and disasters.

Although each disaster presents individual problems, these general guidelines will usually apply to any disaster you may be called to respond to:

1. Don't let yourself become overwhelmed by the immensity of the disaster. Administer aid to those who need it. Carefully evaluate the injuries, and determine which victims should be treated first. Then set about administering the aid, treating victims one by one. This will help you maintain some calm and feel that you are making progress, despite the immensity of the disaster.

2. Assist the rescuers at the scene. Fire, police, and EMS personnel will follow a specific plan. Ask how you can assist. Make sure you are part of a solution—work with the rescuers as they see fit.

3. Encourage victims or bystanders who are able to do necessary chores at the scene. Work can be therapeutic.

4. Identify yourself; stay self-assured, sympathetic, and businesslike, and reassure anxious victims or bystanders.

5. Assess and care for physical injuries immediately.

6. Keep spectators away from the victims, but do not leave the victims alone. If all rescue personnel are busy dealing with physical injuries, assign a responsible bystander to stay with anyone showing unusual behavior.

7. Respect the right of victims to have their own feelings, and accept the physical and emotional limitations of victims.

8. Accept your own limitations; there are limits to what can be done. You will provide more effective care if you establish priorities and refuse to overextend yourself.

Triage

All the medical knowledge in the world and the finest care by a First Aider will not help if priorities are not properly ordered. It is critical that you know which victims of a multiple-victim accident or disaster require first aid care first and that you classify those who need attention and care the most desperately.

Triage, a French term meaning picking or sorting, is a process of sorting and classifying sick and injured victims. Triage is a procedure by which the sick and wounded are classified as to type and urgency of condition and, based on the assigned priorities, are sent to facilities where they can receive care.

Conducting Triage

Learning Objective **14** Describe how to perform triage.

Triage should be conducted by the most experienced First Aider as soon as the scene is secured (traffic is controlled, the fire is out, and so on). Move from victim to victim, performing a limited amount of lifesaving care and tagging the victims for later care. This sets the stage for the next arriving rescuers, who can focus on caring for salvageable victims.

The three-level method of triage uses different tags for life-threatened (highest priority), urgent (second priority), and delayed (lowest priority) (see Table 28-2). Those who are dead are taken to a morgue in a different area of the disaster scene. The two-level method (see Table 28-3) uses separate tags for immediate (first priority) and delayed (second priority).

To conduct triage:

1. Move quickly from one victim to the next; complete a primary survey on each.

2. Correct immediate life-threatening problems. Apply the ABCs (caring for airway/breathing/circulation) on a limited basis, depending on the availability of rescuers who can help with triage and treatment. *You should not spend more than 30 to 60 seconds per victim during the actual triage.*

3. Tag each victim as to priority.

4. Ask for additional assistance if needed.

5. Assign available manpower and equipment to highest-priority victims.

conversion hysteria Converting anxiety to a physical dysfunction, such as blindness or deafness

triage A system of sorting victims into categories by treatment priority

TABLE 28–2	**Three-Level Triage**		
	Highest Priority	**Second Priority**	**Lowest Priority**
Level of emergency	Critically injured but can recover if treated immediately	Seriously injured; may die without further treatment	Noncritical injuries or minor wounds; mortal wounds
Examples	Airway and breathing difficulties, cardiac arrest (treat *if* enough personnel available), uncontrolled or severe bleeding, severe head injuries, severe medical problems (poisoning and diabetes), open chest or abdominal wounds, shock	Burns, major or multiple fractures, back injuries with or without spinal cord damage	Fractures, minor injuries, obviously mortal wounds making death reasonably certain, cardiac arrest if there are not enough personnel

Note: Dead victims will be taken to a morgue in different location. Victims requiring vigorous care for cardiac arrest should be treated as dead.

TABLE 28–3	**Two-Level Triage**
Immediate (First Priority)	**Delayed (Second Priority)**
Includes those who have critical injuries that threaten life but are salvageable; those requiring immediate medical care (within 5 to 15 minutes) to survive	Includes those who are seriously injured but whose lives are not threatened; those whose injuries are minor and whose treatment can be delayed; and those who are very critically injured—nonsalvageable or dead; also includes those with no injuries or only minor injuries requiring first aid care

6. When additional help arrives, arrange for treatment and transport of highest-priority victims first.

7. If possible, notify emergency personnel and/or hospital(s) of number and severity of injuries.

8. Triage rescuer remains at the scene to assign and coordinate manpower, supplies, and vehicles.

9. Reassess victims regularly for changes in status.

PROGRESS CHECK

1. In a mass casualty or disaster, extreme anxiety, sweating, and vomiting are _____ reactions. *(normal/abnormal/delayed)*

2. Becoming blind or deaf after a mass casualty or disaster is a sign of _____ . *(physical injury/conversion hysteria/sensory trauma)*

3. During a mass casualty, you should keep spectators away and _____ . *(give victims privacy/isolate victims/stay with the victims)*

4. A victim with obviously mortal wounds should be classified in the _____ triage priority. *(highest/second/lowest)*

5. A victim with a life-threatening condition that could be saved if treated immediately should be classified in the _____ priority. *(highest/second/lowest)*

6. A victim who is seriously injured and who may die without treatment should be classified in the _____ priority. *(highest/second/lowest)*

Summary

- The goals of psychological first aid care are to help the person begin functioning normally as soon as possible, to minimize psychological disability, to decrease the intensity of emotional reaction until professional help is available, and to keep the victim from hurting self or others.

- A number of physical disorders can create symptoms that mimic psychological disorders; assess the victim carefully to make sure there is not a physical problem that needs to be cared for.

- The most common psychological crises include panic, agitation, bizarre thinking and behavior, danger to self, and danger to others.

- Take every suicide threat seriously; the threat is particularly serious if the victim has a plan.

- Never try to argue someone out of committing suicide, and never challenge someone to go ahead.

- People who are about to become violent manifest certain behaviors, such as clenching the fists, moving in quick and irregular ways, shouting, cursing, and so on. Become familiar with these signs and act quickly to protect yourself.

- Always try to get consent before you care for or transport a victim.

- If you have to restrain a victim who is threatening to hurt someone (including self), use reasonable force based on the victim's size, strength, mental status, and behavior.

- If you arrive at a crime scene, make sure the scene is safe before you enter; take care to preserve the chain of evidence for the police.

- Use professionalism, empathy, and courtesy to help calm the victim of a psychological emergency. Use restraints only when absolutely necessary, and always use soft restraints.

- Victims of a mass casualty or disaster are normally extremely anxious, weak, shaky, and nauseated; they can be helpful if given specific tasks.

- Triage is a system of identifying and prioritizing victims so that the most effective care can be given to the largest number of victims. Those who have life-threatening injuries but who can recover with treatment should be treated and transported first; those with minor or obviously mortal injuries should be treated and transported last.

Key Terms

Make sure you understand the following key terms:

suicide
reasonable force
concealment
cover
conversion hysteria
triage

Critical Thinking Exercise

You are called by a friend who says his roommate seems depressed and has talked about "not wanting to go on any longer." You arrive to find the roommate who seems intoxicated. He says that his girlfriend broke up with him earlier in the day. You note two empty pill containers on the end table near where he is sitting. He admits he has been drinking but denies taking the pills. He does not want to go to the hospital.

Your friend tells you that he may have overreacted and offers to stay and watch his roommate.

1. Do you think the patient took the pills from the containers? Why or why not? How could you find out more information about this?

2. Should you activate EMS?

3. How do you respond to your friend who wants to stay at the dorm with the patient?

Chapter 28 Self-Test

Student: _____ Date: _____

Course: _____ Section #: _____

If you believe the statement is true, circle the T. If you believe the statement is false, circle the F.

T   F   **1.** While talking to a victim, ask questions that are direct and specific to measure the victim's contact with reality.

T   F   **2.** Do *not* leave a victim of a psychological emergency alone.

T   F   **3.** It is appropriate to lie to a victim to protect the victim from unpleasant facts.

T   F   **4.** Suicide threats do not need to be taken seriously.

T   F   **5.** Few people have as much ability to cope with crisis as they think they do.

T   F   **6.** People under severe emotional stress usually feel that they are in complete control.

T   F   **7.** Violent behavior is often an attempt to gain control.

T   F   **8.** Burns are in the highest priority of care in triage.

T   F   **9.** If a person is having a psychological emergency, you do not have to obtain consent to treat because the person is not lucid anyway.

T   F   **10.** It is impossible to tell by a person's behavior whether the person is about to become violent.

For each item, circle the correct answer or the phrase that best completes the statement.

1. In dealing with a mass casualty, you should *not*
   a. remain self-assured and businesslike
   b. feel responsible for treating every victim
   c. assign tasks to bystanders
   d. make clear that you understand the victim's feelings

2. How should you handle the emotional reactions of panic victims in mass casualties and disasters?
   a. show extreme sympathy
   b. douse the person with water
   c. firmly but gently isolate the person
   d. administer mild sedatives

3. A victim who is talking compulsively and joking inappropriately is having what kind of reaction?
   a. normal
   b. panic
   c. overreacting
   d. conversion hysteria

4. Which guideline for psychological care is *not* correct?
   a. establish rapport with the victim
   b. encourage the victim to talk out feelings and fears

   c. slap the victim to bring him or her around
   d. encourage an exhausted victim to sleep

5. Which is *not* a principle of psychological first aid care?
   a. every person has limits
   b. emotional trauma is less serious than physical trauma
   c. every person has the right to his or her feelings
   d. everyone feels emotionally distraught as a result of physical injury

6. What is a sound way to deal with a suicidal person?
   a. trust rapid recoveries
   b. try to shock the person out of a suicidal act
   c. show the person you are disgusted with his or her actions
   d. ask the victim directly about suicidal thoughts

7. What physical illness would most likely appear to be psychological?
   a. cardiac arrest
   b. epilepsy
   c. diabetic coma
   d. insulin shock

8. Which of the following should you *not* do when dealing with a potentially violent victim?

   a. position yourself between the victim and the door
   b. present a comfortable, confident, professional manner
   c. keep a safe distance from the victim
   d. let the victim know what you expect

9. Triage means

   a. giving emotional support to victims
   b. mobilizing available rescue personnel
   c. establishing a community plan
   d. assessing and categorizing the injured so treatment can begin

10. Which of the following is *not* in the highest-priority category of triage?

   a. airway and breathing difficulties
   b. severe bleeding
   c. fracture
   d. open chest wound

Part 3   Matching

Match the type of reaction at the left with the correct definition at the right.

Definition

1._____ Mood may shift rapidly from extreme anxiety to relative calmness.

2._____ The individual remains motionless and looks numbed and dazed.

3._____ The person shows extreme anxiety, including sweating, shaking, weakness, nausea, and sometimes vomiting.

4._____ Judgment seems to disappear completely.

5._____ The person talks compulsively, jokes inappropriately, and races from one task to another, usually accomplishing little.

Reaction

a. Normal reaction
b. Blind panic
c. Depression
d. Overreaction
e. Conversion hysteria

Part 4   What Would You Do If?

You are a pedestrian at a busy downtown intersection where a person is wandering dangerously among the traffic and seems to be oblivious to what is going on around him. He is anxious and withdrawn and is talking to himself. He also seems to be very fearful of something.

29

Lifting and Moving Victims

Learning Objectives

When you have mastered the material in this chapter, you will be able to

1 Discuss the general guidelines for moving victims

2 Identify the situations in which an emergency move must be made

3 Describe and demonstrate the walking assist

4 Describe and demonstrate the blanket drag

5 Describe and demonstrate the shirt drag

6 Describe and demonstrate the sheet drag

7 Describe and demonstrate the firefighter's carry

8 Describe and demonstrate seat carries

9 Describe and demonstrate the extremity lift

10 Describe and demonstrate the chair litter carry

11 Describe and demonstrate the flat lift and carry

12 Describe and demonstrate how to use backboards to move a victim

13 Describe and demonstrate how to use a blanket stretcher

14 List objects that can be used for improvised stretchers

15 Discuss the guidelines for moving a victim on a stretcher

On the Scene

On his way to university classes one morning, 23-year-old Kent Ashby came upon a two-car accident in which one vehicle had broadsided another. Two victims had been ejected from the vehicles. A third, a woman about 30 years old, had unfastened her seat belt and managed to get out of one of the cars; she was leaning against it and cradling her right arm against her chest.

Running to the scene, Kent could see that one of the victims was lying beside a pool of gasoline that had streamed from the ruptured tank of one of the cars. The other victim was quite a distance away. Kent knew that the first victim had to be moved—there was danger of the gasoline igniting.

By this time, two other vehicles had stopped. Kent sent the driver of one to call for emergency personnel. He asked the driver of the other, 46-year-old Judith Sterling, to help in the move. She refused, stating that she had just recovered from back surgery. Kent was on his own.

Because spinal damage was likely, Kent knew he had to pull the victim in the direction of the long axis of the body, to provide the greatest possible protection for the spine. Using his forearms as a support on each side of the victim's head, Kent grasped the shoulders of the victim's shirt firmly. Using the shirt as a handle, he pulled the victim toward him and out of the pool of gasoline.

When emergency crews arrived a minute or two later, Kent was already starting a primary survey and had identified life-threatening problems that emergency medical personnel needed to address immediately.

An injured person often needs to be moved. It is your responsibility to see that the victim is moved in a way that will prevent further injury and will not cause unnecessary pain and discomfort. Improper moving can add to the original injuries, increase shock, and endanger life.

Under normal circumstances, a victim should not be moved until a thorough assessment has been made and first aid care has been given; ideally, you should leave moving a victim to professional emergency teams. Under some situations, however, you will need to move the victim *before* assessment and care in order to remove the victim from a potential hazard or to reach other, more seriously injured people. This chapter discusses the general guidelines for moving victims and details various rescue moves.

29.1 General Principles of Moving

> Learning Objective 1 Discuss the general guidelines for moving victims.

Although speed is important in cases where a victim is exposed to hazards, it is always more important to accomplish the handling and moving of a victim in a way that will not further injure the victim. As a basic rule of thumb, you should not move a victim until you absolutely have to or until you are completely ready to—and, if you can avoid it, you should not try to move a victim by yourself if you can wait and get help.

When moving a victim, follow these guidelines:

- If you find a victim in a facedown position, move the person to an assessment position *after* doing the ABCD assessment and checking for possible neck and spinal injury (see Figures 29-1 through 29-5).

- Generally, you should not move a victim if moving the person will make injuries worse.

FIGURE 29–2. Raise the victim's arm on the side closest to you (the side you will roll the victim to.)

FIGURE 29–1. Perform an assessment, including checking for injuries to the neck and spine.

FIGURE 29–3. Place your hands at the hip and neck/shoulder area.

FIGURE 29-4. Roll the victim toward you. Keep the neck and spine in line.

FIGURE 29-5. Carefully rest the victim on his or her back continue your assessment.

- Provide all necessary emergency care; splint all fractures, especially those of the neck and back.

- Move a victim only if there is immediate danger (see the section that follows). Only when there is a threat to life should a victim be moved before the ABCDs are completed.

- If it is necessary to move a victim, your speed will depend on the reason for the move. For example, a victim who needs to be moved away from a fire should be moved as quickly as possible; a victim who needs to be moved so you have access to another victim should be moved with due consideration to his or her injuries before and during the move.

When to Make an Emergency Move

Learning Objective **2** Identify the situations in which an emergency move must be made.

Normally, top priorities in first aid care are maintaining the victim's airway, breathing, circulation, and spinal status and controlling hemorrhage. But when the scene of an accident is unstable, threatening your life as well as that of your victim, your priority changes—you must first move the victim.

Under life-threatening conditions, you may have to risk injury to the victim in order to save his or her life. *You should make an emergency move only when no other options are available,* such as in situations involving:

- Uncontrolled traffic

- Physically unstable surroundings (such as a vehicle on its side that you cannot stabilize)

- Exposure to hazardous materials

- Fire or threat of fire (fire should always be considered a grave threat)

- Hostile crowds

- The need to reposition the victim in order to provide life-saving treatment (such as moving to a firm, flat surface to perform CPR)

- The need for access (you may need to move one victim to gain access to another)

- Weather conditions (you need to control exposure if the weather is very cold, wet, or hot, or windy enough to turn objects into projectiles)

PROGRESS CHECK

1. In general, you should move a victim to an assessment position only after checking for possible _____ injury. *(head/spinal/chest)*

2. Unless there is a pressing reason, you should move a victim only after _____ . *(necessary first aid care/thorough assessment/ help arrives on the scene)*

3. The speed with which you move a victim depends on _____ . *(the victim's injuries/the victim's desires/your reason for moving)*

4. You should move a victim before assessment or care if the scene _____ . *(is especially unpleasant/threatens life/is crowded)*

29.2 One-Rescuer Techniques

Although two or more people should be available to move injured victims, you might be faced with moving a victim by yourself—usually because of a flood, fire, building collapse, or some other life-threatening situation. Use the following techniques.

Walking Assist

Learning Objective **3** Describe and demonstrate the walking assist.

The **walking assist** (see Figure 29-6) is a method of moving a victim in which a single rescuer functions as a "crutch" in assisting the injured victim to walk.

1. Stand at the victim's side and drape the victim's arm across your shoulders.

2. Support the victim by placing your arm around his or her waist.

3. Using your body as a crutch, support the victim's weight as you both walk.

FIGURE 29–6. One-rescuer walking assist

Blanket Drag

Learning Objective **4** Describe and demonstrate the blanket drag.

The **blanket drag** (see Figure 29-7) is a method of moving an injured victim in which a rescuer places the victim on a blanket and drags the victim to safety.

1. Spread a blanket alongside the victim; gather half the blanket into lengthwise pleats.

2. Roll the victim away from you, then tuck the pleated part of the blanket as far beneath the victim as you can.

3. Roll the victim back onto the center of the blanket on his or her back; wrap the blanket securely around the victim.

4. Grab the part of the blanket that is beneath the victim's head and drag the victim toward you; if you have to move on a stairway, keep the length of the victim's body in contact with several stairs at once to prevent the victim from bouncing on the steps.

Shirt Drag

Learning Objective **5** Describe and demonstrate the shirt drag.

FIGURE 29–7. Blanket drag

walking assist A method of moving a victim in which a rescuer functions as a crutch in assisting the injured victim to walk

blanket drag A method of moving a victim in which a rescuer places the victim on a blanket and drags the victim to safety

The **shirt drag** (see Figure 29-8) is a method of moving a victim in which a single rescuer uses the victim's shirt as a handle to pull the victim.

A T-shirt won't work for a shirt drag because it stretches too much to work well. If the victim is wearing a shirt other than a T-shirt, take these steps:

1. Fasten the victim's hands or wrists loosely together, then link them to the victim's belt or pants to keep the arms from flopping or coming out of the shirt.

2. Grasp the shoulders of the victim's shirt under the head; use your forearms to support both sides of the head.

3. Using the shirt as a handle, pull the victim toward you; the pulling power should engage the victim's armpits, not the neck.

Sheet Drag

The **sheet drag** (see Figure 29-9) is a method of moving a victim in which a single rescuer forms a drag harness out of a sheet, passes it under the victim's arms at the armpits, and uses it to pull the victim.

1. Fold a sheet several times lengthwise to form a narrow, long "harness"; lay the folded sheet centered across the victim's chest at the nipple line.

2. Pull the ends of the sheet under the victim's arms at the armpits and behind the victim's head; twist the ends of the sheet together to form a triangular support for the head. Be careful not to pull the victim's hair.

3. Grasping the loose ends of the sheet, pull the victim toward you.

FIGURE 29–8. Shirt drag

Firefighter's Carry

The **firefighter's carry,** a method of lifting and carrying a victim in which one rescuer carries the victim over his or her shoulder, is not as safe as most ground-level moves because it places the victim's center of mass high—usually at the rescuer's shoulder level—and because it requires a fair amount of strength. However, it is preferred if a single rescuer has to move a victim over irregular terrain.

Unless there is a life-or-death situation, do not attempt a firefighter's carry if the victim has suspected spinal injury or fractures of the extremities.

To perform the firefighter's carry (see Figures 29-10 through 29-13 on page 488):

1. Position the victim on his or her back with both knees bent and raised; grasp the back sides of the victim's wrists (Figure 29-10).

FIGURE 29–9. Sheet drag

shirt drag A method of moving a victim in which a single rescuer uses the victim's shirt as a handle to pull the victim

sheet drag A method of moving a victim in which a single rescuer forms a drag harness out of a sheet by passing it under the victim's arms at the armpits, and uses it to pull the victim

firefighter's carry A method of lifting and carrying a victim in which one rescuer carries the victim over his or her shoulder

FIGURE 29–10.

FIGURE 29–11.

FIGURE 29–12.

2. Stand on the toes of both victim's feet; lean backward and pull the victim up toward you (Figure 29-11).

3. As the victim nears a standing position, crouch slightly and pull the victim over your shoulder. (Figure 29-12).

4. Pass your arm between the victim's legs and grasp the victim's arm that is nearest your body, then stand upright (Figure 29-13).

FIGURE 29–13.

FIGURES 29–10 through 29–13. Firefighter's carry

29.3   Two- and Three-Rescuer Techniques

Seat Carries (Two Rescuers)

Learning Objective **8** Describe and demonstrate seat carries.

A **seat carry** (see Figures 29-14 through 29-16) is a method of lifting and moving a victim in which two rescuers form a "seat" with their arms.

1. Raise the victim to a sitting position; each First Aider steadies the victim by positioning an arm around the victim's back.

2. Each First Aider slips his or her other arm under the victim's thighs, then clasps the wrist of the other First Aider. One pair of arms should make a seat, the other pair a backrest.

3. Slowly raise the victim from the ground, moving in unison. In one variation of the technique (Figures 29-17 through 29-19), the First Aiders make a seat with all four hands; the victim then supports him or herself by placing his or her arms around the First Aiders' shoulders.

> **seat carry** A method of lifting and moving a victim in which two rescuers form a "seat" with their arms

FIGURE 29–14.   **FIGURE 29–15.**   **FIGURE 29–16.**

FIGURES 29–14 through 29–16.   Seat carry

FIGURE 29–17.   **FIGURE 29–18.**   **FIGURE 29–19.**

FIGURES 29–17 through 29–19.   Seat carry variation

Extremity Lift (Two Rescuers)

> Learning Objective 9 Describe and demonstrate the extremity lift.

The **extremity lift** is a method of lifting and carrying a victim in which two rescuers carry the victim by the extremities. Do not use this method if the victim has back injuries.

1. One First Aider kneels at the victim's head; the other kneels at the victim's knees.

2. The First Aider at the victim's head places one hand under each of the victim's shoulders; the second First Aider grasps the victim's wrists.

3. The First Aider at the victim's knees pulls the victim to a sitting position by pulling on the victim's wrists; the First Aider at the victim's head assists by pushing the victim's shoulders and supporting the victim's back.

4. The First Aider at the victim's head slips his or her hands under the arms, and grasps the victim's wrists (see Figure 29-20).

5. The First Aider at the victim's knees slips his or her hands beneath the victim's knees.

6. Both First Aiders crouch on their feet and then simultaneously stand in one fluid motion (see Figure 29-21).

Chair Litter Carry (Two Rescuers)

> Learning Objective 10 Describe and demonstrate the chair litter carry.

If the victim does not have contraindicating injuries and if a chair is available, you can use the **chair litter carry**. Sit the victim in the chair. One First Aider then carries the back of the chair while the other carries the legs; the chair itself is used as a litter (see Figures 29-22 and 29-23). Be sure the chair is sturdy enough to support the weight of the victim.

Flat Lift and Carry (Three Rescuers)

> Learning Objective 11 Describe and demonstrate the flat lift and carry.

The three-rescuer **flat lift and carry,** when three rescuers lift and carry the victim to a stretcher, is an effective way to move a severely injured victim who cannot sit in a chair or when a cot cannot be moved close to the victim (see Figures 29-24 through 29-27). It has the advantage of permitting you to move the victim through narrow passages and down stairs. Use this method only if the victim does not have spinal injury.

1. Three First Aiders line up on the least injured side of the victim; if one First Aider is noticeably taller, that person stands at the victim's shoulders; another stands at the victim's hips, and the third at the victim's knees.

FIGURE 29–21.

> **extremity lift** A method of lifting and carrying a victim in which two rescuers carry the victim by the extremities
>
> **chair litter carry** A method of lifting and moving a victim in which the victim is seated in a chair and two rescuers carry the victim in the chair
>
> **flat lift and carry** A method of lifting and moving a victim in which three rescuers or more lift and carry the victim to a stretcher

FIGURE 29–20.

FIGURES 29–20 and 29–21. Extremity lift

FIGURE 29–22 and FIGURE 29–23. Chair litter carry

FIGURE 29–24.

FIGURE 29–25.

FIGURE 29–26.

FIGURE 29–27.

FIGURES 29–24 through 29–27. Flat lift and carry

2. Each First Aider kneels on the knee closest to the victim's feet.

3. The First Aider at the victim's shoulders works his or her hands underneath the victim's neck and shoulders; the next First Aider's hands go underneath the victim's hips and pelvis; and the final First Aider's hands go underneath the victim's knees.

4. Moving in unison, the First Aiders raise the victim to knee level and slowly turn the victim toward themselves until the victim rests on the bends of their elbows.

5. Moving in unison, all three rise to a standing position and walk with the victim to a place of safety or to the stretcher. To place the victim on the stretcher, simply reverse the procedure.

This move can also be done with four First Aiders: position them at the victim's head, chest, hips, and knees. Support is then given to the head, chest, hips, pelvis, knees, and ankles.

PROGRESS CHECK

1. In seat carries, a "chair" can be formed by a pair of arms or by _____ . *(two hands/four hands/a pair of shoulders)*

2. Never use the extremity lift if the victim has _____ . *(head injuries/back injuries/ fractures)*

3. If you have access to a sturdy chair and the victim does not have contraindicating injuries, use the _____ . *(chair lift/chair carry/ chair litter carry)*

4. If you have at least three rescuers, use the _____ to move a severely injured victim. *(flat lift and carry/extremity lift/chair carry)*

29.4 Equipment

Canvas Litter/Pole Stretcher

Canvas litters (see Figure 29-28) have been used by armies worldwide for at least two centuries. The modern tubular-framed, vinyl-coated nylon version accommodates victims weighing as much as 350 pounds.

Use a canvas litter when a victim can be rolled in a single unit, without moving one end of the body ahead of the other (a method called a *logroll*). Do *not* use one when the victim has to be moved lengthwise or when spinal immobilization is needed.

Backboards

Learning Objective **12** Describe and demonstrate how to use backboards to move a victim.

If you need to immobilize the spine, manually support the victim's head and neck in normal anatomic position until the victim is supine on the backboard; apply a rigid cervical collar to the victim's neck. Figures 29-29 and 29-30 illustrate short and long backboards, respectively.

FIGURE 29–28. Canvas litter or stretcher

FIGURE 29–29. Short backboard

FIGURE 29–30. Long backboard

There are several ways to get a victim onto a backboard; both require two First Aiders. If the victim is sitting:

1. While one First Aider stabilizes the head and neck, approach the victim from behind; slide a short board carefully behind the victim's back.

2. With the victim leaning against the board, secure the torso, then the head, to the board.

3. Slowly lower the board, maintaining manual support of the victim's head and neck. Move in several short steps instead of one long one.

If the victim is supine:

1. Bring a long board to within arm's reach.

2. Kneeling at the victim's side, reach across the victim and grab his or her shoulder and hip. With another First Aider stabilizing the head and neck, roll the victim toward you.

3. With the victim on his or her side, examine the victim's back; then pull the backboard toward you and place it on edge against the victim's back. Roll the victim onto the board.

4. Strap the victim securely to the board, using at least three straps and preferably four.

If the victim is in a prone position, logroll the victim onto a spine board.

Blanket Stretcher

> Learning Objective 13 Describe and demonstrate how to use a blanket stretcher.

When space is limited or you need to traverse stairs or cramped corners, you can use a blanket as a stretcher *if* the victim has no neck, back, or pelvic injuries or a fractured skull.

Use a blanket that is strong, free of holes and in good condition, and large enough to support the victim's entire body.

To use a blanket as a stretcher (see Figures 29-31 through 29-36 on page 494), logroll or slide the victim onto the center of the blanket; tightly roll the side edges of the blanket toward the victim to form handholds. Position as many First Aiders around the victim as needed to distribute the hands evenly. If the weather is cold, use two blankets instead of one, folding one around the victim for warmth.

You can also fold and roll blankets to immobilize the head or other body parts.

Improvised Stretchers

> Learning Objective 14 List objects that can be used for improvised stretchers.

You can improvise a stretcher with any of the following:

- A blanket, canvas, or sheet and two poles (fold the sides of the blanket or other material over the two poles; see Figures 29-37 through 29-40 on page 495).
- Cloth bags or sacks and two poles (cut holes in the bags to accommodate the poles)
- Three or four coats or jackets and two poles (fasten the jackets, turn the sleeves inside out, and pass the poles through the sleeves)

You can move an infant or toddler in an infant car seat; it also acts to immobilize the child.

Stretcher Transportation

> Learning Objective 15 Discuss the guidelines for moving a victim on a stretcher.

Before you use a stretcher, lock the crosspieces in place, test it by placing an uninjured person of the same weight as the victim on it, and pad it with a blanket or similar material. Then move the victim using this technique:

1. Three First Aiders position themselves on the victim's least injured side at the victim's knees, hips, and shoulders; the fourth is positioned at the victim's hips on the opposite side. Each First Aider rests on the knee nearest the victim's feet.

2. The hands of the First Aider at the shoulders are placed under the victim's neck and shoulders; the First Aider at the victim's knees places his or her hands under the victim's knees and ankles; and the First Aider at the victim's hips places his or her hands under the victim's pelvis and small of the back.

3. Moving in unison and keeping the victim's body level, the four slowly lift the victim and rest him or her on the knees of the three First Aiders. The fourth First Aider places the stretcher under the victim, then returns to his or her original position.

4. Moving in unison, the four gently lower the victim to the stretcher and cover the victim with a blanket.

5. The four position themselves, one at each end and one at each side of the stretcher, facing the victim.

6. All four First Aiders grasp and lift the stretcher. The two First Aiders on either side each shift one hand

FIGURE 29–31.

FIGURE 29–32.

FIGURE 29–33.

FIGURE 29–34.

FIGURE 29–35.

FIGURE 29–36.

FIGURES 29–31 through 29–36. Proper use of a blanket stretcher

FIGURE 29–37.

FIGURE 29–38.

FIGURE 29–39.

FIGURE 29–40.

FIGURES 29–37 through 29–40. Improvised stretcher

FIGURE 29–41. Stretcher transportation

and support the end of the stretcher nearest the victim's feet, allowing the First Aider at that end to turn around with his or her back to the stretcher. Then, the First Aiders at the sides of the stretcher move in unison, one to the end near the victim's

head, and one to the end near the victim's feet; all four First Aiders then grasp an end of a stretcher pole. The First Aiders are now ready to transport the stretcher. The victim is transported feet first (see Figure 29-41); the First Aider at the victim's head constantly monitors the victim's condition.

PROGRESS CHECK

1. You should maintain manual support of the _____ until the victim is supine on a backboard. *(backboard/head/head and neck)*

2. Use a blanket as a stretcher only if you do not suspect a _____ . *(pneumothorax/ hemothorax/fractured skull)*

3. Before you place a victim on a stretcher, you should test it with an uninjured person of the same _____ . *(height/weight/gender)*

Summary

- Unless you are facing life-threatening conditions, you should not move a victim until assessment and care are completed. Ideally, leave moving to professional emergency teams.

- You should move a victim before assessment and care if there is a threat to life, such as uncontrolled traffic, physically unstable surroundings, exposure to hazardous materials, fire, or bad weather conditions. You may also have to move one victim to get access to another.

- The speed with which you move a victim depends on your reason for moving the victim.

- Ideally, two or more First Aiders should help move a victim; if you are on your own, you can use any of several one-rescuer techniques, such as the walking assist, blanket drag, shirt drag, sheet drag, or firefighter's carry.

- If you suspect neck or spinal injuries, do *not* use the firefighter's carry, extremity lift, chair litter carry, or flat lift and carry.

- If you do not have a commercial stretcher, you can improvise a stretcher from a blanket, canvas, or strong sheet and two poles. You can also make a stretcher from cloth bags or sacks or several jackets and a pair of poles.

- One of the most versatile pieces of equipment in caring for and moving the victim is the backboard.

Key Terms

Be sure you understand the following key terms:

walking assist
blanket drag
shirt drag
sheet drag
firefighter's carry
seat carry
extremity lift
chair litter carry
flat lift and carry

Critical Thinking Exercise

As you are driving to work, you come across a car accident. You find one person outside of his crashed vehicle on the ground leaning against the back bumper. He is bleeding from the head and says his knee hurts. You notice a strong smell of gasoline. Looking under the vehicle you see a growing pool of what you believe to be gasoline.

1. Is this patient a candidate for an emergency move? Why or why not?

2. If you decide to move this patient, which move would you use if you are alone?

3. Which move would you use if someone came and offered to help?

29 Chapter 29 Self-Test

Student: _____ Date: _____

Course: _____ Section #: _____

Part 1   True/False

If you believe the statement is true, circle the T. If you believe the statement is false, circle the F.

T F **1.** Usually, all necessary care should be provided before moving a victim.

T F **2.** Only when you are facing a threat to life should a victim be moved before the ABCDs are completed.

T F **3.** The extremity lift is a good lift to use if the victim has back injuries.

T F **4.** The three-rescuer flat lift is not a good move to use for a severely injured victim.

T F **5.** A victim should be transported head first on a stretcher.

T F **6.** The blanket drag is an effective way for a single rescuer to move a victim to safety.

T F **7.** The shirt drag cannot be used if the victim is wearing only a t-shirt.

T F **8.** The firefighter's carry is considerably safer to use than most other ground-level moves.

T F **9.** If you find a victim facedown, immediately move the victim into the assessment position before doing any kind of assessment.

Part 2   Multiple Choice

For each item, circle the correct answer or the phrase that best completes the statement.

1. Two or more rescuers can use a blanket to transport an injured victim safely as long as the victim does not have
   a. a fractured pelvis
   b. a spinal injury
   c. a skull fracture
   d. any of the above

2. When carrying a victim on a litter, how many rescuers should ideally lift and carry?
   a. two
   b. three
   c. four to six
   d. eight

3. An injured victim may be moved by a First Aider only if the victim's position
   a. creates the risk of shock
   b. endangers the victim's life
   c. is inconvenient for giving first aid
   d. prevents the victim from receiving first aid

4. If you use a shirt drag to move an injured victim, pull the victim on his or her
   a. back, feet first
   b. back, head first
   c. stomach, feet first
   d. stomach, head first

5. When is it appropriate to move a victim away from the emergency site before giving first aid care?
   a. when there is danger of fire or explosion
   b. when the victim is blocking another victim who needs lifesaving care
   c. when it is impossible to protect the scene
   d. all of the above

6. A victim who is slightly injured may be moved by one rescuer using the
   a. walking assist
   b. logroll
   c. shoulder drag
   d. extremity lift

7. If the move is a nonemergency move, you should
   a. treat for shock before moving the victim
   b. complete first aid care before moving the victim
   c. only move the victim if it is impossible to give first aid
   d. all of the above

8. The primary consideration in an emergency move is protecting the
   a. head
   b. extremities
   c. heart
   d. spine

1. You must move a severely injured trauma victim who is unconscious; other First Aiders are available.

2. You must move an unconscious victim away from a burning automobile.

30

Vehicle Stabilization and Victim Extrication

Learning Objectives

When you have mastered the material in this chapter, you will be able to

1 Discuss how to locate all victims of a vehicle accident

2 Discuss how to deal with dangers at the scene of a vehicle accident

3 Describe how to stabilize a vehicle

4 List the basic tools and equipment needed to rescue a victim from a vehicle

5 Describe how to gain access to a victim who is trapped in a vehicle

6 Describe and demonstrate how to stabilize a victim trapped in a vehicle

7 Describe and demonstrate how to remove a victim who is lying on the seat of a vehicle

8 Describe and demonstrate how to remove a victim who is lying on the floor of a vehicle

On the Scene

Thirty-three year-old Karen Norton was pulling around the corner into the grocery store parking lot when a car struck her from behind with tremendous force. Though Karen was secure in a seat belt, her 6-year-old daughter Amy had unbuckled her restraint in the backseat and was trying to find some crayons at the time of the accident. The impact slammed her into the front seat, then hurled her onto the floor in the backseat.

Twenty-two-year-old Brian Millgate was just loading his own groceries into his car when he heard the impact. He ran to the scene; the driver of the second car was still in his seat belt and appeared to have only minor injuries. Karen, concerned for Amy, had left the car and was running around the smashed vehicle, screaming. Brian could smell gasoline.

Brian immediately enlisted the help of another shopper to calm Karen down. A store employee came running toward them, announcing she had already called 9-1-1. Brian asked her and a middle-aged man to help him reach Amy.

Both rear doors opened, despite damage to the vehicle. Amy was lying across the floor. Brian positioned himself at Amy's head and held her head and neck in alignment; he instructed the store employee to hold Amy's feet and legs in alignment. Finally, he instructed the middle-aged man to lean over the front seat and grasp Amy's clothing at her waist, hips, and thighs. At Brian's instruction and on the count of three, all three lifted Amy to the backseat, maintaining body alignment. Brian had just started a primary survey when paramedics arrived on the scene; his quick action enabled them to begin assessment and care immediately.

E xtrication is the process of removing a victim or victims from a dangerous, life-threatening situation, typically from inside a wrecked car. Ideally, **extrication** should be performed by trained or professional emergency crews. However, if a victim faces danger and emergency crews have not arrived, you may need to extricate the victim from the vehicle yourself.

This chapter explains how to locate victims and deal with dangers at the scene of a vehicle accident, and gives basic guidelines on victim extrication.

FIGURE 30–1. Placing a flare at the accident scene

30.1 Basic Guidelines

The number-one guideline in providing first aid care for victims at the scene of a motor-vehicle accident is the same as in any other situation: your own safety as a First Aider comes first. For example, if you start giving care to a woman trapped in a car before you know that the car has been stabilized, you could get injured when the car shifts—and emergency personnel who respond to the scene will have one more victim to deal with. Make sure you take the time to ensure your own safety; if you're injured, you will not be of any help to the victim.

In addition to making sure that the vehicle is stabilized, as discussed later in this chapter, you need to make sure that you can:

- Safely reach the victim
- Render first aid care without risk of personal injury
- Move any supplies or equipment without risk to your own safety
- Involve others in caring for the victim as appropriate, without risking your own or others' safety

In most cases, a victim will not have to be moved immediately, and you will be able to wait for an emergency team to arrive.

The general rule is to leave the victims where they are unless they are threatened by immediate danger, such as uncontrollable traffic, risk of explosion, risk of drowning, fire, or presence of toxic chemicals or fumes (such as leaking gasoline). If you determine that a victim does not need to be moved before emergency personnel arrive:

- Control the hazards and stabilize the accident scene (see Figure 30-1)—shut off engines, set flares, douse fires, and so on. Allow no one to smoke because of the possibility of spilled gasoline.
- Gain access to the victim if it is possible and safe to do so.
- Perform life-saving care to stabilize the victim.

- Stay with the victim until the emergency team arrives.

If you determine that the victim needs to be moved, there are several basic factors you have to consider before you attempt the move. Considering these factors will help you decide how to proceed, whether you need others to help, and what you should do to secure the safety of the victim, of yourself as a First Aider, of anyone you ask to help, and of other bystanders. Consider:

- Your own physical condition—your strength, stamina, and any injury or illness you have that could affect your ability to move the victim
- The victim's size
- The victim's condition
- The limitations posed by the vehicle itself—jammed doors, jammed windows, broken glass, twisted metal, and so on
- The availability of others who can help
- Any dangers at the scene that need to be controlled or considered

Deciding to Stop at the Scene

If you are involved in a motor vehicle accident, the law in most states mandates that you stop and give help to anyone who is injured. But what if you were not involved in the accident, and arrive shortly after it occurred? The law in most states does not strictly mandate that you must stop and give help, but as a trained First Aider you have a moral obligation to give help if you can. If police or other emergency personnel are

---

extrication The process of removing a victim from a dangerous situation or wrecked car already at the scene, do not stop or give help unless they specifically ask you to.

The first thing you should do when you see an accident is call 9-1-1. Before you begin to assess the scene in detail or make any effort at stabilizing the vehicle or caring for victims, call for emergency medical personnel. While they are on their way to the scene, you can begin to take care of any emergencies that are within your scope and ability. If you don't have a cellular phone, see if any victims or bystanders have either a cellular phone or a CB radio that you can use to call for help. Other options are emergency roadside phones, the phones of nearby businesses or residents, or a nearby pay phone.

Keeping Yourself and Others Safe

To protect yourself, victims, and bystanders, park well off the highway and at least five car lengths away from the crash, leaving plenty of room for emergency vehicles when they arrive. Make sure you do not park in an active traffic lane; if you can avoid it, don't park in the emergency lane, either—a police car or ambulance might need to travel in the emergency lane to reach the crash. Turn on your vehicle's emergency flashers and raise the hood so that passing motorists are alerted to the fact that there is an accident.

Before you start helping any victims, make sure that all bystanders are safe and protected from injury. People are naturally curious and may want to watch what's happening. Even close friends or family members of a victim or victims need to be positioned well off the road or highway so they are not in danger from passing traffic or emergency vehicles. If you have flares or reflectors, light them and place them well behind the crash scene to warn oncoming drivers; a standard distance is *at least* 100 yards, or at least the length of a football field. Make sure you do not ignite flares around leaking gasoline or diesel fuel or any other flammable substance that could cause a fire.

Locating the Victims

Learning Objective 1 Discuss how to locate all victims of a vehicle accident.

Care first for all victims you can locate immediately, using standard triage methods to determine who should be treated first—then scour the area for any victim who might be hidden. Use a systematic approach to increase your odds of finding all the victims:

- Ask coherent, conscious passengers how many were in the car (see Figure 30-2).

- Ask witnesses if someone left the site or took a victim away.

FIGURE 30–2. Gathering information at the accident scene

- In high-impact accidents, search the vehicle and area carefully, especially in ditches and tall weeds. Search a broad area, since a high-impact crash can throw victims hundreds of feet. Remember that victims may also be wedged into what look like impossibly small spaces. A victim may even be wedged under the dashboard.

- Look for tracks in the earth or snow. Accident victims are often disoriented, and it's not uncommon for them to wander away from the scene.

Dealing with Dangers

Learning Objective 2 Discuss how to deal with dangers at the scene of a vehicle accident.

Make sure the ignition is turned off in all involved vehicles. Turn it off yourself if you have to. If a car is on fire and firefighting personnel have not arrived, follow these guidelines:

- If passengers are not trapped, move them before you try to contain the fire. As much as possible, considering the urgency presented by the fire, try to keep victims in alignment and prevent further injury.

- If passengers are trapped, deal with the fire. Many people carry fire extinguishers in their vehicles. Aim the extinguisher directly at the flame and move in a sweeping motion. A small extinguisher may empty in as few as 10 seconds, so aim directly at the largest flame. You might also be able to smother a fire with heavy coats or a blanket.

If you approach an accident with downed power lines:

- Assume all downed lines are live; call for expert assistance.

- Park your vehicle at a safe distance from the power line.

- Warn bystanders to stay clear.

- Tell victims to stay inside their vehicles.

- *Never try to handle a live wire yourself* (see Chapter 24).

30.2 Stabilizing the Vehicle

Learning Objective 3 Describe how to stabilize a vehicle.

After all possible hazards have been controlled, make the rescue setting as safe as possible. Consider any vehicle unstable until you have made it stable, regardless of how it came to rest after the collision.

If the vehicle is overturned, place a solid object—such as a wheel chock, spare tire, cribbing, or timber—between the roof and the roadway (see Figures 30-3 and 30-4).

FIGURE 30–3. Stabilizing an overturned vehicle with cribbing

Hook a chain to the vehicle's axle, then loop the chain around a tree or post.

If the vehicle is resting on all four wheels, place the gear selector in park; on a standard shift, place the vehicle in reverse. Use blocks or wedges at the wheels to prevent unexpected rolling.

If the air bag has not deployed, disconnect the negative side of the battery and the yellow air-bag connector, which in most cars can be found where the steering column meets the dashboard. If the air bag did deploy, expect cornstarch residue in the passenger area. Reassure victims that the powdery residue is completely harmless.

Tools and Equipment

Learning Objective 4 List the basic tools and equipment needed to rescue a victim from a vehicle.

In most cases, you will be able to wait for trained personnel to stabilize the vehicle and safely remove the victims. In some cases, however, you will need to stabilize the vehicle and remove the victim to prevent further injury or to save the victim from risk of fire or drowning, for example. Have the following basic tools

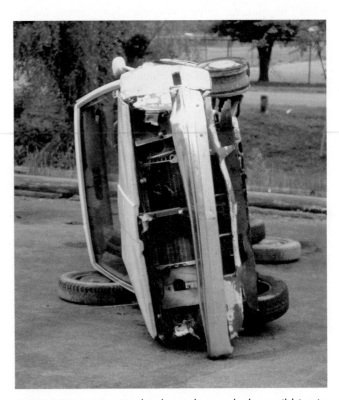

FIGURE 30–4. Spare wheels can be used when cribbing is not available.

on hand for possible vehicle stabilization and victim extrication:

- Hammer
- Screwdriver
- Chisel
- Crowbar
- Pliers
- Linoleum knife
- Work gloves and goggles
- Shovel
- Tire iron
- Wrench
- Knife
- Car jack
- Rope or chain

If you include some or all of these in your first aid kit, you can use them to help extricate victims safely and effectively.

FIGURE 30–5. Gaining access to the victim through a window

PROGRESS CHECK

1. You should consider _____ vehicle unstable. *(an overturned/a stacked/any)*

2. To stabilize an overturned vehicle, chain the _____ to a post or tree. *(frame/axle/door)*

3. If a vehicle rests on all four tires, place an automatic gear selector in _____ . *(reverse/overdrive/park)*

4. To stabilize an upright vehicle that is resting on all four tires, use blocks or wedges at the _____ . *(frame/bumpers/wheels)*

30.3 Gaining Access to the Victim

Learning Objective 5 Describe how to gain access to a victim who is trapped in a vehicle.

To gain access to a victim:

- Attempt to open the door nearest the victim by using the door handle. If that door is jammed or crushed, check all other doors.

- If doors are locked, ask a person inside the car to unlock them; if necessary, slide a coat hanger between the door frame and window to force the lock.

- If the doors cannot be opened, determine the next best point of entry. Remember rear hatches on some cars and rear doors on sport utility vehicles.

- If you have to break a window (see Figure 30-5), wear gloves to protect yourself.

- Always break the window farthest from the victim to avoid injuring the victim with broken glass or with your tools.

- If possible, put strips of broad tape over the glass before you break the window to keep broken pieces of glass from spraying the victim.

- To break a window, give a quick, hard thrust in the lower corner with a spring-loaded punch, screwdriver, or other sharp object.

- Once the window is broken, use your gloved hand to pull glass outside the vehicle.

- Clear all glass away from the window opening.

- Before you crawl through a broken window, drape a heavy tarp, blanket, or coat over the edge of the window and on the interior of the car just below the window. Cover the victim with a blanket to protect against broken glass.

PROGRESS CHECK

1. The first step in trying to gain access to a victim is to try the _____ . *(door nearest the victim/window nearest the victim/window farthest from the victim)*

2. Try to open the door with _____ . *(a crowbar/a tire iron/the door handle)*

3. If you need to break a window, choose the one _____ the victim. *(closest to/farthest from/across from)*

4. If you can, put strips of _____ over the window before you break it. *(tape/aluminum foil/webbing)*

30.4 Stabilizing and Moving the Victim

> Learning Objective **6** Describe and demonstrate how to stabilize a victim trapped in a vehicle.

Note: You should use backboards only if you have been specifically trained in their use; use of backboards and spineboards is not considered a usual first aid skill. As outlined earlier, leave the victim in place unless there is immediate threat to life. You might have to move a victim who is blocking your access to a second victim whose injuries are life threatening.

Once you are inside the vehicle with the victim, follow this procedure:

1. Conduct a quick but thorough primary survey; if more than one victim is involved, perform triage.

2. Stabilize airway, breathing, circulation, and hemorrhage; correct any life-threatening problems, then provide other care as needed. Bandage all wounds, splint all fractures, and give psychological support.

3. If you need to move the victim before you have immobilized him or her because of threat to life or because of blocked access to another victim, take these steps:

- Cut away any jammed seat belts.
- Immobilize the neck with a rolled blanket (see Figure 30-6): Place the blanket behind the victim's head, allowing both long ends to fall across the chest; cross the ends on the chest; applying gentle tension on both long ends, pass them under opposite arms; gather the blanket behind the victim and rotate him or her from the seat into your arms.

4. Once the victim has been stabilized and moved, continue to monitor airway, breathing, circulation, bleeding, and temperature.

FIGURE 30–6. Rolled blanket used as improvised cervical collar

Be aware that during a long extrication procedure, shock combined with temperature extremes can be fatal. Maintain body temperature with blankets if necessary, and provide shade during the summer.

Removing a Victim on the Seat of a Vehicle

> Learning Objective **7** Describe and demonstrate how to remove a victim who is lying on the seat of a vehicle.

1. Have one First Aider maintain stabilization of the head and neck to keep the victim's head in normal alignment with the body.

2. Apply an improvised or rigid cervical collar.

3. Have a second First Aider carefully move the victim's legs and body into alignment while the first rescuer maintains head stabilization. At least one other First Aider should then move the victim slightly away from the seat to allow a long backboard to be slipped beneath the victim's back (see Figure 30-7).

4. Ease the victim against the backboard. On signal from the First Aider at the victim's head, hold the victim snugly against the backboard and push the backboard down until the backboard and victim are flat on the seat. Secure the victim to the backboard and remove from the car.

FIGURE 30–7. Moving the victim onto a long backboard

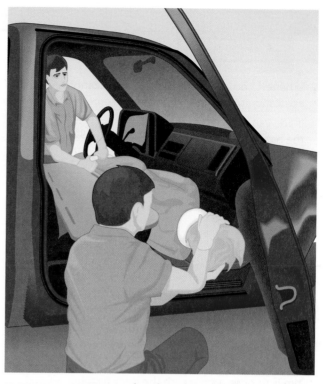

FIGURE 30–8. Keeping head, neck, and legs in alignment in preparation for application of long spine backboard

If the victim is found facedown, give urgent first aid without moving the victim more than necessary.

Removing a Victim Lying on the Floor

Learning Objective 8 Describe and demonstrate how to remove a victim who is lying on the floor of a vehicle.

If the victim is on the floor of the vehicle:

1. Place the backboard flat on the seat.

2. Have one First Aider keep the victim's head and neck in alignment with the body while another First Aider maintains alignment of the feet and legs (see Figure 30-8); if possible, secure the victim's legs together with a bandage.

3. While the body is kept in alignment, have at least one other First Aider reach over the seat and grasp the victim's clothing at the waist, hips, and thighs.

4. On signal from the First Aider at the victim's head, lift the victim onto the backboard, maintaining body alignment. Secure the victim to the backboard and remove the person from the car.

PROGRESS CHECK

1. Your first priority once you are in the vehicle with the victim is to _____ . *(secure the person to a backboard/give psychological support/perform a primary survey)*

2. If more than one victim is involved, _____ . *(send for help/perform triage/stay out of the vehicle)*

3. If necessary, you can immobilize the victim's neck with a _____ . *(blanket/seat belt/bandage)*

4. _____ combined with weather extremes can be fatal during long extrication. *(Bleeding/Shock/Head injury)*

Summary

- Whenever possible, leave vehicle stabilization and victim extrication to trained or professional emergency crews.

- If you can wait for emergency crews to arrive, control the hazards, stabilize the accident scene, gain access to the victim, and perform life-saving care—but do not try to extricate the person from the vehicle.

- Make sure you look for all the victims who could have been involved; look in ditches, tall weeds, and under the dashboard.

- If the vehicle is on fire and the passengers are not trapped, move them first; if they are trapped, deal first with the fire.

- If there are downed power lines at the scene, tell the victims to stay in the vehicle; never try to manage downed power lines by yourself.

- Consider any vehicle unstable until you have stabilized it, regardless of how it came to rest after a collision.

- The first thing you should try in gaining access to a victim is to open a door with the door handle.

- Once you are inside the car with the victim, complete a rapid primary survey, perform the ABCDs, correct life-threatening conditions, provide other first aid care as needed, and continue to monitor the victims.

Key Term

Make sure you understand the following key term:

extrication

Critical Thinking Exercise

You are driving white-knuckled in a heavy rainstorm. Passing semitrucks partially block your vision of the road ahead. Suddenly a car that appears to be filled with teenagers goes zooming by you in the carpool lane. A sudden feeling of "stupid kids" washes over you.

Then you see a slow-motion nightmare begin to form in front of you. The high-speed car cuts in front of you to pass another car in the carpool lane. At the same time, a semitrailer is pulling into the same lane. The car slides into the trailer and skids sideways across the freeway. Coming into contact with the grass in the median causes the car to flip in the air and roll several times, coming to a steaming halt on its roof. Three teenagers are thrown out of the car, and three are still inside the car.

1. What considerations would you make to decide whether to stop and help?

2. What would you do to prevent any further injuries to others stopping to help?

3. What is the first step you would take *before* you left your car?

4. How would triage be used in this situation?

5. Would you try to move victims out of the car?

30 Chapter 30 Self-Test

Student: _____   Date: _____

Course: _____   Section #: _____

Part 1   True/False

If you believe the statement is true, circle the T. If you believe the statement is false, circle the F.

T F   **1.** Suspect any vehicle of being unstable until you have made it stable.

T F   **2.** Part of stabilizing a victim is to splint all fractures.

T F   **3.** A victim's head and neck should be stabilized before a cervical collar is applied.

T F   **4.** When you gain access to an accident victim, you should first establish an open airway.

T F   **5.** *Extricate* means to pull a person quickly out of a wrecked vehicle.

T F   **6.** Do not worry about a downed power line unless it is sparking.

T F   **7.** Stabilize a standard-transmission vehicle by putting the transmission in first gear.

T F   **8.** Break the window nearest the victim so you will have immediate access to the victim.

Part 2   Multiple Choice

For each item, circle the correct answer or the phrase that best completes the statement.

1. Cars that are upside down or lying on their side should be
   a. turned upright
   b. taken apart
   c. stabilized as is
   d. left untouched

2. Once you have gained access to the victim, you should first
   a. check for ABCDs and bleeding
   b. remove victim from vehicle
   c. splint fractures
   d. treat for shock

3. When a victim is lying on the seat of a car, what is the first step involved in removing the victim from the car?
   a. move the legs and body into alignment
   b. stabilize the victim's head and neck to align with the body
   c. drag the victim head first from the car
   d. move the victim to the floor

4. *Extrication* means
   a. picking and sorting the injured
   b. gaining access to the accident scene
   c. moving and transporting the injured
   d. disentangling or freeing a trapped victim

5. What should you do if the victim does not need to be rescued immediately and a rescue team will be arriving soon?
   a. control the hazards and stabilize the accident scene
   b. gain access to the victim if possible
   c. give first aid care to stabilize the victim
   d. all of the above

6. What part of the vehicle should you check first to gain access to a trapped victim?
   a. windows
   b. floor
   c. roof
   d. doors

Part 3   What Would You Do If?

A 65-year-old driver has run his vehicle into a parked car, then skidded sideways into traffic where his car was broadsided on the passenger side. When you arrive, he is unconscious and pale and slumped into the steering wheel. He is not wearing a seat belt. Both doors are jammed, but the window on the passenger side is knocked out.

What two factors concerning extrication would you consider first? How would you gain access to the victim?

Appendix A: Skills Assessment Sheets

SKILLS ASSESSMENT: VICTIM ASSESSMENT

CONDUCT A SCENE SIZE-UP		
Take body substance isolation precautions (gloves, plastic wrap, etc.).	1	
Assess for safety hazards.	1	
Determine the number of victims.	1	
Determine if the victim is injured or ill.	1	
Determine what resources are needed (EMS, fire department, police department).	1	
CONDUCT A PRIMARY SURVEY		
Manually stabilize the victim's spine if spinal injury is suspected.	1	
Ask for the chief complaint.	1	
Assess the airway and open it manually if necessary.	1	
Assess the breathing and provide rescue breathing if necessary.	1	
Assess circulation (assess a radial pulse in a responsive victim and a carotid pulse in the victim with an altered mental status).	1	
Assess for and control any major bleeding.	1	
Assess the mental status.	1	
CONDUCT A BRIEF NEUROLOGIC EXAM		
Reassess the mental status of the victim and assess alertness if talking.	1	
Note speech pattern.	1	
Note ability of victim to obey commands (squeeze fingers or wiggle toes).	1	
Reassess victim's response to voice or pain if victim has an altered mental status.	1	
DETERMINE THE CHIEF COMPLAINT AND OBTAIN THE VITAL SIGNS		
Ask the victim, "Where do you hurt?" or "Are you ill?"	1	

Assess the vital signs: Pulse, respiration (breathing), temperature and color of skin, capillary refill.	4	
Look for medical alert tags or other information devices.	1	

GATHER A HISTORY

Gather a SAMPLE history from the victim or relatives or bystanders if the victim's mental status is altered. S Signs and symptoms the victim is exhibiting and complaining of A Allergies M Medications P Pertinent medical history (major surgeries, history of heart attack, stroke, etc.) L Last time the victim had something to eat or drink E Events prior to the incident	1 1 1 1 1 1	

CONDUCT A SECONDARY SURVEY

Assess the face, mouth, ears, and nose.	1	
Assess the eyes.	1	
Assess the skull and neck.	1	
Assess the chest.	1	
Assess the abdomen.	1	
Assess the pelvic region.	1	
Assess the back of the body.	1	
Assess the lower extremities (check pulses and motor and sensory function).	1	
Assess the upper extremities (check pulses and motor and sensory function).	1	
Total Possible Points.	37	

SKILLS ASSESSMENT: MOUTH-TO-MASK VENTILATION

Take body substance isolation precautions (gloves, plastic wrap, etc.).	1	
Open the airway using the head-tilt/chin-lift maneuver (use the jaw-thrust maneuver if spinal injury is suspected).	1	
Establish breathlessness using the "look, listen, and feel" method.	1	
If ventilations are required, place the barrier device over the victim's mouth and nose.	1	
Position your hands to assure an adequate seal.	1	
Maintaining head tilt and mask seal, administer two slow, full rescue breaths.	1	
Check the pulse.	1	

If a pulse is present, provide one slow, full breath every 5 seconds. If there is no pulse, immediately start CPR.	1	
Recheck the pulse after 1 minute of ventilations.	1	
Total Possible Points.	9	

SKILLS ASSESSMENT: AUTOMATED EXTERNAL DEFIBRILLATION

Establish unresponsiveness.	1	
Activate the EMS system.	1	
Open the airway using the head-tilt/chin-lift method if no spinal injury is suspected.	1	
Look, listen, and feel for breathing.	1	
Provide two slow, full rescue breaths.	1	
Check the pulse.	1	
If no pulse and defibrillator is immediately available, turn on the AED.	1	
Apply the pads to the victim's chest.	1	
Clear the victim and "analyze" the rhythm.	1	
If prompted to deliver a shock be sure no one is touching the victim.	1	
Press the "shock" button.	1	
Follow the instructions of the AED and deliver up to three shocks if advised to do so.	1	
Check the pulse.	1	
If no pulse, perform 1 minute of CPR.	1	
After 1 minute of CPR reassess the victim using the AED; be sure no one is touching the victim and "analyze" the rhythm.	1	
Deliver additional shocks if advised.	1	
Total Possible Points.	16	

SKILLS ASSESSMENT: BLEEDING CONTROL AND SHOCK CARE

Take body substance isolation precautions (gloves, plastic wrap, etc.).	1	
Apply direct pressure to the site of bleeding.	1	
Elevate the extremity.	1	

IF THE WOUND CONTINUES TO BLEED HEAVILY		
Apply additional dressings to the wound.	1	
IF THE WOUND CONTINUES TO BLEED HEAVILY		
Locate and use the appropriate pressure point.	1	
ONCE BLEEDING IS CONTROLLED		
Bandage the wound.	1	
IF VICTIM IS AT RISK FOR SHOCK		
Place the victim in a supine position with the legs elevated.	1	
Cover the victim to prevent heat loss.	1	
Activate the EMS system immediately.	1	
Total Possible Points.	9	

SKILLS ASSESSMENT: CARE FOR WOUNDS WITH IMPALED OBJECTS

Cut victim's clothes away without disturbing the impaled object.	1	
Manually secure the impaled object to prevent movement.	1	
Control bleeding if necessary.	1	
Stabilize the object with bulky dressings.	1	
Tape or otherwise secure the layers of bulky dressings in place.	1	
Calm the victim.	1	
Monitor and treat for shock.	1	
Total Possible Points.	7	

SKILLS ASSESSMENT: MUSCULOSKELETAL INJURIES

Assess for signs and symptoms.	1	
IF A SPRAIN IS SUSPECTED		
Immediately immobilize the joint.	1	
Use the "RICE" method: Rest, Ice, Compression, Elevation.	4	

IF A STRAIN IS SUSPECTED		
Immediately immobilize the body part.	1	
Place the victim in a comfortable position.	1	
Apply cold directly to the strained area.	1	
IF A CRAMP IS SUSPECTED		
Gently stretch the cramping muscle.	1	
Apply steady, firm hand pressure to the cramping muscle.	1	
Apply an ice pack over the cramped muscle.	1	
Decide whether an electrolyte drink is in order.	1	
IF THE INJURY IS A DISLOCATION		
Immobilize in the position found.	1	
Elevate and ice-pack the limb.	1	
Treat for shock (warmth and comfort).	1	
Seek medical attention.	1	
IF A FRACTURE IS SUSPECTED		
Immediately immobilize the injured part.	1	
Without moving the injured area, gently remove clothing and jewelry around the injury site.	1	
Clean and cover any open wound and exposed bone.	1	
Assess blood flow and nerve function.	1	
Gently apply the proper splint.	1	
Apply elevation and cold compresses.	1	
Seek medical care.	1	
Total Possible Points.	24	

SKILLS ASSESSMENT: POISONING EMERGENCIES

IF THE VICTIM HAS INGESTED A POISON		
Take a history to identify the substance.	1	
Identify any signs or symptoms.	1	

Contact the nearest Poison Control Center.	1	
Pursue accepted first aid care, including activated charcoal.	1	
IF THE VICTIM HAS INHALED A POISON		
Take a history and recognize signs and symptoms of inhalation poison.	1	
Activate the EMS system immediately.	1	
Move the victim into fresh air.	1	
Monitor the ABCDs.	1	
Begin CPR if necessary.	1	
IF THE VICTIM HAS INJECTED A POISON		
Recognize the signs and symptoms of toxic injection.	1	
Activate the EMS system.	1	
Prevent vomiting aspiration by placing the victim in a sitting position.	1	
Protect from added injury.	1	
Identify the causative agent of the toxic injection.	1	
IF THE VICTIM HAS ABSORBED A POISON		
Take the necessary protection against the absorption of the poison by wearing gloves.	1	
Recognize the signs and symptoms of absorbed poison.	1	
Remove victim from poison source and contaminated clothing.	1	
Irrigate with clean water, including "hidden" areas (soap, water, and rinsing well, may be necessary).	1	
Reduce swelling, pain, and itching with cold, wet compresses.	1	
Severe reaction necessitates activating the EMS system.	1	
Total Possible Points.	20	

SKILLS ASSESSMENT: FIRST AID CARE FOR CHEST PAIN (RESPONSIVE VICTIM)

Activate the EMS system.	1	
Introduce yourself to the victim.	1	
Perform an initial assessment.	1	
Prevent the victim from moving or exerting himself or herself.	1	

Assess vital signs.	1	
Place the victim in a position of comfort.	1	
If the blood pressure is above 100 systolic and you are allowed to do so, assist the victim in taking a prescribed nitroglycerin tablet. Be sure the medication was prescribed to the victim.	1	
If the chest pain is still present and the blood pressure remains above 100 systolic the victim may take another nitroglycerin after 3 to 5 minutes.	1	
Loosen the victim's clothing and assure the victim's comfort until EMS arrives.	1	
Total Possible Points.	9	

SKILLS ASSESSMENT: FIRST AID CARE FOR HYPERVENTILATING

Activate the EMS system.	1	
Remain calm and try to calm the victim down.	1	
Persuade the victim to control his or her breathing using these methods: • Breathing with abdominal muscles • Breathing through the nose • Holding the breath for a few seconds • Breathing out slowly through pursed lips.	1	
Continue calming and reassuring.	1	
Monitor vital signs.	1	
Total Possible Points.	5	

SKILLS ASSESSMENT: APPROACH TO THE PEDIATRIC ASSESSMENT

Activate the EMS system.	1	
Conduct a scene size-up, primary survey, and brief neurologic exam.	1	
Determine the chief complaint from the child if possible. If not, obtain the information from the parent or primary caregiver.	1	
Assume a confident, calm demeanor.	1	
Take a position at or below the child's level.	1	
Explain what you are doing in terms the child can understand—without "talking down" to the child or using baby talk.	1	
Be honest and gentle.	1	
Palpate painful areas last.	1	

Involve parents.	1	
Perform the secondary survey from the toes to the head.	1	
Total Possible Points.	10	

SKILLS ASSESSMENT: FIREFIGHTER'S CARRY

Position the victim on his or her back with knees bent.	1	
Grab the victim's wrists.	1	
Stand on the victim's toes of both feet.	1	
Lean backward and pull the victim up toward you.	1	
As the victim nears a standing position crouch and pull the victim over your shoulder.	1	
Stand upright with the victim over your shoulder.	1	
Pass your arm through the victim's legs and grab the victim's arm nearest your body.	1	
Carefully walk to safety.	1	
Total Possible Points.	8	

SKILLS ASSESSMENT: VEHICLE STABILIZATION

Locate all victims of a vehicle accident.	1	
STABILIZE THE SCENE		
Use materials at hand to prevent movement of the vehicle.	1	
Deal with fire or other dangers.	1	
GAIN ACCESS TO THE VICTIM(S)		
Attempt to open a door first.	1	
If opening a door is unsuccessful, break a window at the best point of entry furthest from the victim.	1	
Protect yourself and the victim(s) when doing so.	1	
Protect yourself and the victim(s) with heavy materials as you gain access.	1	
STABILIZE THE VICTIM(S)		
Perform a primary survey and triage if necessary.	1	
Stabilize the ABCs and correct any life-threatening problems.	1	

Protect the victim from further injury through proper immobilization.	1	
Continue to monitor ABCs, bleeding, and temperature.	1	
REMOVE VICTIM(S) FROM THE VEHICLE ONLY WHEN NECESSARY TO SAVE A LIFE		
Proper movement of a victim lying on a vehicle seat.	1	
Proper movement of a victim lying on the floor.	1	
Total Possible Points.	13	

Appendix B: Answers to Self-Tests

Chapter 1

PART 1 ▶ TRUE/FALSE

1. F
2. T
3. T
4. F
5. T
6. F
7. F
8. T
9. T
10. F

PART 2 ▶ MULTIPLE CHOICE

1. A
2. B
3. A
4. D
5. D
6. B

PART 3 ▶ MATCHING

Actual Consent—C
Implied Consent—A
Minor's Consent—B

Chapter 2

PART 1 ▶ TRUE/FALSE

1. F
2. F
3. F
4. T
5. T

PART 2 ▶ MULTIPLE CHOICE

1. D
2. B
3. B
4. B
5. D
6. D
7. D
8. D
9. A

PART 3 ▶ MATCHING

1. G
2. A

3. C
4. F
5. J
6. D
7. E
8. I
9. B
10. H
11. M
12. K
13. L

Chapter 3

PART 1 ▶ TRUE/FALSE

1. F
2. T
3. T
4. F
5. T
6. T
7. F
8. T

PART 2 ▶ MULTIPLE CHOICE

1. B
2. D
3. B
4. D
5. D
6. B
7. B
8. B
9. C
10. D

PART 3 ▶ MATCHING

Primary Survey
1. D
2. E
3. G
4. J
Secondary Survey
5. C
6. A
7. F
8. L
9. I
10. H
11. K
12. B

PART 4 ▶ WHAT WOULD YOU DO IF?

Signs: victim has fallen, bluish lips, shallow gasps, confusion. Symptoms: dizziness. Assess ABCDs, conduct a neuro exam, determine the chief complaint, assess vital signs, take a history, and conduct a secondary survey. Phone 911 before beginning assessment.

Chapter 4

PART 1 ▶ TRUE/FALSE

1. T
2. T
3. F
4. F
5. F
6. F
7. T

PART 2 ▶ MULTIPLE CHOICE

1. B
2. C
3. A
4. A
5. B
6. D
7. A
8. C
9. A

PART 3 ▶ FILL IN THE BLANKS

Look for the chest to rise and fall.
Listen for air escaping during inhalation.
Feel for breath against your cheek.

PART 4 ▶ WHAT WOULD YOU DO IF?

Choking (obstructed airway) is the likely cause of the incident. Ask someone to activate the EMS system and then perform abdominal thrusts on the victim until the item is expelled. If the obstruction is not cleared, the victim will eventually become unconscious. If this happens, gently guide the victim to the floor. There you will perform a finger sweep, attempt to ventilate. Reposition the head if ventilations do not go in. If the airway remains obstructed, perform CPR (see Chapter 5).

PART 5 ▶ SKILLS REVIEW

1, 3, 2, 4

Chapter 5

PART 1 ▶ TRUE/FALSE

1. F
2. F
3. F
4. F
5. F
6. F
7. T

PART 2 ▶ MULTIPLE CHOICE

1. D
2. C
3. A
4. A
5. A
6. C
7. D

PART 3 ▶ WHAT WOULD YOU DO IF?

The fact that the man grabbed his chest might indicate but not limit you to suspecting a cardiac problem. Check to see if the victim is responsive (D). Ask someone to activate the EMS system. If the victim remains unresponsive, the ABCs will help you rule out choking as a possible cause of the man's problem. Open the airway (A) and determine if the victim is breathing (B). If he is not breathing, deliver two slow, full breaths. If the ventilations go in, the victim does not have an airway obstruction; check a pulse (C) and begin chest compressions. If the ventilations do not go in, reposition the head and attempt ventilation again. If the breaths still do not go in treat the victim as an unresponsive obstructed airway victim.

Chapter 6

PART 1 ▶ TRUE/FALSE

1. F
2. T
3. F
4. F
5. T
6. T
7. T
8. T
9. F
10. T
11. F
12. F

PART 2 ▶ MULTIPLE CHOICE

1. C
2. A
3. D
4. C
5. D
6. B
7. A
8. D
9. B
10. C
11. D
12. A
13. B
14. A
15. A
16. B

PART 3 ▶ MATCHING
MATCHING #1

1. Activate the EMS system.
2. Place the tourniquet between the heart and wound.
3. Wrap the tourniquet around the limb twice and tie in a half-knot on the limb's upper surface.
4. Place the short stick at the half-knot and tie a square knot.

5. Twist the stick to tighten the tourniquet only until bleeding stops.
6. Secure the stick in place.
7. Make a written note of the location and the time the tourniquet was applied.
8. Do not cover a tourniquet.

MATCHING #2

1. B
2. D
3. F
4. A
5. C
6. E

PART 4 ▶ WHAT WOULD YOU DO IF?

1. Activate the EMS system. Assess ABCDs. Control bleeding and monitor for shock.
2. Activate the EMS system. Assess ABCDs. Secure an open airway, begin rescue breathing if necessary, and use EpiPen if present and local protocol allows.

Chapter 7

PART 1 ▶ TRUE/FALSE

1. F
2. F
3. T
4. T
5. T
6. F
7. F
8. F
9. F

PART 2 ▶ MULTIPLE CHOICE

1. A
2. A
3. D
4. B
5. C
6. B
7. A
8. D

PART 3 ▶ WHAT WOULD YOU DO IF?

1. The impaled object in the chest poses two main problems: stabilizing the impaled object and applying an occlusive dressing. Occlusive dressings are discussed in Chapter 9. Be sure the EMS system is activated and support the victim's breathing.

2. First, be sure the scene is safe and take body substance isolation precautions. Activate the EMS system. There is the potential for significant bleeding. Direct pressure, pressure bandages, and pressure points may be used to control the bleeding. Tourniquets are rarely necessary.

Chapter 8

PART 1 ▶ TRUE/FALSE

1. T
2. F
3. F
4. F
5. T
6. T
7. F
8. T
9. T
10. F
11. F
12. F

PART 2 ▶ MULTIPLE CHOICE

1. A
2. D
3. D
4. D
5. C
6. B
7. A
8. C

PART 3 ▶ MATCHING

1. E
2. B
3. C
4. D
5. F
6. A

PART 4 ▶ WHAT WOULD YOU DO IF?

1. Activate the EMS system. Do not remove the wood fragment. Place victim on his back and stabilize the head. Encircle the eye with gauze if there is bleeding.
2. Activate the EMS system. Assess ABCDs. Maintain a clear airway, control bleeding, and immobilize the neck and/or jaw if you suspect fracture.

Chapter 9

PART 1 ▶ TRUE/FALSE

1. T
2. T

3. T
4. T
5. F
6. T
7. F
8. T
9. T
10. F
11. F

PART 2 ▶ MULTIPLE CHOICE

1. A
2. C
3. D
4. D
5. A
6. A
7. A
8. C
9. A

PART 3 ▶ MATCHING

1. D
2. B
3. C
4. A

PART 4 ▶ WHAT WOULD YOU DO IF?

1. Activate the EMS system. Assess ABCDs. Apply an occlusive dressing and position victim to ease breathing. Provide artificial ventilations if necessary.
2. Activate the EMS system. Assess ABCDs. Immobilize the spine, apply moistened dressings to evisceration and cover with occlusive material. Do not attempt to replace intestines. Treat for shock.
3. Activate the EMS system. Assess ABCDs. Place victim on his back with knees bent; preserve body warmth.

Chapter 10

PART 1 ▶ TRUE/FALSE

1. F
2. T
3. F
4. T
5. F
6. T
7. F
8. F
9. F
10. T

PART 2 ▶ MULTIPLE CHOICE

1. A
2. C

3. A
4. B
5. D
6. D
7. A
8. A

PART 3 ▶ MATCHING

1. A
2. E
3. F
4. C
5. D
6. B

PART 4 ▶ WHAT WOULD YOU DO IF?

1. Activate the EMS system. Assess ABCs, immobilize the spine, use a bandage compress to control bleeding, and treat for shock.

Chapter 11

PART 1 ▶ TRUE/FALSE

1. T
2. F
3. F
4. F
5. F
6. F
7. T
8. F
9. T
10. T

PART 2 ▶ MULTIPLE CHOICE

1. B
2. C
3. A or D
4. A
5. C
6. B
7. D
8. B

PART 3 ▶ MATCHING

1. A, E
2. B, H
3. D, G
4. C, F

PART 4 ▶ WHAT WOULD YOU DO IF?

1. Activate the EMS system. Assess ABCDs, immobilize the spine, check distal pulse on leg, and assess nerve function; apply minimal traction to leg if severe deformity is present or circulation is cut off. Immobilize leg and pelvis.

Treat for shock. If you must transport, splint the entire leg; use traction splint if trained.

Chapter 12

PART 1 ▶ TRUE/FALSE

1. F
2. T
3. T
4. F
5. F
6. T
7. F
8. T
9. T

PART 2 ▶ MULTIPLE CHOICE

1. B
2. A
3. C
4. A
5. D
6. D
7. D
8. C

PART 3 ▶ MATCHING

1. B
2. C
3. D
4. B

PART 4 ▶ WHAT WOULD YOU DO IF?

1. Assess ABCDs, conduct primary and secondary surveys, control any bleeding, immobilize the hip, and transport to a medical facility.
2. Suspect a radial head fracture. Assess by asking victim to open palm and turn her hand over—substantial pain indicates radial head fracture. Splint arm, use a sling and ice, and transport to a medical facility.

Chapter 13

PART 1 ▶ TRUE/FALSE

1. A
2. T
3. F
4. T
5. F
6. T
7. T
8. F
9. T
10. F

PART 2 ▶ MULTIPLE CHOICE

1. D
2. C
3. A
4. D
5. C
6. D
7. D
8. A

PART 3 ▶ WHAT WOULD YOU DO IF?

1. Activate the EMS system. Conduct a primary survey. Maintain an open airway and immobilize the spine. Control bleeding.
2. Activate the EMS system. Conduct a primary survey. Roll him to his side, supporting his head and neck. Maintain an open airway and closely monitor vital signs. Calm the victim and treat for a head injury.
3. Activate the EMS system. Conduct a primary survey. Immobilize the spine and maintain an open airway. Control bleeding and treat for shock.

PART 4 ▶ SKILLS REVIEW

3, 2, 4, 1

Chapter 14

PART 1 ▶ TRUE/FALSE

1. T
2. F
3. F
4. T
5. F
6. F
7. T
8. F
9. T
10. F

PART 2 ▶ MULTIPLE CHOICE

1. B
2. B
3. D
4. B
5. A
6. A
7. B
8. A

PART 3 ▶ MATCHING

1. B
2. B
3. A
4. B
5. B

6. A
7. B

PART 4 ▶ WHAT WOULD YOU DO IF?

1. Activate the EMS system. Move victim far away from the garage. Assess level of consciousness and conduct a primary survey. If victim stops breathing provide artificial ventilation.

Chapter 15

PART 1 ▶ TRUE/FALSE

1. F
2. F
3. F
4. F
5. F

PART 2 ▶ MULTIPLE CHOICE

1. A
2. A
3. A
4. C
5. B
6. B
7. B
8. A
9. D
10. D

PART 3 ▶ WHAT WOULD YOU DO IF?

1. After assuring safety, taking body substance isolation precautions, and activating the EMS system you should open the victim's airway, assist ventilations if necessary, and be prepared for vomiting. Remember that the victim may be suffering from a medical condition that mimics alcohol intoxication. Treat for shock by elevating the victim's legs (if there are no injuries to the legs).

Chapter 16

PART 1 ▶ TRUE/FALSE

1. T
2. F
3. T
4. F
5. F
6. T
7. T
8. T
9. F
10. F

PART 2 ▶ MULTIPLE CHOICE

1. C
2. B
3. A
4. D
5. D
6. D
7. D
8. C
9. C
10. C

PART 3 ▶ WHAT WOULD YOU DO IF?

1. Activate the EMS system. Try to calm the victim and have her cease all activity. Place her in a position of comfort (most likely sitting) but be prepared to assist her ventilations if necessary. She is at risk of going into cardiac arrest so be prepared for CPR and use an AED if available.

Chapter 17

PART 1 ▶ TRUE/FALSE

1. T
2. T
3. F
4. T
5. T
6. T
7. F
8. F
9. F
10. T

PART 2 ▶ MULTIPLE CHOICE

1. C
2. D
3. D
4. D
5. A
6. B
7. C

PART 3 ▶ MATCHING

1. C
2. F
3. A
4. G
5. H
6. B
7. E
8. D

PART 4 ▶ WHAT WOULD YOU DO IF?

1. Activate the EMS system. Calm the victim and loosen restrictive clothing. Be

prepared to assist ventilations if necessary. Monitor the victim's breathing carefully. If the victim has medications for his condition and you are allowed, assist him in taking them.
2. Similar to the previous scenario; if the victim is tiring, you will likely need to assist her ventilations.

Chapter 18

PART 1 ▶ TRUE/FALSE

1. T
2. T
3. F
4. T
5. T
6. T

PART 2 ▶ MULTIPLE CHOICE

1. C
2. D
3. D
4. A
5. A
6. D, then activate the EMS system
7. D
8. A
9. C
10. D

PART 3 ▶ MATCHING

1. A
2. B
3. B
4. A
5. B
6. A
7. B
8. A
9. B
10. A
11. B
12. A
13. B

PART 4 ▶ WHAT WOULD YOU DO IF?

1. Activate the EMS system. Conduct primary and secondary surveys; ask the husband if she is diabetic. Maintain an open airway and treat for shock. Be alert for vomiting.
2. Activate the EMS system. Conduct a primary survey; ask the brother if she is diabetic. If conscious, administer some form of sugar.

Chapter 19

PART 1 ▶ TRUE/FALSE

1. F
2. F
3. F
4. T
5. F
6. F
7. T
8. T
9. F
10. T

PART 2 ▶ MULTIPLE CHOICE

1. C
2. A
3. A
4. C
5. B

PART 3 ▶ WHAT WOULD YOU DO IF?

1. Activate the EMS system. Conduct primary and secondary surveys. Place the victim on the left side to maintain an open and clear airway, act to prevent shock.
2. Activate the EMS system. Conduct primary survey. Maintain a clear and open airway and treat for shock. Suspect ruptured esophageal varices.

Chapter 20

PART 1 ▶ TRUE/FALSE

1. F
2. T
3. F
4. T
5. F
6. T
7. T
8. T
9. T
10. T
11. T
12. T
13. F
14. T

PART 2 ▶ MULTIPLE CHOICE

1. A
2. D
3. A
4. D
5. B

PART 3 ▶ WHAT WOULD YOU DO IF?

1. Activate the EMS system. Assess level of consciousness,

conduct a primary survey, and treat for status epilepticus.
2. Activate the EMS system. Assess level of consciousness, conduct primary and secondary surveys, and treat for shock.

Chapter 21

PART 1 ▶ TRUE/FALSE

1. T
2. F
3. T
4. F
5. T
6. T
7. F
8. F
9. T
10. F

PART 2 ▶ MULTIPLE CHOICE

1. B
2. C
3. D
4. A
5. A
6. A
7. B
8. B
9. B
10. B
11. B
12. A
13. B
14. D
15. B

PART 3 ▶ MATCHING

1. C
2. A
3. B

PART 4 ▶ WHAT WOULD YOU DO IF?

1. Activate the EMS system. Ask the mother if it's a single birth or multiple, estimated due date, and complications with this pregnancy. Conduct a primary survey, use an obstetrical kit if present or sterile materials from first aid kit, take infection control precautions, elevate the woman's buttocks, support her head, and remove clothing. Support infant's head and body when delivered, ensure umbilical cord is not around infant's neck, suction infant's mouth and provide infant care. Transport

mother, infant, and placenta to the hospital.

Chapter 22

PART 1 ▶ TRUE/FALSE

1. F
2. T
3. F
4. F
5. T
6. T
7. F
8. T

PART 2 ▶ MULTIPLE CHOICE

1. A
2. C
3. B
4. C
5. B
6. C
7. D
8. B
9. C
10. A

Chapter 23

PART 1 ▶ TRUE/FALSE

1. T
2. F
3. F
4. T
5. F

PART 2 ▶ MULTIPLE CHOICE

1. B
2. C
3. C
4. C
5. D
6. D
7. D
8. D

PART 3 ▶ MATCHING

1. B
2. A
3. A
4. A
5. A
6. B
7. A
8. A
9. A

PART 4 ▶ WHAT WOULD YOU DO IF?

1. Suspect poisonous snakebite. Conduct a primary and secondary survey; lower and immobilize the affected extremity, activate the EMS system, and seek medical attention immediately.
2. Activate the EMS system and conduct a primary survey. If the victim has a sting kit or EpiPen, assist him/her in administering the medication. Prepare for respiratory arrest.

Chapter 24

PART 1 ▶ TRUE/FALSE

1. T
2. F
3. T
4. T
5. T
6. F
7. T
8. F
9. F
10. T
11. T
12. T
13. F
14. T

PART 2 ▶ MULTIPLE CHOICE

1. A
2. D
3. B
4. C
5. B
6. D
7. D
8. B
9. A
10. C
11. A
12. D
13. B
14. D

PART 3 ▶ MATCHING

1. B
2. A
3. A
4. B
5. C
6. A
7. A
8. A
9. A
10. B
11. C

PART 4 ▶ WHAT WOULD YOU DO IF?

1. Activate the EMS system. Assess level of consciousness, conduct a primary survey, remove the source of the burn, provide irrigation to partial-thickness burns, and cover area while continuing to irrigate. Cover full-thickness burns with a sterile dressing.
2. Activate the EMS system. Assess level of consciousness, conduct a primary survey, remove clothes, dust off lime powder, flush with water.
3. Activate the EMS system. Ensure safety of yourself and victim by moving to cover. Stabilize victim's neck and spine, immediately begin CPR.

Chapter 25

PART 1 ▶ TRUE/FALSE

1. T
2. T
3. T
4. T
5. T
6. F
7. F
8. T
9. F
10. T
11. T
12. F
13. F
14. F
15. T
16. F
17. F
18. F
19. F

PART 2 ▶ MULTIPLE CHOICE

1. B
2. A
3. C
4. C
5. D
6. B
7. B
8. B or C
9. C
10. B

PART 3 ▶ MATCHING

1. B
2. D
3. A
4. C
5. A
6. D
7. B or C
8. E
9. A
10. A

PART 4 ▶ WHAT WOULD YOU DO IF?

1. Suspect heat exhaustion. Conduct a primary survey and a secondary survey; urge the victim to take sips of water and move to the shade for additional cooling. Activate the EMS system.
2. Suspect hypothermia. Conduct a primary survey and a secondary survey; move the victim to warm surroundings, remove any wet clothes, and begin passive external re-warming. Activate the EMS system.

Chapter 26

PART 1 ▶ TRUE/FALSE

1. F
2. F
3. T
4. T
5. F
6. F
7. F
8. F
9. T
10. F

PART 2 ▶ WHAT WOULD YOU DO IF?

1. Activate the EMS system. If properly trained, rescue the victim from the water, immobilize the spine, establish an airway, assist ventilations, and begin CPR if necessary.

Chapter 27

PART 1 ▶ TRUE/FALSE

1. T
2. F
3. F
4. T
5. F
6. F
7. F
8. F
9. T
10. F

PART 2 ▶ MULTIPLE CHOICE

1. B
2. C
3. C
4. C
5. A
6. C

7. C
8. A
9. B
10. D
11. B
12. C
13. A
14. A
15. A

PART 3 ▶ WHAT WOULD YOU DO IF?

1. Assess ABCDs, control bleeding, irrigate wound with sterile water, dress the wound and monitor it.
2. Assess ABCDs, control bleeding, immobilize the spine if needed, stabilize the fracture, realign the bones if necessary, and send two members from your party for help.

Chapter 28

PART 1 ▶ TRUE/FALSE

1. T
2. T
3. F
4. F
5. F
6. F
7. T
8. F
9. F
10. F

PART 2 ▶ MULTIPLE CHOICE

1. B
2. C
3. C
4. C
5. B
6. D
7. D
8. A
9. D
10. C

PART 3 ▶ MATCHING

1. E
2. C
3. A
4. B
5. D

PART 4 ▶ WHAT WOULD YOU DO IF?

In what appears to be a psychiatric emergency, assure your safety from the victim as well as the traffic. Notify EMS and law enforcement. The victim may be experiencing feelings of paranoia. Approach slowly and keep your distance. Do not make quick or threatening moves. Be alert for signs of aggressive behavior developing, which means danger for you. If you feel you cannot manage this person by yourself, wait for law enforcement.

Chapter 29

PART 1 ▶ TRUE/FALSE

1. T
2. T
3. F
4. F
5. F
6. T
7. T
8. F
9. F

PART 2 ▶ MULTIPLE CHOICE

1. D
2. C
3. B
4. B
5. D
6. A
7. D
8. D

PART 3 ▶ WHAT WOULD YOU DO IF?

1. The three-person flat lift would work here. Most importantly, choose a move that is efficient and reduces risk of damage to the spine.
2. A move such as a shirt drag would work once the victim was moved from the vehicle to the ground. While removing the victim from the vehicle, try to maintain the head and neck in a neutral in-line position.

Chapter 30

PART 1 ▶ TRUE/FALSE

1. T
2. T
3. T
4. F
5. T
6. F
7. F
8. F

PART 2 ▶ MULTIPLE CHOICE

1. C
2. A
3. B
4. C
5. D
6. D

PART 3 ▶ WHAT WOULD YOU DO IF?

1. Consider first if the victim really needs immediate extrication and decide what the safest plan is. To reach the victim, stabilize the scene and gain access through the passenger window.

Glossary

A

ABCDs Airway, breathing, circulation (hemorrhage), and disability

abdomen The area of the body between the nipples and the groin

abdominal aortic aneurysm A section of the wall of the aorta in the abdomen that weakens, dilates, and eventually ruptures

abdominal cavity Contains the liver, spleen, gallbladder, small and large intestine, pancreas, appendix, and stomach

abrasion A superficial wound caused by rubbing, scraping, or shearing

abruptio placenta A condition in which a normally positioned placenta separates from the uterine wall usually during the last 3 months of pregnancy

absence (petit mal) seizure A seizure characterized by a blank stare that lasts only a few seconds, most common in children; an absence seizure does not involve convulsions

absorption Taking a substance into the body through the skin

acromioclavicular joint The joint in the shoulder where the clavicle, scapula, and humerus join

activated charcoal A special steam-distilled charcoal that can absorb many times its weight in contaminants because of its porous surface

active drowning Drowning in which the victim is struggling in the water and is still breathing

actual consent Informed consent

acute mountain sickness An altitude-related illness that resembles a severe hangover

air embolism A diving injury in which air bubbles enter the bloodstream

amniotic sac A sac of fluid in which the baby floats

anatomical position Standing erect with the arms down at the sides, the palms facing forward

anatomical snuffbox The area of the wrist through which the radial artery passes

angina pectoris Chest pain caused when the heart's need for oxygen is not met

anterior Toward the front

arcing injury (flash burn) An injury caused when an electrical current jumps from one surface to another; nearby skin is burned, but electricity does not actually pass through the skin

arteriosclerosis A disease condition in which the arteries lose their elasticity

articulate To fit into each other

aseptic Free of bacteria

aspiration Breathing foreign matter into the lungs

ataxia Inability to keep balance

atherosclerosis A condition in which fatty substances and other debris are deposited on the arterial walls

atonic seizure Also called a "drop attack," a seizure in which the legs of a child suddenly and temporarily collapse

aura The first phase of a seizure that lasts only a few seconds and involves a peculiar sensation that may be psychic or sensory in nature

autonomic discharge A stage in a generalized tonic-clonic seizure that lasts for a few seconds and includes hyperventilation, salivation, and rapid heartbeat

autonomic nervous system The part of the nervous system that influences the activities of involuntary muscles, glands, and organs

avulsion The tearing loose of a flap of skin, which may either remain hanging or be torn off altogether

B

bandage Material used to hold a dressing in place

barotrauma A diving emergency in which body cavities are subjected to extreme pressure

basic life support A term that describes the first aid procedures necessary to sustain life in an emergency situation

Battle's sign Bruising behind the ears (mastoid process); a very late sign of skull fracture

billowing Loss of heat inside a tent when the wind flaps the sides of the tent and warm air is replaced with cold air

birth canal The vagina and lower part of the uterus

black widow spider A poisonous spider identified by a red mark shaped like a hourglass on its underside

blanket drag A method of moving victim in which a rescuer places the victim on a blanket and drags the victim to safety

bloody show Pink-tinged mucus in the vaginal discharge that is evident as labor begins

blue bloater A victim of chronic bronchitis

bronchospasm Generalized spasm of the bronchi

brown recluse spider A brown poisonous spider identified by a violin-shaped mark on its back; brown recluse spider bites do not heal and require surgical grafting

C

carbon monoxide An odorless, colorless, tasteless, toxic gas resulting from incomplete combustion of anything containing carbon.

cardiac arrest A condition in which the heart stops beating

cardiac muscle The muscle that makes up the heart

carpopedal spasm Drawing up of the hands at the wrists and knuckles with flexed fingers

carotid pulse The pulse at the groove on either side of the neck

central nervous system The part of the nervous system that consists of the brain and the spinal cord

central vertigo The least common type of vertigo (dizziness), which mimics a transient ischemic attack or stroke; victims do not experience nausea, vomiting, hearing loss, or a whirling sensation

cerebral embolism A clot that forms elsewhere in the body, travels through the bloodstream, and lodges in a cerebral artery

cervix The neck of the uterus

chair litter carry A method of lifting and moving a victim in which the victim is seated in a chair and two rescuers carry the victim in the chair

chronic obstructive pulmonary disease A range of diseases including emphysema, chronic bronchitis, and asthma

colicky pain Cramplike pain that occurs in waves

Colles's fracture A displaced fracture of the forearm caused when the victim falls on the palm of the hand with the wrist extended

compensatory shock The first stage of shock, in which the body attempts to overcome the decrease in tissue perfusion

complex partial (psychomotor) seizure A seizure that starts with a blank stare, then progresses into chewing or other random activity; the victim seems dazed

concealment A place or an object that will hide you, such as shrubbery

conduction The loss of body heat to nearby objects through direct physical touch

condyloid joint A modified ball-and-socket joint

conjunctivae The transparent mucous membrane lining the eyelids and covering the outer surface of the eyeball

contact burn A burn caused by touching either a hot surface or a live electrical circuit

contusion A bruise to the tissue of a muscle

convection The loss of body heat to surrounding air, which becomes warmer, rises, and is replaced with cooler air

conversion hysteria Converting anxiety to a physical dysfunction, such as blindness or deafness

coral snake A type of poisonous snake that does not have a pit or fangs

coronary artery disease A condition in which a coronary artery has been damaged

coup-contrecoup A mechanism of brain injury in which the head comes to a sudden stop but the brain continues to move back and forth inside the skull

cover An object that will both hide you and stop bullets, such as a tree

cramp Uncontrolled spasm of a muscle

cranial cavity Contains the brain

cravat A folded triangular bandage

crepitus A sandpaperlike grating sound made by the ends of a broken bone as they rub together

croup A vital infection that causes swelling beneath the glottis and progressive narrowing of the airway

crowning The emergence of the baby's head at the vaginal opening

cyanosis Bluish discoloration from lack of oxygen

D

decompression sickness A diving injury in which gases (usually nitrogen) enter the bloodstream

deep Remote from the surface

defibrillation The application of electricity to the chest of a victim whose heart has stopped

delirium tremens A life-threatening condition causing delirium that usually occurs within 5 days of an alcoholic's last drink

dermis The second layer of skin, which contains the hair, follicles, sweat glands, oil glands, and nerves

dilation The stage of labor during which the cervix dilates and contractions occur

dislocation An injury in which the joint comes apart and stays apart; the bone ends are no longer in contact with each other

distal Farther from the point of reference

distraction The sudden pulling apart of the spine that stretches and tears the cord

dressing A sterile covering for a wound

drowning Death from suffocation due to submersion

"dry" drowning Drowning in which little or no water enters the lungs

duty to act The legal obligation to give aid or perform first aid care

dyspnea Shortness of breath or difficulty in breathing

E

eclampsia The second stage of toxemia of pregnancy, when life-threatening convulsions or coma occur

ectopic pregnancy A pregnancy in which the fertilized egg is implanted outside the uterus

elliptical pupils Pupils that are vertical slits, like those of a cat

emphysema A respiratory disease characterized by overinflated alveoli

endocrine glands The ductless glands that regulate the body by secreting hormones

epidermis The outermost layer of the skin

epiglottitis A bacterial infection that causes swelling of the epiglottis and blocking of the airway

epilepsy A chronic brain disorder characterized by recurrent seizures not caused by acute problems, with or without loss of consciousness

esophageal varies Bulging, engorged, weakened blood vessels in the lining of the wall of the wall of the lower one-third of the esophagus

evaporation The loss of body heat when perspiration is changed from liquid to vapor

evisceration The protrusion of abdominal contents through a laceration or other wound

exhalation (expiration) The act of breathing air out of the lungs

external Outside

extremity lift A method of lifting and carrying a victim in which two rescuers carry the victim by the extremities

extrication The process of removing a victim from a dangerous situation or wrecked ear

extruded Forced out of position; an extruded eyeball has been forced out of the socket

F

face mask A barrier device that covers a victim's mouth and nose

face shield A barrier device that covers a victim's mouth

fetus The developing unborn baby

firefighter's carry A method of lifting and carrying a victim in which one rescuer carries the victim over his or her shoulder

first aid The temporary and immediate care given to a person who is injured or who suddenly becomes ill

flail chest Instability of a section of chest wall

flat lift and carry A method of lifting and moving a victim in which three rescuers or more lift and carry the victim to a stretcher

foramen magnum The opening at the base of the skull that houses the brain stem

fracture A break in the bone

frostbite Damage to the tissues resulting from prolonged exposure to extreme cold

frostnip Freezing of the skin surface

full-thickness (third-degree) burn A burn involving all layers of the skin as well as fat, muscle, and bone: a third-degree burn is characterized by dry, leathery, charred skin

G

gastric distention Inflation of the stomach with air

gauze pads Commercially manufactured, individually wrapped sterile pads made of gauze

generalized tonic-clonic (grand mal) seizure A convulsive seizure characterized by alternating muscle rigidity and jerking, temporarily suspended breathing, and altered mental state

gestational diabetes Temporary diabetes that develops in a pregnant woman

globe The eyeball

glucose Sugar

golfer's elbow Inflammation in the tendon attached to the inner side of the elbow

Good Samaritan laws Laws that protect health care personnel and provide guidelines for care

H

heat cramps Muscle spasms caused by a disturbance in the electrolyte balance of the muscles; generally seen when the body loses too much salt and other electrolytes during profuse sweating

heat exhaustion A heat-related emergency caused by excessive loss of water and salt through sweating, characterized by cold, clammy skin and a weak, rapid pulse

heatstroke A life-threatening emergency caused by a disturbance in the body's temperature regulation mechanism, characterized by extreme fever, hot and dry or moist skin, delirium, or coma

hematoma A collection of blood beneath the skin

hemophiliac A person whose blood will not clot because of congenital abnormalities in the clotting mechanism

hemoptysis Coughing up of blood

hemothorax An accumulation of blood in the chest cavity

hernia Protrusion of an internal organ through the abdominal wall or into another body cavity

high altitude cerebral edema (HACE) An altitude-related illness that causes swelling of the brain and increased pressure inside the skull

high altitude pulmonary edema (HAPE) An altitude-related illness that causes fluid to go into the lungs from body cells

hyperglycemia A condition that results from too little insulin and too much sugar in the blood

hyperthermia Greatly increased body temperature

hypertonic phase The phase in a seizure that signals the end of continuous muscle contractions, characterized by extreme muscle rigidity and hypertension

hyperventilation A condition characterized by overbreathing or breathing too rapidly

hyperventilation syndrome An abnormal state in which rapid breathing persists

hypoglycemia A condition that results from too much insulin and not enough or lack of sugar in the blood

hypothermia Greatly decreased body temperature

I

implied consent Assumption that a victim of life-threatening injury or illness would give consent

inadequate breathing Breathing that is too slow or shallow to support life

infectious disease A disease that can be transmitted from one person to another or from an insect or animal to a person

inferior Below, or lower than, a point of reference

ingesting Taking a substance into the body through the mouth

inhalation The act of breathing in (inspiration), or the drawing of air or other gases into the lungs

inhalation injury An injury caused by breathing in heat, toxic chemicals, smoke, or carbon monoxide

inspiration The act of breathing in (inhalation)

insulin A hormone needed to facilitate movement of glucose out of the bloodstream, across the cell membranes, and into the cells

internal Inside

involuntary muscle Smooth muscle over which a person has no voluntary or conscious control

irreversible shock The final stage of shock, in which body organs start to die

ischemic stroke A stroke caused by a clot inside the brain

ischial tuberosity The spot where the top of the hamstring attaches

L

labor The process that begins with the first uterine contraction and ends with delivery of the baby and placenta

labyrinthine vertigo The most common kind of dizziness, caused by a disturbance in the inner ear and characterized by nausea, vomiting, and a whirling sensation

laceration A break in the skin, lacerations can have either smooth or rough edges and can be of varying depth

larynx The voice box

lateral To the right or left of the midline (center) of the body; away from the midline

lateral recumbent (recovery, or coma) position Lying on the right or left side with the lower arm in front of the body, with the head dependent

M

mammalian diving reflex A reflex that prevents death after submersion in cold water

mandible The lower jaw

maxilla The upper jaw

meconium The feces of the newborn; greenish or brownish-yellow amniotic fluid indicates that the baby had a bowel movement in the uterus before delivery

medial Toward the midline (center) of the body

minor's consent The right of consent given to a parent or guardian

miscarriage Loss of pregnancy before 20 weeks of gestation, also called "spontaneous abortion"

modified HAINES recovery position Extend the arm, logroll the victim on his side, rest his head on the extended arm, bend the knees to stabilize his body

myocardium The heart muscle

myoclonic seizure A seizure characterized by sudden, brief, massive muscle lerks that involve part or all of the body

N

near-drowning Survival, at least temporarily, of near suffocation due to submersion.

negligence Acting with carelessness, inattention, disregard, inadvertence, or avoidable oversight

nitroglycerin Medication prescribed to ease the pain of angina pectoris

O

occlusive Waterproof and airtight

ocular Having to do with the eye

orbit The body socket that holds the eyeball

P

pallor Paleness

palmar surface method A method of using the size of the victim's palm to estimate the percentage of body surface that has been burned

palpable Able to be felt by the First Aider

paradoxical breathing A condition in which the injured area of the chest moves opposite the rest of the chest during breathing

parasympathetic nervous system The part of the autonomic nervous system that opposes the sympathetic nervous system

paresthesia Pricking or tingling sensation that indicates loss of circulation

partial-thickness (second-degree) burn A burn that involves both the epidermal and dermal layers of the skin characterized by blistering, swelling, and pain

passive drowning Drowning in which the victim is not breathing and is face-down in the water

patella The kneecap

PCP Phencyclidine, a hallucinogenic drug that acts as an anesthetic

pelvic cavity Contains the reproductive organs, urinary bladder, urethra, and rectum

perfusion Circulation of oxygen-rich blood to cells

pericardial cavity The tough fibrous covering that contains the heart

perineum The area of skin and muscle between the vagina and the anus

peripheral nervous system Structures of the nervous system (especially nerve endings) that lie outside the brain and spinal cord

peritonitis Inflammation of the lining of the abdomen

pink puffer A victim of emphysema

pit viper A type of poisonous snake, such as a rattlesnake, characterized by a pit between the eyes and nostril

placenta Structure on the inner lining of the uterus that provides the fetus with nourishment

placenta previa A condition in which the placenta is positioned abnormally

plaque Fatty deposits on the arterial walls

pneumothorax A condition in which air from a lung or from the outside fills the chest cavity, but does not fill the lung

posterior Toward the back

postictal phase The phase following a seizure, during which all muscles relax and the victim slowly becomes responsive but remains exhausted

postseizure phase One of the final phases of a seizure, during which the victim progresses into a coma

preeclampsia A condition in pregnancy associated with high blood pressure and swelling of the extremities; the first stage of toxemia

premature baby A baby that weighs less than $5\frac{1}{2}$ pounds and/or is born after less than 36 weeks' gestation

presenting part The part of the baby that emerges first through the birth canal; in a normal birth it is the head

pressure point A place where an artery is close to the skin surface and lies over a bone

progressive (decompensatory) shock The second stage of shock, in which the compensatory mechanisms have failed the blood pressure begins to decrease, and the organs are beginning to suffer from the lack of perfusion

prolapsed cord The presentation of the umbilical cord at the vaginal opening before the baby

prone position Lying face down on the stomach

pulmonary edema A condition in which plasma seeps out of the capillaries into the lungs as a result of pressure from a failing heart

Q

quadrants Sections: the abdomen is divided into four quadrants

R

raccoon eyes Bruising around the eyes in the absence of trauma to the eyes; a sign of skull fracture

radial pulse The pulse at the wrist on the thumb side

radiation The loss of the body heat to the surface of another object without physical contact

reasonable force The amount of force required to keep a person from injuring self or others

"reasonable-man" test Did the First Aider act the same way a normal, prudent person with similar training would have acted under the same circumstances?

reduce To straighten

respiration Exchange of oxygen and carbon dioxide in the lungs

respiratory arrest Total cessation of breathing or respiratory effort

respiratory distress An abnormal condition where breathing is labored, noisy, irregular, or unusually fast or slow or a combination of these

roller bandage A form-fitting bandage designed to be wrapped around a wound site

Rule of Nines A method of estimating how much body surface was burned by mentally dividing the body into regions, each representing 9 percent (or a multiple of 9 percent) of the body surface

Rule of Threes The rule stating that survival time is considerably reduced if a victim is without all three factors required for survival: shelter, water, and food

S

sclera The white of the eye

seat carry A method of lifting and moving a victim in which two rescuers from a "seat" with their arms

secondary drowning Death from aspiration pneumonia following resuscitation after a water accident

seizure An involuntary, sudden change in sensation, behavior, muscle activity, or level of consciousness that results from irritation or overactivity of brain cells

sheet drag A method of moving a victim in which a single rescuer forms a drag harness out of a sheet by passing it under the victim's arms at the armpits, and uses it to pull the victim

shirt drag A method of moving a victim in which a single rescuer uses the victim's shirt as a handle to pull the victim

shock Inadequate tissue perfusion

signs Things you can observe about the victim, such as bleeding

silent myocardial infarction A heart attack that does not cause chest pain

simple partial (Jacksonian) seizure A simple, partial seizure characterized by jerking in the fingers and toes; the jerking may spread to involve the entire arm or leg, but the victim stays awake and aware. It may progress to a generalized toxic-clonic seizure

skeletal (voluntary) muscle Muscle that is under direct voluntary control of the brain

Smith's fracture A displaced fracture of the forearm caused when the victim falls on the back of the hand with the wrist flexed

smooth muscle The muscles found in the walls of the internal organs and blood vessels, generally not under voluntary control

special pads Large, thickly layered bulky pads used to control bleeding and stabilize impaled objects

spinal cavity Contains the spinal cord

sprain An injury in which ligaments are stretched and partially or completely torn

status asthmaticus A severe, prolonged asthma attack that represents a dire medical emergency

status epilepticus A severe, prolonged seizure lasting longer than five minutes or a series of seizures that occur without the victim's regaining consciousness between them

sterile Free of all microorganisms and spores

stoma A surgical opening in the neck

strain An injury to the muscle that occurs when the muscle is stretched beyond its normal range of motion, causing the muscle to tear

stroke Any disease process that impairs circulation to the brain

sudden infant death syndrome (SIDS) Sudden death of an apparently healthy infant, usually while asleep

suicide Any willful act designed to end one's own life

superficial Near the surface

superficial (first-degree) burn A burn that involves only the epidermis, or outer layer of skin, characterized by pain and redness

superior Above, or higher than, a point of reference

supine position Lying face up on the back

sympathetic nervous system The part of the autonomic nervous system that causes blood vessels to constrict, stimulates sweating, increases the heart rate, causes the sphincter muscles to contract, and prepares the body to respond to stress

symptoms Things the victim describes to you, such as abdominal pain

syncope Fainting

T

tennis elbow Inflammation of the bony protrusion of the elbow

tension pneumothorax A situation in which air enters the pleural space through a one-way defect in the lung, resulting in a progressive increase in pressure in the pleural cavity that causes the lung to collapse and that impairs circulation

thermal burn A burn caused by flames

thoracic cavity Contains the heart, trachea, lungs, large vessels, and esophagus

thrombus A clot that forms in a cerebral artery

tonic phase The early stage of a seizure during which the victim loses consciousness, and the body is completely rigid with continuous muscular contraction

tonic-clonic phase The phase of a seizure characterized by muscular rigidity and relaxation that alternate rhythmically in rapid succession

toxic Poisonous

tracheal deviation Displacement of the trachea to one side or the other

traction Gentle, steady pulling movement of a bone in alignment with its natural position

transient ischemic attack Brief attacks similar to strokes that occur when arterial blockage is partial or brief

traumatic asphyxia Sudden compression of the chest wall that forces blood to flow the wrong way

triage A system of sorting victims into categories by treatment priority

triangular bandage Triangle-shaped piece of cloth used to apply splints and form slings

Type I diabetes Diabetes that results when the body produces little or no insulin

Type II diabetes Diabetes that results when the body does not produce enough insulin or the cells do not respond as well to the insulin

U

umbilical cord An extension of the placenta that resembles a sturdy rope, through which the fetus is nourished

uterus The organ in which the baby grows

V

vagina The passage for childbirth

ventilation The mechanical process of moving (breathing) air into and out of the lungs

ventricular fibrillation A chaotic, unorganized beating effort of the heart that is incapable of producing a pulse or circulation

vernix caseosa The white, cheeselike covering on a newborn's skin

vertigo Dizziness

voluntary nervous system The part of the nervous system that influences activity of the voluntary muscles and movements throughout the body

W

walking assist A method of moving a victim in which a rescuer functions as a crutch in assisting the injured victim to walk

"wet" drowning Drowning in which water enters the lungs

withdrawal syndrome A four-stage syndrome that occurs after a cutback in the amount of alcohol a person is used to or when blood alcohol levels start to fall after severe intoxication

wound An injury to the skin and underlying musculature that disrupts the normal continuity of the affected tissue, organ, or bone

X

xiphoid process The lower tip of the sternum

Index

Credits

PHOTO CREDITS

Grateful acknowledgment is made to the following copyright holders for permission to reprint photos in the figures listed below:

Chapter 1: 1-2 Rick Nye.   **Chapter 3:** 3-9, 3-10 Rick Nye.   **Chapter 5:** 5-23 through 5-35 Rick Nye.   **Chapter 6:** 6-27 through 6-33 Rick Nye.   **Chapter 8:** 8-8 Western Ophthalmic Hospital/Science Photo Library/Photo Researchers, Inc.; 8-9 Dorling Kindersley.   **Chapter 9:** 9-5, 9-18, 9-24 Rick Nye. **Chapter 11:** 11-5 Stock Solution/Index Stock Imagery, Inc.; 11-6, 11-7 Charles Stewart, M.D.; 11-16 Dan Limmer; 11-19, 11-20, 11-24 Rick Nye.   **Chapter 12:** 12-1, 12-14 Rick Nye.   **Chapter 13:** 13-5, 13-25 Rick Nye.   **Chapter 14:** 14-10 Beckman/ Custom Medical Stock Photo, Inc.   **Chapter 15:** 15-14, 15-15 Rick Nye. **Chapter 16:** 16-10 Rick Nye.   **Chapter 19:** 19-2, 19-4 Rick Nye. **Chapter 20:** 20-4 through 20-7 Rick Nye.   **Chapter 22:** 22-8 David Effron, M.D.; 22-9 through 22-13 Robert A. Felter, M.D. **Chapter 23:** 23-1 Dave King/Dorling Kindersley; 23-2 Ed Degginger/Color-Pic, Inc.; 23-3 John Cancalosi/ Nature Picture Library; 23-4 Karl Shone/Dorling Kindersley; 23-8, 23-9 Photo Researchers, Inc.; 23-15, 23-16, 23-18 Corbis; 23-20 Jane Burton/ Dorling Kindersley; 23-21, 23-22 Corbis; 23-23, 23-24 Frank Greenaway/Dorling Kindersley; 23-25 Corbis; 23-28, 23-30 Rick Nye.   **Chapter 24:** 24-15 Andy Crawford/ Dorling Kindersley. **Chapter 27:** 27-2, 27-3 Rick Nye.   **Chapter 29:** 29-1 through 29-27 and 29-31 through 29-40 Rick Nye.   **Chapter 30:** 30-1 Rick Nye; 30-2 Photo Researchers, Inc.

ILLUSTRATION CREDITS

Figures **2–8, 2–10, 2–11, 2–12, 2–15** (brain only), and **2–17** are adapted from Michael D. Johnson, *Human Biology: Concepts and Current Issues,* San Francisco, CA: Benjamin Cummings, © 2001 Benjamin Cummings, an imprint of Addison Wesley Longman, Inc.

Figures **2–13, 2–14** are adapted from William J. Germann and Cindy L. Stanfield, *Principles of Human Physiology,* San Francisco, CA: Benjamin Cummings, © 2002 Pearson Education, Inc.

Figure **3–1** is adapted from "Pyramid of Life" by Ray Johnson, *Jems,* June, 1985, pp. 56–58.

Figure **12–2** is adapted from Scott K. Powers and Stephen L. Dodd, *Total Fitness and Wellness,* 3rd ed., San Francisco, CA: Benjamin Cummings, © 2003 Pearson Education, Inc.

Figure **15–12** is adapted from Martin A. Alpert, M.D., "Modern Management of Delirium Tremens," *Hospital Medicine,* May 1990.

Figure **20–2** is adapted from *Mayo Clinic Health Letter,* November 1988, by permission of Mayo Foundation for Medical Education and Research.

Figure **23–14** is adapted from "Insect Stings—Responding to the Gamut of Allergic Reactions" by Dr. John W. Georgitis, *Modern Medicine.* Reprinted by permission of the Dr. John W. Georgitis, Piedmont Allergy & Asthma Research, 1364 Westgate Center Drive, Winston–Salem, NC 27103.

Figure **24–35** is adapted from *Hospital Medicine,* May 1989, page 85.

Figure **25–11** is reprinted by permission of publisher from James R. Blackman, "Caught in Cold Water," *Emergency Medicine,* January 30, 1985, Copyright © 1985 by Quadrant HealthCom Inc.

Figure **26–3** is adapted from Pat Samples, Spinal Cord Injuries: "The High Cost of Careless Diving," *The Physician and Sportsmedicine,* July 1989.